Lyttle's

Mental Health and Disorder

SECOND EDITION

Edited by

Tony Thompson
MA, BEd(Hons), RMN, RNMH, DipN(Lond), CertEd, RNT
Senior Lecturer, Department of Nursing
University of Nottingham;
College Co-ordinator,
Mid-Trent College of Health
Nottingham, UK

and Peter Mathias
BSc, MA, MSc, PhD
Lead Manager of Joint Awarding Bodies,
London, UK

BAILLIÈRE TINDALL
London   Philadelphia   Toronto   Sydney   Tokyo

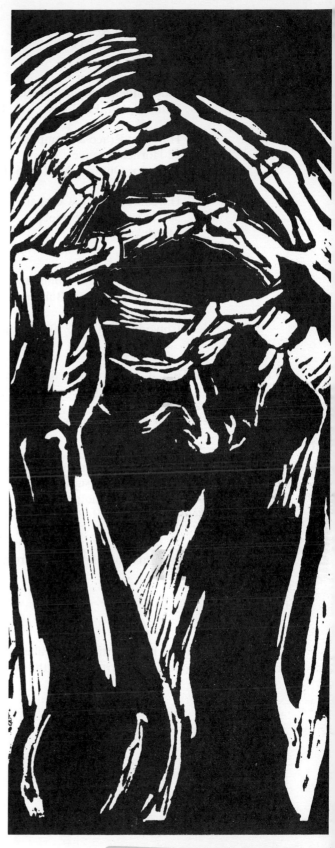

Baillière Tindall   24–28 Oval Road
W. B. Saunders   London NW1 7DX

The Curtis Center
Independence Square West
Philadelphia, PA 19106-3399, USA

Harcourt Brace & Company
55 Horner Avenue
Toronto, Ontario, M8Z 4X6, Canada

Harcourt Brace & Company, Australia
30–52 Smidmore Street
Marrickville
NSW 2204, Australia

Harcourt Brace & Company, Japan
Ichibancho Central Building
22–1 Ichibancho
Chiyoda-ku, Tokyo 102, Japan

A catalogue record for this book is available from the British Library

ISBN 0–7020–1416–8

Typeset by Fakenham Photosetting Ltd, Fakenham, Norfolk
Printed and bound in Great Britain by Bath Press, Bath, Avon

CONTENTS

PART I CORE CONCEPTS IN CONTEXT

PART II THE NATURE AND EFFECTS OF DISORDER

PART III INTERVENTION AND TREATMENT

PART IV **THE ORGANIZATION AND PROVISION OF CARE**

PART V **POLICIES AND PRIORITIES**

LIST OF CONTRIBUTORS

Carol Baxter SRN SCM HV DN FETC MSc

Health & Race Consultant
126 Eccles Old Road
Salford
Manchester
M6 8QQ

Colin Beacock RNMH RGN Cert. Ed

Director of Nurse Education (Acting)
Rampton Hospital
Retford
Nottingham
DN22 0PD

John Brown BSc MPhil

Lecturer in Social Work
Department of Social Policy and Social Work
University of York
Heslington
York
YO1 5DD

Paddy Cooney BA(Hons) CQSW DMS

Development Consultant
Centre for Mental Health Services Development
King's College London
Campden Hill Road
London
W8 7AH

Margaret Elinor Evans BEd Cert.Ed(FE) RGN
NDN Cert OBS RHV RSCN RNT

College Coordinator
Child Health
Mid Trent College of Nursing and Midwifery
A Floor
University Hospital
Queen's Medical Centre
Nottingham
NG7 2UH

Antoine Farine MSc BA (Physiology) RN RNT
RCNT BTTA DN(Lond) Cert Ed

Specialist Subject Leader in Biological Sciences
Mid Trent College of Nursing and Midwifery
Queen's Medical Centre
Nottingham
NG7 2UH

Mary Headley Mb MRCPsych

Unit General Manager
Area Mental Health Unit
St Luke's Hospital
Loughgall Road
Armagh
BT71 7NQ

Frank Clifford Johnson RMN SRN STD RNT

Education Officer
English National Board
BSP House
Station Road
Chester
CH1 3DR

Carys Llewellyn Jones DipSoc. Studies, Post
Grad Dip. Psych Social Work, Member of
Mental Health Act Commission

Lecturer in Social Work
CACS 9th Floor Tower
University of North Wales
Bangor
Gwynedd
LL57 2DG

Christine A. Kirk MA MBBChir RCPsych

Consultant Psychiatrist for the Elderly
Bootham Park Hospital
York
YO3 7BY

Jack Lyttle RMN RGN DN RNT

Formerly Senior Tutor Mental Health
Argyle & Clyde College of Nursing
Royal Alexandra Hospital
Paisley

Sue Marshall BA(Hons) MPhil RGN

Clinical Psychologist
Newton House
20 Health Lane
West Bromwich
West Midlands

Rosaleen Moore Diploma in Social Work
(CQSW)

Unit Director Community Mental Health
Services
St Luke's Hospital
Armagh

Eric Moxham SRN RMN RNT DipEd MEd

College Coordinator—Mental Health Branch
Mid Trent College of Nursing and Midwifery
A Floor
Queen's Medical Centre
Nottingham
NG7 2UH

Aru Narayanasamy BA MSc RGN RMN
Cert Ed RNT

College Coordinator for Common Foundation
Programme
Mid Trent College of Nursing and Midwifery
A Floor
Queen's Medical Centre
Nottingham
NG7 2UH

Kamlesh Patel Dip SW CQSW

Deputy Director
The Bridge Project
Equity Chambers
40 Piccadilly
Bradford
BD1 3NN

Ruth Prime BA SRN QCSW DH Inspector

DH Inspector (retired)

Colin Pritchard MA AAPSW Director Mental
Health

Professor Social Work Studies
Department Social Work Studies
University of Southampton
Southampton
SO9 5NA

Julie Marsh Repper SRN RMN BA(Hons)

Lecturer Nursing/Mental Health
Department of Nursing and Midwifery Studies
Queen's Medical Centre
Nottingham
NG7 2UH

Gerard Rice BA(Hons) CQSW Post Grad. Dip
SW

Project Team Leader
The Bridge Project
Equity Chambers
40 Piccadilly
Bradford
BD1 3NN

David Thomas Sines PhD BSc(Hons) RMN
RNMH PGCTHE RNT FRCN

Professor of Community Health Nursing
Department of Nursing
Faculty of Social and Health Studies
University of Ulster at Jordanstown
Newtownabbey
Co Antrim
BT3 7OQ

Lynne Diane Smith RMN SRN Dip Nurs(Lond)
Cert Ed (FE) RNT

Lecturer in Mental Health Nursing
College of Nursing and Midwifery
City General Hospital
Newcastle Road
Stoke on Trent
Staffordshire ST4 6QG

Paul Tarbuck SRN RMN ON(Lon) TCert, BA
Theol

Director of Advanced Nursing Studies ENB 770
Core
Practice Development Centre
Ashworth Centre
Ashworth Hospital
Magnull
Liverpool
L31 1HW

Enid E. Wright BSc (Econ) Diploma in Applied
Social Studies

Policy Analyst
Central Council for Education and Training in
Social Work (CCETSW)
Derbyshire House
St Chad's Street
London
WC1H 8AD

INTRODUCTION

In the first edition of this book *Mental Disorder, Its Care and Treatment* (1986) Jack Lyttle introduced the basic concepts of mental disorder and identified the therapeutic possibilities which lay in the hands of the helping professions, particularly nursing, at a time when 'the focus of psychiatric care is moving steadily from hospital to community'.

Since 1986 the movement towards provision in the community has continued and been given added impetus by the National Health Service and Community Care Act (1990) and changes in the organization of the health services. Nurse training has been reformed through Project 2000 and nursing has added an emphasis on the promotion of health to its roles of intervening and helping in instances of ill-health and disorder.

The knowledge and understanding described in Jack Lyttle's first edition has continued to be expanded, developed and implemented by practitioners and researchers within a variety of professions and it is clear that there is great potential to provide effective help and services to the diversity of people experiencing problems of mental ill-health in a multiracial society.

In this second edition, which seeks to bring the first edition up to date and demonstrate how effective and sensitive help can be given within the services of the nineties, the contributors provide:

(i) discussion of the core requirements and expectations made of nurses and other mental health practitioners in terms of the values and skills necessary to practice in a multiracial society;

(ii) information about the nature and effects of mental health and disorder;

(iii) analysis of the basic treatments and interventions;

(iv) descriptions of the organization and provision of care from primary to secure settings;

(v) exploration of the practical implications of recent developments in social policy.

The book is organized into five sections:

1	Core concepts in context
2	The nature and effects of disorder
3	Treatment and interventions
4	The organization and provision of care
5	Policies and priorities

The second edition is for nurses taking the mental health branch within Project 2000 training programmes, people involved in programmes of continuing professional development and educationists and managers in the health and social services. In many ways the book can be seen as a partner to *Standards and Mental Handicap* (Thompson and Mathias, 1992) which analyses and describes the potential for therapeutic intervention and support of people experiencing learning disability within services governed by the NHS and Community Care Act. *Standards and Mental Handicap* places the work of nursing into a single framework of competence alongside the work of social work and the remedial professions. This second edition of *Mental Health and Disorder* concentrates on the functions of nursing although the sections on health and disorder, treatment and intervention and the organization and provision of care will be relevant to other professions as well.

The book is based on the assertion that nursing shares key purposes with other professions and that it is possible to identify the specific functions, qualities and knowledge required of practising nurses from these key purposes (see Fig. 1).

Key Purposes	Prevent and diminish the effects of distress and illness Treat, support, rehabilitate, advocate, protect Uphold codes of conduct, be effective in a multiracial society		
Main Functions	Identify, analyse and assess factors causing distress and illness	Promote health, provide direct care and make interventions	Manage care programmes and services
Qualities	Be critical, analytical and accountable, continue professional development	Counter discrimination, inequality and individual and institutional racism	Work within and develop policies, laws and safeguards in all settings
Knowledge	Understand influences on mental health and the nature/causes of disorder and illness	Know the effects of distress, disorder, illness on individuals, families, groups	Understand the basis of treatments and interventions

Figure 1 *Key purposes of nursing related to main functions, qualities and knowledge.*

Figures 2 and 3 show how the main themes of chapters of the book relate to the functions and knowledge performed and required in nursing as described in Fig. 1.

Figure 2 shows which chapters deal in the main with the function: identify, analyse and assess factors causing distress and illness and the related knowledge:

understand the influences on mental health and the nature and causes of disorder and illness; and know the effects of distress, disorder and illness on individuals, families and groups.

Figure 3 shows the chapters which deal with the two functions

Promote health, provide direct care and make interventions;

Manage care programmes and services and the related knowledge. Understand the basis of treatments and interventions.

The relationship of the chapters to Figs 1, 2 and 3 is shown at the beginning of each one as are a statement of chapter aims and a list of key issues.

Unlike the first edition, the second edition features the contributions of people from a variety of backgrounds in practice, education, management and research. Inevitably a variety of opinion is expressed and a number of arguments are developed some of which may conflict, overlap or duplicate. The structure of this edition reveals concepts, models and developmental aspects of mental health promotion and recognizes the importance of established knowledge and practice. It is intended to form part of the contribution to the growing body of work in the area of interdisciplinary practice.

Somewhat revolutionary aspects of change will occur in the next decade regarding the way in which practitioners are prepared to work in mental health. The impact will be all the greater because of the context in which services and policies develop. The major aim of this edition is to help practitioners achieve standards underpinned by the skills, knowledge and attitude needed to take forward the nature and culture of care provision.

> *Function*
> Identify, analyse and assess factors causing distress and illness

> Chapters 1, 4, 5, 6, 7, 8, 9, 10, 11, 12, 13, 16, 19.1, 20

Themes

Mental health may be disturbed by biological or psychosocioeconomic events (1, 6.)		
An understanding of brain function and physiology (20.1) helps to inform treatment particularly with respect to schizophrenia (20.2), depression (20.3) and dementia (20.4)	Psychosocial pressures may vary with lifestage, age, gender, race, class (4, 5, 6, 13). Socioeconomic conditions may play a role in suicide (12)	Disturbances of affect and emotion may be a component of mental ill-health (7)
Mental ill-health or illness may be short-term or have long-term effects. People with enduring problems need carefully planned help (19.1)	Disturbances in affect, behaviour, cognition help in classification and diagnosis—labels can disadvantage (10). Personality disorders require specialized intervention (11).	Behavioural disturbances (eating, sleeping, movement) may accompany ill-health (8) which may also be associated with disorders in cognition (perception, attention, thinking, language, memory) 9.
Prejudice, discrimination and racism can affect mental health and the behaviour of practitioners (4, 5, 13)		

Figure 2 *The relationship of the main themes of chapters to the function: identify, analyse, and assess factors causing distress and illness.*

> *Function*
> Promote health, provide direct care and make interventions
> Manage care programmes and services

Themes

Nurses apply a range of skills and can play a variety of roles within services governed by social policies (2, 28, 29) and influenced by international trends (3). Practitioners in Britain's multi-racial society must possess anti-discriminatory competence (4, 5, 13)	Nurses provide direct care and manage interventions (15) in order to promote health (16) and will work in a range of settings including (i) primary health care (21); (ii) community services (22, 23, 24); (iii) special hospitals (26, 27); and (iv) psychiatric and general hospitals (25)	People with enduring problems require effective services, nurses will work alongside others to provide them in services organized through purchaser-provider separation and care (case) management (19.1, 19.2, 19.3)
Care and treatment programmes will often have a combination of physical (20) and non-physical components (14, 17) and may also require provision of spiritual care (18)	Community nursing involves a range of skill (32) and nurses will work with others to ensure services are available to, and used by, black people and members of minority ethnic groups (23)	Laws (29), safeguards (30) and social policy (28) provide further contexts for practice

Figure 3 *The Relationship of main themes of chapters to the functions (i) promote health, provide direct care, make interventions and (ii) manage care programmes and services.*

As editors, we wish to thank each of the contributors for the energy and effort which they brought to this project. We would also like to acknowledge Jack Lyttle, whose first edition of this book has proved to be an inspiration to almost a generation of nurses and whose insight and compassion into the particular challenges of mental health nursing, we hope to reflect and pay tribute to in this edition.

PART

I

CORE CONCEPTS IN CONTEXT

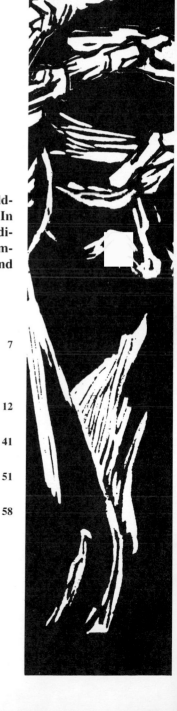

Nurses should consider themselves accountable for their actions and part of a world-wide group of practitioners which shares common ideals, purposes and methods. In Britain, nursing takes place in a multiracial society and one in which public expenditure is under close scrutiny. Practitioners have to be able to identify their competence and persuade those who purchase and manage services of its relevance and effectiveness.

As a registered nurse ... you must recognize and respect the uniqueness and dignity of each patient and client, and respond to their need for care, irrespective of their ethnic origin, religious beliefs, personal attributes; the nature of their health problems or any other factor.

UKCC Code of Conduct 1992

1

THE CORE CONCEPTS OF CARE IN MENTAL HEALTH AND DISORDER

Tony Thompson and Peter Mathias

AIMS

i) To identify trends in the provision of services and the implications for practitioners

KEY ISSUES

Nursing skills and knowledge
Change
Promotion of mental health

Identify, analyse and assess factors causing distress and illness	Promote health, provide direct care and make interventions	Manage care programmes and services
Be critical, analytical and accountable, continue professional development	Counter discrimination, inequality and individual and institutional racism	Work within and develop policies, laws and safeguards in all settings
Understand influences on mental health and the nature/causes of disorder and illness	Know the effects of distress, disorder, illness on individuals, groups, families	Understand the basis of treatments and interventions

TOWARDS MENTAL HEALTH

One of the most rewarding features of professional caring within human services is being aware of skills and knowledge in a combination which helps fulfil the physical and emotional health needs of people. Although this role of fulfilment is not exclusive to nurses or social workers, these two groups particularly have to be competent in order to assist the person and their family to cope with, or prevent, life experience which impedes optimum physical and emotional health. Caring and health promotion go together when professionals strive to be effective against other factors that may hinder a person's ability to function in a well-adapted way. Professional efforts are directed towards helping people to maintain their mental capabilities, to achieve their potential and conserve their integrity.

The provision of mental-health orientated services has undergone substantial change during the past decade. The concepts of care to be undertaken by nurses and others have changed even more dramatically. Nurses working in mental health services, especially with people with a mental illness, have been expected to assume increased responsibility in the areas of (i) comprehensive assessment, (ii) development of skills and adaptive behaviour for achieving quality of life, and (iii) programme design to increase coping abilities and modify problematic or challenging behaviour. Further, they have developed sophisticated counselling services and have co-ordinated services in order to maximize the effectiveness of other agencies and disciplines input. These, and other significant changes to the role and function of professionals in mental health services has led to an expansion of the theoretical basis for practice and role expertise.

The nature of mental illness and the notion of positive mental health are always likely to be controversial. Perhaps one of the exciting aspects of training in this field is the opportunity to contribute to the controversy in an increasingly informed way. The student of mental health soon realizes that there is little consensus regarding the issues that surround present thinking and practice. One major feature of specializing in this field is its association with values tied to social and political constructs, which sometimes encourage a narrow role and function. The ideas contained in this text are those associated with liberating the professional outlook and creating a transdisciplinary view of care provision.

WHO SHAPES THE PROVISION OF CARE?

It is important to recognize that the issues and views about mental health and services are often underpinned by philosophical and political beliefs, not necessarily associated with medicine. It is this mix of ideas, proposition and theory that has shaped the present mental health services and the role and function of both the practitioner and client within these services. The concept of mental health and psychiatric illness and the way in which professional input should meet the challenge of providing an appropriate service, tend to be shaped by the prevailing or dominant views of those who influence the health care agenda.

The prevailing ideology in the UK is one of supporting community care and self-care and originates from a political view that seeks to include economic and social policy interests. Other cultures have a different view and these will be focused on briefly in other sections of this book. Historically, mental illness has confounded those with the task of providing service and preparing practitioners. One reason for this is the attempt to explain physiological illness and psychological illness using the same or similar theoretical perspectives. Whilst this is understandable as parallels can be drawn, the distance between the two remains. This may be helpful if the space between forms a testing ground for ideas which may target the person with a physical or mental health problem. The way in which problems of mental health or illness is viewed by the community as deviating from normal behaviour may make it particularly difficult for practitioners to develop a therapeutic role.

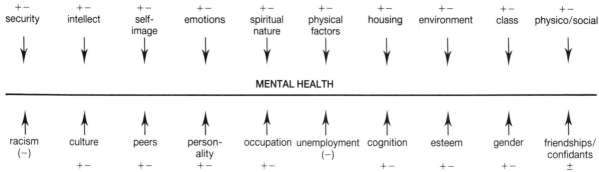

Fig. 1.1 *Factors associated with mental health.*

REFERENCE POINTS

Professionals who work within the field of mental health promotion and mental illness soon become aware of the fickle nature of what is considered to be a sign of mental illness. Those who have worked for over a decade within hospital settings can often reflect on the fact that behaviour associated with bizarre dress may be taken into account when confirming mental illness—yet years on may find themselves buying similar apparel for their offspring. In delusional states patients may, for example, suggest that they are affected by TV monitors or overhead electricity pylons or gases escaping from walls, symptoms sometimes taken to confirm pathological conditions and yet suddenly environmental awareness introduces us to sick building syndrome and research is initiated into the effect on people's health who are stressed by computer monitors or who live near high voltage cables!

Perhaps one of the most important features of mental illness is that it is usually people close to the person exhibiting signs of irrationality who classify signs and behaviour as mental illness. They may use a change in the person's outlook, expression, thought content and rules associated with communication against a 'yard-stick' composed of 'mutual norms'. When the rationality of a behaviour or action is not understood in terms of social acceptance or boundaries, it is not unusual for lay society to deem the person mentally ill. Neither is it unusual for this view to be legitimized by a range of professionals.

A major difficulty for professionals is the fact that the so called 'norms' of expression, mood and behaviour are dependent upon the context and environment in which people function as rational human beings. On top of this is the way in which a person is able to articulate reasons for these phenomena. Society tends to ascribe the term mental illness when there is a breakdown in 'normal' or acceptable human actions. The concept of normality is rather like that of reasonableness, it is dependent to a great extent on the person who undertakes the defining. Generally speaking, our community functions with a shared reality that has constructed mutual value systems, morality, behaviour and beliefs. Figure 1.1 indicates some of the factors associated with mental health and illness. Whatever explanations are given regarding the way in which we perceive or come to understand problems of mental health, all are complex. Unfortunately, sociological explanations have themselves become abused by lay persons and professionals. Much distress can be caused to families when it is suggested that a person's mental state is simply a way in which society classifies or labels its deviant members. Whilst appearing to be acceptable to an extent in academic terms and having a value in explaining some of the experience of a person with problems of illness and ill health, the insensitive and inappropriate application of labelling theory may be of no consolation to those who see before them a loved family member disintegrating in personality and behaviour, and for whom treatment, protection and help is sought.

When considering some of these forces in the field of activity that affects the state of equilibrium in mental health, it becomes obvious that the concept is prone to ambiguity and contradiction. It is these contradictions that rest heavy on the shoulders of professional workers in mental health as psychiatry has in the past and in some cases still is seen as a form of social control. Accounts of its abuse are well recorded both in the Western world and in Eastern European and former communist bloc countries.

When judgements regarding such abstract phenomena as morality and intelligibility are made, those working in mental health have been shown to be faced with two options as to what changes mental health into a mental illness (Ingleby, 1982). Firstly, that those in psychiatry should eliminate value or moral judgements from their criteria and stick only to objective or clinical considerations when assessing or diagnosing—a tall, if not impossible, order as we all have similar forces acting on us. Secondly, we could simply regard psychiatric practice as a legitimate form of social control, like the legal or penal system. Of course, for this to be ethically and professionally acceptable the 'norms' inherent in social order would have to be fair, objective and just in their origin and maintenance. For this kind of social order to be free of all contradiction there would have to be universally constructed and accepted morality and the interests of all members of society would have to be in harmony!

When Symonds (1991) subjects these ideas to analysis he identifies that 'the reality and one of the major concerns of sociology is the nature of the conflicts and contradictions built into the social order'. It is believed, therefore, that the moral norms underpinning the social order are not objective, but 'value-loaded' and generated, transmitted and maintained in accordance with the dictates of particular interest groups. It follows, therefore, that whenever a moral judgement is made, questions must be asked regarding the nature of the person making the judgement, including their beliefs, interests and their objectives. Those working in contemporary mental health services are likely to spend time in their practice doing this not least of all in counselling sessions and team meetings. Simply put, it can be seen throughout our history that 'normality and conformity' have at times been equated with the concept of insanity. Such notions have been manipulated by the lay public particularly through the tabloid press and of course serve as a particularly powerful political slogan when used to describe deviation from policy, for example, 'the loony left'.

The major point here is that in many ways those working within mental health are vulnerable as the boundaries and imperatives of madness can so easily be associated with ideology. Therefore, history has shown us that the system has on occasions been a method of ensuring the maintenance of social order. Of course there are many other 'meanings' that account for a person's experience and behaviour and these are identified in other chapters. These cover more of the deviance theory and socially relative nature of our knowledge regarding mental health and well-being, medical viewpoints which assume a scientific stance and the policy issues which impinge upon both care and prevention and whether this is aimed at individuals or society in general.

PROMOTION AND PREVENTION

Changes in the direction of professional practice within mental health, particularly those associated with community care, will continue to impact upon and challenge skills and knowledge associated with treatment towards those of prevention. However, we need to be aware that such notions as 'promotion and prevention' can become slogans and in-vogue words which are devalued by being euphemisms used in an attempt to reduce the stigmatizing effect of 'mental illness'. This can be seen when treatment units using legitimate ethical means to treat illnesses feel bound to include a reference to mental health in their 'logo'. The real aim in promotion and prevention is a health ethos, and the World Health Organization describes the objectives of this in explicit terms. Our mental health is in a constant flux state. It is ever changing, reflecting responses to the environment. It is intrinsically connected to our physical, emotional and social health (Ironbar and Hooper, 1989).

Several contemporary approaches to the promotion of mental health and their applications have been described by Evans (1992) who draws attention to some of the possible causes of confusion within terms, including:

1 Positive mental health—referring to the adopting of strategies intended to enhance the existing mental health of people. The term uses the notion of maximizing human potential, emphasizing adaptive skills and draws on primary sources of Maslow (1954) and his notion of self-actualization.

2 Mental health awareness and education— referring to the dissemination of information aimed at dispelling myths regarding problems of mental health. Information technology and high-quality, rapid desk-top publishing is a good example of how the profile of issues regarding mental health has been raised in the public arena. The range of options and resources available is included in this strategy and is particularly seen in television or radio public service announcements.

3 Problem prevention and ill-health—the subtle difference between prevention, which is likely to be associated with bio-medical approaches or interventive techniques, is contrasted with the more positive approach of promoting a 'holistic' view of health.

One of the hazards of professional work in these areas is that of confining our attention to narrow concerns of individual problems. This can in turn overemphasize the person's own responsibility for his or her health and lead us to ignore the way in which the community or economic organization of society can adversely affect overall mental health.

A major aim of this book is to ensure that all professionals in mental health, or in therapeutic relationships with problems associated with mental illness, are aware of the wide social and political context. It is in this area of partnership that we can openly promote health and determine strategies of illness prevention. All participants in this process need to challenge both their own and others' assumptions regarding theory and practice. When this occurs we are more likely to achieve a healthy state of promoting the empowerment of those involved in the process of care, reducing the chances of controlling the communities needs and instead adopt practices which lead to effective partnerships for the health of all as promoted by the World Health Organization for the year 2000.

REFERENCES

Evans, J. (1992) Healthy minds. *Nursing Times*, **88** (16).

Ingleby, D. (1982) The social construction of mental illness. In Wright, P. and Teacher, A. (Eds) *The Problem of Medical Knowledge*. Edinburgh: Edinburgh University Press.

Ironbar, N.O. & Hooper, A. (1989) *Self-instruction in Mental Health Nursing*. London: Baillière Tindall.

Maslow, A.H. (1954) *Motivation and Personality*. New York: Harper & Row.

Symonds, R.F. (1991) Sociological issues in the conceptualisation of mental illness. *Journal of Advanced Nursing*, **16**, 1470–1477.

PERSONAL AND PROFESSIONAL ROLES, SKILLS AND BEHAVIOURS
PRESENT AND FUTURE

F.C. Johnson and L.D. Smith

AIMS

i) To analyse the implications for mental health nursing of recent health-related and professional initiatives
ii) To explore the meaning of competence in relation to the management of client problems and its value to those involved
iii) To consolidate previous learning in relation to skills-associated parameters and development
iv) To determine the skills inherent in practising as a first level mental health nurse
v) To promote continuing skill development necessary to enhance practice

KEY ISSUES

Professional change and progression
Influence of society on skill requirement
Roles
Client need
Competence
Skill development
Skills required to practise

Identify, analyse and assess factors causing distress and illness	Promote health, provide direct care and make interventions	Manage care programmes and services
Be critical, analytical and accountable, continue professional development	Counter discrimination, inequality and individual and institutional racism	Work within and develop policies, laws and safeguards in all settings
Understand influences on mental health and the nature/causes of disorder and illness	Know the effects of distress, disorder, illness on individuals, groups, families	Understand the basis of treatments and interventions

INTRODUCTION

On 27 April 1992, while addressing the Congress of the Royal College of Nursing, the Secretary of State, Virginia Bottomley, announced a review of mental health nursing in response to 'considerable changes in the shape of mental health services', it being considered 'vital that mental health nursing continues to keep pace with these developments' (DH, 1992a). The review promises to be comprehensive, involving nurses and other members of the multidisciplinary team in an examination of the education, leadership and clinical practice associated with mental health nursing. Its findings will be of considerable significance in regard to the specifics of roles and practice undertaken. This chapter, however, is founded on the hypothesis that, whilst there may be modifications in the degree or extent to which a particular skill may be employed in any one care setting with any individual client, the skills implicit in mental health nursing and its conduct are both consistent and identifiable.

These mental health nursing skills are analysed and discussed later within the body of the chapter, but initially it would seem appropriate to explore the recent and continuing influences exerted on mental health nursing. Such an exploration finds value in its identification of expectations made by society and its agents upon role and practice.

PROFESSIONAL DEMANDS—INITIAL PREPARATION

The statutory body, the United Kingdom Central Council for Nursing, Midwifery and Health Visiting (UKCC, 1986) has declared that the practitioner of the future should be:

'competent to assess the need for care, to monitor and evaluate care and to do this in a range of institutional and non institutional settings'.

In addition, the UKCC calls for 'a thinking person with analytical skills', competent to 'engage in autonomous practice', a 'doer' and moreover 'a knowledgeable doer'. The statements heralded the introduction of the major programme of reform in pre-registration nurse education, Project 2000, and implicit within them are certain inferences and assumptions that require to be clarified.

In the first quotation, it may be seen that the UKCC calls for a practitioner competent to *manage* client care delivery. This is then expanded to include actual hands-on, clinical *delivery* of care in the requirement for a 'doer', and one who is 'knowledgeable' in relation to the care being delivered. This is not the total expectation for there is, in addition, a requirement for the practitioner to have thought critically about, and analysed, all aspects of this care delivery and be able to apply the principles of competent client care in any setting. Certainly this call for competent practice in a variety of settings is a valuable decontextualization of the nurse's role away from not only an institution-based care but also the sickness-centred care strongly associated with it. However, most important is the demand for 'autonomous practice'—the right to practice independently, to govern oneself and one's own activities. It is the occupation of a definitive role within overall health-related practice in which the individual exerts influence and control and assumes responsibility. It is a role separate and different from those undertaken by other members of the multidisciplinary team, but it is one of equality and validity in relation to the other health professionals. The UKCC's requirement for an autonomous practitioner provides an impetus for increasing efforts towards professionalization and movement towards an independent clinical practitioner.

In providing guidance to nurse educationists in respect of developing courses to meet the requirements of the UKCC and Project 2000, the English National Board for Nursing, Midwifery and Health Visiting (ENB, 1989) identified the need for students to 'utilise a range of learning strategies . . . take responsibility for their learning' and asserted the necessity for 'critical enquiry' and an 'analytical approach to the practice of nursing'. Guidelines facilitated 'shared learning opportunities' which could be conducted on both an intra-professional and interprofessional basis whereby benefiting both client care and student development. There was, in addition, a recognition of the role and value of 'student choice' in relation to both theoretical and practical components of the course, within the constraints of overall course requirements, for example, course length, the need to meet European Community directives (EEC, 1981) and to achieve prescribed learning outcomes.

Such guidelines have significance to student nurses, teachers and course planners. In requiring the student to take responsibility for learning, the ENB acknowledge the individual as an adult learner (Knowles, 1975), capable of assuming this responsibility, or of learning to do so with assistance. This requires a concomitant alteration in the role of the teacher who, now no longer responsible for the learning that does or does not take place, assumes the role of facilitator (Knowles, 1975; Rowntree, 1990).

Again, implicit in the ENB's recognition of the student nurse as an adult learner, is the acknowledgement of the unique life skills and experiences brought by each student nurse to the course. Each will have different ambitions and personal needs to be met. The 'principle of choice', identified by the ENB as desirable wherever possible in both academic and practice aspects of course content and organization, provides recognition and acceptance of the fact that the pathway required to achieve the prescribed learning outcomes will not—and indeed should not—be identical for every student. The needs of the student nurse may be met by individualized planning and negotiation. This was reinforced by the express recommendation that courses should utilize a variety of learning strategies, which facilitates the development of a preferred learning style based on the student's experience of each method employed.

It would appear that the ENB has attempted to fulfil two separate objectives. The student nurse not only gains insight into the beliefs, roles and priorities of action inherent within other professionals, gaining valuable knowledge of other resources available to the client and nurse, but also—and importantly in the quest for auton-

omy—he or she is placed in a position of equality with students of other professions. The shared knowledge facilitates interprofessional understanding and interaction, whilst not diminishing in any way the separateness of each discipline or invalidating the way in which each utilizes the knowledge.

The degree to which shared learning is achieveable within Project 2000 is currently dependent upon locally based initiatives. The supernumerary status awarded within the framework of Project 2000 not only enhances the education of the student nurse but also enables the incorporation of the wide variety of learning opportunities available to the student. The Project 2000 model thus facilitates the development of the autonomous practitioner, knowledgeable and skilled in the practice of nursing, who is able to both manage and deliver care within the variety of settings envisaged and demanded by the UKCC.

However, there is little value in changing the perceptions, expectations and abilities of individuals undertaking pre-registration courses without a concomitant effort to address the needs of registered practitioners. The new student will gain experience of practice and will be influenced by the beliefs, feelings and roles currently utilized by supervisors. To address the needs of one group without simultaneous attention to the other would be paying lip service to the need for change and development within the profession.

THE REGISTERED PRACTITIONER

The UKCC, in its publication of a code of professional conduct (UKCC, 1989) prescribed the standard of behaviour demanded of practitioners in order to:

'justify public trust and confidence ... uphold and enhance the good standing and reputation of the profession, to serve the interests of society and above all to safeguard the interests of individual patients and clients'.

It is important to internalize the 16 target behaviours contained within the code required to be demonstrated in practice, for the UKCC firmly places accountability for the standard and quality of practice on the shoulders of each individual practitioner. Each of the target behaviours is of considerable significance to the nurse.

The practitioner is charged with promoting the safety and well-being of patients, ensuring that no act or omission on the nurse's part is detrimental to the client. There is a requirement for the nurse to take into account the customs, values and beliefs of the client in all aspects of care management and delivery, recognizing and respecting 'the uniqueness and dignity of each patient and client' irrespective of 'ethnic origin, religious beliefs, personal attributes, the nature of the health problems or any other factor'. The code requires nurses to work with patients, clients and their families, fostering, recognizing and respecting their involvement in the planning and delivery of care. Active participation by those individuals significant in and to the care process is to be encouraged, engendering partnerships in care and negotiation regarding outcomes and actions rather than dependency and compliance in response to professional domination.

The nurse is cautioned against abuse both of the privileged relationship with the client, in respect of access to information and property, and also of the professional qualifications held, in regard to promotion of commercial products. In addition, the nurse is urged to refuse any 'gift, favour or hospitality' offered by individuals currently in care 'which might be interpreted as seeking to exert influence to obtain preferential consideration', thus reasserting the principles of equality of care for all, according to individual need.

However, the registered practitioner has other demands imposed by the profession. The UKCC expressly requires continuing development of the nurse to both maintain and improve professional knowledge and competence, and to acknowledge any limitations of competence, refusing to perform any activity in such instances until appropriate education and assessment has been undertaken. This is not an *option* proffered by the UKCC. It is a necessity, a demand, a requirement.

The practitioner is further required to work in a 'collaborative and co-operative manner with other health care professionals', recognizing and respecting their contributions to overall care and service provision. Collaboration means working together in partnerships where all parties are equally important in the activities undertaken. We believe that the statement aims to provoke a reassessment and realignment of attitudes and behaviour and the development of an 'autonomous practitioner' determined by the P2000 model of education (UKCC, 1986).

In order to reinforce this heightened status, it is valid and reasonable for the registered practitioner not only to *have* conscientious objections, but also to *verbalize* these to the appropriate person or authority where these are relevant to professional practice. Having reflected on practice issues, the nurse is entitled to make considered judgements in the light of knowledge, beliefs, values and opinions. This finds extension in the demand for nurses to make professional judgements in relation to the adequacies of resource provision which may jeopardize or mitigate against safe standards of practice, again, making these judgements known to appropriate individuals or authorities.

Finally, the Code of Professional Conduct demands that the registered nurse cares for and assists in the development of both peers and subordinates, taking appropriate action in each instance. The nurse is responsible for ensuring that the workload of, and pressures on, colleagues and subordinates are not excessive, constituting a hazard to, or preventing, safe practice. Similarly, teaching other nurses and facilitating their continuing acquisition of competence in practice is no longer an option—it is a duty, an expectation made of a professional which cannot be ignored or side-stepped. Registered nurses must be willing to impart the knowledge and skills inherent within their spheres of practice to others.

CONTINUING PROFESSIONAL DEVELOPMENT

To reinforce the demands of the Code of Conduct, and in line with the innovations of pre-registration education programmes, in 1989 the UKCC launched a project group charged with 'developing a coherent and comprehensive framework for education and practice beyond registration' (UKCC, 1989). The project group reported in 1990 (UKCC, 1990) and its recommendations were offered for discussion and debate by the profession. Decision on these recommendations is awaited.

However, in reaching their recommendations, the Postregistration Education and Practice Project (PREPP) group reviewed the context of future professional practice, in particular the changes in demographic trends and patterns of disease and the inequalities of health care recognized within UK society (Black, 1980). In addition the group identified the importance of the World Health Organization's emphasis on health promotion (WHO, 1986) and the influence of legislation, in the form of the NHS and Community Care Act 1990.

PREPP report

The nine recommendations embodied within the PREPP report are thought crucial to both the ongoing development of the individual registered nurse and also the profession as a whole. It is recognized, for example, that individuals assuming a new sphere of practice require initial support and guidance to facilitate both consolidation of previous learning and its specific application to the area of care provision. In particular, a period of three to six months is recommended for the support of newly registered nurses by experienced role models, called preceptors, prior to assuming a primary practice role, that is, the acceptance of:

'responsibility with confidence, in co-operation with other practitioners and disciplines as required, for the individual's or group's health care needs. This involves care which is comprehensive, appropriate and, where possible, research based'.
Black, 1980

This recognition of the need for adequate sup-

port reinforces the requirements of the Code of Professional Conduct (UKCC, 1992) for nurses not to undertake activities for which they feel inadequately prepared or practised, without prior instruction and assessment of competence. This is deliberately and specifically applied to those individuals who have returned to practice after a break of five years or more, and who will be required to undertake an individualized programme to update their knowledge and skills base.

PREPP requires all nurses to *demonstrate* that they have maintained and enhanced professional knowledge and performance, and to record developmental activities within a 'personal professional profile'. There is a recommendation that five days' study leave should be taken by each practitioner within every three-year periodic registration period and, to reinforce the importance of such activities, that these should be formalized by appropriate legislation.

The Project Group envisaged a continuum of practice levels and abilities from primary to advanced practitioner roles. The advanced practitioner role is one which incorporates 'high standards of care', 'direct care, education, research, management, involvement in health policy-making and development of strategies'. PREPP envisages a gradual movement from one level to the next via the accumulation of credits towards a recordable qualification, the 'standard, kind and content' of which will be determined by the UKCC. In addition the Group believes that for some, specialist practitioner status will lead to consultant practice level, a standard of performance associated with 'pioneer roles' in health care and treatment, acting as 'an authoritative resource' for others and as an innovator in areas of special challenge.

Community Education and Practice report

In line with the recommendations of PREPP, and again in response to changing expectations and patterns of care provision, a second UKCC report identified proposals for the future of Community Education and Practice (UKCC, 1991); that is, action required to ensure that registered practitioners are prepared to function effectively within the community. The report emphasizes the need for nurses who are 'responsive and relevant to the needs of society and to the health services', and, whilst recognizing the increasing emphasis within Project 2000 (UKCC, 1986) of gaining experience in institutional and non-institutional settings, calls for specific preparation for the specialist community health care nurse. There is a recommendation for an educational/practice programme which provides all registered practitioners with the core skills required for community practice plus additional requirements to meet the needs of the nurse in a specific area of practice, for example, mental health and occupational health nursing. The proposals recommend that credit should be given for prior experience and learning, courses be both flexible and based on shared inter/intradisciplinary learning, and lead to a recordable qualification.

The community health care nurse of the future, if proposals are enacted, will be an individual who is competent to:

---

1 Provide skilled nursing care in differing environments with varied resources
2 Support informal carers
3 Search out and identify evolving health care needs
4 Make informed judgements to distinguish between health and social needs
5 Advise on services available and access to them
6 Stimulate awareness of health needs
7 Empower people to influence health policy
8 Provide leadership, management and teaching skills to ensure quality and continuity of care
9 Provide health data to employing authorities through health profiles
10 Inform them about the provision of health policies
11 Undertake quality assurance activities.

The Community Education and Practice group have in their report reaffirmed the value and role of primary health care provision in total client care, linking it with both the aims of pre-registration education and those envisaged within post-registration nurse education outcomes.

ENB framework for continuing practice

The framework provides ten key characteristics and their detailed learning outcomes which may be utilized by the practitioner in any or all of three activities. Used by the nurse alone, they may be valuable in the reflective processes accompanying a review of development to date or in identification of current learning needs and activity required. When based on 'a constructive partnership between the practitioner, manager and educationist', the ten key characteristics may be utilized to discuss the individual's role within the organization and the professional development needs associated with it. Each individual participating within the partnership must be committed to enabling needs to be met, and again credit accumulation and transfer (CNAA, 1986) is the basis for the programme of study. When utilized formally in this way, the programme leads to the Higher Award, a professional and academic qualification that will be at a minimum of first level degree. During activities undertaken, the registered practitioner is required to maintain a professional (profile) portfolio, to serve both as a record of achievement and also as a vehicle to facilitate the development of critical thinking and reflective skills. The ENB further recognizes the value of the framework in identifying the development needs of those individuals returning to practice after a break in service by assisting in the construction of individualized learning schedules relevant to need and thus avoiding repetition and duplication.

It is appropriate at this point to recap on the demands of the Profession upon its members, and the following words and phrases spring readily from this text:

---

thinking ... analytical ... critical ... competent ... autonomous ... knowledgeable doer ... variety of practice settings ... range of learning strategies ... adult learner ... choice ... responsible for learning ... shared learning ... opportunities ... accountability ... judgement ... continuing development ... primary/specialist/consultant practice ... specific preparation ... leadership ... resource person ... empowering agent ... influencing health care provision ... flexible programmes to meet specific practice needs ... support for development activities.

These are important facets of *what* nurses will be doing and *how* they will do it. There are even indications of *where* nurses will practice but who will be the recipients of nurses attention? Government legislation and the activities of other national and international agencies may offer some insight into this area (see also Chapter 3).

GOVERNMENT INFLUENCES

Caring for People

The White Paper, *Caring for People*: *Community Care in the Next Decade and Beyond* (DH/DSS, 1989) provided a framework designated to assist people 'to lead, as far as possible, full and independent lives', and to 'secure the services they need', 'stimulating public agencies to tailor services to individual needs'. The Government affirmed its commitment to provide both services and support to those affected by the problems of 'ageing, mental illness, mental handicap or physical or sensory disability', enabling independent living either in their own homes or 'homely' settings within the community. The White Paper promotes the concepts of 'achievement of full potential' and 'choice', with individuals having a greater say in 'how they live their lives and the services they need to do so'. There is a call for services that 'respond flexibly' and that 'concentrate on those with the greatest need' and 'key changes' are identified to facilitate the development of the services envisaged. The White Paper determines that local authorities will become responsible—with assistance from others—for 'assessing individual need, designing care arrangements and securing their delivery within available resources'. Local authorities are required to 'produce and publish plans' relating to the development of community care services and

these should be consistent with those of health authorities and other interested parties. There is a requirement for 'making maximum use of the independent sector' and for inspection/registration units which monitor standards of care within residential homes to be developed 'at arm's length' from the authority, to ensure objectivity in function. The White Paper further proposes a new funding structure for those requiring financial assistance for residential or nursing home care, with local authorities becoming responsible for this support, and, in addition, proposes specific grants towards the 'development of social care for seriously mentally ill people'.

The White Paper clearly differentiates between social care and health care. Social care includes '... help with personal and domestic tasks such as cleaning, washing and preparing meals, with disablement equipment and home adaptations, transport, budgeting and other aspects of daily living'. Health care 'covers investigation, diagnosis, treatment, rehabilitation and continuing care together with—most importantly—community health services, including community nursing'. It is envisaged that health care within the community will continue to be provided by the primary health care team, but that where health care needs are exceeded by social needs, social services authorities will be required to assess the individual's needs for community care, with assistance from 'all agencies and professionals involved'. The White Paper recommends that one individual should be responsible for co-ordinating action—'a case manager' and whilst recognizing that this individual may often be employed by a social service authority, identifies that for some clients community nurses may be particularly suitable to fill this role because they are the professionals in most regular contact with the client.

Indeed, the White Paper recognizes the significant contribution of community nurses, their 'skills and expert knowledge', and their ability to assist people with 'social, psychological and health care problems which may affect their quality of life'. There is also an acceptance of the degree and variety of neighbourhood networks available for mobilization by nurses and that therefore they have an 'important contribution' to make in assessment of the client's needs, the development of care arrangements and their subsequent delivery. The White Paper also highlights, however, the Government's wish to:

> 'ensure that nurses's time is deployed to the best effect on work which requires their special skill, leaving work which does not require those skills to be done by others'.

It appears to us that the care described within the White Paper as 'health care' may be interpreted as active, health-enhancing and therapeutic in nature, whilst that referred to as 'social care' may be viewed as that required in longer term maintenance of that health status achieved; a more supportive, general assistance not requiring higher level skills associated with the nurse. Traditionally, nurses have undertaken a variety of tasks not specifically or strictly incorporated within the term 'patient care', particularly outside of office hours when, in the absence of appropriate staff, they run errands, perform secretarial/clerical duties and the roles associated with off-duty therapists (Davies, 1977). The nurse's ability to 'cope and get things done'—whatever the nature of the work required within the overall care setting—is not that envisaged within the White Paper. The nurse will utilize specific roles and skills within definitive areas of client care, deferring all other aspects of care required to more appropriately qualified staff.

Viewed at this point, Government influence would appear to be of positive benefit to the nurse, building upon this vision of the autonomous professional with a definitive role. A Department of Health Circular (DH, 1990) however, issued in 1990, charged district health authorities, in collaboration with social services authorities, to design and implement local care programme policies for all in-patients considered for discharge and all new patients accepted by the specialist psychiatric services. This circular too differentiated between social and health care, obviously building on the White Paper (DH/DSS, 1989), and whilst one may argue as to the unrealistic and artificial division between the two within mental health care (White and Brooker,

1990a,b; Townsend and Davidson, 1982), when the circular confirms that those individuals discharged into the community will continue to be 'patients of the consultant psychiatrist', the inference may not be so supportive of the autonomous nurse.

During the last decade, community psychiatric nurses (CPNs) have forged stronger links with general practitioners and the primary health care team. The latter have found nurses a valuable source of help in relation to the care required by clients with temporary psychological problems and CPNs have increasingly concentrated their attention on these individuals who are 'responsive to intervention and concomitant job satisfaction' (White, 1991). White considers that, whilst not 'universally popular with some CPNs', they will need to re-align themselves with closer working relationships with psychiatrists to assume the role of key worker/case manager for those discharged from hospital, who frequently have more long-term and persistent mental health problems. He points in addition to studies on the role and function of practice nurses, and suggests that the care of 'minor' mental health problems may be incorporated within their remit, or that perhaps general practitioners will directly employ CPNs or other counselling services to meet their needs in this direction. White is concerned that some CPNs may have 'inadvertently deskilled themselves' in relation to the care required by the client experiencing chronic mental health problems by their emphasis on the clientele with acute, short-term problems and considers that resettlement and rehabilitation would seem to be a major function of CPNs in the future.

In 1993, the White Paper (DH/DSS, 1989) was implemented as legislation and we can only infer from our analysis that there is a definitive role envisaged for nurses in that the focus of attention will be those clients who exhibit the challenging behaviours associated with mental health problems. This role appears to incorporate that of key worker/case manager and would seem to demand active intervention rather than low-level support and maintenance. Care will be planned and delivered in collaboration with others, utilizing all available resources, whether statutory, voluntary or independent in nature, to assist the individual.

The element of partnership and collaboration is reiterated by the Government in its child protection legislation (DH, 1991), and also by those reviewing the services required by the mentally disordered offender (DH and Home Office, 1992). The latter calls for prisoners to have the right of access to medical and nursing care of the same standard as that available to other citizens, that is, the standard set by the National Health Service. 'Contracting in' of National Health Service mental health care services would, the report states, enhance case management and the subsequent transition from prison to the community. The report calls for diversion and removal of mentally disordered offenders from the criminal justice system, highlighting problems associated with self-harm, violence towards others, chemical abuse and HIV and AIDS, in addition to the longer-term problems associated with persistent mental health disorders. The report advises that services for this group should be included in local authority plans in 1993–1994, and this, plus the desire to contract in mental health services from district health authorities, reaffirms our belief in the role of the mental health nurse as a 'collaborator' in care planning and delivery and an interventionist in strategies to prevent, minimize and eradicate problems associated with challenging behaviours.

The Health of the Nation

One more aspect of recent Government action requires to be identified, not in relation to the role envisaged for the mental health nurse within it but, quite the contrary, because of the role which we believe mental health nurses *should* have within it. The action referred to is, of course, *The Health of the Nation* (DH, 1992b) which aims to promote healthier lifestyles and which is developed from *Targets for Health for All* (WHO, 1986).

It calls for a co-operative and co-ordinated approach towards reductions in deaths from coronary artery disease and stroke, cancers, accidents and suicide, and in addition a reduction in the incidence of HIV, AIDS and other sexually transmitted disease, and unwanted pregnancies.

The role of stress in relation to susceptibility to auto-immune disease and cancer is identified (Borysenko and Borysenko, 1982), as is the relationship between stress and coronary heart and cerebro-vascular disorders (Lazarus and Folkman, 1984). The individual experiencing the effects of stress is more accident prone in general because of poor concentration and attention levels (Powell and Enright, 1990) and coping mechanisms commonly employed include excessive use of alcohol and cigarettes (HEA, 1988). Cigarettes are linked with cancer (Doll and Peto, 1981) and alcohol with accidents (Godfrey *et al.*, 1989). We also believe that the mental health nurse has significant value in the assistance required by at-risk groups in relation to sexually transmitted diseases and sex education, generally as part of education for living programmes.

In relation to suicide, it seems strange that there are still so few twenty-four-hour crisis intervention services provided by professional nurses and, whilst voluntary organizations such as the Samaritans provide a very valuable assistance to society, this would appear to be a role that mental health nurses are admirably qualified to fill. The mental health nurse of the future should be actively involved within health promotion and problem prevention, and this will be recognized by regional- and district-level working groups in their activities to meet targets prescribed.

ROLES AND PARAMETERS

The previous discussion identifies the roles and responsibilities which the registered practitioner is required to assume within overall care provision. These may be incorporated within the following designations:

1 *Care manager*—requiring the practitioner to assess an individual's need for care, differentiate between social and health care needs and identify those health care deficits that are amenable to nursing intervention, referring others to the appropriate agency. In addition, the nurse will plan nursing strat-

egies, monitor the care delivery processes and evaluate the effectiveness and acceptability of provision.

2 *Care collaborator*—involving the nurse in teamwork with other nurses and support workers to deliver nursing care prescribed and also with other disciplines and agencies, to compile a comprehensive plan to meet an individual's total need for health and social care.

3 *Interventionist*—relating to the delivery and implementation of specific nursing strategies and interventions by the practitioner, to assist the individual towards health recovery and the achievement of optimum health status.

4 *Resource manager*—necessitating efficient and effective use of temporal, material and personnel resources, including self, in health care provision, where these fall within the practitioner's sphere of authority and influence. This includes the continuing development of existing individuals, services and facilities, and the creation of new instruments and vehicles to assist in meeting health requirements.

5 *Health promoter*—requiring the nurse to design, implement, monitor and evaluate educational programmes and strategies to assist individuals to adopt healthier lifestyles. In addition, there is a requirement to create opportunities, to enhance the desire and motivation of individuals towards optimum health and wellbeing.

6 *Facilitator*—requiring activities and strategies to enable smoother transitions, achievement and acquisitions by others towards specific goals and intentions. These should assist, guide, enhance and support the individual in endeavours rather than providing the answers or actions required, thus create dependency and remove responsibility for the task.

7 *Researcher*—demanding logical and systematic investigation and examination of all aspects of health care need and subsequent care provision and delivery, utilizing appropriate criteria, such as effectiveness, efficiency and levels of consumer acceptance

and satisfaction as a basis for judgements made.

8 *Adviser*—encompassing all activities aimed at informing, enlightening or appraising others of relevant facts, findings, opinions, beliefs, feelings and intentions associated with professional activity.

9 *Energizer*—incorporating skills and behaviours that encourage and motivate individuals—including self—towards analysis of current performance and, where appropriate, generate desire for development, change, innovation and attainment. The role includes activities associated with creation of an environment conducive to, and expectant of, critical self appraisal and positive peer evaluation.

The parameters of the above roles, it may be remembered, were identified in the statement that health care described 'investigation, diagnosis, treatment, rehabilitation and continuing care' of the individual. We believe that the mental health nurse can assume a position unavailable to those colleagues within other branches of nursing.

HEALTH CARE

The nurse's role in health care differs substantially within each branch speciality because it is dependent upon the nature of the problems that prompt the individual to seek assistance. Where somatic discomfort, disturbed body function or distorted body contours form the basis of complaints, whether in a child or adult, investigations are conducted via specialist departments, for example, radiography, haematology and electrocardiography. These are dependent upon the complaints of the individual, a detailed medical history and physical examination, and from the results, diagnosis is formulated and treatment prescribed.

In these initial stages, the role of the nurse is primarily organizational, educative and supportive but once treatment commences, responsibilities transfer to the areas of specialist preparation and other care required, including maintenance of the therapeutic programmes initiated by medical and paramedical colleagues. The goals of nursing care at this time are towards sustaining and enhancing previous healthy function, facilitating the achievement of optimum benefit from treatment regimes and promoting health awareness and psychosocial well-being. Rehabilitation and continuing care finds extension of these activities to include those relating to maintenance of the individual's motivation towards realistic short-, medium- and long-term goals and of facilitating the utilization of appropriate resources to assist both the individual and the family during the extended care situation.

Where intellectual disability and its associated problems prompt assistance to be sought, the nurse assumes a different role. Medical examination and a comprehensive individual and family history may elicit the aetiology of the problems and this is of great value—as it is in somatic disease and disorder—in the development of services aimed at prophylaxis, promotion of health-orientated lifestyles and in prevention of continuing exposure to causative agents, for example, non-accidental injury and biopsychosocial deprivation. However, the damage is permanent and the diagnostic element of the impairment is of little value in predicting the health care requirements of the individual, for ultimate performance and optimum levels of function need not be limited by it.

Treatment is based on a comprehensive assessment of behaviour, skills and abilities, limitations and needs, that is, a multidisciplinary, multisituational analysis of every facet of the performance associated with life and living. Within treatment, there is a requirement for multifocused activities and strategies, with simultaneous attention towards biologically based sequelae, the cognitive, affective and behavioural effects and sociocultural implications of the original impairment whilst maximizing skills and abilities. The nurse's role is central within the treatment schedule, both as a therapist and as an overall manager of care, giving appropriate assistance throughout the changing needs encountered, whether in the initial treatment period or in rehabilitation and continuing care phases. A focus for family involvement, the nurse fulfils valuable roles as collaborator, resource manager, facilitator and adviser, in addition to intervening where necessary to provide counselling and support in times of distress and difficulty.

MENTAL HEALTH NURSING

However, in any review of the basis for psychiatry and mental health care, there is likely to be excessive vagueness, inconsistency and conflicting ideation and yet, for the most part, it is the area of nursing in which the nurse is able—if so desired—to relate to and identify with most closely. It is difficult, if not impossible, to appreciate fully the thoughts, feelings and behaviours of the individual whose length or quality of life is continuously threatened by neoplasia, heart disease or AIDs. Similarly, it is difficult to envisage a world in which an individual is unable to share the quality and quantity of experience readily encountered and expected by the vast majority of the society in which he or she resides; independence, recognition for achievements valued by that society, acceptance and integration are examples.

Yet everyone has felt depressed. Anxiety is a common experience and many express what they know to be irrational fears. Some have experienced feelings of guilt at a level well beyond that warranted by the stimulus which provoked the feelings, while others have been unable to experience remorse for some past action that society has labelled bad, wicked or unacceptable. It is not uncommon for individuals to develop a headache or some other somatic symptomatology when called upon to do something they do not wish to do. It seems relatively simple to relate to delusional ideation when listening to heated discussions on subjects such as politics, economics and religion. Most of us will have experienced a hallucination. Illusions are relatively commonplace as are misperceptions relating to personal skills and limitations, presentation of self to the world, and body image. Temporary loss of the ability to differentiate between reality and fantasy is another common experience. We recognize the idea of total absorption in a horror film, jumping and screaming as the victim is grabbed by a vampire! Compensation, by overeating or overspending, or denial of self worth by food refusal or other deprivation tactics, are also features of 'normal life' and living. In fact, the majority of symptomatology associated with 'mental illness' finds expression to a lesser degree, lower intensity, or in a more acceptable form or situation within 'normal' mental functioning parameters.

Mental health nursing may be considered therefore to relate to assisting individuals who exhibit thoughts, feelings and behaviours that are unacceptable to, or inappropriate in, current society and yet which are in essence merely extensions of everyday functioning. It is relatively simple to identify with such experiences even though the degree, extent or depth of them may be beyond the nurse's comprehension. Such an analysis may also assist in the implementation of strategies to ameliorate, eradicate or prevent problems in some individuals as will be discussed.

MENTAL HEALTH CARE

We stated earlier that the basis for psychiatry is vague and full of inconsistencies, and this in itself is of significance to the role of the nurse within mental health care.

Theories provide descriptions, explanations, predications and methodology to control phenomena. They are utilized to guide and determine action, education and research and provide a base-line for professional practice and development. Whilst there is disagreement in regard to the need or value of one all-encompassing perspective (Jacox, 1974; Chinn and Jacobs, 1979), Stevens (1984) provides a measure of compromise by suggesting that the degree of complexity of a subject area may dictate the broadness or narrowness of theories. Whichever position is assumed on this continuum, some generality is necessary.

In psychiatry, little is proven or able to be generalized but this should not evoke complete dismissal. It is an area of study fraught with difficulties and ambiguities and heavily dependent both on society itself and other branches of medicine.

The parameters of the field alter dramatically with the views and expectations of society. We have demonstrated the relative 'normality' of symptomatology which, in excess, may be regarded as requiring assistance. However, the dividing line is drawn by the society in which it occurs and is therefore culturally bound. Behaviour considered unacceptable in Great Britain may be the norm in Papua New Guinea or some other culture. Similarly, acceptability in London may be construed as inappropriancy in a rural village elsewhere in the country. In any society where geographically generated diversity is further compounded by the introduction of a variety of different ethnic, religious or other social groupings, setting these parameters becomes even more difficult. Integration and cross-culturalization blurs previous boundaries and in addition creates problems for those cultures introduced.

Distortions of parameters also occur in response to relaxation of the degree of liberality demonstrated within a society and, whilst the treatment of dissidents in other countries may automatically spring to mind, nearer to home compulsory admission and treatment of individuals exhibiting promiscuity, homosexuality and alcoholism were, at one point in history, relatively common. Views of antisocial and aberrant behaviour alter, mirroring the changes within a society. These may generate increased expectations in relation to the amelioration or eradication of previously accepted or disregarded symptomatology. Feelings associated with depressed mood or anxiety were considered an everyday part of life which were expected and tolerated, whilst little expectation—and even less discussion—centred around sexual function and therefore problems were not acknowledged. In some areas of modern-day living, the requirement for assistance has increased in line with expectations and awareness.

The limited discussion above indicates the fluidity of the parameters of the field, but when the nature of the problem area is examined, an understanding of the difficulties surrounding psychiatry increases. Thoughts, feelings and behaviours are not the most tangible or concrete of human function in terms of their origin, there is still more of the brain that is unknown than known and advances continue to influence theories of aetiology. New technology continues to reveal the intricacies and minutiae of body composition and function, enabling study of areas of potential influences and value, previously unavailable for examination. However, when one considers the myriad of factors that may provoke or exacerbate mental health problems, for example, prenatal, perinatal, postnatal, physiological, psychological, sociological, genetic, biochemical, structural—to identify but a few—it is not surprising that the origins of such problems continue to be described as multifactoral in nature. Certainly no one theory has generality or, even in relation to a specific diagnosis, is consistently relevant. Aetiology is vague.

Investigation too is often less than scientific for whilst appropriate technology may be utilized to exclude or assess the degree of somatic influences as causation of problems; subjective observations of behaviour frequently form the basis of diagnosis. Differentiation between diagnostic categories of neurosis and psychosis is usually made with relative ease, with predominant symptomatology providing the diagnostic 'fine tuning'.

Medical treatment is limited in many instances, with medication promoting insight into the inappropriacy of bizarre thoughts and perceptions, and thereby reducing their frequency or verbalization, or providing symptomatic relief, thereby reducing stress. Electroplexy is utilized in some selected clients to good effect in stabilizing mood. However, both methods of intervention are the subject of continuing and intense debate with regard to their actual value and place in client care, and whether their use is more advantageous or damaging to the individual because of the side-effects of administration.

It may be seen that psychiatry—for all of the above reasons and more—is able to provide only a small proportion of assistance required by the individual experiencing problems associated with their mental health. A dearth of concrete information regarding aetiology makes 'curative' treatment difficult and whilst research continues in this area, the mental health nurse, in conjunction with other members of the multidisciplinary team, provides a major role within health care.

The nurse within mental health care assumes a significant role within the investigation phase of care, for many problems associated with cogni-

tion, affect and behaviour may not be spontaneously exteriorized on initial contact. A differentiation between symptomatology required for diagnostic purposes and medical treatment, and the problems to be identified for a nursing assessment and subsequent care planning, may be of value at this juncture to prevent later confusion. Psychomotor acceleration is a sign, and 'feeling very low' a symptom, but the problems associated with these relate their effects on health and well-being, on the safety of the client and others within the care situation and potential sequelae on the usual roles and responsibilities of the individual. The effects of all of these on those significant in the care process is of considerable importance, for what may not be a problem as perceived by the client, may be adjudged a considerable problem by carers or other interested parties.

Where people have insight in relation to the problems they are currently experiencing, ventilation of these problems in their entirety and with complete honesty may, quite naturally, require feelings of trust to have been established—beliefs regarding personal and psychological safety, acceptance and recognition as someone worthy of attention and assistance—and this is rarely achievable on first contact or within minutes. Time, availability and attention are required, in addition to the skills and characteristics of the nurse, to promote a milieu conducive to exploration.

Efficient collection and collation of relevant data is time consuming. It is multicontextual and involves a variety of individuals, including other clients, significant others and health personnel, as behaviour in, and reactions to, such interactions may provide information of considerable value in relation to diagnosis.

Nurses administer medical treatment in the form of medication and often, by the sheer nature of their role as the health care professional in most regular and frequent contact with the client, are best able to judge the response to, and effects of, these preparations. In addition, the nurse undertakes preparation and after-care of individuals receiving electroplexy and, again, frequently participate during actual treatment. Response to electroplexy is very individual and may take days to be fully elicited, and therefore the nurse assumes an ideal position to monitor and advise on the benefits or otherwise gained.

The majority of the remaining treatment required to assist the individual to eradicate or ameliorate symptoms of mental health disturbance, and associated rehabilitation and continuing care, fall within the remit and skill base of the mental health nurse, in conjunction with other professional and lay health care personnel. The position of the nurse within mental health may be considered unique, in relation to the significant role undertaken within all aspects of health care.

THE PHILOSOPHY OF MENTAL HEALTH NURSING

Whilst we will not undertake an in-depth discussion in relation to this area, there are aspects that require to be analysed and considered in relation to the roles and skills of the nurse within quality mental health care provision. For example:

Is the individual truly unique?

The word 'unique' is frequently applied to people and situations and even the UKCC in its code of conduct (UKCC, 1992) refers to the patient/client as such, but is its meaning fully comprehended and acted upon? Is it understood that the individual's skills and limitations, experiences, expectations, hopes, fears, beliefs, prejudices, responses, reactions and needs are as idiosyncratic as fingerprints? If the individual is truly unique, then to provide assistance that meets specific needs and deficits, the nurse must be aware that every interaction, strategy and schedule has to be modified and specially tailored to be appropriate. For the individual to join in a pre-set day centre five-day programme when only three half-day sessions within it are of any value to specific problems and needs experienced is a poor use of resources as well as superficial care planning. Similarly, joining an anxiety management group once each week is of little use to the individual experiencing severe problems if no other inter-

ventions are employed. Care has to be specific to the individual's needs if it is to be of optimum benefit. Creativity and flexibility are characteristics of great value.

There is also the question of individual worth, that is:

Are some people worth more than others? Or do some deserve more or less of the nurse's time, effort or skill?

This may provoke a cry of indignation but considered further, the value of the question may become clear. Mental health nurses see people at their most distressed and vulnerable. Nurses, like all human beings, experience feelings ranging from anger to sadness, pity to apathy, empathy to disgust and fear to pleasure. Should an individual's value or degree of merit be based on words verbalized or behaviours exhibited, the quality and quantity of health care and skilled attention may be affected. It is therefore of great importance that the nurse is able to differentiate between what the individual is and what he or she does. If the nurse is unable to accept individuals as they are at that moment, the nurse's moralistic and judgemental attitude will inhibit the development of any therapeutic relationship (Egan, 1990), not only with this nurse but perhaps with others within the care setting. Should the nurse feel unable to interact with a client from the basis of trust and respect, this needs to be recognized by asking for assistance to deal effectively with feelings generated. This is a developmental issue and not something that the nurse should feel ashamed of or vulnerable to admit.

Nomenclature

What do we call the person seeking mental health care—a patient or a client?

This is not merely pedantry. By definition, a 'patient' is someone who receives medical treatment whilst a 'client' is an individual who employs a professional as an agent (Hanks, 1979). There is a significant difference.

A patient *receives*, is given to and is done at, for and to, by someone who knows best what is needed. In somatic disease, for example, a patient needs an appendicectomy, needs an intravenous infusion to rehydrate or restore electrolyte balance or needs a fracture immobilized in plaster of Paris. In most instances the causation of the problem is clearly defined and, by trial and error over years of practice, the best treatment found to date has been identified and can be applied. However, even where there is dispute about the best method of treatment, the doctor has his preferred strategies and will advise in view of these. The patient takes the advice and is done at, to, or for, his illness, for otherwise the doctor may refuse to accept responsibility for the outcome. In psychiatry there is no certainty in regard to either aetiology or treatment and therefore the 'patient' may be at a great disadvantage within such a system.

A client, on the other hand, directs the interaction and subsequent activities, whilst taking advantage of the specialist advice and skills of the professional. Solicitors, for example, are not given *carte blanche* to do as they please on behalf of clients. They will inform about facts, opinions and the potential sequelae of such options, but the client will make the decision on future action based on informed judgement. Certainly if, at a later date, clients feel badly advised, they may take appropriate action to address their grievance.

The client within the health care system has an entitlement to the same service. There is a right to be provided with a professional analysis of the problem, the choices available to assist in problem resolution, an objective assessment of the value of each choice, and advice based on experience of the treatments offered. The client has the right to accept or reject that advice based on information given and request the 'service' that he, as a customer, has the right to expect. Should a service not be available to meet the client's expectations, there are two options—to settle for what may be considered as second best or to take custom elsewhere. Either way, the client remains in control. To return to the analogy of the solicitor–client relationship, who would dream of allowing a solicitor to make the final decision on a particular house purchase or on the specific details within a 'last will and testament'? It would not be sensible to leave such decisions to others and it can be argued that those relating to health and wellbeing are of greater importance to the individual. Should the individual seeking assistance be called a patient or a client?

One final question in relation to philosophy and nursing must be:

Should the parameters and limitations of socially acceptable behaviour be extended or distorted to accommodate mental illness?

A tangible example may assist in the consideration of this. The nurse walks past a client in the corridor who is exhibiting grossly antisocial behaviour. At a later point in the day, when off duty, the nurse visits the supermarket and sees another shopper behaving in a similarly antisocial manner. Is the nurse's reaction and response the same in both instances? If the answer to this is 'no', then how useful is this re-setting of expectations to the client, who remains significantly different to the rest of society; to the client's family, who continue to find the problem unacceptable; to the nurse, who sees no improvement in the client's 'condition' or to society, which loses the potential of an entire human being and which continues to bear a financial burden for care provision?

THE SKILLS OF THE MENTAL HEALTH NURSE

A skill may be considered as an ability to use 'knowledge effectively and readily' ... in performance, a 'learned power of doing a thing competently' or a 'developed or acquired aptitude or ability' (Gore *et al.*, 1981). It may also be expressed as an 'ability coming from one's knowledge, practice, aptitude to do something well' (Stein, 1967). Both definitions refer to a prescribed standard, that is 'doing something well' or 'competently', and indeed the reader may recall this continuing demand of the UKCC for a 'competent' practitioner (UKCC, 1986). Wood and Power (1987) drew a distinction between competence and performance, concluding that competence 'refers to what a person knows and can do under ideal circumstances', incorporating knowledge and abilities, whilst performance describes 'what is actually done under existing circumstances', which may be influenced by a variety of factors, including mood, motivation, attention and style. Tuxworth (1991) concurs with this view but, in addition, describes the difficulties of defining competence within an occupational field, due to the nature of activities undertaken. Activities may be process-, product- or people-orientated, or combine all three dimensions and therefore must be field specific to be of value. Whilst we admit to its lack of technical description, we assert that competent health care provision and nursing activity is that which is of a quality and quantity, appropriacy and breadth, depth and frequency which the nurse would approve of being given to the people held most dear to him or her as an individual.

Learning to learn

Perhaps one of the most basic skill requirements needed by the nurse is that of learning—learning *is* a skill. Problem-solving techniques will be required within many activities associated with both personal and professional performance. Defining the goal to be achieved, identifying the limitations within current status that prevent achievement of the goal and then generating solutions to remove these limitations, provides a plan of action. Solutions selected may later be evaluated with regard to success in meeting objectives, and activities modified in response.

Learning what to learn is also a skill, and whilst individuals consider 'learning' to be those activities carried out prior to an examination, the experiential learning that takes place during life and activities of living goes unrecognized and undervalued (Steinaker and Bell, 1979). Concrete experience generates awareness and curiosity with regard to issues. Reflection and analysis of cur-

rent knowledge highlights areas of deficit and special interest. Asking questions of 'what if . . .?' 'is there an alternative to this?' 'why?' and 'who says so?' assists in this process, and facilitates the formulation of hypotheses. These may then be tested, leading to further concrete experience and a continuing cyclical motion (Kolb, 1976). Learning how to learn may significantly improve performance in learning and problem solving (Ramprogus, 1988) and advanced cognitive skills are vital in nursing.

Skills of self awareness

The nurse is required to exert positive and therapeutic effects on the client and others involved within the care situation and yet, as is any other individual, is only a human being. As such, nurses hold values and beliefs, attitudes and prejudices, assumptions and feelings that significantly affect their ability to respond to and meet the needs of clients. An awareness and acceptance of these as potential problems may be a difficult learning experience for it requires reflection, introspection, analysis and honesty. Questions may be asked consciously for the first time—'what are my thoughts and feelings in relation to?' and 'which experiences of life have provoked or supported these?' and at times the answers are not forthcoming, irrational or perfectly well justified. Exploration may provoke the desire to examine alternatives or conflicting viewpoints but an *awareness* of these issues and their potential effects on the nurse–client relationship is the important factor. Difficulties require an early declaration, ventilation of problems encountered and a willingness to accept assistance of the nature required.

As with any skill, time, practice, guidance and appropriate role-modelling assist the nurse during a period of intense vulnerability. However, it is a very necessary experience for nurses must learn to separate personal from professional self, not just because the nurse may exert a detrimental or less than helpful influence on the client, but also because the nurse cannot select individuals to care for or work with who they like or have an affinity for; professional behaviour must override personal issues. In addition, the client may respond less than positively to the nurse at times and subsequent exploration may exclude specific behaviour or characteristics of the nurse as causative of the response. Transference and counter-transference, based on unconscious identification, may exert positive and negative effects on the therapeutic relationship and may be seen to occur in both directions—nurse to client as well as client to nurse—and hence awareness of this may facilitate exploration of problems.

An awareness of strengths and weaknesses associated with performance facilitates areas of limitation to be addressed and improved whilst aptitudes are maximized to their full potential. A plan of action may then be constructed, identifying realistic goals and objectives, appropriate resources to assist in development and criteria on which to judge the degree of success attained. Involvement of a personal mentor/supervisor/preceptor may faciliate opportunities being created to assist in the activities and the advantage of another's expertise and networks.

A significant aspect of the 'strengths and weaknesses' activities above is that which relates to the effect of the way in which the nurse presents to others. Verbal and non-verbal communication may evoke adverse and undesirable responses without any such intention on the part of the nurse. On occasions it may be that body language exposes personal feelings or beliefs that are out of place in a professional interaction. However, at other times the nurse may consistently present in a manner adjudged as 'disinterested', 'hassled', 'pre-occupied', 'threatening' or 'intimidated', without conscious intention or awareness. A similar reaction emanating from several clients/visitors/colleagues may prompt further self exploration and assistance in a plan of action, which may usefully include role play and video exercises.

Looking at self is not easy. Learning about self can be intriguing, astounding, depressing and uplifting but it is always enlightening! Accepting the positive as well as negative aspects of self maintains balance and self esteem, providing 'positive strokes' as well as developmental areas. It is exactly the process utilized with clients, so it must be worth a try!

Care management skills

The role of the care manager relates to those activities that facilitate assessment of the client's need for health care and analysis of the amenability of such needs to nursing intervention. Referral to other more appropriate agencies in regard to those needs—whether health or social in nature—which do not fall within the nurse's area of expertise is included within this role, as are those activities that relate to planning, monitoring and evaluating all aspects of health care delivery.

Assessment is, in essence, a comparison between the yardstick provided by the concept 'normality' of function, and the picture presented by the client. An in-depth knowlege therefore of this 'normal' function is required prior to any activity taking place. This encompasses the accepted parameters associated with all aspects of physiological, cognitive, affective, behavioural and socio-cultural performance.

Successful data collection required to make this comparison, and hence elicit areas of problem and need, is heavily dependent upon the relationship initially developed and subsequently sustained with those individuals significant in the situation. This includes other professional and lay colleagues, as well as the client and those central to his or her life.

The nurse's attitude to the individuals involved and the characteristics displayed during periods of contact are of major importance. Quiet, calm and measured interaction provoke optimism and trust in the professional's abilities. Good utilization of time and other available resources facilitates unhurried interactions and the impression of primary attention and focus of concentration upon the current activities. Confidence in the care team displayed by the nurse is a professional duty. With regard to this, demonstration of the acceptance of people as they are, by recognizing and affirming their continuing control over life and of the care activities, is paramount. Client assistance is available on a basis of partnership which relates only to areas of need and difficulty and only for a period perceived as necessary by that partnership.

Actual data collection requires a variety of skills to be utilized. Cognitive skills of knowing the potential sources of information available, of comprehending their relative value to current requirements and of the methodology to be used to access information available is vital to the assessment. A major source—but by no means the sole one—are the clients themselves. The perceptual skills of the nurse, whether visual, auditory, olfactory or tactile in origin, provide valuable insight into the individual's performance at that specific time within the current situation. Responses, reactions and other initial observations may not prove consistent as the milieu changes but useful indicators are provided to elicit details that may confirm or refute those observations.

Communication skills—the effective use of verbal and non-verbal behaviour—forms a major element in all aspects of care, and activities related to assessment are no exception. Interviewing, counselling, reading and report writing are all aspects requiring skilled performance to achieve optimum benefit and effect. An appreciation of the manner in which data collected may be distorted—whether by emotional, cultural, linguistic or environmental factors or those associated with the subjective interpretation of material—also facilitates maximum value of data. Data collected may be to the detriment of the client and his family as well as benefit, and strict adherence to the maintenance of confidentiality coupled with this awareness assists in activities aimed to help the individuals involved. The appropriacy and preparation of the environment, good use of temporal resources and consideration and acceptance of the client's right to reticence, support the verbal and non-verbal communication strategies that aim to inform, elicit information and encourage and support the individual. Closing interviews on a positive note and making arrangements for further action assist in this activity. A clear knowledge of legal, administrative and procedural aspects relating to the specific client's situation is of major importance in the subsequent care delivery and hence warrants special attention.

The perceptions of all individuals—the client, family, other professional and lay colleagues—are collated and, in discussion with the client, the comparison activities ensue. Specific identification of 'deviations from the norm' is required,

with discussion regarding what seems to be the areas of need, remembering that what may be seen as a problem by the nurse or relatives, may not be perceived as such by the individual client.

Professional judgements are then required with regard to the differentiation between social and health needs, and the aspects of the latter which fall within the areas of expertise and remit of the nurse. Liaison with others to generate the necessary assistance in relation to other problems is required, utilizing appropriate communication strategies and networks. Data required in relation to health care needs are then made available to the care team for discussion and comment, in a process designed to gain assistance and generate potential solutions to problems. The potential strategies arrived at may then be discussed with the client in relation to their viability and acceptability. Once agreements have been reached, the planning element of care activities may commence.

Planning initially involves the client and nurse in prioritization activities to identify those problem areas of prime concern and those of a secondary importance. In addition, the generation of short-, medium- and long-term objectives is required and again professional judgement is required to engender realistic expectations and time parameters.

Planning documentation is required to be accurate, clearly legible and in a format and terminology easily understood by all involved. Contents need to be comunicated to those significant in care organization and delivery, and again confidentiality of data must be assured.

Monitoring of care delivery is reliant on several factors. Time management skills facilitate an appropriate period to be set aside with peers and other agents to review professional views, feelings, beliefs and actions related to client care and professional performance. The 'comforting skills' referred to earlier are as valuable within interactions with colleagues as with clients and their families. Positive attitudes towards self disclosure should be inculcated, thus facilitating free and frank discussion and continuing self development via constructive comments and suggestions from co-workers. Effective time management ensures that time available is of maximum benefit to the client, care team and its individual members. Communication skills ensure the appropriate strategies are utilized in information giving, taking feedback, recognizing and valuing successes, and supporting and assisting in developmental issues and challenges which present. Again documentation of reviews should be relevant, accurate and understandable, identifying progress attained and modifications suggested in relation to continuing care from mmm the professional perspective.

Discussion with the client and family to review the progress of care delivery to date from their perspective may then be conducted from an all-round position. Levels of satisfaction, or otherwise, will significantly add to the information gained from the professional involved, facilitating modification of the continued care delivery where necessary by negotiation and compromise strategies at times. Recording and communicating the client's perceptions to care delivery and liaison with colleagues to effect the necessary modifications to plans completes the process.

Evaluation activities are those of assessment and comparison discussed at an earlier point. However, this time the yardstick provided is not that of 'normality' and its associated parameters, but the very specific short-, medium- and long-term objectives set by mutual assent by client and professional. The degree to which success has been achieved in relation to problems considered in need of priority attention, perceived limitations and obstacles that have influenced achievement and areas of continuing need are judged by the client, the nurse and the team. Reassessment of client needs and problems may then be required in order that new yardsticks may be identified or modified plans be drawn up and agreed.

Care management requires innumerable skills: perceptual, communication, comforting, organizational and presentational. Skills of logic, cognitive analysis, integration and reflection, in addition to the breadth and depth of the knowledge base necessary to deal with people in a wide variety of situations, experiencing a myriad of problems, in relation to very different backgrounds and expectations are essential to the role of the manager.

Care collaborator

This role involves the individual professional with teamwork with other nurses and support workers to deliver prescribed nursing care. In addition, the role encompasses those interactions and activities conducted within intraprofessional and intra-agency teams aimed at planning and delivering comprehensive health and social care.

Much has been written recently with regard to groups: development, cohesion, roles, communication value and limitations, uses and abuses. Wide reading on the subject is invaluable. Subsequent critical analysis of material and integration of selected principles into patterns of activity provide the foundations upon which group and team working spirit develop.

In collaboration, knowledge and understanding play a pivotal role and not only in the areas of theories of group development and function. The autonomous professional envisaged by the UKCC (1986) requires knowledge and comprehension in relation to both the role and functioning parameters of all individuals, including self within the team. An appreciation of the remit of each, the skills inherent within that remit and an overview of the objectives and priorities of the parent organization from which each emanates, may help to provide a realistic view of what each is able to bring to the team.

'Comforting' skills play an important role in group work. Facilitating ease and relaxation within co-members promotes trust, openness and honesty. When individuals feel threatened or insecure in their position, interactions are strained and negotiations impaired.

Communication skills, as utilized in other professional roles, facilitate clarification, accuracy of information transfer and general understanding. Appropriacy of terminology, avoidance of jargon and clear enunciation facilitate discussion and decision-making processes for all participants, regardless of background and are therefore to be applauded. The ability to negotiate and influence is far more effective in generating favourable responses than confrontation and demands and this skill should be developed.

The ability to separate personal and professional issues and a primary goal of optimizing client assist, are useful points to remember in all care collaboration activities. High standards of professional knowledge, skills and integrity; positive and co-operative attitudes; flexibility, and a willingness to compromise where possible, are of great value in care collaboration.

Interventionist

The interventionist role encompasses the delivery and implementation of activities associated with specific nursing interventions and strategies aimed at assisting clients to manage problems and meet their own needs. Interventions are necessarily problem-centred, and frequently develop from the theoretical perspectives put forward to explain the symptomatology of mental health deviations. Examples are behaviourism and behaviour modification techniques, psychoanalytical theory and regression techniques, and humanistic theory and counselling strategies.

The principles of utilization of intervention are identical in all cases. The nurse requires an indepth knowledge of the theories underpinning activity, the aims and expectations associated with its use, the indications and parameters of utilization, and contra indications and potential repercussions that may ensue. At this point professional judgements may be made in relation to its value and limitations, but the client has the right to make informed judgements based upon the most objective data available. The nurse should be thoroughly competent in the skills associated with the strategy/intervention and perform them professionally and to the highest possible standard despite personal feelings if the client's decision favours use.

The nurse has the right and professional responsibility to voice conscientious objections to the *appropriate person or authority* (UKCC, 1992). Professionalism ensures that this appropriate person is *not* the recipient of care.

Strategies and interventions should be evaluated in relation to the degree to which objectives associated with initial implementation have been attained. Factors which may have influenced achievement levels must be identified and removed/ameliorated at the earliest possible review point.

Objectivity is required in relation to care delivery. The design or utilization of existing measurement tools and instruments should be incorporated in all areas of care delivery possible. Actual value to specific client problems may then be provided in a more scientific format available for comparative studies.

Resource manager

The role is associated with the skills of efficient and effective use of temporal, material and personnel resources, including self, in provision of health care, where these fall within the sphere of the individual's responsibility. In addition, continual development of resources available, new and existing services, and instruments and vehicles to achieve efficient health care is needed.

The organization identifies the specific role of the area or department within the overall plan of service provision and delivery. Objectives and goals of care are developed in relation to this role, and the target population identified within appropriate limits. Numbers of staff and the skill mix considered necessary to achieve objectives are also areas decided by the organization and its representatives, although some negotiation may be possible following the presentation of reasoned and well-proportioned evidence to the contrary. Standards relating to the quality of care provision may be generated by the care team for negotiation with, and approval by, the appropriate authority, on behalf of the organization. Yardsticks should therefore be available, and clarification of their continued appropriacy and accuracy should be undertaken prior to action. Changes uncovered or agreed via review must be communicated to all involved within service and care provision both as information of relevance and to facilitate review of current activity and function.

Personnel represent the most valuable resource available and therefore efficient, effective and appropriate utilization of each individual is a primary objective within management activities. The quantity, quality and diversity of skills required to achieve goals is inherent within the yardstick utilized and an analysis of current availability and use may elicit disparity. The nature and skill levels of current activities may demonstrate individuals functioning outside of their abilities or experience. Inappropriacy in this area may promote anxiety in some, and boredom and feelings associated with being undervalued by others. Individuals may be under-utilized or overstretched with regard to workload and responsibilities for a variety of reasons and this too requires identification, and subsequent action. Skills may be unavailable in the appropriate quantity or quality to meet the goals associated with care delivery, and it requires initiative to address deficits. In addition, an individual's needs, desires and ambitions must be balanced against organization needs and development areas, and a match or accommodation reached wherever possible. Implementation of strategies to assist within areas of time management and prioritization are invaluable with regard to personal and professional organization, though the majority of planning activities will depend upon the specific findings of the exploration undertaken.

Material resources available may be investigated using the same principles. These include delivery, and equipment and materials provided to support activities. Questions related to the details of provision, current location and ease of access are of value in this process. Details of who uses the resource, how often and for what purpose(s) may prove enlightening, as is information regarding the perceived appropriacy of that which is available for use in relation to the need generating it. Cost of resources is an important factor in this analysis of use, for greater value for both client and care team may be available following negotiation with appropriate agencies. Resources that are unused, under-used or overstretched require attention. Where value is reduced because of location, limitations or difficulties in relation to accessibility or inappropriacy due to size, quality or amenability to function, replacement may be the preferred course of action following appropriate negotiation.

Areas of omission or deficit require the same planning in relation to short-, medium- and long-term goal generation and the identification of strategies to assist in meeting goals. Time for the attainment of realistic goals is an essential feature of the planning activities, as is the identification of resources to assist.

A major exercise in relation to the above may engender feelings of anxiety, insecurity and disease. Rather more effective is the development of an expectation of continuing review and improvement of facilities, services to clients and own abilities. This may be initiated by problem-airing activities with each individual being provided with the time, opportunity and 'permission' or approval to identify areas of difficulty or problems that exert a detrimental effect on care provision, organization or role development. A thorough analysis of factors associated with each problem may then be undertaken on either an individual or group basis, and solutions generated and selected to achieve desired goals.

Communication skills of influencing and negotiating achieve less opposition and negativity towards activities than coercion, imposition and confrontation. Team support for activities and subsequent strategy implementation provide impetus and feelings of vested interest in attainment of goals, and therefore enhance chances of success. Continuing problem identification and analysis, generation and implementation of planned activities, and evaluation of attainment represent the cyclical nature of service and personnel development as an integral and expected—and therefore more acceptable—part of role.

Health promoter

This aspect of professional role incorporates activities associated with design, implementation, monitoring and evaluation of health promotion programmes and strategies. The nurse is also required to create opportunities to enhance the desire and motivation of individuals towards adoption and healthier lifestyles and the attainment of optimum health status.

The skills associated with assessment of need, planning of strategies to meet identified needs, and evaluation of strategy success have previously been discussed within the roles of care and resource manager.

The knowledge base required to underpin activities is exceedingly broad, as it incorporates all areas of healthy function—physiological, psychological, social and spiritual—and the factors believed to influence its development and maintenance. In addition a detailed knowledge of resources available to assist in the promotion of health and vehicles via which information is regularly publicized are necessary.

Self-awareness skills are required to analyse the appropriacy of one's own behaviour and performance in relation to role modelling health and health-orientated lifestyles. The values of adopting strategies to maximize health must be a personal choice by the nurse. The difficulties associated with promoting health, when the professional does not demonstrate a belief strong or sincere enough to incorporate it within his/her own lifestyle, are obvious.

Assessment of client need for health-promotion activities is an integral part of the total assessment of the client's need, and forms part of the negotiation process relating to goals and strategies designed to meet needs. However, assistance may be required by others who may not be the direct focus of care activities. Individuals significant to the client, care workers and colleagues, the professional's own family and friends, are examples to be remembered. The nurse also may have access to other groups—children and adolescents at school, students in universities, parents at play centres and groups associated with other roles and occupations.

The client or individual participating in activities needs to feel in control of these activities and events, and that amendments in lifestyle are advantageous or necessary for continuing or improved health and wellbeing. Decisions relating to the extent and nature of changes to be implemented and the speed of goal achievement envisaged are the individual's alone. Options may be put forward by the nurse, with a concomitant and objective analysis of the values and limitations of each to facilitate informed judgements. Short-, medium- and long-term goals may then be generated, with strategies designed to assist in attainment. Rewards which are specific to the values and interests of the individual may be incorporated within the programme as with any relating to behaviour modification. These must be of sufficient worth to enhance motivation to adhere to the programme.

Difficulties experienced in attainment of goals require the implementation of comforting skills to provide support and reassurance of continuing value, and reduce levels of guilt or inadequacy associated with 'failure'. Replanning of strategies and review of targets may be appropriate at this point, with an associated evaluation of rewards. All achievements must be recognized with progress towards optimum health providing the yardstick against which specific attainments may be judged by the individual client.

Health promotion activities may, with nursing assistance, become self perpetuating and motivating in nature. Secondary gains in areas of presentation of self to others, enhanced self esteem and improved general functioning may provide impetus to continue towards goal attainment and subsequent further problem/goal identification and related action.

Facilitator

The role encompasses activities and strategies designed to assist in smoother transition, achievements and acquisitions towards specific goals and intentions. These serve to assist, guide, enhance and support the individual concerned rather than provide answers or actions for him, thus creating or maintaining dependency. Individuals are encouraged to take responsibility for their own achievements.

Prior to undertaking activities towards any goal or target, an individual has a variety of needs that require to be addressed. An interest and desire to make changes in current circumstances or situations is vital, and thus may be aroused by skilful publication of options available. Bombardment of an individual with information rarely succeeded in promoting activities. More effective is the 'personal touch' which evokes feelings of recognition and value. Statements such as 'I've been thinking about our discussion and wondered whether this may be of help/what you've been looking for/of interest to you', are more likely to promote sufficient interest to at least read, or listen to, whatever is being proposed.

A positive reaction on the part of the individual then heralds full discussions relating to the implications, benefits and limitations of the course of action, enabling informed judgements to be made. Communication skills relating to informing stimulating interest, decision making and problem solving have been utilized. The comforting skills associated with generating feelings of ease, optimism in relation to success and recognition or personal value and abilities support verbal and non-verbal interactions to good effect. Ventilation of doubts surrounding the activities envisaged, within the safe environment, and the development of strategies to ameliorate the effects of such doubts with realistic planning activities, restores or enhances confidence, thus generating optimism and comfort. Comfort and ease within the situation is a necessary factor, with positive attitudes displayed in relation to decisions made and continuing expression of worthiness of attention and assistance. Exteriorization of thoughts and feelings related to activities may enable solutions to be highlighted and therefore problems reduced.

Resources to assist in decision-making activities are available and the facilitator needs to be aware and knowledgeable in regard to these. Printed materials, videos, and individuals who have already experienced the realities of the course of action considered may all be of value to the individual within the process.

To function effectively within the facilitator role a great deal more knowledge is required. Appraisal, analysis and comprehension of options available is required to be continuously updated and reviewed to maintain accuracy. Networking skills may elicit personnel who demonstrate advanced levels of expertise or experience within a wide variety of contexts. Consolidation of contact-relationships via the utilization of appropriate interpersonal skills may encourage assistance from these sources.

A knowledge, too, of those seeking assistance in efforts towards development is a necessary factor. Time utilized to cultivate relationships conducive to openness, honesty and ease of approach is well spent. Interest shown in an individual's ability, performance or personal/professional characteristics lays foundations for subsequent interactions and activities. Presentation of self is therefore an integral part of facilitation. A genuine interest and warmth displayed within all situations and interactions engenders approach-ability. Positive responses and reactions elicit feelings associated with safety and trust, consistency and acceptancy, awareness of the needs of others, and value of each irrespective of the presence of cues to the contrary!

Continuing to assist the individual to generate a plan of action towards realistic and achievable goal achievement requires logical analysis of problems and development of potential solutions. Strategies elicited may then be examined and explored in relation to advantages and limitations inherent in their use and appropriate activities determined. Resources available to assist in attainment of goals may then be identified and gathered or approached for involvement in the plan. The activities may then be initiated and the plan operated.

Conjoint review of progress and activities on a regular basis may provide a boost to motivation, an impetus to continue and recognition of attainment to date. In addition it provides the opportunities to ventilate difficulties and successes, to modify activities and plans in the light of continuing knowledge acquisition and to explore further resource availability. The facilitator may also provide objectivity in contrast to the subjective feelings generated by personal involvement, assisting the individual to view positive aspects accrued to date rather than over-emphasizing problems experienced. Evaluation of the degree or extent to which goals have been attained and re-planning for subsequent continuing development completes the activity undertaken.

All of the above is achieved via negotiation, and is the result of communication strategies which serve to prompt consideration of various areas for inclusion and promote exploration of thoughts, feelings and behaviours which may influence activities. Role modelling a variety of strategies that assist in rational planning, for example brainstorming techniques, enables skills to be acquired and subsequently utilized in self-directed activities, thus promoting independence and self-reliance. The employment of skilled questioning, paraphrasing and reflective techniques engenders confidence as the individual discovers knowledge of his/her own abilities to generate material for utilization and direction of activities. The ability to control the pathway and speed of activities, from initiation of a course of action through to its evaluation, promotes feelings of enhanced satisfaction and self-esteem.

Researcher

This role requires logical and systematic investigation in relation to all aspects of health care, utilizing appropriate criteria, such as efficiency, effectiveness and levels of consumer satisfaction, as a basis for subsequent judgements.

Research activities may be viewed by some as a special event, something done occasionally for a specific, designed purpose, perhaps as an integral part of a course or some similar requirement. The role of the nurse as a researcher should not be viewed in such a manner, for research is an integral part of everyday practice.

The description of the role of resource manager within care provision may have given an indication of this element of integration in relation to that specific focus of attention. A major proportion of our knowledge and skill base should have its foundation within research activities. An idea or piece of information is presented and, to ascertain the veracity and generality of the item, we undertake appropriate investigation, via a literature search, observation, or by asking questions. The information and impressions are collated and potential bias accounted for, or removed, where possible. Judgements relating to the individual piece of information may then be made on the balance of the investigation undertaken and from the viewpoint of greatest degree of objectivity possible.

There may of course be a personal bias or a vested interest in the outcome of the enterprise. This may provoke difficulties and dilemmas in regard to selection of material, inclusion of all findings and evidence relevant, or in the manner in which findings are presented or interpreted. Statistics, for example, are notoriously open to manipulation.

The optimum course of action may be that of declaration of the presence of potential bias—honest, open and professional—and to undertake the activities with assistance where necessary from a mentor/supervisor/preceptor, thus eliciting an awareness for personal and professional growth, facilitating demonstration of the adherence to professional standards, utilizing resources to the full and displaying confidence in self and one's own abilities. In this way control and responsibility for activities are maintained and the greatest degree of growth achieved.

This objectivity is of prime importance in relation to research, as in so many activities undertaken by the nurse. It is too easy to become totally accustomed to the environment, to the existing methods and quality of health care provisions and the nature of standards associated with everyday activity and functioning. To provide efficient and effective care, the nurse needs to be able to 'see' clearly and, by this, we mean to be able to view the situation as if for the first time, every time. It also requires an ability to perceive the situation or activity with the expectations associated with a 'professional outsider', someone unbiased and dispassionate and yet possessing preconceived ideas of standards applicable and appropriate to the occurrence. In addition the action of 'stepping back' for one moment—on a regular basis—and attempting to view the scene from the client's perception or from the lay visitor's standpoint, is of great value. Appraisal from such a situation, whilst difficult, provides information relating to the impressions which may be generated in others and, by viewing this from the 'worst possible scenario' position, may be enlightening. The question 'would this be good enough for my mother?' may be the one that evokes the most definitive reply.

Once identified, areas considered in need or worthy of interest, further exploration or remedial attention, require considerable reflection and analysis prior to initiating any course of action. Initially, a definitive identification of outcomes required at the termination of activities is required—in other words, what is the individual setting out to do? Is it to describe what is actually happening, or to explain why it is happening in this way? Perhaps the individual wishes to solve a problem, or analyse reaction to events or change. Exploration of the options available in a certain situation may provide another reason for activity, as may examination of the continuing validity of an aspect of health care provision or organization. From this definitive identification of intention or outcomes desired, a research statement or hypothesis may be generated.

Data collection and collation skills have been analysed at some depth within the discussion appertaining to the care manager role. 'Comforting', self awareness, communication and perceptual skills, and those cognitive aptitudes and abilities associated with knowledge, understanding, reflection, analysis and decision making are prerequisite for effective and efficient performance in this sphere of the researcher role.

Evaluation of the study requires the utilization of analytical skills and the yardstick of measurement is that provided by the original goals and intentions underpinning and focusing activities. Comparisons drawn between these goals and the resultant fundings of the investigation may serve to satisfy needs in relation to provision of information required to meet a research statement or may validate or repudiate assertions within a hypothesis.

However, activity has not been completed until an analysis of the values and limitations of the focus of study, planning activities, methodology utilized and findings is subsequently conducted to identify areas requiring further investigation and exploration. Re-planning activities may then commence.

Publishing results and findings is of the utmost importance, for there is little value in such activities if appropriate individuals and authorities are unaware of their existence and are therefore unable to utilize information gained. Communication must be sensitively approached, with any individuals directly involved within the study given first knowledge wherever possible and appropriate. Discussion may then be generated and reactions and responses made, underpinning subsequent activities and direction of continuing exploration.

Investigations undertaken may evoke sensitive material and the duties and parameters relevant to confidentiality of information must be enacted and maintained. Indeed some areas of research may require permission to be sought in relation to conduct, and publication of findings may then be specified and agreed by negotiation. Adherence to these limitations is paramount if professional standards and trust within the relationship is to be maintained. Dilemmas encountered within this area are, of course, provided for within the Code of Conduct (UKCC, 1992), and guidance in relation to subsequent professional activity is offered.

Adviser

The role is associated with those activities that aim to inform, enlighten or appraise others of materials relevant to professional practice. It is a role that may be assumed by the professional or that may be ascribed to the nurse by others. However, prior to an analysis of the skills and aptitudes necessary to accomplish the objectives inherent within this role successfully, it may be valuable to differentiate between being an 'adviser' and 'giving advice'. We would assert that the term 'advice' equates with opinion, a suggestion proffered as a specific course of action in a particular situation. On occasions, nurses may be asked for their personal or professional opinion but it may be wise to analyse the specific situation in which the request is made before the professional accedes.

The adviser provides factual information, for example statistics, analysis of care services or an identification of potential resources available within a specific situation. In addition, the individual may provide explanations to enhance understanding, perhaps in relation to a particular activity, aspect of care delivery, or methods by which one service may enmesh with, or support, another in function. A broad spectrum of options available may be suggested, perhaps in regard to meeting a specific need and at times, the adviser may play 'Devil's advocate', in order to elicit hindrances or objections which may be raised in regard to an activity or course of action. The adviser may frequently be asked to affirm or explain issues relating to professional standards operating, but all of the above relate to facilitating decision making, not making decisions for the individuals concerned.

The knowledge base required to perform efficiently and effectively as an adviser is broadly based and detailed in relation to the individual's specific areas of practice and responsibility. In addition, associated but more peripheral spheres of activity need to be known and thoroughly understood, facilitating continuing integration across subject/speciality boundaries and a more effective advisory capacity. Reflection on, and analysis of, continuing inputs and experiences is required on a regular basis and the nurse needs to maintain awareness of the sources of these regular inputs whilst appreciating the value of serendipity and vicarious learning opportunities. Maintenance and expansion of current knowledge and understanding is vital.

'Knowing' is important, too, in relation to the parameters applicable to ascribed advisory roles undertaken. A clear knowledge and understanding of expectations and limits associated with specific situations or remits, both in relation to self and other participants, is necessary. This facilitates efficient performance but also assists in the development of relationships which are of a harmonious nature and of mutual benefit. The nurse gains new experiences, with all of the values implicit in these, whilst the partner(s) of the interaction gain information to assist in decision making.

The 'comforting' skills previously discussed are the basis of professional relationships, engendering feelings of safety, acceptance, value and respect. This in itself promotes openness and honesty and encourages extra efforts towards funding optimum value for all participants from the relationship. Self presentation is an all important aspect within initiation and maintenance of relationships. The nurse should represent a useful resource; one that is warm, approachable, knowledgeable and willing to impart such information to assist where possible.

Communication strategies—both verbal and non-verbal—utilized with skill, facilitate non-threatening, effective, professional interactions. Clarity of enunciation, the utilization of appropriate language and provision *only* of the information necessary, form the strategies on which advisory function pivots. Accuracy of material is vital, as is currency and continuing validity of such material. Printed aids provided to support discussions should also show these characteristics. The value of a relaxed and open-body stance cannot be overestimated, with its impression of unhurried, unpressurized communication which is free of conflict.

The role of adviser is integral to all other roles discussed within this work. However, we believe the role is currently undervalued and will emerge as an important aspect of continuing professional activity in relation to health and social care provision.

Energizer

The energizer utilizes skills and behaviours that encourage and motivate individuals, including self, towards analysis of current performance and, where appropriate, generates desire for development, change, innovation and attainment. The role includes those activities associated with creation of an environment conducive to, and expectant of, critical self-appraisal and positive peer evaluation. Skills relating to the development of a belief in the ability to succeed, those that empower individuals to act and those that facilitate recognition of success are also necessary. Participation in, support for, and incorporation of, activities that result from the 'energizing' process is important.

Knowledge of a variety of subjects, issues, theories and activities, provides a firm foundation for the role. The theories of motivation provide an awareness and appreciation of the broad factors associated with reduced and enhanced performance, of the elements that hinder and assist optimum function and the methodology by which interest, ambition and enthusiasm may be generated. However, this knowledge alone is insufficient, for the nurse must be open and able to recognize these factors operating and evoke the appropriate strategies to assist.

To achieve this, the individual requires an overall detailed knowledge of the people who are currently providing the focus of such activities. Reflections on their current responses to situations, their skills and limitations, their potential and perceived needs are integral to the situation. Awareness of each person's ambitions and desires in relation to performance is essential, as is the reasoning behind such drives. A substantial appreciation of the nature of the individuals concerned and of 'what makes each tick' is developed via perceptual skills and cognitive aptitudes utilized within all interactive processes.

The environment within which activities are set is of great importance and value to the nurse energizer, for it may be seen to stimulate or inhibit activities required. Physical characteristics, for example the provision of areas conducive to discussion which are comfortable and private, or areas which support reflection, peace and solitude, are valuable. If there is no facility to sit down and discuss elements of practice with colleagues, it is unlikely this will occur. In relation to publicizing opportunities available, material that is well presented is an attractor to the senses and may provoke thought and subsequent action.

Opportunities made available to facilitate both individual and group involvement in activities are advantageous. Individually centred activities are valuable but the use of, and encouragement of, paired and group undertakings has a positive effect in many instances. Role modelling strategies have a benefit, as involvement of another individual in activities may be of value in relation to analysing one's own performance, and identifying learning opportunities. Pairings may promote a useful competitive edge to some proceedings and necessary support in others. Groups may provide a common cause/activity that galvanizes all towards maximum effort. Creativity in the utilization of all resources available to maximum advantage, whether in the short-, medium- or long-term development phases, promotes variety and stimulation with regard to overall function.

Rational planning activities and the skills utilized in their performance have previously been discussed within several role analyses and hence require no further explanation or attention here. Suffice it to say that realistic objectives and goals and a staged plan-of-action is required to be negotiated on an individual basis.

Awareness of self and one's own skills, characteristics and responses to innovation, change and ongoing developmental activities is vital. Acceptance and welcome of these challenges is only a small proportion of the needs of the effective, efficient energizer. The nurse is required to recognize and exteriorize own feelings and ideation associated with such situations and the actions and strategies by which these will be ameliorated or eradicated within personal plans to initiate the course of activity required. A willingness and ability to ventile areas of vulnerability within self and performance should be viewed as positive by all, for it indicates the nurse's feelings of safety and acceptance by others within the situation and the recognition that all individuals possess growth points.

CONCLUSIONS

This chapter has addressed many issues in its aim of identifying and analysing roles, skills and behaviours implicit in efficient and effective practice—both present and future—within mental health nursing. Each aspect discussed is worthy of a chapter in its own right and the brief attention here, whilst necessary in regard to the length of this work, may hopefully generate further interest and exploration.

Mental health nurses need to maintain an up-to-date and accurate knowledge of current events and their influence on, and implications for, the profession. Skills utilized in practice require to be of the highest level possible to assist the client in recovery. Above all, however, a constant analysis of practice, performance and self presentation, an honest evaluation of the effectiveness of these in care delivery and the subsequent initiation of a plan of enhancement will aid both client and nurse in the attainment of optimum health.

We consider that there are many events in life that are *worse* than dying—living in prolonged pain is a useful example. Intense psychological distress, alienation and feelings of profound worthlessness equate with this physiological pain.

The skilled mental health nurse has the knowledge and aptitudes necessary to assist the client to make life worth living.

FURTHER READING

Bynum, W.F., Porter, R. & Shepherd, M. (Eds) (1985) *The Anatomy of Madness: Essays in the History of Psychiatry*, Vols 1–3. London: Tavistock.

Thompson, T. & Mathias, P. (Eds) (1992) *Stan-

dards and Mental Handicap: Keys to Competence. London: Bailliere Tindall.

REFERENCES

Black, Sir Douglas (Chair) (1980) Inequalities in Health: Report of a Research Working Group. London: DHSS.

Borysenko, M. & Borysenko, J. (1982) Stress, behaviour and immunity. *General Hospital Psychiatry*, **4**, 59–67.

Chinn, P. & Jacobs, M. (1979) A model for theory development in nursing. *Advances in Nursing Sciences*, **1**(1), 1–11.

Council for National Academic Awards (CNAA) (1986) *Credit Accumulation and Transfer Scheme*. London: CNAA.

Davies, C. (1977) Continuities in the Development of Hospital Nursing in Britain. *Journal of Advanced Nursing*, **2**, 479–493.

Department of Health, Department of Social Security, Scottish Office and Welsh Office (DH/DSS) (1989) *Caring for People: Community Care in the Next Decade and Beyond*. London: HMSO.

Department of Health (DH) (1990) *The Care Programme Approach for People with a Mental Illness Referred to the Specialist Psychiatric Services*. HC (90) 23/LASSL (90) 11. London: Department of Health.

Department of Health (DH) (1991) *The Children Act 1989—An Introductory Guide for the National Health Service*. London: HMSO.

Department of Health (DH) (1992a) Press Release, H92/139. London: HMSO.

Department of Health (DH) (1992b) *The Health of the Nation*. London: HMSO.

Department of Health (DH) and Home Office (1992) *Review of Health and Social Services for Mentally Disordered Offenders and Others Requiring Similar Services: Report of the Staffing and Training Advisory Group*. London: HMSO.

Doll, R. & Peto, R. (1981) *The Causes of Cancer*. Oxford: Oxford University Press.

Egan, G. (1990) *The Skilled Helper*. Pacific Grove, CA, USA: Brooks/Cole.

English National Board for Nursing, Midwifery and Health Visiting (ENB) (1989) *Project 2000—'A New Preparation for Practice', Guidelines and Criteria for Course Development and the Formation of Collaborative Links Between Approved Training Institutions within the National Health Service and Centres of Higher Education*. London: ENB.

European Economic Community (EEC) (1981) *The Report of the European Community Advisory Committee on Training in Nursing*. Brussels: EEC.

Godfrey, C., Hardman, G. & Maynard, A. (1989) *Priorities of Health Promotion—an Economic Approach*. University of York: Centre for Health Economics.

Gore, P. *et al.* (1981) *Webster's Third New International Dictionary of the English Language*. Massachusetts: Mirriam-Webster.

Hanks, P. (Ed.) (1979) *Collins Dictionary of the English Language*. Glasgow: Collins.

Health Education Authority (HEA) (1988) *Stress in the Public Sector*. London: Health Education Authority.

Jacox, A. (1974) Theory construction in nursing: An overview. *Nursing Research*, **23**, 4–13.

Knowles, M. (1975) *Self Directed Learning*. New York: Associated Press.

Kolb, D. (1976) *Learning Style Inventory Technical Manual*. Boston: McBer.

Lazarus, R. & Folkman, S. (1984) *Stress, Appraisal and Coping*. New York: Springer.

National Health Service (NHS) and Community Care Act 1990. London: HMSO.

Powell, T. & Enright, S. (1990) *Anxiety and Stress Management*. London: Routledge.

Ramprogus, V. (1988) Learning how to learn nursing. *Nurse Education Today*, **8**, 59–67.

Rowntree, D. (1990) *Teaching Through Self Instruction: How to Develop Open Learning Materials*. London: Kogan Page.

Stein, J. (Ed.) (1967) *The Random House Dictionary of the English Language*. New York: Random House.

Steinaker, N. & Bell, M. (1979) *The Experiential Taxonomy*. New York: Academic Press.

Stevens, B. (1984) Nursing theory: Analysis, application, evaluation. Boston: Little, Brown.

Townsend, P. & Davidson, N. (Eds) (1988) *Inequalities in Health (The Black Report)*. Harmondsworth: Penguin.

Tuxworth, E. (1991) Beyond the basics—higher level competence. In Thompson, T. & Mathias, P. (Eds) *Standards and Mental Handicap, Keys to Competence*. London: Baillière Tindall.

United Kingdom Central Council for Nursing, Midwifery and Health Visiting (UKCC) (1986) *Project 2000: A New Preparation for Practice*. London: UKCC.

United Kingdom Central Council for Nursing, Midwifery and Health Visiting (UKCC) (1989) Minutes of the 59 Meeting of the Central Council held on 17 March 1989, CC/89/31, London.

United Kingdom Central Council for Nursing, Midwifery and Health Visiting (UKCC) (1990) *The Report of the Post Registration Education and Practice Project*. London: UKCC.

United Kingdom Central Council for Nursing, Midwifery and Health Visiting (UKCC) (1991) *Report on the Proposals for the Future of Community Education and Practice*. London: UKCC.

United Kingdom Central Council for Nursing, Midwifery and Health Visiting (UKCC) (1992) *Code of Professional Conduct*. London: UKCC.

White, E. (1991) *The Third Quinquennial National Community Psychiatric Nursing Survey*. University of Manchester: Department of Nursing.

White, E. & Brooker, C. (1990a) The future of community psychiatric nursing: What might the 'Care Programme Approach' mean for practice and education? *Community Psychiatric Nursing Journal*, **10**(6), 27–30.

White, E. & Brooker, C. (1990b) The Care Programme Approach. *Nursing Times*, **87**(12), 66–67.

Wood, R. & Power, C. (1987) Aspects of the competence—performance distinction: Educational, psychological and measurement issues. *Journal of Curriculum Studies*, **19**(5), 409–424.

World Health Organization (WHO) (1986) *Targets for Health for All*. WHO Regional Office for Europe.

INTERNATIONAL DIMENSIONS OF NURSING

Tony Thompson and Peter Mathias

AIMS

i) To identify the role of the World Health Organization in the promotion of health
ii) To identify world targets for health
iii) To describe nursing initiatives in Europe

KEY ISSUES

Nursing as an international activity
Participation in world organizations and world trends
Measurable targets

Identify, analyse and assess factors causing distress and illness	Promote health, provide direct care and make interventions	Manage care programmes and services
Be critical, analytical and accountable, continue professional development	Counter discrimination, inequality and individual and institutional racism	Work within and develop policies, laws and safeguards in all settings
Understand influences on mental health and the nature/causes of disorder and illness	Know the effects of distress, disorder, illness on individuals, groups, families	Understand the basis of treatments and interventions

INTRODUCTION

The international profile of the function of nurses working within the mental health field is increasing. Nurses are participating effectively in strategies that are aimed at attaining the major aim of 'Health for All'. As important and valued members of health and social care teams, they are able to provide a highly competent workforce in an expanding range of communities.

In recent years the World Health Organization (WHO) has made pointed reference to the importance of mobilizing nurses in the efforts to attain health for all (WHO, 1978). This feature of WHO's initiative is highly appropriate to nurses in mental health because of their wide range of contemporary skills as direct care givers, managers of services and promoters of health. The World Health Assembly (WHA, 1989) adopted Resolution WHO 42.27. This resolution reinforced nursing's involvement in primary health care; further it urged Member States to take the necessary action in order to develop strategies to recruit and retain, educate and re-orientate and improve the qualifications of nursing personnel in order to meet national needs.

WHO's impact on evolving services is significant, although not always appreciated by busy practitioners. The history of psychiatric care is laced with evidence that humane governments are best able to help people with a disorder or mental health problem. Unfortunately, the converse is also true and events which have recently unfolded in eastern European countries offer testimony to this fact.

It will be necessary for all health care workers to appreciate the influence that WHO has on governments and it is likely that nurses preferring to work in mental health or pursuing programmes of professional development will be required to identify the WHO role quite specifically.

The World Health Organization is a specialized agency of the United Nations with primary responsibility for international health matters and public health. Through this organization, which was created in 1948, the health professions of some 170 countries exchange their knowledge and experience with the aim of making possible the attainment by all citizens of the world by the year 2000 of a level of health that will permit them to lead a socially and economically productive life.

'By means of direct technical co-operation with its Member States, and by stimulating such co-operation among them, WHO promotes the development of comprehensive health services, the prevention and control of diseases, the improvement of environmental conditions, the de-velopment of human resources for health, the co-ordination and development of biomedical and health services research, and the planning and implementation of health programmes....'. *WHO, 1992*

Of course, these aims are ambitious and they endeavour to encompass a range of activities concerning whole aspects of health for the population of member countries; this includes improving mental health and the training of health personnel. Progress towards meeting these aims relies on international co-operation in establishing standards not only for health but those associated with the design of training programmes.

An excellent example of such collaboration can be seen in the ten recommendations of the first WHO European Conference on Nursing convened in 1988 (ECN, 1989). The basis of many chapters of this book is to convey these features as they apply specifically to mental health and disorder, and to remind the nurse and others working in mental health services of the type of influence behind many of today's programmes of professional preparation and continuing professional development.

TEN RECOMMENDATIONS FOR THE FIRST WHO EUROPEAN CONFERENCE ON NURSING (1988)

1 All nurses, their professional associations, non-governmental organizations and volunteer groups should be strong advocates for policies and programmes for health for all at national, regional and local levels.

2 Innovative nursing services should be developed that focus on health rather than disease; patterns of work should be appropriate, efficient and conducive to primary health care. Governments, health authorities and nurses' professional organizations should take urgent steps to remove factors that inhibit this process and should draw up or modify legislation and regulations to

ensure that nurses are able to meet their responsibilities as frontline workers in primary health care.

3 In keeping with European policies for health for all, the nurse's practice should be based mainly on the principles inherent in the primary health care approach. The focus should be on:

(a) promoting and maintaining health, and preventing disease;

(b) involving individuals, families and communities in care and making it possible for them to take more responsibility for their health;

(c) working actively to reduce inequities in access to health care services and to satisfy the needs of whole populations, especially the underserved;

(d) multidisciplinary and multisectorial collaboration; and

(e) assurance of the quality of care and the appropriate use of technology.

4 All basic programmes of nursing education should be restructured, reoriented and strengthened in order to produce generalist nurses, able to function in both hospital and community. All specialist knowledge and skills subsequently acquired should be built on this foundation. Nursing education should include ample experience outside the hospital. Candidates for nursing education should have completed a full secondary education (which may vary from country to country) and have qualifications for admission that are equivalent to those required by a university or other institute of higher education. The directors of schools of nursing or departments of nursing education, and teachers and supervisors of nursing programmes must all be nurses.

5 Nurses managing care and services must base care on the health needs and participation of the population in accordance with the regional strategy for health for all, and must take account of:

(a) demographic and epidemiological trends;

(b) the social and physical environment;

(c) lifestyle issues;

(d) cultural values and beliefs and ethical considerations;

(e) economic choices and alternatives; and

(f) the qualified personnel available.

Nurse managers must have professional autonomy so that they allocate resources in accordance with the principles of the health for all strategy.

6 To ensure the full co-operation of the nursing community, nurse researchers should be appointed to all national and regional research councils dealing with health or related research, including bodies such as the European Advisory Committee on Health Research. WHO should urge nurses to start community care demonstration projects that produce measurable improvements in care and promote the efficient use of resources in selected communities. To permit the development of community-oriented nursing practice, education and leadership, nursing research must be a part of all fields of practice. An equitable share of existing funds should be made available for nursing research projects.

7 WHO, its collaborating centres, intergovernmental and non-governmental organizations, and national nurses' associations should set up information systems and increase communication and the dissemination of information and research results through national, regional and international networks. Modern technology should be used to strengthen links between consumer and other groups, organizations and institutes.

8 Nursing should be included as one of the essential elements of national health plans now being developed based on the regional strategy for health for all, and nurses should take part in the debate on health policy. Legislation on nursing practice should recognize the nurse's contribution to the organization, development and delivery of health care. It should be formulated in a way that promotes nurses' ability

to meet the health needs of the population.

9   In the light of demographic trends and their implications for the development of primary health care, health manpower policies should be based on health for all and should include:

   (a) a plan to recruit nursing personnel, drawn up in collaboration with nurses, administrators and politicians and using current manpower data bases;

   (b) terms and conditions of service that attract and retain qualified nurses, ensure the appropriate use of nursing personnel, and recognize continuing education as a part of career development;

   (c) a programme of continuing education accessible to all nurses; and

   (d) counselling programmes for personal and career development.

10 In view of nurses' strong influence as role models for the population, individual nurses and nurses' organizations have a special responsibility to exemplify a healthy lifestyle and, more specifically, to support the concerted European action against tobacco by promoting smoke-free working environments. Cessation counselling should be made available to all nurses who smoke.

Since these aims were first identified, the world of work for all health care workers and the mental health nurse specifically has continually changed, sometimes unpredictably and with increasing speed. Hence, the topics contained in this book are intended to assist in reflecting on the WHO targets for Health for all by the year 2000 and to help anticipate and respond in a competent way to change in order to enhance practice.

TARGETS FOR HEALTH FOR ALL—2000

Target 1 By the year 2000, the differences in health status between countries and between groups within countries should be reduced by at least 25%, by improving the level of health of disadvantaged nations and groups.

Target 2 By the year 2000, all people should have the opportunity to develop and use their own health potential in order to lead socially, economically and mentally fulfilling lives.

Target 3 By the year 2000, people with disabilities should be able to lead socially, economically and mentally fulfilling lives with the support of special arrangements that improve their relative physical, social and economic opportunities.

Target 4 By the year 2000, there should be a sustained and continuing reduction in morbidity and disability due to chronic disease in the Region.

Target 5 By the year 2000, there should be no indigenous cases of poliomyelitis, diphtheria, neonatal tetanus, measles, mumps and congenital rubella in the Region and there should be a sustained and continuing reduction in the incidence and adverse consequences of other communicable diseases, notably HIV infection.

Target 6 By the year 2000, life expectancy at birth in the Region should be at least 75 years and there should be a sustained and continuing improvement in the health of all people aged 65 years and over.

Target 7 By the year 2000, the health of all children and young people should be improved, giving them the opportunity to grow and develop to their full physical, mental and social potential.

Target 8 By the year 2000, there should be sustained and continuing improvement in the health of all women.

Target 9 By the year 2000, mortality from diseases of the circulatory system should be reduced, in the case of people under 65 years by at least 15%, and there should be progress in improving the quality of life of all people suffering from cardiovascular disease.

Target 10 By the year 2000, mortality from

cancer in people under 65 years should be reduced by at least 15% and the quality of life of all people with cancer should be significantly improved.

Target 11 By the year 2000, injury, disability and death arising from accidents should be reduced by at least 25%.

Target 12 By the year 2000, there should be a sustained and continuing reduction in the prevalence of mental disorders, an improvement in the quality of life of all people with such disorders, and a reversal of the rising trends in suicide and attempted suicide.

Target 13 By the year 2000, all Member States should have developed, and be implementing, intersectoral policies for the promotion of health lifestyles, with systems ensuring public participation in policy-making and implementation.

Target 14 By the year 2000, all settings of social life and activity, such as the city, school, workplace, neighbourhood and home, should provide greater opportunities for promoting health.

Target 15 By the year 2000, accessible and effective education and training in health promotion should be available in all Member States, in order to improve public and professional competence in promoting health and increasing health awareness in other sectors.

Target 16 By the year 2000, there should be continuous efforts in all Members States to actively promote and support health patterns of living through balanced nutrition, appropriate physical activity, healthy sexuality, good stress management and other aspects of positive health behaviour.

Target 17 By the year 2000, the health-damaging consumption of dependence-producing substances such as alcohol, tobacco and psychoactive drugs should have been significantly reduced in all Member States.

Target 18 By the year 2000, all Member States should have developed, and be implementing, policies on the environment and health

that ensure ecologically sustainable development, effective prevention and control of environmental health risks and equitable access to healthy environments.

Target 19 By the year 2000, there should be effective management systems and resources in all Members States for putting policies on environment and health into practice.

Target 20 By the year 2000, all people should have access to adequate supplies of safe drinking-water and the pollution of ground water sources, rivers, lakes and seas should no longer pose a threat to health.

Target 21 By the year 2000, air quality in all countries should be improved to a point at which recognized air pollutants do not pose a threat to public health.

Target 22 By the year 2000, health risks due to micro-organisms or their toxins, to chemicals and to radioactivity in food should have been significantly reduced in all Member States.

Target 23 By the year 2000, public health risks caused by solid and hazardous wastes and soil pollution should be effectively controlled in all Member States.

Target 24 By the year 2000, cities, towns and rural communities throughout the Region should offer physical and social environments supportive to the health of their inhabitants.

Target 25 By the year 2000, the health of workers in all Member States should be improved by making work environments more healthy, reducing work-related disease and injury, and promoting the wellbeing of people at work.

Target 26 By the year 2000, all Member States should have developed, and be implementing, policies that ensure universal access to health services of quality, based on primary care and supported by secondary and tertiary care.

Target 27 By the year 2000, health service systems in all Member States should be managed cost-effectively, with resources being distributed according to need.

Target 28 By the year 2000, primary health care in all Member States should meet the basic health needs of the population by providing a wide range of health-promotive, curative, re-habilitative and supportive services and by actively supporting self-help activities of individuals, families and groups.

Target 29 By the year 2000, hospitals in all Member States should be providing cost-effective secondary and tertiary care and contribute actively to improving health status and patient satisfaction.

Target 30 By the year 2000, people in all Member States needing long-term care and support should have access to appropriate services of a high quality.

Target 31 By the year 2000, there should be structures and processes in all Member States to ensure continuous improvement in the quality of health care and appropriate development and use of health technologies.

Target 32 By the year 2000, health research should strengthen the acquisition and application of knowledge in support of health for all development in all Member States.

Target 33 By the year 2000, all Member States should have developed, and be implementing, policies in line with the concepts and principles of the European health for all policy, balancing lifestyle, environment and health service concerns.

Target 34 By the year 2000, management structures and processes should exist in all Member States to inspire, guide and co-ordinate health development, in line with health for all principles.

Target 35 By the year 2000, health information systems in all Member States should actively support the formulation, implementation, monitoring and evaluating of health for all policies.

Target 36 By the year 2000, education and

training of health and other personnel in all Member States should actively contribute to the achievement of health for all.

Target 37 By the year 2000, in all Member States, a wide range of organizations and groups throughout the public, private and voluntary sectors should be actively contributing to the achievement of health for all.

Target 38 By the year 2000, all Member States should have mechanisms in place to strengthen clinical considerations in decisions relating to the health of individuals, groups and populations.

The targets and their components remain important and the tasks for governments, particularly in developing countries, remain formidable. Whilst many targets remain to be achieved, their very existence offers an invaluable yardstick for all participants to measure relative success. Further, the concept of health is itself a stimulus to co-operation. It has an appeal to our common humanity which has no equivalence in any other area (Robinson, 1987).

The principles that underpin the themes of the latest targets (WHO, 1991) reflect important facets of the mental health nurse role and function. Examination of these highlights many areas for discussion by the practitioner in all aspects of mental health services:

---

1   Health for all implies equality, so the present inequalities in health between countries should be reduced as far as possible.
2   When people are healthy, they are able to mobilize their physical, mental and emotional capabilities, and in this sense they are able to promote their own health. Emphasis in health care must be on the *promotion of health* and the *prevention of disease*.
3   The people themselves will achieve Health for All. A well-informed, well-motivated and actively *participating community* is essential to the attainment of the common goal.
4   Because the health authorities can deal with

only part of the problems to be solved, multisectorial co-operation, involving all sectors of government and the society concerned is the only way of ensuring the prerequisites for health, promoting healthy policies and reducing the risks in the physical, economic and social environments.

5 The focus of the health care system should be on primary health care: meeting the basic needs of each community through services provided as close as possible to where people live and work, readily accessible and acceptable to all, at an affordable cost.

6 Lastly, some health problems transcend national frontiers; pollution and trade in health-damaging products are obvious examples of problems whose solutions require international co-operation.

Another way of considering these principles is by realizing that a person's health status must be viewed in a holistic way, yet another feature of the contemporary preparation of the nurse in the field of mental health. The following declaration of the European Conference on Nursing in 1988 (ECN, 1988) offers further insight into the role in which mental health nurses may contribute and are developing in order to influence the targets and make these operational. It also reflects the commitment of nursing as a whole within Europe in supporting the targets.

VIENNA DECLARATION ON NURSING IN SUPPORT OF THE EUROPEAN TARGETS FOR HEALTH FOR ALL

The participants at the European Conference on Nursing, meeting in Vienna from 21 to 24 June 1988, expressed the need for urgent action by governments and national health decision-makers to help nurses make the changes that were required in nursing if the regional targets for Health for All were to be achieved, and made the following declarations:

---

1 Health, which is a state of complete physi-

cal, mental and social well-being and not merely the absence of disease or infirmity, is a fundamental human right. The attainment of the highest possible level of health is a most important social goal, whose realization requires the action of many professions.

2 The persisting inequalities in people's health status, both between and within countries of the WHO European Region, are politically, socially, economically and professionally unacceptable and are therefore of common concern to all nurses.

3 Having provided nurses from the 32 countries in the Region with their first opportunity to re-examine their role, education and practice, the conference reaffirms the status of nursing as a major force that can make a major contribution to achieving the 38 targets adopted by the Member States at the thirty-fourth session of the WHO Regional Committee for Europe in 1984.

4 The participants pledge to bring the new role of the nurse in the era of Health for All to the attention of ministries of health, the organizations and trade unions of all health professions, regulatory bodies and other groups throughout the Region. Nurses should develop their new role by: acting as partners in decision-making on the planning and management of local, regional and national health services, playing a greater role in empowering individuals, families and communities to become more self-reliant and to take charge of their health development, and providing clear and valid information on the favourable and adverse consequences of various types of behaviour, and on the merits and costs of different options for care.

5 New attitudes and values need to be fostered among all health professionals, health care consumers and related groups that are consistent with the directives and principles of Health for All and the primary health care approach. Nursing can best fulfil its potential in primary health care when nursing education provides a sound foundation for nursing practice, especially work in the

community, and when nurses take account of the social aspects of health needs and have a broader understanding of health development. Policies should be adopted and activities identified to enable nurses to practise with sufficient autonomy to carry out their new role in primary health care.

6   Research to improve nursing practice along these lines should be encouraged through the creation of research policies and financial support. Such research should use human resources efficiently, and ensure the evaluation and use of its results. Nurses should also be involved in the research process.

DIMENSIONS OF MENTAL HEALTH

The mental health practitioner will appreciate that many illnesses and disorders may be more appropriately viewed as social rather than medical disorders. Health, like illness, has a number of social dimensions which makes any unambiguous definition difficult. This is particularly true of mental health. Nevertheless, an attempt must be made to outline the suggested dimensions of mental health if any clarity of perspective is to be achieved.

Wright and Taylor (1970) list some commonly used criteria for 'normality' or mental health. These were quoted in the first edition of this book as follows:

Happiness

Unhappiness is often the presenting feature of mental disorder and the gravity of the disorder may be assessed in terms of the degree of unhappiness it causes in the sufferer. There may be a close relationship between unhappiness and other evidence of mental disorder.

Unhappiness may be a necessary and acceptable response to the life situation of the individual—for example in grief and sympathy for others. It can, however, be regarded as evidence of disorder if it is disproportionately increased in quantity or quality—to the point of causing incapacity and enduring feelings of misery.

Efficiency

The mentally healthy person is said to display efficiency in applying his drives to fulfilling his needs satisfactorily, whether the needs are physical, psychological or social. In mental disorder, much mental energy is often directed inwardly in a way that creates internal friction and tensions at the expense of efficiency. Efficiency may be noticeably lacking in the common disorders of depression and anxiety.

Lack of anxiety

Anxiety is probably the chief component of a wide range of mental disorders, particularly the neuroses, and is often accompanied by well-marked and distressing physical symptoms. These symptoms include sweating, tension with tremors, visual disturbances, headache, 'palpitations', gastric disturbances and impairment of sleep and appetite.

Anxiety may be considered as 'fear spread thin' and, like unhappiness, may be justified—for example, examination anxiety in students or the anxiety evoked by an impending visit to the dentist.

Anxiety becomes abnormal when it permeates the inner life of the individual in a lasting and incapacitating way that cannot be explained by simple reference to external events. For example, anxiety may be generated by previously unthreatening objects or situations (phobic anxiety) or when the sufferer is unaware of the reason for his anxiety (free-floating anxiety).

The mentally healthy person copes with the anxieties of everyday life without disintegration or lasting incapacity.

Lack of guilt

Guilt may reflect a need for self-punishment which may eventually become socially incapacitating if uncontrolled. Guilt is again a natural response to many situations and only becomes a problem if it becomes so pervasive as to cause incapacitating tensions with associated loss of efficiency. Equally abnormal is the individual who is incapable of guilt responses. This may be a distinguishing feature of the psychopath who lacks internal controls and is incapable of feeling guilt or remorse for his antisocial actions.

Maturity

Freud suggested that we develop from an early stage of inner disorganization in which we gratify our needs and drives without an awareness of the effects of our actions on other people. He suggested that this infantile stage was governed by the 'Pleasure Principle'. Maturity suggested movement towards the development of internal controls, of a 'conscience', as we become aware of the fact that our behaviour affects other people. We learn to forego or postpone instinctual gratification as our social awareness develops and we mature to live according to the 'Reality Principle'.

Maturity is not synonymous with the dissipation of self-seeking infantile drives but with their regulation—they linger on in the mature adult but are controlled.

The frustrated or stressed adult may revert to immature behavioural patterns, reminiscent of his childhood behaviour; that is, he may show *regression*. Excessive dependence and immaturity may be a feature of neurosis.

The sociopath (psychopath) does not seem to have developed those internal controls which give rise to behaviourally regulating feelings of guilt and remorse. His behaviour may be considered as immature insofar as he has not made an effective transition for Pleasure to Reality Principle and thus remains locked in impulsive and self-gratifying patterns of behaviour without regard for the consequences of his actions on other people.

Adjustment

Adjustment refers to the individual's capacity to adjust to the demands of society in a flexible and resilient way. This criterion implies the capacity to adjust to the demands of society in a productive and adaptable way.

Loss of adjustment and adaptability may be very apparent in the social disintegration of psychosis.

Autonomy and self-esteem

Autonomy implies independence; self-control, self-sufficiency and self-esteem imply a healthy awareness of one's positive attributes and a realistic feeling of a confidence in these attributes. The two contribute to a positive image of self.

Lack of self-sufficiency and self-esteem may be very noticeable in depression and many other mental disorders.

The ability to establish adequate emotional bonds with others

This is perhaps the cement that holds together the fabric of society and it may be noticeably lacking in the emotional impoverishment and social isolation of schizophrenia. The capacity for love and friendship is perhaps central to effective social functioning.

The psychopath is often shallow and insincere in the area of relationships and may simply 'use' others in a very manipulative way.

Contact with reality

The individual can be expected, if 'normal', to cope adequately with the realities of his group and of society and to perceive these in an undistorted way. However, the psychotic may withdraw into an inner 'reality' in which he loses touch with the world of the observer. The boundaries of reality may become blurred and indistinct to the sufferer of psychosis and he may be unable to distinguish aspects of inner reality from external or 'true' reality; that is, 'reality testing' may be impaired.

This major symptom of mental disorder may be revealed by the disordered thought processes of the sufferer of psychosis, which indicate disordered perceptions of reality. The psychotic may express false, unshakeable beliefs which are quite unamenable to logic, these being known as *delusions*. He may, for example, express the belief that he is the victim of a conspiracy to murder him—the nurses and medical staff perhaps being considered as parties to the conspiracy—or he may believe that he is suffering from incurable illnesses, despite medical evidence to the contrary, the illnesses being imagined as punishment for imagined past misdeeds.

Thus mental health, like mental illness, has many dimensions, none of which is fixed.

CONCLUSIONS

The central message contained within the contemporary health policy initiatives is that people need education in order to take responsibility for their state of health including healthy behaviour.

Professionals are parties who share responsibility for the fight against illness and promotion of the healing process (Cmich, 1984). The fitness concept is equally applicable to mental health and physical health. When considering the attributes of a mentally healthy person (Farrell, 1991) emphasizes:

Problem solving with maturity
Coping and handling crises
Utilizing family and social networks.

Throughout this book these and other important factors are reinforced. All together the means to achieve mental health relies on basic needs being met and that means access to life's necessities, food, water and shelter. It includes access to information and shelter to interpret information and maximize its use (Seedhouse, 1986).

FURTHER READING

Aggleton, P. (1990) *Health*. London: Routledge.

Clarke, A.C. (1991) Nurses as role models and health educators. *Journal of Advanced Nursing*, **16**, 1178–1184.

Hugman, R. (1991) *Power in Caring Professions*. London: Macmillan Education.

Robertson, C. (1991) *Health Visiting in Practice*, 2nd ed. Edinburgh: Churchill Livingstone.

REFERENCES

Cmich, D. (1984) Theoretical perspectives of holistic health. *Journal of the Society of Health*, **54** (I), 30–32.

ECN (1988) *European Conference on Nursing*. Summary Report. Vienna: WHO Regional Office for Europe.

ECN (1989) *European Conference on Nursing*. Copenhagen: WHO Regional Office for Europe.

Farrell, E. (1991) *The Mental Health Survival Guide*. London: MacDonald Optima.

Robinson, J. (1987) Working towards the targets. *Senior Nurse*, **16** (3).

Seedhouse, D. (1986) *Health: the Foundations for Achievement*. Colchester: Wiley.

Wright, D.S. & Taylor, A. (1970) *Introducing Psychology, An Experimental Approach*. Harmondsworth: Penguin.

World Health Assembly (WHA) (1989) *Handbook of Resolutions and Decisions of the World Health Assembly and the Executive Board*. Geneva: WHO.

WHO (1978) *Primary Health Care*. Health for All Series No. 1. Geneva, Alma-Atal: WHO.

WHO (1991) *The Health Policy for Europe—Summary of the Updated Edition*. Copenhagen: WHO Regional Office for Europe.

WHO (1992) *The I CD-10 Classification of Mental and Behavioural Disorders, Clinical Descriptions and Diagnostic Guidelines*. Geneva: WHO.

4

ANTIDISCRIMINATORY PRACTICE

Tony Thompson and Peter Mathias

AIMS

i) To draw attention to the effects of unfair discrimination and social disadvantage on mental health
ii) To explore antidiscriminatory competence

KEY ISSUES

Variety of discrimination
Discrimination interacts with mental health
Antidiscriminatory competence

Identify, analyse and assess factors causing distress and illness	Promote health, provide direct care and make interventions	Manage care programmes and services
Be critical, analytical and accountable, continue professional development	Counter discrimination, inequality and individual and institutional racism	Work within and develop policies, laws and safeguards in all settings
Understand influences on mental health and the nature/causes of disorder and illness	Know the effects of distress, disorder, illness on individuals, groups, families	Understand the basis of treatments and interventions

DISCRIMINATION AND DISADVANTAGE

Members of the caring professions practise in a society in which people may experience social and economic disadvantage as a result of unfair or unjust discrimination. Practitioners must equip themselves to understand, recognize and counter the effects of such discrimination and disadvantage on mental health and the provision of services.

Unfair discrimination interacts with mental health in a variety of ways and may affect people's willingness to use the services, the diagnosis given once the service has been engaged, the treatment which follows and willingness to maintain treatment programmes.

Unfair discrimination and its disadvantageous effects on quality of life, opportunity, independence, control over life events, housing, education, work and leisure brings its own pressures and stressors which may threaten mental health. The interaction between culture, cognition, beliefs and values may result in differing concepts of mental health and different ways of showing distress and it is important that practitioners know when and how to pay attention to these factors.

It is not possible to provide formulae which show the relationship between discrimination, disadvantage, stress, poor mental health and mental illness. Nevertheless, it is possible to identify some of the interactions and many of the subsequent chapters include references to the experience of different groupings within British society with respect to the mental health services and these provide a basis from which to evaluate personal practice.

ANTIDISCRIMINATORY COMPETENCE

It follows that practitioners must build these understandings into their practice if they are to be able to offer effective services to those seeking help. In Chapter 2 Johnson and Smith show that the UKCC's Code of Professional Conduct makes specific mention of the need to take into account the customs, values and beliefs in all aspects of care management and delivery. Added to this demand for sensitivity to varying needs is the emergent idea that practice should be actively antidiscriminatory. The incorporation of antidiscriminatory perspectives into statements of competence was one of the key achievements in the development of National Vocational Qualifications in Care, a set of qualifications available to people who work alongside nurses, social workers and remedial therapists in the health and social services. The achievement was an important one

because it involved agreement amongst employer and staff in the public, private and voluntary health and social services about the central features of the value base which should apply to the provision of services across sectors. It is therefore relevant to the Charters and Equal Opportunity policies issued by the services and may have some relevance to the codes of conduct which apply to members of the professions.

The value base is expressed as a unit of competence called Promote Equality for All Individuals and its components or elements are:

Promote antidiscriminatory practice

Maintain the confidentiality of information

Promote and support individual rights and choice within service delivery.

Acknowledge individual's personal beliefs and identity

Support individuals through effective communication

The full version of the unit with its underpinning knowledge requirements can be found in the National Occupational Standards for Care (1992) and can be used by practitioners and their colleagues to evaluate their practice and the standards reached by their services.

The unit (Promote Equality for All Individuals) is sometimes referred to as the value base unit and is based on the following principles of good practice.*

PRINCIPLES OF GOOD PRACTICE

---

1   The rights of all individuals within society should be promoted and supported so that

---

* Note that everything in bold type which follows is taken directly from the National Occupational Standards for Care produced by the Care Sector Consortium (1992). The National Standards are under Crown Copyright and the extracts are reproduced here with the permission of the Employment Department.

equality and quality of life is available to each individual within the service. This is regardless of their age, class, caste, colour, creed, culture, gender, health status, marital status, mental ability, mental health, offending background, physical ability, place of origin, political beliefs, race, religion, responsibility for dependents, sensory ability, sexuality or other specific factors which result in discrimination.

2 Each individual should be treated as a person with a variety of individual needs.

3 Antidiscriminatory practice should be developed and promoted so that each individual is guaranteed the same quality of service.

4 The confidentiality of information and its sources should be respected and disclosed only to those who necessarily require it and after agreement with the individual concerned.

5 All involved in the delivery of care are essential and integral to the care team (consistent with client choice) and therefore clients and their partners, relatives, friends and community should be involved at all stages.

6 The health and safety of workers, clients, their partners, relatives and friends is of paramount importance and therefore all actions should be consistent with health and safety guidelines while not imposing unnecessary restraints on individual action.

7 Every individual should be encouraged to be as independent as possible and to exercise informed choice in relation to her/himself, her/his belongings and service requirements taking into account any risk involved.

8 Individual choice, wishes and preferences should be confirmed with the individual and respected in actions taken.

9 Communication (verbal and/or non-verbal) should be that most appropriate to the individual.

Each of the unit's five elements (1–5 above) carries with it statements of the knowledge and skill necessary for competence and descriptions of the things which can be done in order to put the value base into practice. For example, element 'promote antidiscriminatory practice' has the following implications for the worker or practitioner:

1 Antidiscriminatory practice is promoted in ways that are consistent with the worker's role and legislation and charters concerning individual rights.

2 The worker's behaviour in the work setting demonstrates recognized good antidiscriminatory practice and is not exploitative or abusive.

3 Where the worker is unsure of appropriate forms of behaviour for specific individuals or has discriminatory feelings towards an individual, the appropriate advice, guidance and support is sought.

4 Where an individual directs discriminatory behaviour to the worker, the appropriate action is taken to the behaviour or support is sought.

5 Where an individual makes inappropriate or discriminatory actions or remarks, the effects or consequences of her/his actions are explained in a manner, and at a level and pace, appropriate to her/him.

6 Where an individual is at risk of abuse, exploitation and discrimination by others, the appropriate action is taken to support the individual.

7 Discriminatory behaviour from others is responded to in an appropriate manner and consistent with agreements made with the work team.

8 Where an individual wishes to make a complaint about discriminatory practice, he/she is appropriately supported in doing so.

The types and forms of discrimination with which the element is concerned include direct (public/evident/obvious) and indirect (hidden/subtle) discrimination against people on the basis of age, class, caste, creed, culture, gender, health status, HIV status, marital status, mental ability, mental health, offending background, physical ability, place of origin, political beliefs, race, religion, responsibility for dependents, sensory ability, sexuality or other specific factors which result in discrimination.

In order to practice in an antidiscriminatory way practitioners need an adequate knowledge base and this is also identified in the standards. With respect to the element 'promote antidiscriminatory practice', for example, practitioners will need knowledge of:

1 The difference between inappropriate, unfair and unjust discrimination in contrast to appropriate, fair and just discrimination (such as when it is necessary to select individuals from a large number and explicit criteria are used to do so).
2 The forms that discrimination may take (overt and covert, such as tone used, language, body language, etc.) and the behaviours that may be expressions of these and that discrimination is not restricted to particular groups in society.
3 The assumptions and oppressions that surround different groups (such as sexism, ageism, heterosexism) the ways in which this is built into society and organizations and how the expression of discrimination may differ from social context to social context.
4 The effects which the worker's own beliefs may have on her/his behaviour and the methods which he/she can use to identify his/her own prejudice and challenge it.
5 The role of the worker in the setting, the limits which are set on the actions that they may take and their relationship to other members of the work team.
6 The different behaviours which may be confusing and the effects that behaviour may have, for example, dress, appearance and the limits to which workers should restrict their own behaviour for fear of being misinterpreted.
7 The other sources of information that may be available to the worker or that may have a bearing on their behaviour, such as guidelines, policy and law.
8 The limits that various environments impose on behaviour and the particular limits that

are imposed in the worker's environment.
9 The legislation and charters that are applicable to the setting/client group and particularly those that govern the way in which the individual relates to others.
10 Possible effects of stereotyping, prejudice and institutionalization on the delivery of care.
11 How an individual's rights may be, but should not be, affected by other's behaviour.
12 Methods of challenging discriminatory behaviour and attitudes.
13 The support services available to the worker.

Practitioners will also need to understand why:

1 No assumptions should be made about an individual.
2 An individual's requests for information should be referred to the appropriate member of the care team if the worker cannot answer them.
3 The language used should be consistent with the individual's own form of expression and why the worker should not resort to terminology of little or no relevance to the individual concerned, for example, clinical.
4 The worker's behaviour should be consistent and non-exploitative.
5 Misleading behaviours should be minimized.
6 Support should be sought from other members of the care team.
7 Some relatives, friends, the worker and other members of the care team may have difficulty altering their behaviour and how individuals can be supported in coming to terms with their own feelings.

ACKNOWLEDGEMENT OF PERSONAL BELIEFS AND IDENTITY

As well as being able to understand and counter the effects of discrimination, practitioners will need to develop practice which is sensitive to the cultural and ethnic background of the client and which will acknowledge personal beliefs and identity. The National Occupational Standards for Care again go into some detail on this issue identifying the following as components of good practice:

---

1 Individuals' beliefs and identity are promoted in ways that are consistent with the worker's role and any relevant legislation and charters.
2 The worker's actions in the work setting represent equal recognition of each individual's personal beliefs and identity.
3 Individuals are addressed and described in their preferred manner.
4 Individuals are encouraged to express their personal beliefs, wishes and views provided that this does not adversely affect the rights of others.
5 Individual's views are sought, listened and responded to, in a manner that is supportive of her/him as an individual.
6 Actions of the worker acknowledge the individual's expressed personal beliefs, wishes and views.
7 Where the worker is unsure how to act appropriately for that individual, support and guidance is sought from an appropriate person.
8 Where necessary, individual's personal beliefs, wishes and views and the way in which they are expressed, are legibly, accurately and completely recorded.

Personal beliefs will relate to ideas of self and religious, cultural, political, ethical and sexual behaviour and in order to work in an appropriate way practitioners will need the following knowledge:

---

1 Legislative requirements and the organizational policies and procedures relating to the recognition of personal beliefs.
2 The role of the worker in acknowledging personal beliefs, the limits and boundaries of her/his work role and the worker's relationship to others in the care setting.
3 The boundaries of identity, self-image, etc. and how personal beliefs and preferences (including the worker's own) may affect her/his ways of dealing with people (e.g. the inappropriate use of the term 'Christian name' to those who are not of the Christian faith rather than using 'first name').
4 How there may be a possible conflict between the worker's and individual beliefs.
5 The different needs that individuals may have.
6 How behaviour is related to stages of development, what these are and the relationship of an individual's behaviour to these.
7 The effect that beliefs and preferences may have on aspects of daily living (such as diet, clothing, transport, worship and access to others).
8 The possible effects of stereotyping, prejudice and institutionalization and the ways in which care is provided.
9 The ways in which the questions asked of individuals may reflect the role of the worker and the power invested in that role.

Practitioners will also have to understand why:

---

1 It is important to encourage individuals to express their personal beliefs and preferences provided that this does not adversely affect the rights of others.
2 An individual's personal beliefs and preferences are important.
3 Recognition and support of individual beliefs is important.

The previous paragraphs have made extensive use of the National Occupational Standards for Care (1992) in order to illustrate the point that it is possible to go beyond general exhortations to apply Equal Opportunities Policies and examine the implications for practice. However, it must be emphasized that the National Occupational Standards do not formally apply to nurses and other professions in care at the time of writing as they are outside the structure of National Vocational Qualifications and anyway have their own codes of conduct and statements of good practice.

EXPERIENCE OF THE MENTAL HEALTH SERVICES

There is a growing literature relevant to the knowledge and skills associated with antidiscriminatory practice in mental health. Ahmad (1992), for example, after reviewing the literature argues that black people are over-represented in those aspects of the mental health services to do with control and under-represented in those concerned with welfare type provisions such as mental health promotion. Crowley and Simmons (1992), in a retrospective case note study of 152 discharged psychiatric patients in London, found significant differences between Afro-Caribbean subjects and others with respect to areas of diagnosis, status on admission and length of stay. Public health statistics for 1991 (HMSO, 1992) show that both physical and mental health experience varies by group—a finding that has prompted the Government to devise strategies against discrimination manifested 'either in the provision of services which are inappropriate or insensitive or through staff applying racial stereotypes'.

Similarly MIND (1992) calls for a major review of the mental health services to make them more appropriate to women arguing that there is growing evidence of harassment and abuse of women within facilities such as wards and day centres. Again issues of diagnosis and treatment are raised with suggestions that GPs and other health workers may fail to recognize the relationship between distress and domestic violence, sexual abuse and problems such as miscarriage and infertility. The MIND report says that women are twice as likely to be diagnosed as suffering from depression as men and two-thirds of prescriptions for psychotropic drugs are written for women. Practitioners therefore need to be aware of the particular pressures and likely experiences of women, be able to challenge approaches to mental health based on stereotypical views of women and men, and find ways to make the provision of services appropriate.

Difficulties in gaining access to appropriate mental health services can also be encountered by other groups. For example, the Central Council for Education and Training in Social Work and the Royal College of Psychiatrists published a report in 1992 (CCETSW, 1992) that considers issues involved in working with people who have both learning difficulties and a mental illness. The report contains case studies that illustrate the difficulties which people with a learning difficulty may have in obtaining suitable help when they experience mental illness or distress.

Health care workers may find that they themselves experience discrimination or find themselves working in situations where colleagues are subject to prejudice and discrimination at either the individual or institutional level. Discrimination may come from clients or staff or the institutional practices of the organization and may be crude and overt or more subtle. The Ashworth enquiry (DH, 1992) received evidence of extensive racism where racism combined with the particular features of special hospitals some of which Beacock describes in Chapter 32 resulted in horrifying experiences for those involved.

CONCLUSION

In finding and developing strategies to recognize and counter discrimination, practitioners are backed by legislation that includes the Race Relations Act, the Sex Discrimination Act, the Disabled Persons Act and the Fair Employment Act (Northern Ireland) which clearly legislate against discriminatory practices on the grounds of race, gender and religion respectively. In addition the Children Act and the National Health Service and Community Care Act lay a special responsibility on those who work with patients, clients and their families to be particularly aware of the needs of those groups of people who are likely to experience discrimination.

An understanding of discrimination should therefore underpin and inform the activities and interventions of members of the caring profession. Carol Baxter, Ruth Prime, Kamlesh Patel and Gerard Rice address these issues directly in later chapters whilst other contributors examine them in relation to the main themes of their contributions. We hope that they will all contribute to a growing understanding of how practice can become truly antidiscriminatory.

FURTHER READING

CCETSW (1991) *One Small Step Towards Racial Justice*. London: Central Council for Education and Training in Social Work.

CCETSW (1991) *Setting the Context for Change*. London: Central Council for Education and Training in Social Work.

CCETSW (1992) *Improving Practice with Elders*. London: Central Council for Education and Training in Social Work.

Miles, A. (1989) *Women and Mental Illness: The Social Concept of Female Neurosis*. Harvester Wheatsheaf.

Phillipson, J. (1992) *Practising Equality. Women, Men and Social Work*. London: Central Council for Education and Training in Social Work.

Sefafica, F.C. (1991) *Mental Health of Ethnic Minorities*. Praegar.

Ussher, J.M. (1991) *Women's Madness: Misogyny or Mental Illness?* Prentice Hall.

REFERENCES

Ahmad, B. (1992) *Black Perspectives in Social Work*. London: Venture Press in association with the Race Equality Unit, National Institute for Social Work. London: Care Sector Consortium.

CCETSW (1992) *A Double Challenge Working with People who Have Both Learning Difficulties and a Mental Illness*. CCETSW Paper 19.27. London: Central Council for Education and Training in Social Work.

Crowley, J. & Simmons, S. (1992) Mental Health, race and ethnicity: a retrospective study of the care of ethnic minorities and whites in a psychiatric unit. *Journal of Advanced Nursing*, **17**, 1078–1087.

DH (1992) Report of the Committee of Inquiry into Complaints about Ashworth Hospital. HMSO.

HMSO (1992) *On the State of the Public Health for the Year 1991*. London: HMSO.

LGMB (1992) *The National Occupational Standards for Care*. Luton: Local Government Management Board.

MIND (1992) *Stress on Women; Policy Paper on Women and Mental Health*. London: MIND.

5

PROVIDING CARE IN A MULTIRACIAL SOCIETY

Carol Baxter

AIMS

i)   To examine the implications of working in a multiracial society
ii) To provide an understanding of personal and institutional racism
iii) To lay the foundations of antiracist practice

KEY ISSUES

Origins of racism
Racism and rights
Poor health experiences
Stereotypical views
Personal racism
Institutional racism
Discrimination in hospitals
Double discrimination
Comparative stereotyping

Identify, analyse and assess factors causing distress and illness	Promote health, provide direct care and make interventions	Manage care programmes and services
Be critical, analytical and accountable, continue professional development	Counter discrimination, inequality and individual and institutional racism	Work within and develop policies, laws and safeguards in all settings
Understand influences on mental health and the nature/causes of disorder and illness	Know the effects of distress, disorder, illness on individuals, groups, families	Understand the basis of treatments and interventions

INTRODUCTION

'The message to all who choose to care for others is that, unless their actions are guided by a sense of importance of every human being, their competence and professionalism will remain questionable.'
Nirza (1986)

People who experience distress and illness come from all sections of society and from different racial and cultural backgrounds. If we are to maintain professional standards, then we must have the appropriate attitude, knowledge and skills to meet the needs of all individuals regardless of their racial or cultural background.

We are often quite unaware of the impact of our own social background on our individuality and professional performance. Very rarely do we appreciate the differences in perspectives which can result in our unwittingly accepting some of our attitudes, ideas and ways of doing things as the 'right' way.

We only need take a look around us to appreciate that white people in Britain enjoy more privileges and have more opportunities and power than black people. Whiteness confers rights that are often denied to black people. Recent figures show that black people are more likely to live in run down inner city areas and in substandard housing, to be found in semi- and unskilled jobs, to be disproportionately affected by unemployment and are economically worse off than their white counterparts (Brown, 1984). There is also evidence that black people have poorer health experiences and less access to appropriate health care (McNaught, 1985). Black people also consistently receive less than their entitlement in benefits or services (Gohil, 1987).

These inequalities have their roots in racial discrimination. Racism is an ideology and an institution developed out of imperialism. Westerners needed to see African and Asian people as inferior and even sub-human in order to rationalize slavery and colonization and the furtherance of economic wealth and gain. Racism is based on the myth of the superiority of the white race. Stereotyping is one way in which racism is perpetuated.

Think back to your childhood and identify images you have learnt about white and black people. These images come from personal experience, family, school friends, literature, radio, television and newspapers. Spend a few minutes jotting down these images, it will become apparent to you that the words which are used to describe white images often reflect what you have learnt about the British Empire. They are generally positive images such as discoverers, powerful, inventors, scientific researchers, responsible, civilized, intelligent. Words that are used to describe black images are generally negative in contrast to the images of white people—poor, needy, primitive, unreliable, helpless, incompetent, aggressive, subservient.

These racist stereotyped views are prevalent in our society. Black people who live in Britain today continue to be seen through this myth and continue to be discriminated against socially, politically and economically. This is reflected in all institutions, including health and social welfare services.

Racism is a complex phenomenon. The way in which it operates can be categorized at two different levels—personal and institutional. Although there will be incidents of personal racism, most people in the caring professions do not deliberately withhold care or treat people differently on the basis of their colour. Institutional racism is the more common and damning form of racism. This happens in a variety of ways. Firstly, by default where the way things are done within organizations does not take account of the needs of black people. For example, despite the fact that not all patients speak English as a first language, services are on the whole provided through the English medium only. Secondly, it happens where people in positions of power base their decisions on racist assumptions and stereotyping. An example of this is the assumption that black people do not need services because 'they prefer to look after their own'. Another very common form of racial discrimination within services is where the rules and regulations apply equally to all, but they have the effect of excluding black and ethnic minority people while maintaining the privileged position of white people. McNaught (1985), from his analysis of a variety of reports, identified some practical ways in which racial discrimination against black patients in hospital has occurred:

1 *Patient's reception and handling.* Ethnic minority patients kept waiting unnecessarily; staff making racist comments in earshot of the patients; addressing patients in a derogatory manner.
2 *Clinical consultation.* Poor or no explanations offered to ethnic minority patients. Assumption that many are 'faking' or hypochondriacs. Inadequate or no examination before diagnosis and prescription of treatment. Delayed, inappropriate or even experimental treatment.
3 *Patient's consent to medical procedures.* Inadequate explanations. Exceeding the procedures that the patient was advised were necessary without further consultation. Unnecessary procedures, said to be racially motivated.
4 *Nursing care.* Offhand treatment. Racist slurs or comments to patients. Unnecessary medication, particularly of the mentally distressed.
5 *Health surveillance/diagnosis.* Utilization of parameters and behavioural models that are culture-specific to white British people, for example, in mental health diagnosis, child health surveillance, social and medical assessment for special education.

DOUBLE DISCRIMINATION

Black people with mental health problems are particularly vulnerable in a racist society.

As is the case with mental illness, racism is also a form of devaluation and oppression. Parallels can be drawn between social role perceptions of people who are mentally ill and people who are black. Two of the most prevalent such role perceptions are that of being a *menace* and that of being *objects of dread*. Even today people with

mental health problems are sometimes viewed as menacing or a threat. Attempts to establish community living are met with objections based on the *notions of danger* to local people, property and property values. Housing policies and practices aimed at keeping black people out of white neighbourhoods are commonplace. The National Association for the Care and Resettlement of Offenders highlighted that black people are more likely to be locked away in mental institutions and to receive custodial sentences and imprisonment (NACRO, 1986).

People with mental health problems are also largely still dreaded in society, often being avoided and denied social intercourse and conversation. Black people are also viewed as socially undesirable and unattractive. Many people will admit to fear and anxiety when there are large numbers of mentally ill people and (in the case of white people) black people around.

The relationship between black people and mental illness has increasingly been discussed in psychiatry. Classical psychiatry, having developed in the colonial era, reflects notions that emerged during the period of 'scientific racism'. Psychiatry prides itself in its scientific background based on anatomy and physiology and more recently in the social sciences. Within it can be found many of the simplistic assumptions of a racist society. Fernando (1988) states that:

'Historically speaking two important sets of ideas came into psychiatry from the basic sciences. First, the view that black people are born with inferior brains and limited capacity for growth; and secondly, that their personalities tend to be abnormal or deviant because of nature (genetic endowment) and/or nurture (upbringing). The influence of these themes ... was overt in the nineteenth century, but, although less obvious since the war, shows a tenacious persistence into the present.'

The ongoing debates concerning the genetic background to mental illness have implications for the ways in which 'races' are perceived. This background, as well as the medical model within which much of psychiatric research is approached, can explain the concern with the incidence of mental illness among black people. Although black people comprise less than one-fifth of the population, they make up a quarter of all inner city mentally ill patients. The widely debated study by Glyn Harrison in Nottingham (Harrison *et al.*, 1988), which is based on estimated populations of black people, reports a considerably higher incidence of schizophrenia among black people in Britain, especially among those born here.

There is a failure of general practitioners to detect early signals of distress and minor forms of mental disorder such as depression and anxiety. Consequently, traditional models of diagnosis are often inappropriate. Lack of recognition of the different experiences, pressures and lifestyles of black people within the method and process of diagnosis often leads to misdiagnosis.

There is considerable concern that some black populations are being over-diagnosed with certain conditions (e.g. schizophrenia among Afro-Caribbean communities) (Burke, 1984). Other ethnic minority populations appear to be under-represented in mental health services.

Black people are four times as likely as their white counterparts to reach a psychiatric hospital through the involvement of the police and to be compulsorily detained in hospital under the Mental Health Act legislation.

There are also measurable differences in the treatment that black patients receive compared to white patients. For black service users, there is greater reliance on physical treatment such as major tranquillizer and electro-cardiotherapy and they are less likely to be offered psychotherapy (Littlewood and Lipsedge, 1982).

The commonly held view that all black people have self-supporting family networks and prefer to look after their own can have serious consequences for the aftercare of black people experiencing mental distress. Many patients are discharged into situations where the aftercare and support is not forthcoming. Carers usually do not have access to information about important issues such as the benefits and side-effects of medication, and about their rights as carers (Christie and Blunden, 1991).

Racism is also considered as a contributory factor in the onset of illness among black people.

Burke (1986) refers to the impact of racism on mental health as follows:

'The evidence points to the conclusion that racism does lead to mental illness; firstly, by fermenting and maintaining social deprivation and so impairing chances of attaining mental health; secondly, by institutional factors which have the effect of withholding care; thirdly, by bully-boy/girl strategies of humiliating blacks into subordination and inflicting sado-masochistic attacks on them; and finally, when this fails, by implementing methods of social/medical control.'

Fernando (1986) states: 'Racism causes depression by promoting blows to self-esteem, inducting experiences of loss, and placing individuals in a position of helplessness,' and he continues '. . . racism is not just an added stress to black and ethnic minorities, but a pathogen that generates depression in the individual.'

Even within the present climate of reform in services, it is still very questionable as to whether the very philosophies that underpin the changes will not in reality further work against black users of services.

One change which has had a great impact on people who experience mental disorder is the move towards care in the community. Under the Community Care legislation voluntary organizations are playing an increasing role in providing services. This move could have severe effects on services for black people. Mainstream white voluntary organizations do not cater adequately for the needs of black people (Dungate, 1984) being mainly based on the needs of the white majority population. However, the few black voluntary organizations that exist are too grossly underfunded and under-resourced to take on this role. There will therefore be an increased burden on black families.

Criticism about other concepts and philosophies underpinning services are based on these very same principles. Services must recognize and address the effects of racism on the users and providers of services. Since service planners and managers are largely white it is possible that it is only those needs, wants and wishes of the white society that will be considered as 'normal' or 'valued' experiences. A simple exercise carried out by a community mental handicap team in Harlesden, for example, demonstrated that what white staff would value for themselves would, in many cases, conflict with what black service users valued (Baxter *et al.*, 1990). The same can be expected in services for other client groups.

What then, you may ask, about the response of black service providers? Should their presence in services not avoid such negative interpretations? Black staff, especially those from backgrounds similar to service users, are indeed vital in providing services to a multiracial clientele. Experience shows that employing staff who can communicate with people in their own languages and who understand their cultures and share their experience of oppression can result in a dramatic increase in the take-up of services by potential clients who are from a similar background.

However, many black staff feel that their particular perspectives, experiences and skills are often not valued and that the initiatives and methods that they develop as more appropriate to the needs of black clients are seen as unprofessional by their colleagues and managers. Others feel that they are viewed as the 'expert' in caring for black service users and that black clients are 'dumped' on them to relieve white service providers of their professional responsibility. Furthermore, since service providers all undergo the same white-client oriented training, not all black service providers therefore will have the necessary skills or feel confident and supported to work from an antiracist perspective. The majority of black staff tend to occupy low grade positions and their presence in services is not reflected at a managerial level. Very rarely, therefore, are black service providers in a position to become involved in informed decision-making.

People with mental health difficulties often have to rely on others to plan their lives. Accordingly, the care programme approach enables service providers to recognize and meet individual needs. However, in many black communities the collectivity of the family and community takes precedence over the more self-centred individualism encouraged in majority white families. This difference in emphasis may be very important when working with users and carers from black communities.

Assessment of an individual's abilities is often based on white British norms which bear little relationship to the everyday life of black people. Many standard assessment procedures involve approaches based on white middle class lifestyle and experiences. A social worker who was herself from the Afro-Caribbean community expressed these concerns as follows:

'The approach brought to assessment can be very Eurocentric. This can be very dangerous. A social worker I know was prepared to recommend that her Afro-Caribbean client was still very depressed and was not making progress. She based her decision on the fact that during a home visit the client offered her tea but had made her a cup of coffee instead. I had to explain to her that this was perfectly rational behaviour in many people of her generation, many of whom will use the term tea to refer to a warm drink.'

At this time of great change when important decisions are being made and new systems and patterns of support and care are being formulated, we should not miss this opportunity to design services to meet the needs of the whole community. The needs of black service users should not be considered as an afterthought or as additional or special, but should be enshrined within the concept of good professional practice. Connelly (1988) puts forward the following arguments in support of an antiracist perspective in services:

1 We all share a common humanity. To preserve this, all people should be given the opportunity to work for and enjoy all improvements in our society. Taking account of individual, racial and cultural diversity of needs is part of this process.

2 As tax and charge payers, black and ethnic minority people have a right as a matter of

course to expect equal access to services which are appropriate and relevant to their needs. Planning and policies to enable this are crucial to social justice.

3 To maintain professional integrity, the competence of service providers hinges on their readiness, willingness and ability to apply existing and increasing knowledge to new situations.

4 Statutory and voluntary organizations have obligations under the Race Relations Act of 1976 to eliminate racial discrimination in employment and the provision of services.

5 Providing services which are appropriate to the needs of the population is making efficient and effective use of scarce resources. The multiracial community is indeed itself a resource and an opportunity to be utilized and cherished.

When looking at competency and practice issues for nurses and social workers, attempts are made to focus on the situation of the most vulnerable black people—those in hospital lead as an area of priority.

For inpatients, first and foremost, the issue of human rights should be addressed. It is now well recognized in services that all service users will need assistance in exercising their rights. As products of Western societies, we are all socialized into a racist culture and therefore have unwittingly accepted some of its attitudes, ideas and ways of doing things. We cannot change the past, but by recognizing its effects we can work towards developing higher professional standards in our future practice.

For black users, therefore, attention should be focused on their right to be treated with dignity and respect as equal human beings. Those involved in providing services should address the following questions:

1 Is your relationship with black service users influenced by unhelpful racist stereotypes?

2 What measures have you taken to learn about and understand the nature of racism and how it affects your work practice?

3 Do you challenge racist jokes or slurs from other patients or colleagues?

4 What types of policies are there to ensure that where the client's rights are violated, the appropriate action takes place?

5 Black clients will need assistance to minimize destructive self-criticism and focus on their positive self worth.

FREEDOM OF CHOICE

Freedom of choice is an integral part of clients' rights. However, as professionals, we have the tendency to make assumptions about users' wants and wishes. This is particularly true for black users where white professionals are less likely to feel confident or take the time to get to know them as individuals. Even where there is some appreciation of the need to provide more individual and culturally specific forms of care, service providers often have difficulties in gaining information relating to a person's culture or racial origin. Such conversations are often viewed as impolite. There are others who may wish to ask such questions, but do not know where to start or what questions to ask. Further difficulties can arise when the service provider and service user do not speak the same language.

If freedom of choice is to become a reality for black service users, then it is important that the options and range of wants and needs are recognized. A priority must be to develop a closer working relationship with families. Included in this approach will be greater priority and confidence in working and taking on board the views of a wider range of people, balancing the individuality, the position of the family and the long-term relationships between them. Some ideas which will help to pave the way in developing a good partnership are listed below:

1 Black and ethnic minority people in this country are most often British citizens by birth. To start off with questions about people's country of origin could give the

impression that you feel that they do not belong in Britain.

2 Do not be blinded in your search for differences. Build up a rapport by acknowledging that you have things in common.

3 Build up a mutual trust and liking by reassuring patients and family members that you do not see their differences as a problem and that their differences will not detract from your ability to plan appropriately for their care.

4 Questions based on some existing knowledge indicate your interest and professional competence will increase as the client's and the family's confidence in you increases. For example, 'I know you are of the Muslim faith. Can you guide me on how I need to take account of this while caring for you?' Do not rely too heavily on the cultural information in books that you have read because this could stereotype your clients. Use the information only as a guide to asking questions.

Unless they have a lot of experience in doing this, everyone has difficulty analysing what is second nature to them. Ask yourself the same question to make sure that you are not asking questions that are difficult to answer. There should be access to good interpreter services in those situations where there are language differences.

Personal hygiene, hair and skin care are very important to a person's feeling of wellbeing. It is important that staff are able to give the appropriate attention to these areas. The personal care and hygiene routines adopted at home should be followed:

1 Choice of either showers or baths should be available as not everyone would feel happy about sitting in a bath.

2 Support workers of the same sex may be preferred when carrying out intimate forms of care.

3 Differences in hair texture and skin colour have implications for routine physical assessment and care procedures. To use white hair and skin as the norm is dangerous.

Appropriate hair and skin care is still an area of gross neglect for black clients. Nurses and care assistants will need to appreciate that some people require their skin (and hair) to be moisturized, especially after procedures that deplete the body of moisture, such as a shampoo or a bath.

CULTURAL AND RELIGIOUS DIMENSIONS

Black service users in hospital will need assistance in maintaining their religious and cultural identity. Service providers should consistently work to the following criteria:

1 All clients should be addressed by their preferred name. Attempts should be made to pronounce accurately and record clients' names. These should not be changed to more English-sounding ones.

2 Clients should have the opportunity to have personal possessions which reflect their culture.

3 Appropriate and preferred dress is important in helping service users to maintain personal appearance. For example, nurses should be able to help an Asian woman to wrap her sari or a young sikh man to wrap his turban.

4 Wall hangings, books, magazines, television programmes and other artefacts that portray positive images of a multiracial society should be utilized. Videos from most ethnic minority communities are now widely available and would be helpful.

5 The service user's religious beliefs (if any) should be established and respected. Assistance to make available places for those who may wish to practise their religion should be given. Mosques, Afro-Caribbean churches and Sikh gudwaras and temples

are welcoming to anyone who wishes to support members of their communities.

6 Catering arrangements should ensure the availability of a choice and range of foods to suit individual preferences. This should include those normally eaten at home. For example, vegetarian, halal and kosher meals should be available if required.

7 Service users should be encouraged to speak in their first language and be assisted in finding situations where this is possible.

8 Daily routines should be of sufficient variety to promote positive identification with people's own racial and cultural background.

FURTHER READING

Baxter, C. (1985) *Hair Care of African, Afro-Caribbean and Asian Hair Types*. Cambridge: National Extension College.

Commission for Racial Equality (1976) *Afro-Caribbean Hair and Skin Care and Recipes*. London: Commission for Racial Equality.

Fryer, P. (1984) *Staying Power. The History of Black People in Britain*. London: Pluto Press.

Katz, J. (1978) *White Awareness*. Oklahoma, USA: University of Oklahoma Press.

Mares, P., Henley, A. & Baxter, C. (1985) *Health Care in Multiracial Britain*. Cambridge: National Extension College/Health Education Council.

Shackman, J. (1985) *The Right to be Understood—A Handbook on Working with, Employment and Training Community Interpreters*. Cambridge: National Extension College.

RESOURCES

'Being White'—a video. 35 minutes. White people from different backgrounds talk about their understanding of the roots of racism and how they take account of it in their daily lives and work situations. Available from Albany Productions.

'Black'—a BBC film, 1983. 50 minutes. Examines the history of black and white relations and features young people talking about their experience of racism. Concord Films Council, 201 Felixstowe Road, Ipswich, Suffolk, IP3 9BJ. Tel. 0473 715 754.

'The Right to be Understood'—a video about working interpreters. Available from the National Extension College, 18 Brooklands Avenue, Cambridge, CB2 2HN.

'Black and In Care'—in this video children talk about their experiences of being in care and how they have and are trying to overcome their difficulties. Available from Black and In Care Steering Group, c/o Children's Legal Centre, 20 Compton Terrace, London, N1 2UN. Tel. 071 359 6251.

REFERENCES

Baxter, C., Poonia, K., Ward, L. & Nadishaw, Z. (1990) Double Discrimination—Issues and Services for People with Learning Difficulties from Black and Ethnic Minority Communities. London: Kings Fund Centre/Commission for Racial Equality.

Brown, C. (1984) *Black and White Britain. The Third PSI Survey*. London: Gower.

Burke, A. (1984) Racism and Mental Illness. In Cox, J. (Ed.) *Transcultural Psychiatry*, pp. 135–157. London: Croom Helm.

Burke, A. (1986) Racism, Prejudice and Mental Illness. In Cox, J. (Ed.), *Transcultural Psychiatry*, pp. 139–157. London: Croom Helm.

Christie, Y. & Blunden, R. (1991) Is race on your agenda? Improving mental health services for people from black and minority groups. London: Kings Fund Centre.

Connelly, N. (1988) *Care in a Multiracial Community*. London: Policy Studies Institute.

Dungate, M. (1984) *A Multicultural Society, the Role of National Voluntary Organisations*. London: Bedford Square Press.

Fernando, S. (1986) Depression and Ethnic Minorities. In Cox, J. (Ed.), *Transcultural Psychiatry*, pp. 107–138. London: Croom Helm.

Fernando, S. (1988) *Race, Culture and Psychiatry*. London: Croom Helm.

Gohil, V. (1987). DHSS Service Delivery to Ethnic Minority Claimants. *Leicester Rights Bulletin*, June/July, No. 32, pp. 7–8.

Harrison, G. *et al.* (1988) A prospective study of severe

mental disorder in Afro-Caribbean patients. *Psychological Medicine*, **18**. 643–657.

Littlewood, R. & Lipsedge, M. (1982). *Aliens and Alienists*. Harmondsworth: Penguin.

McNaught, A. (1985) *Race and Health Care in the United Kingdom*. Occasional Paper 2. London: Health Education Council.

NACRO (1980) *Black People and the Criminal Justice System: Summary of the Report of the NACRO Race issues Advisory Committee*. London.

Nzira, V. (1986) Race: The ingredients of good practice. In Philpot, T. (Ed.) *The Residential Opportunity? The Wagner Report and After*. Wallington: Reed Business Publishing/Community Care.

PART

II

THE NATURE AND EFFECTS OF DISORDER

The purpose of this section is to explore the nature of mental health, disorder and illness. The section opens with a general examination of mental health problems and then analyses the relationship between mental health and affect and emotion, behaviour and cognition. The use of a common language and understanding of mental ill-health is explored. Two special topics are introduced: the link between mental illness and suicide, and the experience of elders in the context of prejudice, discrimination and racism.

The mind is its own place,
and in itself can make a heav'n of hell,
a hell of heaven

Milton

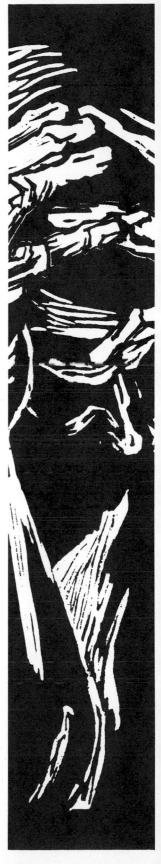

6

MENTAL HEALTH PROBLEMS

F.C. Johnson and L.D. Smith

AIMS

i) To explore the extent to which mental health problems are experienced within the general population

ii) To examine the potential implications of such problems on the individual, significant others and society

iii) To investigate the degree to which mental health problems are preventable

iv) To introduce the reader to the format of the following chapters relating to specific mental health problems

KEY ISSUES

Overt incidence
Covert incidence
Resource utilization
Living with mental health problems
'Cost' incurred
Problem differentiation
Education for living
Sociology ⎫
Psychology ⎬ of relevance
Anthropology ⎭

Identify, analyse and assess factors causing distress and illness	Promote health, provide direct care and make interventions	Manage care programmes and services
Be critical, analytical and accountable, continue professional development	Counter discrimination, inequality and individual and institutional racism	Work within and develop policies, laws and safeguards in all settings
Understand influences on mental health and the nature/causes of disorder and illness	Know the effects of distress, disorder, illness on individuals, groups, families	Understand the basis of treatments and interventions

INTRODUCTION

'Oh, sir, I never saw a face like it! It was a discoloured face—it was a savage face, I wish I could forget the roll of the red eyes and the fearful blackened inflation of the lineaments! ... This, sir, was purple; the lips were swelled and dark; the brow furrowed; the black eyebrows widely raised over the bloodshot eyes.'
Bronte, 1977

Jane Eyre was describing the features of Bertha Rochester, the violent and unpredictable prisoner–wife of the man she had planned to marry in the classic nineteenth-century love story.

Such descriptions of individuals who perpetrate aggressive, irrational and grossly antisocial behaviours are evident throughout literature. Homer (1992), for example, described the torture of Ajax by the Furies, until the man fell upon his own sword, and also wrote of Ulysses (Homer, 1965) who feigned 'madness' to justify his absence from the Trojan War. Shakespeare detailed the distresses of King Lear (1935) and Lady Macbeth (1935), amongst others; Dickens (1991) described that of Miss Haversham; Edgar Allan Poe (1992) explored the 'House of Usher' and even Lewis Carroll's (1992) *Alice in Wonderland* featured the Mad Hatter and the bloodthirsty Queen of Hearts. However, it is not a phenomenon solely associated with past writings, for some of the modern day cinema productions, for example, 'Silence of the Lambs' (1991) and 'Fatal Attraction' (1987) terrify and astound the observer by the visual impact of the ferocity, impulsiveness and sheer unexpectedness of the behaviours exhibited.

The images are not merely the products of creative imagination either, for history has recorded the antisocial behaviours of, for example, Caligula and the Borgias. Lady Caroline Lamb's description, in 1812, of the poet Lord Byron as 'Mad, bad and dangerous to know' casts a new perspective on his works. John Clare was certified insane in 1841, and spent 23 years writing his poetry whilst in St Andrew's Hospital, Northampton. The Russian Tsar, Peter the Third (1728–1762) conducted a full military court martial against a mouse that had eaten one of his beloved wax soldiers. The mouse was ceremoniously executed following a guilty verdict. Indeed, the nineteenth-century economist and critic, Bagehot felt obliged to declare that 'it has been said, not truly, but with an approximation to the truth, that in 1802 every hereditary monarch was insane'.

Perceptions relating to the effects of mental health problems upon the individual within society alter slowly, despite protestations of enlightenment and understanding. Personal experiences and anecdotal evidence confirm the continuing misconceptions and apprehensions surrounding contact with individuals experiencing such problems. Student nurses, for example, within the period of preparation prior to placement in mental health care facilities and service provision, commonly verbalize extreme concern in relation to their abilities to cope with the excessive levels of violence which they expect to encounter. Fears are also expressed with regard to 'what to say to them' and 'what to talk to them about', as if 'they' are somehow different to the 'us' of the professional. Recruitment evenings elicit similar queries from all age groups within the audience, as do educational sessions with a wide variety of special interest groups. These fears, whilst saddening, are understandable in the light of popular media portraiture.

The beliefs and feelings of the general population are of vital importance when considering deviations from health status, whether somatic or psychological in nature. The readiness and rapidity of any request for health care assistance depends upon those significant individuals within the specific situation recognizing the existence of a problem and the amenability to, and availability of, appropriate assistance. Problems associated with somatic health provide a frequent topic of conversation in a variety of settings—the office, the hairdresser's, the pub and the bus queue are examples of this. Whilst 'nervous breakdowns' continue to be discussed within the intimate circles of the family's adults or very close and trusted friends only, awareness of, and the ability to recognize, the prodromal indicators that may herald the onset/exacerbation of mental health problems remains limited at the level of most public value—that of 'common knowledge'. Many individuals within the population—if not all—would be aware of the potential dangers to somatic health and survival of severe chest pain or stertorous respiration and would, therefore, summon urgent medical assistance. A similar level of awareness and knowledge is necessary in the domain of mental health to facilitate assistance being sought at the earliest possible opportunity. The relevance of such action is realized when the extent and implications of problems of mental health are analysed.

BEYOND THE STATISTICS

In the financial year 1989/90, an estimated 194,500 people—of all ages—were admitted to National Health Service Hospitals under mental illness specialties.
DH, 1991

For each of the individuals above, admission alone may have provoked a variety of traumas or facilitated great benefits being accrued. There may be positive advantages in withdrawal from an environment or situation that may have created conflicts. Sometimes inappropriate or ineffectual response patterns have been endorsed or encouraged. Perhaps societal roles, and their related expectations and commitments, limit or inhibit attention being awarded to self and one's own difficulties, feelings and desires, the individual being swept along by day-to-day routines and the necessities associated with life and living.

For the remaining members of the household, too, such a temporary absence may be a great advantage. A loved one experiencing—and exteriorizing the effects of—mental health problems may create feelings of impotence, distress, anxiety, guilt, frustration and anger, in varying amounts and combinations in observers. Distance may facilitate exploration of such feelings in a milieu of rest and temporary relief from the pressures and tensions created by close proximity. Appropriate education at this juncture may engender a new perspective upon the situation

and enable the development and operation of management strategies to assist the family to deal more successfully with problems that are experienced. The fact that such strategies may be introduced at a time when responsibility for the loved one's health and wellbeing has been transiently passed to the professions, and there is the relative safety and security of supervision during their initial utilization, may add confidence to the participating family. The combined effects of the above may create the comprehension, renewed ability and volition to participate more effectively in activities designed to assist the individual towards recovery.

Admission to hospital may be seen to validate the individual's experiences and problems. You must be aware of the perceptions of the population in relation to the hierarchy of action initiated in the face of a health problem, that is:

1 A minor irritant—no action undertaken
2 A slight functional nuisance—a visit to the chemist
3 Continuing/exacerbating symptomatology or significant functional problems—general practitioner consultation
4 Unresponsive/confusing symptoms or those giving rise to mild concern—'tests' at a variety of hospital-based departments and return to the general practitioner
5 Unresponsive/deteriorating status or giving rise to some/increasing concern—outpatient appointment
6 Major problem, highly significant, deserving of only top level, highly skilled attention and analysis—admission to hospital.

Hospitalization is a significant event. The lay population, exposed to increasing media attention on National Health Service functioning and organization, hears of hospital closures and rationalizations, increasing pecuniary problems, staff shortages, bed unavailability, waiting-list excesses and the like. They perceive it to be only a problem of major proportions which will supersede all of the above influences and warrant admission to one of these rare and increasingly pressurized beds. The value of the adage 'a stitch in time saves nine' may not be considered by the lay population as an option in the prevailing climate. The values of a short, intensive and dynamic period of hospitalization within the early phase of a problem, in apposition to a more prolonged and protracted admission at a later date, which may require more radical and extensive intervention, and which would therefore be more distressing for all concerned and more expensive in terms of resource utilization, is unconsidered. It must be a serious problem—and genuine—to warrant admission! Ideation relating to the possibility of 'faking' the symptomatology of health deviation, exaggeration and 'making a mountain out of a molehill', or of creating 'excuses' for lack of conformity or accession to demands, disappear, often to be replaced by feelings of guilt and associated statements such as 'he really was ill!' There may be feelings of relief—in both the individual and significant others—that there really is a problem and that this problem is amenable to intervention, a fact inferred by hospitalization, for rarely are resources utilized for purely observational or palliative activities. This in itself engenders feelings of hope and optimism in relation to a favourable outcome of the current distress, which is, in itself, a necessary and valuable element of the health care assistance initiated.

This 'validation' process may find extension in regard to the affirmation of the individual—and the family—as worthy of attention and assistance. The feelings generated by thoughts of 'non-one cares', 'no-one's listening' and 'no-one is willing or able to help', are of isolation, valuelessness and increasing distress. Negative thoughts and emotions may assume a vortex-like motion, which further continues and enhances the decline in mental health status and ability to respond effectively to the pre-existing situation. The interest, activity and confidence of professional attention may provide a sense of significance which will at least serve to halt this downward spiral, if nothing more. Hospitalization may infer 'permission' to be fragile, human and subject to the occasional limitation or need for assistance. Admission may be viewed as a form of security during a period of perceived weakness and vulnerability, or as a protective device against initiation, or continuation, of actual or potential damage which the individual may feel capable of inflicting upon self or loved ones. Similarly potentially negative effects of the family up on the individual may be minimized, or the family's fears of continuing deleterious influences, represented by the individual's current behaviour, may be significantly reduced.

Hospitalization may denote a safety net, beyond which the individual and family are actively prevented from falling. Asylum—that is, a sanctuary, a retreat, refuge or safe-harbour—may be perceived to be of great value and hence advantageous within the experience.

For others, the elements interpreted as positive above may prove detrimental, with admission to hospital often creating more problems than are solved. 'Hospitalization', for example, may be viewed as effective avoidance of problems and responsibilities which may have represented a precipitating factor or a resultant feature of the individual's current departure from health status. Instead of a temporary transfer of responsibility to the assisting professionals, there may be a refusal of further contact or substantial involvement in care. Admission to hospital may rarely be the instrument by which the family removes an unwanted burden, though the relief experienced by temporary absence of an individual may prompt dubiety in regard to the desire, wisdom or ability to resume previous roles, responsibilities or obligations in relation to that individual. Similarly, once away from what may be perceived as a controlling, restrictive, personally dissatisfying or positively detrimental environment and/or relationships, the individual may have no wish to return to the *status quo*, eagerly anticipated by the family. Yet again, rather than positively affirming the value and worthiness of the individual, admission to hospital may serve to reinforce one's own perceptions—or those of others—of weakness, inability to 'cope' with life and living, or of unreliability. Thus it may be utilized as a further stick with which to beat oneself or a potent weapon for utilization within the family circle as a whole.

The above analysis could, for the most part, apply to any individual experiencing admission to any hospital, for any aspect of health care, of any cause, whether somatic or psychosocial in origin, a fact frequently forgotten by health care workers of all designations. The fact that an individual is experiencing admission to a hospital dealing with mental health problems may merely serve to compound the issues.

Despite the changing designation from 'mental hospitals' to 'mental health units', the altered perceptions of the population served by the facility may be approximated to a veneer that is wafer-thin and similarly durable. As if in recognition of the paucity of attempts to convince otherwise, the residents of the hospital's locality reject the lip service provided by a new title, assured that mental health units still mean mental illness hospitals/centres that treat 'lunies', 'nutters', 'weirdos', and 'the bewildered, be-fuddled and confused' of society. It is a sensible deduction, when considered, for such units do not cater or assist the mentally healthy at all, and hence there has been little effect on the stigma associated with admission to such units. Therefore, in addition to those problems inherent in admission to hospital, there may be added problems because of the nature of the hospital and continuing misperceptions related to the 'clientele' of the establishment.

For the individual and the family—who will also be aware of the above perceptions—there may be added fears and anxieties in relation to the behaviours of others within the ward. Many have seen the horrors of 'One Flew Over the Cuckoo's Nest' (1975) and other similar film productions and have fears of being unable 'to get out' once in, or of the treatment being more distressing than the original problems—'chemical strait-jackets', 'straight' electroplexy and leucotomy were all depicted in the film referred to. Visiting may be viewed with apprehension by the family—anxiety about entering the facility and encountering other 'inmates' and of witnessing profound and distressing alterations in their loved one's health. Although frequently dispelled after just one visit, such thoughts and feelings need to be addressed and explored prior to admission to minimize the potential problem.

Any of the above may present as problems, merely because an admission form has been completed in a ward of a specifically designated hospital. It may also be that the age of the individual on admission may create significant and different problems that need to be considered and accounted for within the preparation, initial and continuing management of the individual and the family.

Children

It is estimated that, in 1989/90, of the total number of admissions to National Health Service Hospitals under the mental illness specialties, 1,100 were children under the age of 10 years.
DH, 1991

Admission to hospital may represent the child's first experience of separation from those individuals who have hitherto comprised this total world and who have, therefore, wielded significant influence and power in relation to the development of his or her self identity. It should be remembered that home and the family may not always be perceived as a place of safety or security, love and acceptance by the child and that in such circumstances, removal from the environment may be viewed as a positive event. Children who feel threatened or vulnerable in the home—and it is their feelings and beliefs that are important here rather than adult or professional carers' perceptions—may see the hospital as a protective shelter from those whom they feel may inflict harm upon them. Children who believe significant adults to be disinterested in their welfare may react favourably to the attention and apparent concern of professional carers for their health and wellbeing, whilst those who feel lonely or isolated may benefit significantly from the company of others and the interactions that ensue and that are often based upon a common understanding and shared experiences. Children who perceive themselves to be 'different', 'oddities' or 'out of tune' with siblings and peers, or with adult demands and expectations, and who therefore feel rejected and ill at ease, may find great comfort within an environment that emphasizes a primary acceptance of them as individuals and yet where there is a consistent and acknowledged unwillingness to accept antisocial or inappropriate expressions and behaviours. Such a consistency of approach may be strongly contrasted with the ambiguities and ambivalences that may have characterized their previous child–adult interactions and may therefore provide the necessary framework and parameters required by the children to both recognize problems and participate in action to achieve their resolution or minimization. A reduction in levels of conflict within the environment and removal from what may have been perceived as a 'battle situation', between parental power and control and the child's intense desire to disregard or overtly refute this, has to be of considerable benefit to all involved within the situation.

Conversely, admission may represent the antithesis of all of the above. The sudden loss of all that the child has previously adjudged to be a safe and familiar environment and where he or she occupied a recognized position within the hierarchy of those comprising its population, may be devastating to the child's beliefs about his or her world, identity and relative security. Loss of specific members of the extended family and peer group may create intense distress as 'normal' routines, rules, expectations and relationships are replaced by unfamiliar faces, places and demands. Grief and confusion may be understandably demonstrated by the child, as his or her world metamorphoses within a short span of time and due to forces beyond his control or influence. The child may interpret admission to hospital and removal from those he or she loves as a punishment for his/her previous or current behaviour. Indeed, who has not heard the despairing parental threats of 'sending a child away' or 'not loving' the child anymore? Memories of the 'cottage homes', 'orphanage' or 'home for naughty children' may persist long after the statement has been made, to be resurrected when insecurities and fears of removal to a strange environment become a reality for the child.

There are, of course, those situations where children are not admitted from the family home as such, but from another care environment, for example, a foster home, children's home, special school or other hospital facility. It may be that, because of their perceptions of past experiences, removal to a different and strange environment may have become the 'norm', and an expected lot in life. As such, hospitalization may evoke feelings of resignation, acceptance, or of determination in relation to yet another system which requires 'beating', within what may be perceived as their fight for survival and supremacy. There are examples within clinical practice—far too numerous to engender comfort—where children have lost that innocent trust in adults which, in the past, has prompted them to look in an adult's direction for protection and safety, for assistance and nurture. Such an absence of trust comprises an integral part of the child's current problems and prevents any progression from the existing mental health status. Management of this problem is fundamental to the successful attainment of the overall outcomes of care and therefore the development of the therapeutic relationship assumes an even greater importance. The care team must repair previous damage to the adult image before any other intervention may be initiated and this may require protracted and strenuous activity.

It may be remembered that the child rarely makes the decision which results in admission to hospital. This is the prerogative of adults and it is parents, doctors, social workers, teacher, nurses and other professional and lay individuals who will pool information, observations and opinions to plan action. The child is relatively impotent in this decision-making process. When one recalls that the child is not a miniature adult as such, but an immature individual requiring significant bio-psychosocial development to achieve adult status, it may become clear that the child's reality is necessarily dissimilar to that of the adult. The logical, conceptual thought processes associated with adulthood are not demonstrated in the child until approximately eight years of age and even then they are limited. Thinking is egocentric and animistic, whilst the child's emotional world is characterized by black and white extremes, with no intermediate shades of grey. Emotional transition from love to hate may be extremely rapid, ambivalence evident when the child's desires are thwarted. In the area of moral development, the very young child acts upon impulse, with immediate action or gratification demanded and sought in response to thoughts and feelings. The child's view of 'bad' behaviour is limited to those actions that result in externally applied punishment until around the age of seven years, when the child begins to internalize parental standards, and experiences 'bad feelings' about certain activities regardless of the likelihood of punishment. As a result, the child begins to inhibit behavioural responses that would previously have found free expression. The specific degree of biopsychosocial development attained—regardless of chronological age—is an important consideration therefore in the assessment of the child's reaction to hospitalization, and requires specific attention by the caring team (Mussen *et al.*, 1990).

The child's family is also likely to be in need of care and attention on admission. Parental reaction may centre on a variety of emotions and these may be conflicting in nature. There may, for example, be strong feelings of inadequacy, as parents reflect on the reasons for hospitalization. Parenthood may be viewed as a role that is more or less successfully performed by the vast majority of the adult population, and therefore thoughts and feelings relating to an inability to understand, assist, manage or control one's own child during this period may be extremely distressing. The admission of children to mental health care facilities is not a common occurrence, as the stated statistic reveals, and therefore it is relatively unlikely that parents' peers have had similar experiences which may be shared and hence engender amelioration of such feelings of inadequacy in role performance. Indeed, shame and embarrassment may be experienced by parents in relation to the need for professional mental health care for their child, which prevents open discussion with friends and relatives, and therefore inhibits utilization of available support systems. Further, disagreements relating to child-rearing practices between peers may be evidenced and create further conflict between parents and their social circle.

Anxiety and concern regarding their own role in the child's development of current problems may be exteriorized. Child-rearing practises, including the relative strictness or laxity of regimes and the handling of this, and previous, difficulties may all undergo close and detailed parental scrutiny. An intense need to apportion blame and responsibility for the child's behaviour may find focus on a wide variety of individuals. Parents may blame each other, their specific or general handling of, or attitude towards, the child and even genetic transmission of faulty material via one 'side' of the family! The child's peers, the school and teachers, the residential environment and the detrimental influence of the media may all be utilized as scapegoats for problems being experienced. Children themselves, may not be excluded from this activity. Parents may be angry and this anger may be directed at the child, who may be perceived as 'deliberately' creating the situation to hurt, embarrass or punish. Similarly, there may be feelings of pain, in response to this interpretation of punishment by the child, in his or her overt expression of what may be considered as private, family problems. Parents may assume the role of helpless victims, rather than that perceived as the only other option—that of causative agents. Fear of criticism by professional carers may also be evident, and may relate to role performance or, on occasions, exposure of their personal weaknesses or unacceptable conduct.

Parents may, of course, be relieved at the child's removal from the family home and this, in itself, may provoke guilt. There is often an expectation that parents must *like* as well as love their children, and whilst this may appear laudable, it may be seen, at times, to be an unrealistic and inappropriate sentiment. Children who require admission to hospital are often perceived by parents as disruptive, challenging and generally difficult to manage. The introspective or withdrawn child, is commonly described as 'studious', 'well-behaved', and 'no problem' to parents and therefore whilst 'antisocial' as such, requires no assistance to 'manage'. The child described by parents as 'obtuse', 'non-conforming', 'aggressive' or 'disturbed' may be difficult to like and affirmation may be sought in regard to the appropriacy and acceptability of such feelings. In addition, approval may be required in relation to the actions undertaken within this admission period, and validation of child-rearing practices and attitudes desired. All are areas to be addressed by the care team utilizing educative strategies and supportive counselling as indicated.

The effect of the child's admission to hospital

upon siblings should not be underestimated and again requires professional attention and intervention. The specific attainments reached towards biopsychosocial maturity will be, yet again, of paramount importance to the degree of understanding of the need for removal from the home environment, but it would not be unreasonable for fears for their own security within the family group to be raised. Guilt may be evoked where other children perceive that they have played a part in provoking or compounding the sibling's problems or difficulties, due to rivalry behaviours. Sadness and grief at their perceived loss, and distress in regard to the lack of concreteness of the duration of this loss may also feature strongly. Misconceptions in relation to what actually happens within the hospital environment may provoke fears and concerns for the safety and wellbeing of their brother or sister and again beliefs relating to a 'punishment' being applied to stop 'naughtiness' may be revealed. Children may be unsure of how to respond and react to the event created by admission, to their sibling and to professionals participating in the care programme. They may be afraid of 'saying the wrong thing', of exposing what they perceive as their own problems—particularly 'bad' behaviours—or family secrets, all of which may bring someone's wrath down upon them. Children who have admired and attempted to emulate the behaviours exteriorized by their sibling may be at greater risk of such a fear and hence may exhibit increased trauma.

Children may, of course, react on, what may be interpreted as, a purely selfish basis. The disruptive child may have been perceived as gaining an unfair—and unwarranted—proportion of parental attention. Removal of the child may therefore be viewed as advantageous, with a greater degree of interaction with parents as a result. Sibling rivalry may have been a predominant feature of the children's relationship and hence 'one upmanship' may be asserted when one competitor is removed from the game. Again the absence of a perpetual conflict between family members may be seen to be a direct consequence of one child's withdrawal or removal from the home, and scapegoating the missing child may fulfil a need in all members of the group. Conversely, the absent child may be considered as gaining of the family's attention and as such represents a lack of parity for and appreciation of the 'well-behaved' children of the family. Resentment may therefore be a feature.

The potential scenarios are limitless and one will, it is certain, be able to identify others which may arise. The importance of the examples above is to provoke consideration of the benefits and limitations of admission as perceived by each individual child and the specific family members and group concerned. Any assessment conducted that precludes this aspect of health care needs and problems will be less than effective in meeting overall objectives of action.

Adolescents

An estimated 1,700 children, aged between 10 and 14 years, and 5,900 young adults, 15 to 19 years of age were admitted to hospitals under the mental illness specialties during 1989/90.
DH, 1991

Whilst a marked increase in biopsychosocial development early in adolescence is an expected feature of growing up, the specific degree of maturity attained by each individual upon the child–adult continuum is a highly variable feature, and peculiar to each adolescent entering the ward facility. This has significant influence on the manner in which hospitalization will be perceived, and hence the response to the event by the individual.

Intellectual development facilitates a more abstract mode of thinking, and reveals abilities to plan logically for the future, reason and analyse events. As new learning reaches a peak, the youngster is capable of endless speculation and theorizing, creating a situation where long-standing authority figures and 'gurus' no longer fulfil intellectual needs and hence the individual searches for a new role model or idol, nearer to his own age and current outlook or beliefs. The teenager often presents as rebellious and nonconforming in relationships with those who represent the 'no longer infallible' adult authority. Indifference, rejection and outright hostility are seen to alternate with periods where there is an intense and overwhelming need for security and comfort, which may only be provided by the family hearth (Kroger, 1989).

It represents a phase where insecurities, uncertainties, indecisiveness, confusion and anxieties are the predominating feelings. There is frequently delight in shocking the 'wrinklies' and pushing every parameter to its limit and beyond, and, simultaneously, guilt in regard to their own behaviour. Reactions may be exaggerated and based on emotion rather than logic, and fantasy life is often vivid. There is no socially defined role—the adolescent neither fits into childhood dependency nor the world of the relatively autonomous adult—and the individual may perceive that the reactions to, and expectations of him, demonstrated by the adults within his world, are inconsistent, situationally based and defined— and enforced—by those adults. At one moment, the adolescent is considered 'too old' to be exhibiting certain behaviours and the next 'not old enough' to participate in particular activities. This confusing and protracted transition, which characterizes Western cultures, predisposes the need for the teenage social group which provides an identity, recognized by others. Affiliation to the group represents an important feature of adolescent life and acceptance into the 'gang' is often 'paramount' in the desires of the individual. Such acceptance is, of course, dependent upon the internalization and demonstration of the groups 'norms' and culture. Parents often seem to have little insight into the devastation inherent in being coerced to wear the 'wrong' clothes, having to be in at night an hour before everyone else or being unable to attend a distant pop concert. To the young, it seems that adults frequently forget the excitement, traumas and anxieties of growing up, amidst the rigours and responsibilities of daily routine and 'grown up' activities (Paton and Brown, 1991).

Peer group inclusion brings elements of comparison and competition, in addition to affiliation. There is conflict between the need to assert individuality and the desire for acceptance; a requirement to be the best and yet be 'one of the gang' and to balance parental-humouring activities with group demands and expectations. It is, of course, the time for sexual maturity and, leaving aside for one moment the thoughts and feelings associated with this aspect of development, the relative success of interactions and relationships with opposite sex members may be viewed as another source of potential conflict. Uncertainty in relation to the individual's acceptability to a desired contact and relative dis-ease and discomfort within these interactions in comparison to same sex activities may be anxiety-provoking. Balancing the needs and expectations of self, parents, the social group and the potential 'partner', is bound to create difficulties within a situation where 'success' with the opposite sex is viewed as a status symbol.

School and the demands for academic attainment, bring added pressures, as adults attempt to focus young people's ideation and attention on future needs at a time when the 'here and now' of life is more than sufficient to contend with. Certainly the transition from school to work ethic, which is necessary during this period, including the inherent changes in role, responsibilities, expectations and 'rules' governing behaviours, must represent a further challenge to the developing self identity, whether perceived as advantageous or limiting in essence. Disappointment in relation to the inaccessibility of a chosen career or job pathway and the prevailing high levels of unemployment, due to recessional influences, may also create disillusionment and rejection of adult values, in addition to anxiety, or apathy in relation to alternatives available.

Set against this background, how may admission to hospital be viewed? The relative fragility of the self concept and the importance of the perceptions of others—peers, colleagues at school or work, teachers and employers for example—in respect of the stigma associated with admission to a mental health care facility, may create distress and uncertainty with regard to his continuing acceptance as an individual. Responses to such feelings may range from withdrawal to hostility and all shades in between, and nurses need to be aware of this in making their assessment of attitudes and behaviours exhibited. Certainly, the commonly encountered communal living facilities provided within ward accommodation may engender embarrassment and anxieties in the mind of the shy and modest, physically maturing youngster. Interruption of school work, whilst minimized to the greatest extent possible by utilization of in-house or peripatetic tutors, may again precipitate anxieties, as may the implications of hospitalization on current and continuing prospects at work. Concerns in relation to either may exacerbate existing problems, as well as precipitate them.

Again separation from the family, home and, importantly, significant social roles and individuals, may be viewed as a punishment, indicative of the power differential between the youngster and parents in particular, and adults in general. Admission may therefore be considered a weapon to engender conformity within an adult-orientated world, and, as such, may evoke overt or covert hostility towards professionals who are perceived as conspiratorial—or at the very least supportive—of parental power. Personnel offering assistance may be greeted with abuse, non-compliance, openly negativistic or introverted behaviour as a result. The individual's feelings of lack of control or choice within the current events may precipitate or exacerbate depressed mood to a degree of sufficient significance to warrant concern for continuing health and wellbeing. Contact with family and peers may be shunned as a result of the feelings of shame or embarrassment at the need for professional assistance.

Conversely, feelings evident on admission may be indicative of the relief experienced at the recognition of the need for help. Young people may believe that, at long last, they are being taken seriously and that hospitalization reinforces the 'real-ness' of their problems and difficulties, rather than an overreaction on their part, or a figment of their imagination. There may be an expectation of light at the end of a dark tunnel and that there will be an almost immediate resolution to their traumas. The 'magic wand' assumption may reflect an implicit faith in, and reliance on, professional opinion and ability—an almost child-like perception of the competency of personnel to 'cure' them of all ills—in contrast to parental bungling and mishandling of them as individuals. The comfort of shared experiences and

professional attention previously discussed is of similar relevance here. Relief may also be the response where the youngster has previously felt unable to deal effectively with the levels of responsibility or degree of expectations imposed upon him by others. Admission to hospital may result in a suspension of, or at the very least, a substantial reduction in, the individual's ability to meet these demands, even if only for a temporary duration. A 'legitimacy' may therefore have been provided for the individual's perceived inadequacies and the hospital ward may represent a refuge from an increasingly unmanageable situation.

There is, of course, the reaction of peers to consider in relation to their significant influence on the teenager's perception of, and response to, admission to hospital. It would be a consolation to believe that the automatic reaction to the knowledge of their friend's problems would be one of concern and support, but it may be that fear and anxiety, provoked by the nature of the problems exteriorized prevent this. Such emotions may be indicated by avoidance of the hospital, and therefore the individual, at a time when there may be a desperate need for familiar faces and reassuring contact. Ridicule and outright rejection may also be a feature, with the teenager assuming the focus of group torment and abuse, though this is rarely conducted in the actual presence of the individual. Negative reactions may provoke guilt in members of the group upon individual reflection, and sadness and despair on the part of the youngster. However, it may be that the worst possible response may be the group's indifference to the problems experienced by the individual, for this may represent his lack of inclusion in, or alienation from, the group's culture and hence isolation from a major element of social identity.

Adulthood

An estimated:
14,500 individuals aged 20 to 24 years,
33,100 aged 25 to 34 years
and 30,500 people of 35 to 44 years of age

were admitted to mental illness specialty hospitals in the financial year 1989/90.
DH, 1991

Adulthood is commonly perceived as the phase of life which is spent acquiring the elements which comprise 'stability and comfort'—whatever that means for the specific individual—and then enjoyment of the fruits of those efforts. Although more individuals choose to remain single and live alone from choice, or opt for cohabitation, marriage remains a popular institution. Despite high levels of attrition at the first attempt, marriage for a second- and third-time points to the continuing belief in, and support for, the activity, with the total number of marriages conducted remaining relatively stable over recent years. The advent of increasingly efficient birth control and the availability of legal and safe abortion may have assisted those who opt for a childless partnership or a reduced family size in comparison to their family of origin. Yet, whilst there has been a considerable overall reduction in the birth rate in the United Kingdom in comparison to the pre-1920 era, there has been a consistent increase in the number of births since the 'trough' of 1977. Again, whilst the number of babies born to single mothers has trebled over recent years, three-quarters of all babies born arrived to married parents (Central Statistical Office, 1992).

Unemployment is currently rising, and yet the vast majority of the available workforce are undertaking paid pursuits. At a time when some expectations have steadily increased—for example, accessibility to higher education, holidays abroad, home and car ownership, and life expectancy—the majority of individuals have expectations of the same milestones as their predecessors—work, separation from the family of origin via marriage, and parenthood (Central Statistical Office, 1992).

The problems that may be associated with the hospitalization of the adult therefore frequently relate to the social roles, behaviours and expectations of these institutions. Employment represents more than financial remuneration for many individuals. It may be seen to provide a period of useful—if enforced—occupation, exteriorization of creativity, social contact and interaction, and social status and identity. To receive these, the employee is required to attend for the prescribed number of hours and days per week, and number of weeks per year. Whilst 'on site', the employee has to perform duties to a more or less defined standard and within the rules laid down, whether by legal instrument or employers' policies, guidelines and regulations. Absence from work due to admission may therefore potentially deplete finances, despite welfare safety nets provided by employers and the state, and in addition reduce social contact and an individual's concept of his or her continuing value to, and status in, society. Boredom may be a feature where significant vacuums occur within a day previously programmed; unfilled with prescribed duties and responsibilities. Anxieties and concerns in regard to the projected or anticipated duration of the current absence from work may be elicited by the above. More likely, however, in the current, recessionary, economic climate, it may be a response to fears of job loss, or reduced future status because of displacement by others in the intervening period of enforced absence. Fears in relation to a continued ability to perform at the level previously demanded, and those associated with the ability to achieve future prospects and ambitions, may arise because of the nature of the problems experienced. Conversely, of course, a sigh of relief in response to removal from the pressures and people associated with work may be the perceived reaction to an even short respite from the 'treadmill'. Distance may facilitate realistic appraisal of the relative role and value of employment activities within current life experiences, the degree of satisfaction expected and attained in relation to activity levels and the opportunities for redressing imbalances perceived.

Similar thoughts and feelings may be elicited by the partner and family, for whom the dividing line between the importance of maintaining employment, and therefore continuing economic stability, and that of addressing health care needs, may resemble a tightrope. Indeed, colleagues and employers within the work place may exhibit similar ambivalances, with concern for the individual's health having to be weighed against the implications of his or her absence. All may identify very closely with the problems experienced and wish to support and assist the individual and yet may be limited by a variety of constraints from doing do. Partnerships, in particular, and relationships in general, may undergo significant attenuation, where because of the inabilities of one, others are implicitly expected to shoulder extra roles, responsibilities and obligations and 'cope' with the repercussions of admission. Resentment may be evident, whether in response to the expectation itself, the potential inability or unwillingness on the part of those who are 'well' to accept these added 'burdens' or, indeed, as a response to the need for such a transfer at all.

There may be a major alteration in the previously perceived degree of dependent–independent status of each partner, within a variety of social relationships, 'strength' and power being seen to pass from one to another as a direct result of the withdrawal of an individual from the home, or other interactive situation. Examples of the previously dominated or heavily 'protected' wife at home assuming a new confidence in her own abilities to organize her life—and that of others—in the absence of the dominant and controlling husband, are frequent. Similarly, children, previously perceived as unable to look after themselves or be assistive generally in the home situation, may respond well to the responsibilities incurred by the temporary loss of a parent. Conversely, of course, in the absence of such a transfer, relationships may be substantially weakened and vulnerable because of the temporary loss of the individual.

Perceptions of the individual may be transformed because of his or her current problems and need for hospitalization. The individual previously adjudged to be always 'on top of things', 'never letting anything get on top of them' or having the 'constitution of a horse' may now be viewed as susceptible to the human frailties and limitations affecting the rest of the population. The child's picture of a parent—almost omnipotent, all-knowing and always there—may be destroyed almost overnight. Sadness, anger, rejection and feelings of betrayal may all be evident in such situations. The role of fear—in regard to the nature of the causation for withdrawal—should not be forgotten. Embarrassment, too, may result in effective avoidance of the individual and hospital. However, all are amenable to modification with appropriate forethought, education and support by professionals.

Where the *status quo* is not represented in the above scenario of the relative security of a heterosexual, formalized and socially acceptable relationship, other and different problems may ensue. Single parents may experience added concerns related to the reduced level of support which may characterize their personal and home situation. An increased need to rely on others, often 'outsiders' with little or no vested interest in the family, may provoke anxieties. Involvement of statutory social services may be viewed as a mixed blessing, with the knowledge that children are safe, and being well looked after, being balanced against the fears that professionals may negatively view the abilities and suitability of the individual to continue in the parental role. Visions of an anticipated prolonged period of attention from these professionals may generate feelings associated with resentment of interference, and lack of future control. Where the individual provides the sole financial support within the home, worries over money, mounting bills and added expenses incurred through hospitalization may be a feature. Certainly, where relationships were already fragile and strained, withdrawal from the situation may elicit advantageous results, by engendering solidarity and support, or significant exacerbation of difficulties, with the ventilation of previously restrained feelings and observations.

Those involved within same sex relationships may encounter added problems because of the unwillingness of significant individuals to accept the nature of the partnership wholeheartedly. In a society that continues to evince a retarded level of activity in the area of equality *despite* sexual orientation, individuals may find the relationship utilized as a scapegoat for problem development or severity. Parents and friends who have difficulty in accepting either homosexuality as a whole, or their loved one's orientation specifically, may find it easy to blame the 'unnaturalness' of the activity and hence may reject the individual or pressurize for change, at a time of considerable vulnerability. Relatives who refuse, for example, to visit whilst the individual's partner is present, merely compound the mental health problems experienced. Other clients within the care environment may demonstrate equally intolerant attitudes should they become aware of the individual's sexual orientation. Such awareness is likely to result from honesty and disclosure within group activities and hence may become an integral element of the educative processes. Other individuals may experience similarly negative attitudes because of widespread prejudices and fears. The prostitute, the transvestite or transsexual may evoke similar responses from those within the mini-society formed by the ward environment. It appears strange that sexual behaviour, above many other 'deviations from the norm', is able to elicit such strong attitudes from people, but it is seen to be so in many instances.

Those who live alone may experience different concerns relating to admission. Where there is only one income into a household, anxieties in relation to finance and continuing employment are obviously likely to be high. Fears for the security of property left temporarily vacant, and for the contents of that property, which frequently represent the individual's self-identity, are understandable when record levels of crime are evident. Worries in relation to the care and safety of pets are frequently voiced, for many individuals find that it is much easier to arrange a baby sitter than a dog-minder. Social services will automatically care for children where there are difficulties, but there is no similar statutory safety net for the pet. Also, roles that may have been acquired by an individual may create concerns. Single people who maintain regular contact with elderly or house-bound individuals living nearby is an example, for they may be more concerned at the implications of their absence upon them, than by their own health and problems. The failure to meet the perceived dependence of other, informal contacts may evoke guilt in many. The importance of the individual person and situation cannot be overestimated if needs on admission are to be met.

Middle Age

An estimated 22,400 individuals aged between 45 and 54 years and 19,300, between the ages of 55 and 64 years, were included in the figures for total admissions to mental illness specialty facilities in the financial year 1989/90.
DH, 1991

This period of life may be perceived as one characterized by consolidation and, yet, simultaneous adjustment activities in relation to all spheres of life. It is a time when individuals may expect to have realized occupational ambitions and have been relatively successful in maintaining that position until retirement from paid employment. However, it is also a period when the individual is required to accept the fact that younger, better qualified and often more energetic and motivated 'whiz kids' may threaten position or indeed overtake them on the ladder. Increased opportunities, advances in technology and greater accessibility to information via the media will always benefit the generation following. Whilst it is almost impossible for such achievements to be made without the assistance of the more experienced person, and therefore there should be positive feelings in response to their role, older employees frequently feel inadequate and outstripped by younger people. Society, of course, may tend to reinforce the perception that older individuals are less valuable than their youthful counterparts by its disregard for the more mature individual. 'Secretary, aged 18 to 24 years . . .', 'Dynamic executive, 30 to 40 years . . .' and 'Divisional manager, probably aged in their early to mid-thirties . . .' are actual examples of advertisements utilized to attract staff. The vast majority of individuals employed in product adverts by the media are young, slim and good looking, unless directly appealing to the older members of society, with a denture fixative or retirement-orientated savings policy.

Mature individuals within society are often financially more secure than young adults, and therefore have money to spend in a variety of ways. The children, an acknowledged expense, have frequently completed studies and apprenticeships, have left the parental nest and have found a tree of their own. Whilst financial assistance may still be a valued part of the relationship, the costs are usually nowhere near as great as when they lived at home. Mortgages, where a previous commitment, are by this time nearing surrender, and there is often not the same expense in furnishings and other major household fixtures and fittings as was necessary when the family was young. Individuals expect to be relatively comfortable at home by this time. Finances and time freed from child rearing provide a basis for the pursuit of hobbies and leisure activities previously not possible. Whilst 'fleeing the nest' and reducing occupational demands and expectations may create difficulties for those who have 'over-invested' in one aspect of life, whether it be the job or the children, others who have maintained a happy equilibrium between all elements, will find this a positive and optimistic phase. Neglect of self-identity, personal growth and the partnership from which the 'family' developed as a by-product, may result in individuals sharing a house, but having little in common and being bored with life once the children or work recedes. Hopefully, continuing education and media attention with regard to the 'quality of life' may engender more effective balance between the various elements involved.

It is a period when individuals may compare their current physical status and abilities to those of their 'peak' performance, 20 years before. Something of relative insignificance may prompt the general review but the minor changes which have, until now, been imperceptible, may suddenly assume gigantic proportions. Taken individually, needing spectacles for reading, the dentist's inference that major work is required and having to ask the shop assistant to 'speak up a bit' are innocuous. If all occur in the space of two days, they can develop the significance of encroaching 'old age'! There may be the realization that the stairs are taken at a slower speed and that there is less flexibility in the joints when undertaking specific activities, as well as wrinkles that are no longer able to be dismissed as 'laughter lines' in the skin. Physiological changes characteristic of the menopause may provoke preoccupation with ageing, signified by the lost ability to bear another child, and the approach of retirement age for working women at 60 years of age may reinforce feelings associated with fast diminishing value. Retirement and its potential implications are discussed in greater detail in the next section, and whilst no-one would dispute the reality of the physical changes noted, it would appear that the attitude demonstrated towards growing older is of significant influence in the differing perceptions of 'getting old' and 'maturing'. It is possible to identify with individuals who present as 'elderly teenagers' and others who resemble 'adolescent grandparents'. It is a useful exercise to reflect on those individuals who, at 50 plus, may be considered as 'growing older' and, yet, who show no signs of 'getting old'. Individuals who keep themselves fit and looking good, adopt current trends and fashions, show a zest for life and abundant energy, drive and enthusiasm for a project, seem to belie their chronological age.

This may represent a period of intense concern regarding somatic health. Cancers, circulatory and respiratory diseases are responsible for a large number of deaths during this age span (Central Statistical Office, 1992). In addition, they often account for protracted and painful illnesses prior to death. Physical suffering, a major reduction in overall function and intense psychological distress are implicit within such a situation, and treatment may be as traumatic as the disease itself. Any individual who has attempted to support and assist a loved one through radical—and often deforming—surgery, chemotherapy or radiotherapy will concur with this, and yet to be offered no treatment creates such despair and feelings of hopelessness in all involved. Whilst self and the partner carry a great risk in relation to the debilitating diseases identified, parents are often becoming increasingly fragile and the health of siblings and peers may also give rise to concern. No parent expects to outlive his/her children and yet, unfortunately, when one views the figures relating to deaths occuring in the younger age groups (DH, 1991), this appears to be a relatively common scenario. This may be a period of life, therefore, associated with major adjustments.

Admission at this point may involve many of the thoughts, feelings and behaviours previously discussed within the potential situations of other age groups. However, in addition, there may be intense relief on the part of the individual that the burdens and stresses implicit in the illness have been removed from the partner's shoulders, although this may mean leaving the partner alone in the marital home. The individual admitted to hospital may be more concerned for the safety and security of the loved one, and the relative capabilities of the partner to manage alone, than about self and the outcomes of the current problems experienced. Practical details associated with living alone, after having been accustomed to the presence of a spouse, may assume major proportions. The disruption to both partners' employment and family commitments may create significant problems, not only of a financial nature but also in the sphere of necessary reorganization of previous duties and responsibilities. Where the health status of the partner remaining at home is precarious, assistance from family and outside agencies may be vital to maintain appropriate care. Therefore, guilt may also be generated.

Those who have, hitherto, lived alone may feel gratitude in being removed from a solitary existence and its loneliness. The company of others may engender tranquillity and relaxation, and provide a warm, comforting, 'cared for' feeling. Often these individuals find great pleasure and a sense of self worth in being able to assist others within the care environment, sometimes being described as 'no nursing problem', needing little care themselves and as providing valuable help to both professional personnel and clients alike. Should an obvious mental health improvement threaten discharge, relapse prior to, or immediately after the event, may be a feature. It may often be seen that children pay a great deal of attention to a lone parent whilst in hospital, but that following discharge they are unable, or unwilling, to maintain the same level of input, expecting the parent to resume his or her previous lifestyle on return home. The attention acquired during hospitalization may provide motivation for maintenance of the sick role or excessive dependency upon others. Health care personnel should be aware of this as a potential response and include strategies and interventions within the plan of care to address problems associated with increasing social isolation and reduced levels of self-esteem and confidence.

Retirement

In the financial year 1989/90 and of the total number of admissions to National Health Service hospitals under the mental illness specialty, an estimated 24,400 individuals were aged between 65 and 74 years, and 41,600 were aged 74 years and above.
DH, 1991

A phase of life characterized by continuing change and readjustment, the more mature members of society would be hard pressed to ignore the stereotype commonly associated with ageing in Western culture. 'Grandma' is often caricatured as unsteady on her legs, profoundly deaf and exceedingly forgetful. 'Grandpa' is frequently portrayed as 'pottering' about the garden or watching the world go by from an armchair in front of the fire. Often 'Grandpa' loses his masculinity and previously dominant role by the depiction of him as 'hen-pecked', incapable of performing simple tasks or conducting himself appropriately and, hence, eccentric or 'doddering'. Generally, the older members of society are represented as relatively inactive, unproductive individuals who, whilst still breathing and eating and therefore technically alive, are rarely associated with living life to the full and having positive expectations for the future, or related to love, laughter, novelty, excitement or achievement.

There are, of course, always exceptions to the 'rule' and a glance at recent television listings provides valuable examples of differing perspectives on ageing. Estelle Getty's interpretation of the part of 'Sophia' in the 'Golden Girls' (1992) and that of the late Joan Sanderson as 'Eleanor' in 'After Henry' (1992) provide an alternative view of the older woman as mischievous, manipulative of others, capable of lively interest, logical and cogent debate and very active participation in social activities and events. Whilst often portrayed as dogmatic or obtuse in relationships with daughters and peers, there are indications of the, very often forgotten, wisdom associated with learning from life and its varied experiences. 'Last of the Summer Wine' (1992) and the outlandish antics of 'Compo' (Bill Owen) and his pals, 'Foggy' (Brian Wilde) and 'Cleggy' (Peter Sallis) must rate very highly on any scale applied to dispelling illusions in relation to inactive, staid or pottering old men being the norm. The escapades of the three rogues are characterized by love of adventure and risk, creativity in both thought and general problem-solving activities, great humour and adolescent fun and a total disregard for the socially generated rules relating to the behaviours appropriate for their age group. The persistent attempts on the part of Compo to achieve romance, love and a sexual encounter with 'Nora Batty' (Kathy Staff) are representative of the fact that expectations in these areas of life need not be ignored or rejected as inappropriate or unrealistic on the grounds of increasing age. 'Compo's' retort following yet another rejection by 'Nora' of 'Thou wanst t' grab me while I'm up to British Standards!' is indicative of the hope, optimism and confidence he feels in regards to his ultimate success!

In the comedy scripts of 'Waiting for God' (1992) Michael Aitken's characters of 'Diana', played by Stephanie Cole, and 'Tom' (Graham Crowden) are two of the residents of Bayview Retirement Home, which is managed by the inept 'Harvey Bains' (Daniel Hill) and his doting and rather simplistic assistant Jane (Janine Duvitski). Tom is prone to expression of his delusional ideation at the drop of a hat and Diana is a caustic and authoritarian character, obviously accustomed to being obeyed. Each script serves to dispel the myth that the older members of society are quiet, well-behaved, nicely spoken and courteously bland individuals who sit placidly waiting to die. The following abridged extract may provide enlightenment, both in regard to the beliefs and attitudes of the younger elements of society towards its older members, and the poten-

tial realities of the needs and desires of the group themselves.

Harvey: I don't know what's got into you all.

Tom: Whisky mainly, and a spot of champers.

Harvey: You're senior citizens. But you're behaving like teenagers. Not just here and now either ... at nights too ... I know what goes on, I'm not stupid. (*the mob get pantoish*)

All: Oh yes you are!

Harvey: Oh no I'm not.

All: Oh yes you are!

Jane: Oh no he's not.

All: Oh yes he is!

Harvey: That's enough! You can't pull the wool over my eyes. I hear the zimmer frames clanking up and down the corridors in the dead of night. I know. But I do nothing. I'm a nice guy.

All: Oh no you're not!

Harvey: Oh yes I ... (*he gets enough control not to get into that one again*). This is the dining room. The focal point of the haven of gentility we call Bayview. This is not a place for carousing ... you are supposed to be at the reflective stage in your lives, you are supposed to be setting an example to the next generations, so if you don't mind could we please have a bit of dignity and decorum. Hmm?

Diana: Oh God ... (*Diana reaches out with her stick and hooks it round Harvey's neck*)
Come here.

Harvey: Arrgh! (*she yanks Harvey backwards onto a chair just in front of her and then leans forward and talks into his ear as he gets over his choking*)

Diana: Listen, you dismal little Gucci pustule, how many times does it have to be dinned into your sieve-like brain that we are the paying customers. You are the staff and as such you do not talk to us like naughty children.

(*she clips him over the head*)

Harvey: I just think you should know where to draw the line.

Diana: You tell us where and when Harvey. What age are we supposed to stop enjoying ourselves? What is the final hour for drinks? What is the date of the last good rumpy pumpy? Eh?
(*she tightens her pull on the stick nearly choking Harvey backwards*)

Harvey: Arrgh!

Diana: Precisely. There is no such time. We are here out of choice or grim necessity but it does not mean we have resigned from the human race. We are still allowed to do whatever the hell we please, be that going catatonic with our memories or revelling o' nights with our chums. Yes?

Harvey: Yes Diana.
(*Diana lets him go. Diana smiles at the company*)
Carry on.
(*the resident at the piano starts playing a conga*)

Basil: Conga time. Conga time. Dada de dah dah.
(*Basil grabs the back of someone else to start the conga line ... The resident's conga line is snaking down the drive with those who are capable doing the leg kicks and yells. Tom is rattling along behind in some slightly squiffy dance of his own*)

Jane: Oh dear ... they're going to end up all over the town again ...

Diana: At least they've got their clothes on this time.

Broadcast on 15.10.92

Reaching the age of retirement need not be the signal to reduce activity, expectations or one's own assessment of value to society. No one would dispute the potential hiatus caused by a drastic reduction in income, the ensuing limited interactions with previous colleagues or the loss of status associated with the post and with being a productive member of society. Neither is the initial disorientation created by the absence of an enforced routine and focus for the day's activities, surprising when it is recalled that the habits of what may represent as much as 50 years of life are often ingrained and almost automatic in nature. However, what does appear surprising is the lack of awareness in relation to the potential role of the indvidual following retirement from full-time occupation. The maximum value of the individual to the society in which he/she resides may only at this point find free expression via the increased opportunities and relative freedom of a workless week. During the employment years, selective elements of the individual's knowledge and skills are utilized to the benefit of a sole organization. Retirement frees the individual's focus and therefore the entire abilities accumulated from a myriad of life's learning experiences may be made available to a broader base of people.

Whilst new learning and that achieved by vicarious means may be reduced at this point (Garrel, 1991) numerous individuals help other less skilled people in a variety of very valuable ways. Older people skilled at a craft may participate in workshops aimed at several different groups, for example, individuals with learning disabilities, people on community work schemes and day hospital users, to the benefit of all involved. People have all sorts of skills, from gardening to hairdressing, from engineering to teaching foreign languages, that may be utilized within the community. Older people may help in playgroups, providing a little extra attention, or participate in supervision of activity groups for children, with great effect. Personal, leisure and occupational skills are valuable to someone, somewhere within the community of residence and a proportion of time spent thus, creates a new sense of worth and value within the provider. The award of a 'gold watch' along with an 'old age pension' and a concessionary travel permit does not mean that time has to lie heavily.

People are generally living longer, owing to a variety of factors. Men and women today, aged 70 years, can expect to live another 10.9 and 14.2 years respectively, which represents a considerable increase since the turn of the century (Central Statistics Office, 1992). Loss of loved ones and gradual decline in physical health are factors of greater relevance here and therefore physical and social isolation are of significance. Geographical and social mobility, the increasing expectations of women to undertake a career of their own rather than solely child-raising and home-making activities, and the financial instabilities of a recessionary economic climate create difficulties for children who would otherwise wish to support older parents. At such a time, admission to a mental health care unit may therefore be viewed as a necessity, no matter how unwelcome, a foregone conclusion or a welcome intervention. Company, care and attention may relieve fears of living alone or feelings of isolation. Inability to manage within the home situation or excessive pressure perceived as falling upon a partner may also engender relief. Conversely concerns about leaving home—never to return—security and the love of a partner at a time of increasing feelings of fragility and vulnerability may indicate added traumas experienced. Anxieties about being 'a nuisance', disrupting the children's lives and work, and 'taking charity' are relatively common. Certainly the continuing association of an old building as the 'workhouse' or 'lunatic asylum' may create significant distress, both for the individual, his partner and his peers.

THE TIP OF AN ICEBERG

The statistics that have been utilized are estimates. An accurate figure for such admission rates is currently unavailable due to the incompatibility of material generated at local and regional levels and processes utilized to collate information at national government level—a problem that is being rectified. The figures utilized, accurate or otherwise, relate solely to admission and are therefore only one aspect of the total picture relevant to the incidence of mental health problems within the population. Hospitalization is an experience that is encountered by only a proportion of those individuals affected and therefore the analysis above of the implications for, and effects on, the individual, his family and the society in which he resides and interacts, is merely one aspect of living with mental health problems. The inference of the

analysis is that all individuals understand the need for admission and are willing to comply. Clearly this is not always so and some individuals are unable to recognize that problems exist or may feel treatment to be inappropriate in the light of—or because of—their current beliefs about themselves, their behaviours or value to society. Indeed:

Of the total number of formal admissions to N.H.S. facilities of patients under the Mental Health Act 1983, 15,145 were categorised as suffering mental illness and 119 as suffering psychopathic disorder.

The vast majority of these formal admissions—13,828 relating to mental illness and 45 in the category of psychopathic disorder—were non-offenders.

1,103 individuals included within these figures for mental illness category and 2 within that for psychopathic disorder were considered in need of a place of safety.
DH, 1992a

The largest proportion of the above, by far, was representative of those requiring assessment, with or without treatment—that is, admission via Section 2 of the Mental Health Act 1983 (DH, 1992a). What would be your response to formal admission if you were convinced that you were healthy or at least had no need for assistance? The potential for 'logical argument' as a method of defending one's own sanity may be rejected as a 'lack of insight' by professionals and yet sitting quietly, waiting for someone to recognize the error made, may be taken as compliance and recognition of the need for help. Certainly a heated reaction, exhibiting anger or expansive gestures may only serve to reinforce the beliefs of health personnel that care is needed! How would you respond to the situation? A variety of reactions may be shown by the individual, adjudged as in need of care, and hence should be expected.

As previously stated, admissions to hospital, whether voluntary or compulsory in nature, are only one indicator by which the prevalence of mental health problems within the population may be discovered. Goldberg and Huxley (1980) suggest that psychiatrists treat three out of four of their clients as out-patients:

In the financial year 1989/90, total out-patients' attendances numbered 1,638,800 of which 206,800 were new patients.
DH, 1991

Even the additional information gained from the above is insufficient to accurately reflect the incidence sought, for Rawnsley (1968) clearly identified the different figures that could be obtained for the prevalence rate of affective disorders in England and Wales depending on material utilized. That rate which had been derived from admission figures alone represented only one-fifth of the rate indicated by combining out-patient and other specialist facilities, and only one-tenth of the rate found via general practice studies. This may indicate that the most accurate figures available relating to incidence may be via such GP studies and yet these show that only one in twenty of those diagnosed as experiencing mental health problems is referred to specialist services. Indeed, with regard to general practitioner recognition and subsequent diagnosis of mental health problems, research both in America and the United Kingdom supports the finding that more than 50% of individuals presenting to the family doctor complain primarily of physical symptoms (Goldberg and Huxley, 1980), which appears to significantly influence diagnosis. Comparison between the GP diagnosis and that of experienced psychiatrists revealed an over-emphasis on somatic complaints and an under-emphasis on depression (Goldberg, 1984; Mann *et al.*, 1981). Beaber and Rodney (1984) found a great reluctance to record a psychological basis for somatic complaints. Surveys consistently reveal that whilst utilizing strict operational criteria, 25 to 30% of individuals presenting to the family doctor do so exteriorizing primarily mental health problems, but that detection and diagnosis at that time demonstrates a 10% lower level of recording. Where mental health problems are diagnosed, doctors

are unlikely to communicate the fact to the attending person. The doctor is more likely to 'reassure' the patient and prescribe a psychotropic drug (Marsh, 1977).

Goldberg and Huxley (1980) indicate that of a general population of 1,000 people, 250 individuals will experience mental health distress. Of these, 230 will visit the GP and 140 will be identified as needing assistance, usually in the form of tranquillizers or antidepressant preparations. Referrals to specialist practitioners will be undertaken on behalf of 17 individuals and six will require admission. Utilizing these figures, admission and out-patient statistics provide merely the tip of the iceberg when analysing the prevalence of the problem.

EXPERIENCING THE PROBLEM

The potential effects of admission to a mental health care unit have been considered in some breadth and length. However, it is only one event within the potential extent of the experience of living with mental health problems, for the individual and his significant others.

Human beings are 'integrated units'—they come as a total package of thoughts, feelings and behaviours, wrapped in a protective waterproof skin and packed with the various organs necessary to maintain existence. As a stone thrown into a pond will create a disturbance in the water as a whole, so one problem area—no matter the site or origin—within the individual's total functioning will have repercussions on other areas. The degree and nature of such repercussions experienced is dependent on the extent of the problem experienced. Again, using the analogy of the stone thrown into the pond, a boulder may create waves reaching the shoreline whilst a pebble may only cause localized and almost insignificant ripples. As an individual, it is possible to be aware of the mind–body interrelationship from everyday life experience. Something as commonly experienced as influenza may be seen to affect total activity—the individual finds difficulty in attending or concentrating, feels lethargic and apathetic, does not really want to be bothered with anything or anyone and behaves, wherever possible, accordingly. A poor night's sleep will commonly cause irritability and lowered 'thresholds' in many instances. People are more awkward, more effort is needed to achieve a task, more time is utilized to seemingly achieve less than usual, and more things go wrong. These thoughts and feelings generated affect psychomotor activity and behaviours, the individual often displaying clumsiness, impulsive actions when thwarted and exaggerated responses to the environment.

A problem in one area of psychosocial function will have similar implications for the individual's overall health and performance. Where mood, for example, is substantially disturbed, a concomitant change in the nature, focus and quality of thought processes may be elicited, which in turn may result in impaired perceptual and memory functions. Behaviours, previously considered characteristic of the individual, may exhibit significant variance. Interactions and social relationships may suffer and social roles undergo considerable distortion. General health may suffer via a number of associated problems. Inadequate or inappropriate nutrition, sleep and exercise will take their toll on the overall ability to function, as will neglect of self-care in bodily hygiene and safety measures. The excessive employment of substances, such as tobacco, alcohol and a variety of chemical preparations, to assist in the management of the situation, carries potential sequelae for biopsychosocial health and wellbeing which are well known and publicized (DH, 1992b). Damage to health status due to injury should not be overlooked, and may be intentional or accidental in nature. Certainly, psychomotor activity may be seen to reflect mood, thought processes and perceptions, and hence may be retarded, accelerated, purposeless or intense in character.

The above example may be reproduced utilizing any specific problem of affect, behaviour or cognition, which in total are indicative of the current mental health status. No matter the primary problem experienced, significant repercussions in all spheres of human function will feature. The intermeshing nature of the individual may be likened to the picture produced by a jigsaw puzzle, for all pieces have to be correctly positioned and interlocked to produce the picture intended. One piece incorrectly placed will prevent the desired product being achieved (see Fig. 6.1). The interplay of the individual 'parts' to

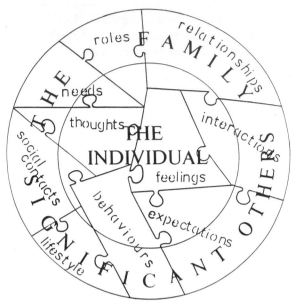

Fig. 6.1 *Integration of client need (from Mental Health Student Handbook produced by North Staffs College of Nursing and Midwifery, Stoke-on-Trent).*

form the corporate 'whole' is clear to see. There is no facility for compartmentalization. We can understand, therefore, that the experience of mental health problems will intrude on all aspects of life and living.

Where lacking insight into the existence of a problem, or its extent, individuals may see only that others are determined to thwart their every action, argue their every utterance and generally deny their reality. Their preoccupation with their thoughts and perceptions may provoke, of course, a total withdrawal from contact with others for periods of varying length. Hallucinations and delusional ideation may create terror and intense fear for their own safety, or their conduct towards others. Antisocial behaviours directed by, or in response to, these perceptions may place them—or others—in danger, whether through disregard or intention. For the family, it is hard to watch a loved one's disturbed behaviour and know that they are impotent to assist. To listen to strange beliefs, or observe reactions to hallucinations, may create considerable distress, as well as fear. Constant assurance and reassurance necessary to allay fears prompted by such symptomatology may be the focus of daily interactions. Shock, shame and sadness relating to the nature and content of the individual's dialogue or exhibited activities may increase distress. Agitation and 'irrational' behaviours may prompt the family to follow the individual everywhere to ensure his or her safety. Routines, including sleep patterns, become disturbed as the days revolve around the individual, his or her actions and need for care and attention. Out-patient departments and general practitioner consultations often provide the only break in the tedium of the daily efforts to maintain the *status quo*. Improvement is often slow, and, of the total number of out-patient attendances, a relatively small proportion represented new patients. Many attend with monotonous regularity as psychiatrists attempt to discover the regime appropriate to need.

For those who have insight into their disturbed mental health status, the feelings associated with being a nuisance, and disrupting the routines and duties of others may create further distress. Being unable to 'snap out of it' or 'pull oneself together' may exacerbate anxieties, depressed mood or guilt feelings. Fears of the problems experienced, their intense nature or their prolonged duration may compound the issue, as may concerns regarding the family's continued willingness to cope. Anxieties about 'going mad' and having to be 'put away' may become a preoccupation. Guilt associated with current inability to perform previous roles and undertake regular responsibilities may prompt a deeper decline.

However, regardless of the presence of insight or otherwise, mental health problems are often poorly understood and hence may create less than beneficial responses from those who care for the individual at home or who are in regular contact. Initial support from significant others may begin to dwindle away when it becomes obvious that 'cure' is not to be effected easily and with speed, thus leaving the immediate family to manage alone. 'Treatment' in the form of medication may take time to achieve any observable improvement, and may need to be adjusted, replaced or added to, several times in the quest to relieve distressing symptomatology. Side-effects and toxic reactions to preparations employed may generate added problems for the individual and to the family's worries. Electroplexy may be feared and hence refused as a potential aid, often because of hearsay or media portrayal. If such 'treatments' are not offered, however, there may be an equally strong reaction on the part of all involved. A lack of understanding in relation to the value of ventilation of problems and subsequent generation of problem-solving activities and strategies may be reflected in statements such as 'Talking to him is no good—can't you give him tablets, or something?' A failure to prescribe chemical preparations to 'cure' the problems may be perceived as inadequate treatment, disinterest or neglect.

The dissimilarity between somatically orientated care and that focusing upon psychosocial function creates difficulties in comprehension for other professional groups, never mind the inexperienced lay individual. Should a skin laceration be the problem, treatment would be observable and anticipated, with cleansing, suturing and dressing the wound being the immediate and skilled response. The lack of amenability of mental health problems to the application of a similar 'plaster' or soothing salve is frequently beyond previous levels of experience and therefore necessitates education.

THOSE AT RISK

Mental health problems represent an extension of 'normal' phenomena (see Chapter 2) and are considered 'pathogenic' only when there is a significant impairment to everyday activities and functions, or—and importantly—when they adversely impact on the lives of others. One in four individuals within the general population may have experienced such problems (Goldberg and Huxley, 1980) but are some individuals more likely to be 'at risk' than others? Where indications of increased susceptibility to impaired mental health status are identified, resources may be focused in an attempt to reduce the risk of problem development by the utilization of mental health promotion strategies.

Community surveys show distinct demographic variations with regard to the experience of mental health problems. Bebbington *et al.* (1981) following interviews with a random sample of 800 people living within the Camberwell area of London and aged between 18 and 64 years, found that:

---

1 Women experienced problems at a rate more than twice that of the male population—15% as opposed to 6%.

2 Married women were four times more likely to have mental health problems than were single women.

3 Women with children aged 15 years and under living at home were twice as susceptible as women without young children at home.

4 Working class women with children at home were particularly prone to 'minor' problems related to mental health status.

5 Married men experienced problems at a rate of half that of single men—3% in comparison to 8%.

6 Men with young children at home experienced a very low rate of mental health problems.

7 There was an increased rate, in both sexes, where unemployment was a factor. Twice the number of unemployed individuals experienced problems as did employed people.

8 A high incidence was associated in both sexes following loss of the marital relationship, whether due to death, separation or divorce.

Whilst actual figures vary considerably, other studies (Dohrenwend and Dohrenwend, 1969; Surtees *et al.*, 1983) have also found the increased incidence within these sections of society.

Reliable data on the incidence of mental health problems in older adults are more difficult to obtain, for unless admission to institutional care becomes a necessity, they exert little demand upon mental health care services. Cooper and Sosna (1980) report that 27% of individuals within their study demonstrated mental health problems—12% with regard to organic psycho-syndromes, with cognitive problems forming the foci, and 15% classified as functional in nature. The majority had been seen by their general practitioner within the three months prior to the investigation (78%), but only 10% had been seen by social workers or community nurses as a follow up or support strategy.

The most extensive and well-known community survey relating to the incidence of mental health problems in children, is that conducted by Rutter (1979) which identified and compared prevalence rates between the Isle of Wight and South London. The inner city area showed a rate of twice that of the Isle of Wight. Factors associated with the development of mental health problems, that is, family discord and disruption, parental illness and criminality, were all found to be of a higher incidence in London than the Isle of Wight and hence the greater degree of child mental health problems. Whilst unable to discover *why* there should be such elevated rates of marital disharmony or depression within the population of women in the London borough, the facts were clear with regard to the children studied, that is:

---

1 Children in severely discordant homes had a higher incidence of mental health problems.

2 Children who had spent at least one week in the care of the local authority were at an increased risk.

3 Where fathers had spent time in prison, there was a higher risk in children of mental health problems.

4 Mothers who experienced depressive or other neurotic problems themselves were more commonly seen to have children with problems.

5 Children in large families were at greater risk than those in smaller ones.

6 Mental health problems were more common in children of labouring or semi-skilled manually employed fathers.

7 Children educated in schools which demonstrated high:
   (a) teacher turnover;
   (b) pupil turnover;
   (c) percentages of free meal provision;
   (d) absenteeism;
   (e) percentages of non-indigenous children; and
   (f) low pupil/staff ratios were more at risk.

Other factors are of significance within the topic area as a whole, for example, one study (Mullen, 1988) reported a three-fold incidence of mental health problems in those exposed to sexual abuse as a child, and another, conducted on in patients, found that almost half had histories of physical or sexual abuse (Carmen *et al.*, 1984). Homelessness and problems with regard to housing increase the likelihood of both psychosocial and somatic disorder Pashley (1991) suggests that 1,100 individuals experiencing mental health problems sleep out or utilize direct access hostels in central London. Fernando (1988) reports that the application of the diagnostic label of schizophrenia is ten times more likely to occur in young men of Afro-Caribbean extract than in their white peers, and Lipsedge and Littlewood (1982) found that the black population has higher rates of admission to hospital, and is, in general, given larger doses of major tranquillizers.

Home and school environment, age, sex, marital status and race all appear to influence the development and maintenance of mental health status and yet, utilizing Goldberg and Huxley's figures of the progress of individuals experiencing problems in this sphere of function, a vast number of these will either go unrecognized or unseen by specialist practitioners (Goldberg and Huxley, 1980). The degree of success of any programme to promote health and prevent problems in the area of psychosocial status, no matter how effective, would make little impact on reducing numbers of individuals seen or admitted by the psychiatrist, and hence no reduction in service costs from that perspective. Indeed, more insight within the general population, and more effective and accurate diagnosis within the GP centre would likely result in more referrals to specialists not less, and hence create an overload of existing services. As health care personnel, the cost–benefit of such activities must be taken into account, for whilst personal and professional instincts lie within the direction of quality health status and maximization of the individual's potential for life and living, this has to be achieved within an overall focus on 'value for money' criteria. Perhaps an analysis of the 'cost' of mental health problems both to the individual and society in general may facilitate benefits being uncovered.

THE COST OF THE PROBLEM

Thompson and Pudney (1990) state that, in 1989:

1 8% of total revenue spending in the National Health Service—some £2,011 million was spent on the care and treatment of those with mental health problems.

2 71% of this figure—that is, £1,575 million—was allocated to in-patient beds—£30,000 per bed per year.

3 Mental health care in-patient facilities represented 20% of all NHS beds.

4 Local authority personal social services and social security sickness and invalidity benefits accounted for £1,046 million.

Social Services total net expenditure in the same year represented 1.7% of total gross expenditure, that is £78,694,000 (Office of Health Economics, 1990). The Health and Safety Executive (1988) suggests that 30–40% of all sickness absence from work is due to mental health distress of some nature, whilst Thompson and Pudney (1990) state that in 1989, 71 million working days were lost. Of the £100 million per year drugs budget in the NHS, some 25% is spent on psychiatric drugs

(DH, 1992b) but there are also, of course, costs that cannot be counted.

Wertheimer (1991) suggests that, every two hours, someone in Britain commits suicide and for each of these individuals, there will have been intense personal distress prior to the act, and family grief after it. The potential skills of each are lost to a society which can ill-afford such a loss. The impact upon individual members and the corporate family group may be both devastating and prolonged. For every individual experiencing problems of mental health status, there may be a similar distress and an accompanying inability to achieve potential personal and occupational skill-levels. For each family, there may be significant repercussions and implications. Continuing fears for mental health status may persist for years and the effects of the mind on somatic health are well documented (Selye, 1956). The personal costs may far exceed those which may be expressed in purely monetary terms.

Whilst mental health promotion and prevention strategies may not significantly reduce the numbers of individuals referred to specialist facilities and services, such a programme may have visible, though necessarily long-term, advantages in relation to a reduction in psychotropic drug costs, admissions to hospital for a range of somatic illnesses associated with mental health problems, and in the number of days lost per year to industry. This in itself would represent an investment in the future. If it were only possible to halt the adverse effects of parental mental health problems on their children, or reduce the levels of isolation and feelings of valuelessness in the older members of society, that must be advantageous to society as a whole.

PROBLEM DIFFERENTIATION

The aetiology of mental health problems is vague and considered to be multifactorial in nature. However, it appears to us that a distinct differentiation may be drawn in relation to the characteristics of the problems experienced and that this differentiation will influence strategies and inter-ventions directed towards promotion, prevention or amelioration of mental health problems.

Some individuals demonstrate a maintenance of contact with reality, whilst others, considered as experiencing 'major' mental health problems, or 'psychoses', exhibit a loss of contact or distortion of that contact with the environment and its events. Considering, logically, the situations when hallucinations or delusions may be exteriorized, it may be possible to draw conclusions in regard to the nature and causation of mental health problems characterized by such symptomatology. Appropriate health promotion and problem prevention may then be viewed as a realistic proposal.

Many of us may have experienced hypnagogic hallucinations, as thoughts become images, seen as actual events, just before falling asleep and similarly hypnopompic hallucinations, which occur just prior to wakening from sleep. The traveller in the desert, deprived of food, water and rest, and exposed to the heat of the day and bitter cold of the night, reports 'mirages', and pilots experience hallucinations at high altitude due to lack of oxygen. Nurses within somatic health care will observe hallucinations in hyper-pyrexial and post-anaesthetic patients. Hypothyroidism commonly causes perceptual problems, and damage to the temporal lobe, whether as the result of trauma or a space occupying lesion, may create similar problems. It is recognized that a wide variety of chemical substances—alcohol, solvents and drugs, both prescribed, therapeutic preparations as well as those utilized unsanctioned—may provoke hallucinatory and delusional experiences. In addition, it is recognized that atrophy of the brain may be a secondary manifestation following a variety of disorders, dysfunctions and diseases—for example, central nervous system pathology, vitamin deficiency, toxin exposure, metabolic and endocrine problems—and hallucinations and delusions may feature. These examples are intended to show that hallucinations and delusions may occur because of a physiological imbalance of the body's finely calibrated internal environment. It would seem a logical extension therefore to assume a biological basis for many of the mental health problems labelled as 'psychotic', and whilst the answers are not available in total yet, it would appear sensible that sooner or later, specific factors will be found to be responsible for symptomatology.

Health promotion currently must be directed towards support of those who have experienced such problems and prevention of further episodes, until successful identification of aetiology has been achieved. An example of support of value to individuals who have experienced 'major' mental health problems is available via studies on the course and progression of clients diagnosed as schizophrenic. Environments which are understimulating will promote withdrawal and regression and rapidly changing social situations, which engender pressure from overindulgent or hypercritical family members, may provoke an acute response from the individual. Environmental management has been found to reduce the risk of relapse, associated with florid symptomatology, especially when combined with appropriate medication.

Leff and his colleagues (1982) identified those relatives exteriorizing high or low levels of expressed emotion and attempted to moderate their potentially detrimental effects on the individual via education. The nature, course and treatment of schizophrenia, the negative effects of change, criticism and over-involvement upon the individual's mental health status, and specific strategies to deal with commonly encountered problems, formed a proportion of the educative contents of the programme. Group discussions demonstrated more effective methods of interacting with individuals, in an attempt to moderate the effects of high/low levels of expressed emotion, and ways in which contact time could be reduced were explored and employed. The study showed considerable reduction in relapse rates where high levels of expressed emotion and over-involvement demonstrated by relatives had been significantly modified and where concurrent medication was maintained. Similar results have been achieved in other studies (Leff *et al.*, 1985; Falloon *et al.*, 1985) and hence the value of family therapy and education in maintenance of the mental health status achieved by the individual would appear proven.

Test and Stein (1978) developed an intensive community support programme wherein individuals maintained residence in their own neighbourhood—though not necessarily within the family home—and received intensive treatment and rehabilitation within the hospital on a daily basis. Following a gradual reduction of this hospital care and the completion of a work-skills related course, individuals were assisted to find open employment. Individuals who, whilst stabilized, had a prolonged history of severely psychotic symptoms, were introduced to a community care programme, whereby a member of the mental health care team was available on a 24 hours a day, seven days a week, basis. Participation in intensive social and daily living skills programmes, life planning and crisis management activities revealed a re-admission rate of 6% in this group in comparison to 58% in a control group receiving traditional mental health care routine practices. However, the improvement was maintained only whilst intensive support continued, with clients reporting greater satisfaction with life and enhanced self-esteem, in addition to fewer symptoms. After 14 months, the individuals were transferred back into routine care facilities and practices, and within months had shown considerable deterioration both clinically and socially. Comparison with the traditionally treated control group at this juncture showed no appreciable distinction. With support, the relapse–re-admission cycle can be interrupted and much effort is needed to create innovative and yet cost-effective—in all meanings of the term—strategies to assist the individual to remain relatively mentally healthy. Family therapy must, of necessity, be employed by all registered health care workers to facilitate effective primary support mechanisms. This requires education and supervised practice, for it is an area currently considered the realm of the specialist. The difficult and challenging behaviours of individuals experiencing protracted, 'psychotic' problems will represent the major focus of many nurses' practice (White, 1991) and, as such, require attention now.

We must also consider that group of individuals for whom contact with reality is relatively unimpaired or intact, and the nature of assistance available to promote mental health, prevent problems and ameliorate the effects of actual problem experience in this group. Again it appears that this group of people have something in common.

Situations that evoke sadness may be associated with failure to meet one's own or society's expectations—lack of achievement or success in a project, acknowledgement of limitations of skills, characteristics and image, or acceptance and recognition of individual value in significant interactions and relationships. 'Loss' also figures strongly—loss of something or someone who has become an integral part of self, representing security, safety or status. In many instances, it is a loss of a 'possession', an entitlement or deserved reward. Considering those events that create anxiety and apprehension in self, it may be that these are related to fears of failure to achieve a prescribed or personally desired objective, of the implications of such a failure and the perceptions of self relating to lack of success. Many of these desired objectives relate to norms—position, possessions and prospects—whilst others relate specifically to the degree of approbation of others applied to self. Similarly guilt is experienced in relation to actions, desires or motives that would engender social disapproval, and being considered a 'not very nice person'. All of these revolve around the expectations of individuals to meet socially induced and constructed values and being unable in some way to achieve them.

Partnerships have evolved considerably from their initial focus of breeding and care of the offspring. Individuals expect to love their partner, be compatible with another individual and the *raison d'être* for the other's living. There is an expectation of 'living happily ever after', 'roses around the door' and 'till death us do part' and an intense disappointment when partnerships do not live up to the 'ideal'. The rationality and logic of a process that takes two individuals of different backgrounds, expectations, needs and experiences and expects these two to live contentedly together until death would have to be questioned. Age, continuing personal growth and development, changing needs, experiences, situations, perceptions and expectations continue in both individuals, and at different rates and phases of life. To achieve a sufficiently acceptable, long-term

'match' would appear the result of a lot of good fortune and a great deal of compromise, and yet it is expected where marriages fail, there may be guilt, sense of failure or inadequacy, sadness and despondency.

And, of course, sexual intercourse, no longer primarily focused upon procreation, has evolved into an activity full of expectations and norms. Improved contraception and lowered infant mortality, plus ecological pressures relating to overcrowding the Earth and its resources, sociological expectations of family size mirroring the couples ability to provide adequately on a financial basis and the demands encapsulated in women's rightful quest for a new role within society have all assisted in this evolution.

Such pressures exist and exert significance on the individual's expectations of the experience of life and living, on the perceptions of self, needs and aspirations and therefore the goals chased and the resultant contentment attained. The aims of life are no longer related to survival but relate to a socially constructed 'quality of life'.

Mental health promotion and prevention programmes may be seen to be of value in three distinct areas. The first may be viewed as a programme of education for living, and commences with 'parents in waiting' and culminates with post-retirement groups. Increased knowledge of, and preparation for, challenges associated with life, including enhancing management strategies and identifying 'coping' mechanisms, which are both effective and yet will not damage health, represent major elements of any such programme. Development of personal, social and daily living skills prepares individuals for living with confidence, and reduces the likelihood of acting from necessity rather than choice. Being content with self and one's own company may reduce situations where relationships are entered into from a standpoint of weakness and vulnerability, rather than equality. Certainly, relationships require to be viewed as one element of the whole individual rather than the sole reason for living, as does work and employment. A promulgation of the importance of self in apposition to achievement, of maximizing current skills and the introduction of problem-solving strategies, which build in, and on, successes, in activities to address areas of limitation perceived as requiring attention by the individual, are vital to enhance feelings of self-esteem, confidence and empowerment. Increased awareness of support systems available to assist where specific difficulties are encountered in a variety of areas of life, serves two purposes. 'Forewarned is forearmed' and therefore such information already available to the individual may reduce anxieties in relation to where to go and who can help within a specific situation.

In addition, however—and importantly—there is a validation of the individual by the recognition that others have such problems, hence the support facility, and therefore the individual is not odd, alone, or particularly inadequate, within this area. Increased value may be engendered by the removal of labels associated with 'mental health' and referring to facilities and services as education centres or community resource units, thus removing, to some extent, the stigma associated with problems associated with living. Misuse of the term 'mental health units', as previously discussed, precludes a positive interpretation of facilities so termed. Personal growth, whether achieved via such assistance or under one's own steam, and the value of one's own attainments—despite the degree of success attained by others—require a re-emphasis. Balancing one's own needs and desires with those of others, deriving status and worth via assorted spheres of life rather than putting all of one's eggs into a single basket, and maintaining equilibrium between own values and those of society may be far more useful and health orientated than two hours of physical 'torture' in the gymnasium once a week.

A second area of attention requires specific interventions with those individuals considered at greater risk of problem development. Compensatory education programmes directed at children, who are both socially disadvanted and demonstrate early signs of disturbed behaviour, aimed at reduction of such behaviour, may engender long-term benefits. Shure and Spivak (1982) developed an eight-week, pre-school educational programme to improve 'interpersonal cognitive problem-solving skills', to assist disadvantaged children to consider and solve interpersonal problems and so reduce behavioural problems prior to entering school. The initital eight-week programme was followed by 12 weeks of formal scripted sessions within each of the first two years of education, and results of this study demonstrated that, in comparison to a matched control group, children improved in areas of focus and consequent behaviour. Previously well-adjusted children included within the study were less likely to demonstrate aberrant behaviour than their matched peers in the control group and where such behaviour was demonstrated, it was less likely to persist. Whilst other studies reveal conflicting evidence of the value of such pre-school learning programmes (Durlak and Jason, 1984) considerable research is required to ascertain benefits that may be accrued from intensive compensatory programmes. Certainly, Durlak and Jason's own research, based on identification of high-risk children via mass-screening techniques and subsequent provision of a behavioural- or relationship-orientated para-professional worker—that is, a specifically trained volunteer, housewife or student—to work with the children, both in groups and on an individual basis, appeared to reveal positive benefits. Prompt attention to dysfunction detected at an early stage of development appeared to both improve behaviour and the ability to adjust, which has been maintained over several years. Long-term evaluation is necessary to reveal its full use, but it is a relatively inexpensive preventative programme because of its reliance on para-professional personnel and its integration within the school programme. It may be a significant 'value for money' activity, should the problems of childhood, which often persist into adolescence and adulthood, be amenable to intervention at this point.

Programmes directed toward parents and pre-school children have revealed that, on a range of indices and outcome measures, positive effects were not only evident, but appeared to be either maintained or to increase with time even though interventions had ceased. Parental and child education in communication, positive reward for desired behaviours, expression of anger, resolution of conflicts and discipline (Rickel *et al.*, 1984) appeared to engender maturation in cognitive and social–emotional development in children to a level appropriate and demonstrable in those of a low risk but otherwise matched control group. Kolvin *et al.* (1981) utilized three types of intervention in their study. For high risk seven-year-olds, a nurture group, a play group and parent counselling and teaching support group, and for maladjusted eleven- and twelve-year-olds, behaviour therapy, group therapy and parent counselling–teacher support group were employed and found to be highly successful in both short- and long-term evaluation.

The value of mother-focused support and education programmes, utilizing a befriending system, appears to be significant. The Leicester, community-based family support scheme, 'Homestart', indicated positive attitudinal changes, increasingly qualitative relationship formation and enhanced levels of parental self-esteem, as well as social and material improvements evident following inclusion in the programme (Eyken, 1982). 'Newpin', in South London, is a similar organization, providing befrienders from corresponding backgrounds and experiences to offer support, practical assistance and friendship. Pound *et al.* (1985) described one of the major aims of the project as a reduction in the high incidence of maternal depression, child abuse and neglect, and therefore the target population was those mothers who were isolated, had problems within the parenting role or who exhibited depressed mood. Evaluation—though based on self-assessment and therefore open to bias—indicated improvements in confidence, self-esteem and significant relationships, in addition to improved social contact and feelings of support. Difficulties overall had appeared to reduce. The Child Development Project (1984) utilized modified health-visitor–mother relationships and interactions to enhance parental confidence and self-reliance, to develop and implement strategies to assist with problems associated with child-rearing practices and experiences, and to improve parent–child relationships and communication in general. Short-term feedback provided positive data in regard to improvements within the home environment at a socio-economic level, with more books evident, more intellectual activities utilized and increased educational ambitions observable. Improved language content and cognitive abilities were also evident. The values to the parent of fostering a

sense of control in previously isolated or helpless individuals should not be under-estimated and may provide principles for employment on behalf of other, similarly perceived individuals, for example, voluntary groups which campaign for higher status of specific groups in society—women, children, the older generation, ethnic and religious minority groups and those of a non-heterosexual orientation. Empowerment is an antidote to depression (Harris *et al.*, 1987) and prevention is far more effective than cure. Indeed Rodin's (1985) study, of the effects of empowering elderly residents within a convalescent home by promoting choice and returning responsibility for many aspects of living back to them rather than concentrating decision-making in the remit of personnel, resulted in her questioning the degree to which biologically determined decline in the elderly has been over-emphasized. Her findings in regard to the detrimental effects engendered by loss of control associated with environmental and personal experiences, suggest these significantly contribute to physical disease and deterioration, psychological withdrawal and even death. Meichenbaum's (1977) study and that of Schulz (1976) within similar areas replicated findings, but the latter showed disturbing evidence in relation to the need for continuing input once begun. Visits by undergraduate students to nursing home residents had been shown to be of great benefit—less medication needed, more activity undertaken, improved health status and increased levels of self-rated happiness and value in residents. However, two years after cessation of the visits, and in comparison to other groups, there was evidence of a greater decline in health and also a higher mortality rate within this group. Positive interventions introduced should not therefore be withdrawn.

The studies above offer insight into the values and limitations of selected health promotion and mental health status maintenance programmes. More research is required, both with regard to the specific aetiology of mental health problems and the methodology by which effective and prolonged—and yet cost effective—prevention may be effected. Those studies of befriending systems within the community identifying a symbiotic value observable—that is, both befriender and befriended gain considerable levels of self-esteem and feelings of usefulness and value from the interactions. It may be, therefore, that effective social organization within the community aimed at education and support of the vulnerable members may be of greatest benefit in prevention of such problems and that the mental health nurse's role within this will be in initial education and organization, and continuing advice and support. Empowering individuals and creating an environment conducive to taking responsibility for self is a major element of health care provision and as such requires a significant proportion of time, effort and high level skills to be utilized in that direction.

CONCLUSION

We have differentiated between overt and covert incidence of mental health problems within the population and identified that the vast majority of resource availability is utilized upon the care of a small minority of those in need, that is on the 6 per 1000 of the population requiring in-patient attention. Thompson and Pudney (1990) make the point so eloquently: 'While we spend £72 per day—the price of a four-star hotel room—on each psychiatric in-patient, we spend just 29 pence a day—the price of a cup of tea—on the rest'. The appropriacy of a major re-allocation of finances towards the seat of the problem must be a priority, with community care viewed as the area where the greatest number may be provided with the greatest good.

Problems of identification and recognition of deviations in mental health status must be addressed via medical training and appropriate experience within client care. Early and effective interventions may then be initiated and an over-reliance on psychotropic medication as a first—and often only—line of assistance offered may then be minimized. One may, in the light of discussions related to the continuing stigma associated with mental health problems and that related to the differentiation between the aetiology of those problems diagnosed as 'neurotic' as opposed to 'psychotic' in nature, wonder whether medicalization may be more of a hindrance than a help to some individuals. 'Neurotic symptomatology' may be considered in essence to be the external indicators of problems of adjustment to life and the demands of living it. They may be the sequelae which herald a problem, but are unlikely to be the problem itself. An over emphasis on a medical label and cure may be a waste of valuable resources, when education to assist in adjustment may, in reality, be what is required and necessary. A 're-assignment' of such clients away from the department of psychiatry may witness more individuals admitting their problems and the need for help, and subsequently seeking and accepting it. In addition it may reduce 'sick role behaviour' observed with a number of individuals experiencing care, which complicates and prolongs health care needs. Whilst the value of medication cannot be ignored within overall care requirements, the major impetus must surely be towards re-education and consequent adjustment to life for these individuals' problems.

A higher profile for mental health issues and education for living is necessary, and may be achieved via the media and—more importantly— via health care personnel in an educative and non-medicalized form. Movement away from predominantly client-focused care towards a greater involvement in family and community activities, designed to engender and organize supportive and therapeutic systems and structures, to promote mental health status and prevent deterioration of those currently experiencing problems, may appear a more effective use of highly skilled personnel. Evidence would indicate the value of these activities to the individual and his family, and hence mental health nurses should be active within this area, increasing accessibility to such services, by assisting in their development.

In regard to those individuals who demonstrate an impaired contact with reality, more effort and resources are required to identify the aetiology of problems experienced and hence develop both effective preventative and therapeutic care. The total income for all United Kingdom mental health charities from the voluntary sector amounts to £9 million per year, in comparison to £73 million for animals, £116 million for cancer and £160 million for overseas aid (Thompson and

Pudney, 1990). AIDS is far less common—3,000 times less common than mental health problems—and yet its high profile guarantees research funding at a high level. Four times the number of individuals who die on the roads each year die as a result of mental health problems (Thompson and Pudney, 1990) and yet there will no comparable health warning on television or on poster boards over Christmas—or at any other time of the year. With one-quarter of the population likely to experience problems in mental health to some degree, intensive research into the area as a whole, but particularly in relation to 'psychoses', is urgently required.

The effects of mental health problems on the individual have been explored in order to demonstrate the importance of early problem detection, efficient and intensive health care provision and the need for the utilization of hospital-based care as a carefully and thoroughly considered strategy within overall service availability. In addition, the highly individualized nature of the experience of mental health problems cannot be overemphasized—there is no such thing as a routine programme of care. Every home situation, every admission to hospital and every visit to an outpatient department or by a community nurse will feature a unique person with specific circumstances which heavily influence his or her response to the problems experienced, and will therefore dictate health care needs. Individualized care is therefore of prime importance to clients, their families and society as a whole.

Individualized client care greatly resembles the jigsaw puzzle previously referred to (Fig. 6.1, p. 89). A variety of problems may be seen to be experienced by the person concerned and hence a variety of reactions and repercussions. The art of nursing the individual experiencing mental health problems lies in compiling an accurate jigsaw and then facilitating effective strategy and intervention implementation. The following three chapters may assist in compilation of the jigsaw.

FURTHER READING

Bynum, W.F., Porter, R. & Shepherd, M. (Eds) (1985) *The Anatomy of Madness: Essays in the History of Psychiatry*, Vols 1, 2 & 3. London: Tavistock.

Doerner, K. (1981) *Madmen and the Bourgeoisie: A Social History of Insanity and Psychiatry*. Oxford: Blackwell.

Scheff, T.J. (1984) *Being Mentally Ill*. Chicago: Aldine.

Szasz, T. (1987) *Insanity: The Idea and its Consequences*. New York: Wiley.

REFERENCES

After Henry—Scriptwriter Simon Brett, Producer Peter Fraser Jones (1992). Transmitted by Thames Television.

Allen Poe, E. (1992) *The Fall of the House of Usher*. In *Complete Stories*. London: Everyman.

Beaber, R.J. & Rodney, W.M. (1984) Under Diagnosis of hypochondriasis in family practice. *Psychosomatics*, **25**, 39–46.

Bebbington, P., Hurry, J., Tennant, C., Sturt, E. & Wing, J.K. (1981) Epidemiology of mental disorders in Camberwell. *Psychological Medicine*, **11**, 561–579.

Bronte, C. (1977) *Jane Eyre*. London: Collins.

Carmen, E.H, Rieker, R.P. & Mills, T. (1984) Victims of violence and psychiatric illness. *American Journal of Psychiatry*, **141** (3), 378–383.

Central Statistic Office (1992) *Social Trends 22*. London: HMSO.

Child Development Project (1984) *Child Development Programme*. Booklet produced by the University of Bristol.

Carrol, L. (1992) *Alice in Wonderland*. London: Everyman.

Cooper, B. & Sosna, V. (1980) Family settings of the psychiatrically disturbed aged. In Robins, L.N., Clayton, P.J. & Wing, J.K. (Eds) *The Social Consequence of Psychiatric Illness*. New York: Brunner/Mazel.

Department of Health (DH) (1991) *Health and Personal Social Services*, England. London: HMSO.

Department of Health (DH) (1992a) *Statistical Bulletin*. London: Government Statistical Office.

Department of Health (DH) (1992b) *The Health of the Nation*. London: HMSO.

Dickens, C. (1991) *Great Expectations*. London: Longman.

Dohrenwend, B.S. & Dohrenwend, B.S. (1969) *Social Status and Psychological Disorder: A Causal Enquiry*. New York: Wiley.

Durlak, J.A. & Jason, L.A. (1984) Preventative programs for school aged children and adolescents. In Roberts, M.C. & Peterson, L. (Eds) *Prevention of Problems in Childhood*. New York: Wiley.

Eyken, W. van der (1982) *Homestart: A Four Year Evaluation*. Leicester: Homestart Consultancy.

Falloon, I.R.H., Boyd, J.L., McGill, C., Williamson, M., Razani, J., Moss, H.B., Gilderman, A.M. & Simpson, G.M. (1985) Family management in the prevention of morbidity of schizophrenia: clinical outcome of a two year longitudinal study. *Archives of General Psychiatry*, **42**, 887–896.

Fatal Attraction—Screenplay James Dearden, Producers Jaffe and Lansing (1987). Paramount Films.

Fernando, S. (1988) *Race and Culture in Psychiatry*. London: Tavistock/Routledge.

Garrel, G. (Ed.) (1991) *Healthy Ageing: Some Nursing Perspectives*. London: Wolfe Publishing.

Goldberg, D. (1984) The recognition of psychiatric illness by non-psychiatrists. *Australian and New Zealand Journal of Psychiatry*, **18**, 128–133.

The Golden Girls—Scriptwriter Susan Harris, A Witt–Thomas Harris Production (1992). Transmitted on Channel 4 Television network.

Goldberg, D. & Huxley, P. (1980) *Mental Illness in the Community*. London: Tavistock.

Harris, T., Brown, G.W. & Bifulco, A. (1987) Loss of Parent in Childhood and Adult Psychiatric Disorder—The Role of Situational Helpless. MS.

Health and Safety Executive (1988) *Mental Health at Work*. London: HMSO.

Homer (1992) *Iliad*. London: Award Publications.

Homer (1965) *Odyssey*. London: Collier Macmillan.

Kolvin, I., Garside, R.F., Nicol, A.R., MacMillan, A., Wolstenholme, F. & Leitch, I.M. (1981) *Help Starts Here*. London: Tavistock.

Kroger, J. (1989) *Identity in Adolescence—The Balance Between Self and Others*. London: Routledge.

Last of the Summer Wine—Scriptwriter Roy Clarke, Producer Alan J.W. Bell (1992). Televised by British Broadcasting Corporation.

Leff, J., Kuipers, L., Berkowitz, R., Eberlein-Vries, R. & Sturgeon, D. (1982) A controlled trial of social intervention in the families of schizophrenic patients. *British Journal of Psychiatry*, **141**, 121–134.

Leff, J., Kuipers, L., Berkowitz, R. & Sturgeon, D. (1985) A controlled trial of social intervention in the families of schizophrenic patients: two year follow-up. *British Journal of Psychiatry*, **146**, 594–600.

Lipsedge, M. & Littlewood, R. (1982) *Aliens and Alienists*. Harmondsworth: Penguin.

Mann, A.H., Jenkins, R. & Belsey, E. (1981) The twelve month outcome of patients with neurotic illness in general practice. *Psychological Medicine*, **11**, 535–550.

Marsh, G.N. (1977) 'Curing' minor illness in General Practice. *British Medical Journal*, **2**, 1267–1269.

Meichenbaum, D.H. (1977) *Cognitive Behaviour Modification: An Integrative Approach*. New York: Plenum.

Mullen, P. *et al.* (1988) The impact of sexual and physical abuse on women's mental health. *Lancet*, **1** (8590), 841–845.

Mussen, P. *et al.* (1990) *Child Development and Personality*. New York: Harper & Row.

Office of Health Economics (1990) *Mental Health in the 1990s—From Custody to Care*.

One Flew Over the Cuckoo's Nest—Screenplay Hauben and Goldman, Producer Milos Forman (1975). Fantasy Films.

Pashley, D. (1991) *Homeless Mentally Ill People in Central London*. Community Care Office, N.W. Thames Regional Health Authority.

Paton, D. & Brown, R. (1991) *Lifespan Health Psychology*. London: Harper Collins Nursing.

Pound, A., Mills, M. & Cox, T. (1985) A Pilot Evaluation of Newpin. A Home Visiting and Befriending Scheme in South London. MS, summarized in the October *Newsletter of the Association of Child Psychology and Psychiatry*.

Rawnsley, K. (1968) Epidemiology of affective disorder. In Coppen, A. & Walk, A. (Eds) *Recent developments in affective disorders*. *British Journal of Psychiatry*, Special Publication, No. 2.

Rickel, A.U., Dyhdalo, L.L. & Smith, R.L. (1984) Prevention with preschoolers. In Roberts, M.C. & Peterson, L. (Eds) *Prevention of Problems in Childhood*. New York: Wiley.

Rodin, J. (1985) Health, control and ageing. In Baltes, M.M. & Baltes, P.B. (Eds) *Ageing and the Psychology of Control*. Hillsdale, NJ: Lea.

Rutter, M.L. (1979) Protective factors in children's responses to stress and disadvantage. In Kent, M.W. & Rolf, J.E. (Eds) *Primary Prevention of Psychopathology*, Vol. 3. *Social Competence in Children*. Hanover, New Hampshire: University Press of New England.

Schultz, R. (1976) Effects of control and predictability on the physical and psychological well-being of the institutionalised aged. *Journal of Personality and Social Psychology*, **33** (5), 563–573.

Selye, H. (1956) *The Stress of Life*. New York: McGraw-Hill.

Shepherd, M., Cooper, B., Brown, A.C. & Kalton, G.W. (1986) *Psychiatric Illness in General Practice*. Oxford: University Press.

Shakespeare, W. (1935) *King Lear*. In *Complete Works of Shakespeare*. London: Odhams Press.

Shakespeare, W. (1935) *Macbeth*. In *Complete Works of Shakespeare*. London: Odhams Press.

Shure, M.B. & Spivak, G. (1982). Interpersonal problem solving in young children: a cognitive approach to prevention. *American Journal of Community Psychology*, **10** (3), 341–356.

Silence of the Lambs—Screenplay Ted Lally, Producers U11, Saxon and Bosman (1991). Orion Films.

Surtees, P.G., Dean, C., Ingham, J.G., Kreitman, N.B., Miller, P. & Sashidharan, S.P. (1983) Psychiatric disorder in women from an Edinburgh community: associations with demographic factors. *British Journal of Psychiatry*, **142**, 238–246.

Test, M. & Stein, L. (1978) Training in community living: research design and results. In Stein, L. & Test, M. (Eds) *Alternatives in Mental Hospital Treatment*. New York: Plenum.

Thompson, D. & Pudney, M. (1990) *Mental Illness: The Fundamental Facts*. London: Mental Health Foundation.

Waiting for God—Scriptwriter Michael Aitkens, Producer Gareth Gwenlan (1992). Transmitted by British Broadcasting Corporation.

Wertheimer, A. (1991) *A Special Scar—The Experiences of People Bereaved by Suicide*. London: Routledge.

White, E. (1991) *The Third Quinquennial National Community Psychiatry Nursing Survey*. Department of Nursing, University of Manchester.

AFFECT AND EMOTION

F.C. Johnson and L.D. Smith

AIMS

i) To review the basis of the experience of human emotion
ii) To formularize a continuum of the emotional responses associated with healthy living
iii) To determine the characteristics of the variety of human emotions
iv) To identify anomalies in the above that may indicate the presence of mental health problems

KEY ISSUES

Physiology
Role of higher cognitive function
Analysis of each emotion
Content, duration, quality and appropriacy
Verbal and non-verbal cues to determine problem
Depression
Elation
Apathy
Blunting
Lability
Inappropriacy

Identify, analyse and assess factors causing distress and illness	Promote health, provide direct care and make interventions	Manage care programmes and services
Be critical, analytical and accountable, continue professional development	Counter discrimination, inequality and individual and institutional racism	Work within and develop policies, laws and safeguards in all settings
Understand influences on mental health and the nature/causes of disorder and illness	Know the effects of distress, disorder, illness on individuals, groups, families	Understand the basis of treatments and interventions

INTRODUCTION

Emotional feelings and responses are an integral and all-pervasive aspect of daily life. From the moment of wakening to the last one before sleeping, the individual is constantly bombarded with mood-altering stimuli which, in turn, colour and influence thoughts, perceptions and behaviours.

An example may be of value:

'Good morning, and here is the 8 o'clock news from your local independent radio station'.

'Six people died and 18 others were seriously injured in a multiple pile-up on the motorway this morning. A police spokesman at the scene said that drivers had ignored warnings of freezing fog and had been driving well in excess of speed limits advised. The injured are being treated at the City Infirmary'.

'200 more jobs are to be lost with the closure of Bainbridges Tiling Company. This brings total job losses in the area in the last month to 2,500'.

'There is to be a further 0.5% interest rate reduction. Major building societies have reported record receipts from savers, who are ignoring Government calls to spend their way out of the recession'.

'On the international front, sporadic fighting between Serbs and Bosnians continues to prevent United Nations relief forces' efforts to provide urgent food and medical supplies to the besieged town of Sarajevo'.

'In Somalia, local militia have agreed a cease-fire, enabling United Nations forces to reach feeding centres in the north of the country. Aid workers believe supplies will have no significant impact on death rates for several weeks'.

'Arms reduction talks continue today and both superpower spokespersons believe an agreement is imminent'.

'And now the weather. Temperatures will remain low—in the region of 4°C for the remainder of the day. Fog will continue to be a major hazard to drivers. A low of 2°C is expected overnight'.

The feelings evoked by the morning news may be various in nature. There may be a great sadness that so many people were killed and injured on the motorway, but also anger, at the senselessness of such an accident, and the stupidity of those driving too fast in such appalling road conditions. There may be fear and anxiety for the safety of a loved one, who was expected to be travelling on that stretch of the road at about that time of the morning, or a sigh of relief breathed that one's own car is still safely tucked up in the garage, out of harm's way. The news of more job losses in the area is likely to engender sadness for those involved and an anxious concern for any specific acquaintance who is to be affected. Should a partner or close member(s) of the family be amongst those being given redundancies, the emotion experienced may be one of despair, with fears for future security. Of course, there is great news for home-owners, with a half of 1% reduction in the interest rate. It may bring a feeling of relief—almost joy—to those struggling to make the monthly repayments, but for those who have already experienced the repossession of their home and the break up of the family unit, there may be anger and bitterness that reductions are coming too late to be of help to them. Some will be indifferent, or apathetic, to the news, with half a percentage point not being significant enought to get excited about one way or the other. Of course those people who don't have mortgages may experience resentment, at what are effectively 'rent reductions' for home owners whilst the actual rent payers never get any relief.

The international headlines may again evoke both anger and sadness. The hatred, greed and wanton disregard for human life and suffering inherent in war may engender feelings of despair for the state and progress of civilized society. The knowledge that some people in the world are cold, hungry, hurt or in fear for their continuing safety may provoke feelings of guilt, in individuals who are sitting toasting their feet by the fire and enjoying breakfast. Feelings of shame and embarrassment may be associated with impotency or a previous lack of willingness to do more to assist the starving in the world. There may be feelings of frustration towards the powerful people in the world who appear to be loathe or slow in stepping in to prevent such carnage, or anger that innocent, uninvolved people have been sent to a place by a government who, they believe, has no right to interfere, no matter what is happening. There may be disgust felt towards countries who spend years arming different factions and militia, and then expect applause for reducing the risk of damage to their own people by agreeing to destroy their own weapons.

Of course, there may be no such acute emotional response to any of the news items. The individual may have become so accustomed to hearing such distressing news that he or she fails to be stimulated by it, absorbing details and yet experiencing no qualitative feeling as a response. For some, the weather forecast will provoke the strongest reaction, as they envisage the day's planned activities severely curtailed or made extremely difficult by the continuing foggy conditions.

'That concludes the news report and, with the time coming up to three minutes past eight, we ask you to drive safely and have a nice day!'

It is not, however, the end of the emotional content for the day. Whether the individual's taste is for the popular music of the day or something a little more timeless and classical in nature, the potential is there for a change of mood. It is not only music, of course, that can evoke or engender emotion and mood in this way. There are artists, poets, scriptwriters and authors who spend a lifetime trying to stimulate people to pleasurable feelings and moods. The theme parks of the nation charge an entrance fee to individuals for the use of the rides and amusements. Often people are terrified but really enjoy the experience. Similarly, people wallow in the floods of tears evoked by a sad film or book, and some gain genuine pleasure from being scared to death by a horror story. The 'arts' rely on such emotions to sell the product for if a book bores the reader, there is the likelihood that the story will neither

be finished nor recommended to friends and certainly the reader will not buy any more of that author's work.

Everyday life creates emotional rollercoasters for the individual. The pleasures associated with touching the fingers of a newborn baby and admiring its wonderful perfection; of wandering unhurriedly by the river or seashore within an environment of peace, tranquillity and absence of demands upon self; or the success associated with the attainment of a hard-fought objective, may be experiences of emotional significance for some. The fears and anxieties associated with any potential or actual threat to wellbeing, no matter the biopsychosocial factor generating such fears, have been experienced by everyone. Anger is a frequent response to the behaviour exhibited by others and sadness and unhappiness may be experienced as a result of the argument which resulted from one's own anger. Remorse and guilt may be exteriorized in trying to compensate for verbal damage—or worse—inherent in any disagreement, or pain may be deep-seated and too intense to eradicate. Emotions and moods are an integral part of life and living, a daily occurrence and something unavoidable for the vast majority of the population. So, what are these moods and emotions? How do they arise and how are they exteriorized?

DEFINING TERMINOLOGY

There is a tendency to use the terms 'emotion', 'affect' and 'mood' interchangeably. However, there are differences between them and whilst overlap may be a feature, it may at times be important to differentiate between the concepts.

The term 'emotion' relates to those consciously perceived feelings and their manifestations which occur in response to external stimuli (Campbell, 1989). For example:

'I feel anxious and apprehensive. My mouth is always dry and my heart races uncontrollably. My hands are sweating and yet I'm cold'.

'I'm happy—I feel fit and well, lively and enthusiastic—everything's going well'.

'I'm so angry, my blood's boiling and I really can't think about anything else'.

'Affect' is the term reserved for the experience of the emotion plus the drive energies that are presumed to generate the conscious and unconscious feelings associated with it. It is the subjective, personal, fluctuating aspect of the individual's experience and relates to the here and now; not the past observations made (Campbell, 1989). Examples may help:

'I've tried so hard to be everything she wanted me to be. I've tried to be a good husband; I've worked hard and we have a nice home and two lovely kids. Now she says she's leaving me and I'm worried that she means it. I feel anxious and apprehensive. My mouth is always dry and my heart races uncontrollably. My hands are sweating and yet I'm cold'.

'I'm successful. I have everything I've always wanted and needed. I feel safe, secure and fulfilled. I'm happy; I feel fit and well, lively and enthusiastic—everything's going well'.

'How dare he belittle me in front of everyone. He made me look stupid and incompetent—and it was his error not mine. He's always treating me like this. I'm so angry; my blood's boiling and I really can't think about anything else'.

The differences between the three are of relevance, for individuals may report that, whilst they have been depressed for quite some time (mood), they now really have gone beyond this point. They do not care for anyone or anything; they are totally apathetic (affect), disinterested in life and living. They believe themselves beyond feeling (emotion) and their world is dark and drab. These are important elements within individual's descriptions of this experience, for whilst they feel apathy, they are likely to be too disinterested to take their own lives. When they feel despair, however, with thoughts associated with the pointlessness of life and being better off dead, they may be motivated to self-harm and present therefore as at greater risk and in need of modi-

fied care and attention. The nurse needs to be posing appropriate questions to elicit important details of the individual's current experience to be of most value in the care process, and to enable judgements to be made in relation to the efficacy of health care.

The focus of concentration in this chapter will, therefore, be on affect and emotion, on the premise that mood may be elicited by appropriate questioning, where affect and emotion rely on accurate observations being made to elicit those appropriate questions. In analysing one, it is hoped to provide insight into the successful exploration of the other.

THE BASIS OF EMOTION

In any analysis of the theoretical perspectives applied to emotion, it would be inconceivable not to include the words of William James (1842–1910), the American psychologist, who made the first real attempt to link the experience of emotions with physiological function. In his work *What is Emotion?* published in 1884, James analysed the role of emotion in life:

'Conceive yourself, if possible, suddenly stripped of all the emotion with which your world now inspires you and try to imagine it as it exists, purely by itself, without your favourable or unfavourable, hopeful or apprehensive comment. It will be almost impossible for you to realise such a condition of negativity and deadness. No one portion of the universe would then have importance beyond another; and the whole collection of its things and series of its events would be without significance, character, expression or perspective. Whatever of value, interest or meaning our respective worlds may appear imbued with are thus pure gifts of the spectator's mind'.

James' work centred around the *order of events* that occur within the emotional state. Utilizing the ideas of a Danish psychologist, Carl Lange, he proposed what has become known as the James–

Lange Theory of Emotions. The theory asserts that the overt responses and bodily changes associated with an emotion *precede* the conscious feelings accompanying the stimuli. The feelings of fear or rage were viewed as the awareness of the inner and outer changes created by the stimuli. An example may be useful:

> 'We feel sorry because we cry, angry because we strike, afraid because we tremble'.
> *James, 1884*

For James, the physical sensations *were* the emotion. He asserted that each emotional experience was the result of its own specific set of physiological activities and hence emotions were perceived as discrete entities, unlike each other, psychologically and physiologically speaking.

In 1927, Walter Cannon's studies cast doubts upon the James–Lange theory, for he 'proved' erroneous the assumptions of discrete physiological activities occurring within each emotion. Cannon discovered that the same pattern of physiological arousal accompanies a number of different emotions. To cast further doubt upon the theory, Cannon, in experiments on dogs and cats, severed the sympathetic nerves that James had considered to arouse the body changes preceding the emotional awareness. The animals were unaware, therefore, of physiological reaction because none was possible, and yet they demonstrated the expressions and emotions appropriate to the stimuli presented. Cannon asserted that emotional feelings do not depend upon the receipt of sensations arising from within the body, turning attention back to the brain.

As a result of his studies, Cannon constructed an alternative explanation for emotion, which was later modified by Phillip Bard, and became known as the Cannon–Bard theory. In essence, the theory asserts that a *simultaneous reaction* from both psychological experience and also physiological reaction to the stimuli is necessary to produce emotion. The individual facing an emotionally arousing event is subject to nerve impulses passing to the thalamus, where they split into two; half travelling on to the cerebral cortex and the other half to the hypothalamus. Those impulses arriving at the cortex produce the subjective experience of anger, fear, joy, etc., whilst the hypothalamus initiates the physiological changes associated with the feeling.

In 1937, James Papez proved that no specific brain centre assumed responsibility for emotional experience as Cannon had asserted. Instead, the anatomist suggested that a 'stream of feeling' and a 'stream of movement' provided a circuit—the Papez circuit—of relay stations via which sensations travelled and merged to create emotion. Papez believed the 'stream of thought' to relay sensations through the thalamus to the major areas of the cortex, whilst the 'stream of movement' involved impulse transmission through the thalamus to the corpus striatum. Papez (1937) believed that as a result of the merging of the two streams 'sensory expectations ... receive their emotional colouring' (see Fig. 7.1).

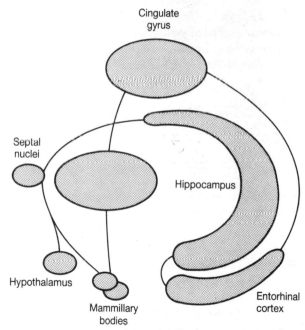

Fig. 7.1 *The Papez Circuit.*

The work of Papez provided the foundation for today's knowledge relating to the neuroanatomy of emotion. The structures that he referred to became known as the Papez Circuit, and are included within the area referred to today as the limbic system. However, in addition to those limbic stuctures it is now known that areas of the brainstem—the reticular formation, the locus coeruleus or 'blue area' of the pons, and the substantial nigra of the midbrain—plus the frontal lobes of the cerebral cortex and the autonomic nervous system, are all involved within emotion generated (Tortora and Anagnostakos, 1984). Exactly how they function remains a matter, largely, of guesswork and inference but it is believed that:

WWhen faced with an event which requires mobilization, a two-fold response occurs. Impulses are transmitted along neural pathways from the sensory receptor, via the reticular system and the thalamus, to the cortex. Motor responses required are initiated immediately, but in the meantime, impulses pass, via the neural connections, from the thalamus to the hypothalamus and, via the amygdala and hippocampus, to the frontal lobe of the cortex. The arousal of all structures provokes the initiation of automatic nervous system mechanism, and an effect is elicited within one to two seconds of perception of the provoking event. By this point, the pituitary gland is activated and provides assistance via blood-borne hormonal influences.

Neuroanatomy and physiology is provided in considerably more detail in other chapters and hence no further attention will be awarded to the subject at this juncture.

INTENSITY OF EMOTION

Previous reference has been made to Cannon's (1927) experiments with cats and dogs, where sympathetic nerve fibres had been severed and yet expressions and emotions displayed were appropriate to the stimuli presented. Whilst this may have proved the case in animal studies, there is some dispute of the fact with regard to humans.

A great deal of anecdotal evidence—often based upon the impressions of physicians—existed to suggest that no alteration in the ca-

pacity for experiencing intense emotion occurred in those individuals unfortunate enough to have severed their spinal cord in accidents. George Hohmann (1966), himself a victim of spinal cord injury, compared the emotional reactions of individuals with varying levels and sites of cord injury, reported before and after their injuries. He found a diminution in the intensity of their emotions and that individuals with injuries high on the spinal cord reported the greatest difference in the before and after emotional experience. The higher the damage, the less visceral sensation the person is able to feel. Individuals reported that the 'heat' had gone out of emotion and that feelings were more 'mental' than whole body experiences. Whilst able to 'react' emotionally, the individuals did not 'feel' emotional.

'It's a sort of cold anger. Sometimes I act angry when I see some injustice. I yell and cuss and raise hell, because if you don't do it sometimes, I've learned people will take advantage of you; but it doesn't have the heat to it that it used to'.

'I say I'm afraid, like when I'm going into a real stiff exam at school, but I don't really feel afraid, not all tense and shaky with the hollow feeling in my stomach, like I used to'.
Hohmann, 1966

Whilst the reporting of remembered emotions and comparing them with current emotional experiences is not particularly objective as a method of scientific study, Jasmos and Hakmiller (1975) provided a less subjective but similar analysis. Men with spinal cord damage were presented with photographs of both clothed and nude women, and asked to imagine being alone with each woman. Thoughts and feelings reported were analysed in relation to expressed emotion, and results demonstrated that those individuals with higher spinal lesions reported less sexual excitement than those with lower sited injuries. In 1985, Lowe and Carroll repeated Hohmann's original study and found no evidence of diminution of emotional intensity in paraplegic subjects. The role of feedback from the autonomic nervous system in the experience of emotion is therefore still an area of dispute, so many years after the studies of James (1884) and Cannon (1927).

PHYSIOLOGICAL DIFFERENTIATION OF EMOTION

Again, Walter Cannon (1927) asserted, that only one pattern of autonomic arousal occurs in response to a wide number of emotional stimuli. More recent studies by Ax (1953), in which he was able to reliably evoke emotions of fear and anger in his subjects, reported differing patterns of peripheral physiological activity for each of the two emotions elicited.

More recently, Ekman *et al.* (1983) demonstrated distinct autonomic patterns of activity for each of six emotions—surprise, sadness, anger, fear, disgust and happiness. Whilst actor subjects held an emotional expression for ten seconds, heart rate, skin temperature and other indicators of autonomic arousal were recorded by researchers. Results showed that the heart rate experienced during the emotions of anger, fear and sadness was higher than that related to the more positively judged emotions of happiness, surprise or disgust. In anger, skin temperature was higher than shown in fear or sadness, and hence a fine differentiation of emotional states is seen via autonomic nervous system patterns of arousal. However, there is a general belief, that such differences identified cannot be totally responsible for differentiation of an individual's emotional experiences. Cognitive appraisal of the presenting stimuli has been considered a potential factor in this differentiation for some years.

EMOTION AND COGNITION

In 1924, Gregorio Marañon published a largely anecdotal study on emotions, which centres on the subjective reports of a group of individuals to whom he had administered epinephrine by injection. About one-third of the subjects reported an experience 'something like' an emotional state, 'as if' something exciting were about to happen or 'as if' they were afraid. The remaining subjects reported that whilst they had experienced no emotion, they felt symptoms associated with arousal. In later discussions with the group members who had reported the 'as if' emotional experiences, Marañon talked with them about emotionally significant events experienced in the recent past. He reported the exteriorization of the full emotional response in regard to these events—the 'as if' status had disappeared.

Utilizing Marañon's work and other available evidence, Stanley Schachter (1971) theorized that, in order for an emotion to be experienced, both cognitive evaluation and physiological arousal must be available to the individual. In a widely cited experiment, Schachter and Singer (1962) administered a placebo—a saline injection—to control subjects whilst subjects were given epinephrine. Both groups were informed that the substance given was a vitamin preparation, but then subjects from both groups were, in essence, treated in one of three ways. Some were informed—without naming the drug—of the physiological effects of epinephrine and warned of feelings such as palpitations, tremors, etc. A second group was given no information and a third group were misinformed. Each subject was then placed in a room with another person, who, whilst claiming also to be an experimental subject, was in fact a 'stooge' and part of the experimental team. Some confederates assumed a euphoric type of behaviour, whilst others were irritable and feigned increasing anger, until they left the room, totally 'enraged'. Researchers made observations via a one-way mirror and also questioned subjects about their experience. Correctly informed, epinephrine-injected subjects reported the least effect to the stooge's behaviour, whilst misinformed subjects, experiencing physiological symptoms unlike those they had been informed to expect, were most affected by the confederate's antics. This latter group mirrored the behaviour exhibited by the stooge and also reported feelings of great happiness or intense anger, according to the behaviour exteriorized by the stooge. Individuals given no information after the injection showed behaviour of neither excess, but responses were seen to be in the middle band of a no-reaction/excessive reaction continuum.

Schachter and Singer (1962) appeared to prove their hypothesis, namely that an emotion is jointly determined by cognitive appraisal and physiological arousal, and that arousal would be interpreted as non-emotional where subjects had received the correct information with regard to the effects of epinephrine. They asserted that those subjects who had either been misinformed or uninformed would experience an arousal for which they could not find a reason, and therefore that they would seek an explanation for their behaviour in the context provided by the stooge. For those given a placebo, the social context on its own—that is, the stooge's behaviour—would not generate emotion. Whilst many criticisms have been levelled at Schachter and Singer's interpretation of results, replications of the study since by Erdman and Janke (1978) have produced a broad agreement with regard to the basic assertion that it is a combination of physiological and cognitive factors that produces the experience of emotion.

George Mandler (1982) asserts the importance of a sense of control with the cognitive analysis of the event evoking emotional experiences and certainly one may be able to differentiate the emotions inherent within two different situations:

1　During a ride on a rollercoaster or other theme park amusement, the individual feels the support beneath him, in the form of the rail, fall away suddenly
and

2　Whilst sitting in an aeroplane at the start of a holiday, the plane suddenly drops in an air pocket.

The cause of the arousal is similar in each scenario, and due to a release from the effects of gravity. In the former example, the reader has *chosen* to ride the rollercoaster and is able to anticipate some of the sensations that may be experienced. He has a sense of control therefore. However, in the second scenario there are feelings of *helplessness* and fear in response to the lack of control over the situation experienced. Two different emotions are perceived, in response to a similar stimulus, where, in essence, a sense of control is the only real variable. Mandler

argues that there is an *interruption of ongoing behaviour and thought* which serves as a trigger, for appraisal processes, to analyse the exact nature of the interruption. Whilst autonomic activity is also triggered at this interruption, Mandler believes that it is the nature of the situation, as determined by cognitive appraisal, that determines the quality of the experience.

AN ANALYSIS OF THE EMOTIONS

Emotion is a derivative of the Latin word, 'movere', meaning to move or to stir, and certainly some sources may consider an emotion to be defined variously as 'a state of agitation'; 'disturbance of equilibrium'; or 'an intense random and disorganized response to a stimulus' (Sperling, 1960). *Roget's Thesaurus* (1982) lists dozens of states, all purported to be emotions and it is possible to spend hours attempting to decide which are actually emotions. Wise people have already addressed the subject and have created much dispute and argument in the process.

Two approaches have been taken in relation to the identification of the specific nature of emotions. One theory assumes that there are a relatively small number of *primary* emotions and that each of these is associated with a specific event which triggers its arousal. For example, Plutchik (1980) identified eight emotions and their triggers which, he observed, were evident universally within every human culture and throughout the animal world.

Emotion	Trigger
Grief (sorrow)	Loss
Fear	Threat
Anger	Impediment
Joy	Potential partner
Trust	Group membership
Disgust	Unpleasant stimulus

Anticipation	New territory
Surprise	Sudden novel experience

Certainly studies by Ekman (1982), Izard (1984), and others would support the universal recognition of facial expressions associated with happiness, anger, disgust, sadness and a combined notion of fear and surprise and there tends to be support for a theory in which, initially at least, emotional reactions occur without cognitive appraisal. Zajonc (1984) and Ekman and Oster (1982) argue for such 'ontogenetic primacy' of emotion over cognitive appraisal, suggesting the newly born infant's facial expression of disgust in response to a nasty taste, as an example. Whilst cognitive elaboration may ensue as part of the development process, Zajonc believed it likely that these universally recognized emotional reactions may be linked reflexly to the perception of a limited range of stimuli.

The role of cognitive appraisal within emotional development is also threatened via the experiments by individuals such as Garcia and Rusiniak (1980) who demonstrated that successful conditioning (classical conditioning) can occur, even when the unconditional stimulus is administered—and has its effect—under anaesthesia. Animals demonstrated nausea when presented with food that had been utilized as a conditioned stimulus, even though the nausea-provoking agent had been presented and had its effect during anaesthesia. Animals were able to respond adversely to a stimulus at an unconscious level and, therefore, without cognitive appraisal.

A second approach, taken by Roseman (1979) and others, asserts that it is the cognitive appraisal of a situation or event that generates the emotion and that if, for example, an experience is desired and occurs, the emotion felt will be one of joy. However, if the event is dreaded (i.e. not desired) and it occurs, the emotion experienced will be one of distress. There are four potential emotional experiences available from the differing combinations of these two elements:

Selection of emotion		
/////////////	*Desired*	*Undesirable*
Occurring	Happiness	Distress
Not occurring	Sadness	Relief
After Roseman (1979)		

The approach asserts that there is a myriad of such aspects taken into consideration within any situation or event prior to the arousal of any specific emotion. 'Selection' of emotion appropriate to any event is, therefore, a little like manipulating a 'Rubik's cube', with the various elements combining to form an overall picture or response.

THE INFLUENCE OF AFFECT ON COGNITIVE PROCESSES

Whilst discussions will continue in relation to the relative role of cognition in the nature of the emotion experienced, there would seem little doubt that affect—the current emotional experience including drives—influences cognitive processes, and particularly memory.

Bower (1981) believes that each emotion occupies a specific node or niche within memory and is linked with the memories of specific events or experiences during which that emotion was aroused. 'Affect nodes' are connected to all other nodes in a sort of semantic network, facilitating the spread of any activation of one node through others nearby. Bowers believes that it is by such means that selective retrieval of congruent memories occurs during an emotion, with nodes in semantic memory being activated, thus eliciting associated memories of a similar emotional quality and nature to that currently being experienced.

Whether or not the above explanation is the 'correct' one, we cannot say but we are aware that the emotional state of an individual is not the sole factor at work in relation to memory processes. The retrieval of material would appear to be dependent both upon the emotion currently experienced and on the affective content of material to be retrieved. Individuals in a positive mood show a tendency to retrieve positive memories, whilst negative mood subjects tend towards negative past event material. It has long been recognized that individuals who are experiencing a depressed mood will recall sad life episodes in excess of those recalled by control subjects and, indeed, Beck (1974) suggests these biased cognitive processes play an important part in both causing and maintaining a depressive episode. Studies by Johnson *et al.* (1983) have found that depressed subjects recalled more tasks associated with failure, or lack of project completion, than did the non-depressed control group.

Blaney (1986), in a review of many such studies, suggests that such mood congruence is a genuine occurrence, but that, whilst all point in a similar direction, the specifics of whether a depressed individual actually recalls *more* negative events or *fewer* positive ones is dependent upon the study format utilized and therefore not clear. Certainly it would be of interest—and value—to ascertain at which level within the lowering of mood, such congruence comes into effect. Should a specific threshold need to be reached to see its occurrence, intervention at such point may prevent the adverse effects of biased cognitive processes described previously by Beck (1974).

The effects of emotion on thinking processes are well known. When too anxious, the individual 'can't think straight' and finds attention and concentration difficult. Feeling 'too happy'—if there can be such a state!—may evoke disinterest in routine events and activities preferring 'to go with the flow'. Sadness and anger are similarly pervasive, causing preoccupation of thoughts and reducing levels and quality of performance. Hebb (1972) suggested a relationship between the level of arousal and efficiency of performance, and that this differs with each task or behaviour (Fig. 7.2).

It is suggested that a mild level of arousal will evoke an alert interest in a current event or situation, whilst intense emotional feelings will disrupt thoughts and behaviours and, hence, reduce effectiveness of performance. Of course, the nature of the task will be significant in regard to the degree of disruption experienced, for many 'routine' aspects of life may be performed quite

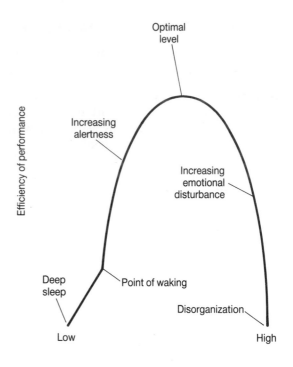

Fig. 7.2 *Relationship between the level of arousal and efficiency of performance.*

adequately whilst thoughts are preoccupied elsewhere. Complex tasks requiring attention and reasoning to achieve completion would be significantly impaired. Selye's (1956) work in relation to the potentially damaging effect of prolonged, intense emotional arousal on body systems and general health is well known and lies at the heart of theories of psychosomiasis (the relationship between stress and illness).

RECOGNIZING EMOTION

It is valuable to be aware of the nature of emotion, the manner in which it is evoked and of the body's mechanisms that are involved in the experience. It is of importance, too, to have an understanding of the various perspectives applied to the experience of an emotion and the factors that may influence that experience. The effect of emotion and mood on the processes involved in cognition and performance is a necessary part of overall management of emotion in everyday life and the mental health nurse must recognize the prevailing mood of an individual and elicit the current affect operating.

One may observe an individual and conclude within a fraction of a minute that he/she is happy, sad, angry, hurt or embarrassed. The clues are easy to see. Happy individuals wear a smile, have sparkling eyes and are bouncy and lively in their movements, showing energy and vitality. The sad person wears an 'unhappy face', eyes are dull (maybe full of tears) and often directed towards the floor. There is little movement, the individual often preferring to sit huddled in a chair, and where movement is observed it is slow, heavy and deliberate. Anger finds expression in expansive movements, the individual utilizing an increased amount of space to perform sharp and sudden activities. Facial expression is characteristically 'like thunder', with skin red and warm from the exercise and eyes wide open and acute in their observations. The pale, tearful face of the individual who feels hurt, bottom lip trembling as he or she cowers from the source of the emotion, and the red-faced fidgety individual standing with head hung low are all characteristic behaviours associated with specific affective experiences. The mental health nurse's observations are important but equally vital is the recognition of what is seen. An increased activity in the eyes of individuals who are depressed, with apparently surreptitious observations of the movement of others within the environment may just indicate their increasing interest in life and elevation of depressed mood. However, in the absence of other cues, it is more likely that they may be awaiting an opportunity to slip quietly away, whether to harm themselves, absent themselves from the care facility, or merely withdraw from therapeutic interventions. The smile that does not reach the eyes, the hollow, forced laugh and the 'miraculous cure' evinced by the individual as 'But I feel much better nurse, really!' are shams and the care worker needs to be aware of their potential.

The mental health nurse not only has to observe and recognize cues available, but also needs to analyse their meanings both as individual pieces of information and within the overview of all available data. Only by these activities may an accurate insight into an individual's affect be gained, prompting effective exploration towards total assessment of need.

PROBLEMS OF EMOTION

There should be little need to affirm the 'normality' of emotional expression but one should be aware of the potential problems associated with somatic disease. Selye (1956) identified the General Adaptation Syndrome, a physiological degeneration of body tissues as a direct result of intense and prolonged emotion, and therefore the relevance of psychosocially directed care within overall health plans for many individuals should be the norm. Coronary artery disease, hypertension, migraine, ulcerative bowel conditions and many other somatic disorders may be precipitated or exacerbated by such prolonged emotional experience and hence warrant the mental health nurse's attention and expertise.

In addition to being implicated within causation and maintenance of somatic dysfunction, problems of an emotional nature may be seen as sequelae in a wide variety of experiences of somatic ill-health. Depressed mood and anxiety feelings may, quite naturally, be evoked where an individual feels his life or lifestyle is threatened in any way and may be prolonged. The same is true for partners and family members involved within the experience. On occasions reactions may be severe with loss of contact with reality, perceptual disturbances and delusional ideation, and those caring for such individuals need to be aware of such strong mental health responses.

Emotional problems may form an integral part of an individual's somatic disease/dysfunction complaints and may indeed prompt medical assistance being sought. Endocrine glands, presumably because of their direct role in the generation of emotion, are particularly prone to emotional symptomatology. In Addison's disease (Primary Adrenal Insufficiency) for example, what would normally be considered a minor problem may evoke a *catastrophic reaction* with the individual rapidly bursting into tears, extremely sad and anxious in mood. Phaochromocytoma, a neoplasm of the adrenal medulla, may cause individuals to experience the 'as if' feelings discussed within Marañon's (1924) epinephrine tests, being edgy, nervous, tremulous and anticipatory of something about to happen. Anxious, apprehensive feelings are commonly experienced by individuals who have hyperthyroidism (((Thyrotoxicosis) whilst those experiencing the reverse, hypothyroidism (Myxoedema) may complain of always feeling low, emotionally lethargic and disinterested in surroundings.

Neurological disorders may create emotional problems for the individual. Within multiple sclerosis, for example, *emotional lability* where emotions are uncontrolled and mobile, and hence unpredictable, may be a feature, as may an unwarranted and excessive level of optimism and happiness, termed *euphoria*. Parkinson's disease may show emotional detachment, and *anhedonia*, that is, the inability to feel plesure. Some, indeed, experience an 'on–off' syndrome, where pronounced changes in affect occur, being anxious or depressed when 'off' and aroused and elated when 'on'. This may be a feature of prolonged treatment. Similarly, according to position and extent, cerebral neoplasia and trauma may engender similar problems of mood and emotion for the client. The brief overview above suggests the extreme importance of a thorough physical examination prior to any diagnosis of a primary mental health problem being made. Indeed, the client's health history is of great importance for a variety of medications may similarly create problems, including certain antibiotic, cardiovascular-acting and steroid preparations, and should therefore be excluded as causative agents.

Within mental health care, individuals may be seen to experience a variety of different problems associated with emotion. *Depression*, a lowering of mood and profound sadness, may be a problem for many, but to be considered 'pathological', that is, in need of treatment, certain characteristics tend to be associated with the experience. Whilst frequently a response to a traumatic life event, it may be that the mood is lowered for no apparent reason. The individual may then be seen to have relinquished contact with reality and also be experiencing a variety of perceptual and thought-related problems. Where contact with reality is maintained, depressed mood may have been of an excessive depth, in relation to the

nature of the precipitating event, or may be of a prolonged duration. Such depression will always feature some degree of physical disinterest and self-neglect on the part of the individual and therefore somatic health may suffer. Self-harm and injury to others may be behaviours exhibited during the individual's experience of lowered mood.

Elevated mood, in the form of *elation* or where it is of a lower level, *euphoria*, may also be experienced and is problematical where it arises when not justifiable in relation to the individual's circumstances. Hold on reality is tenuous initially as mood begins to rise and is subsequently lost. Such elation and euphoria is accompanied by some degree of complete psychomotor acceleration and hence presents other problems for both client and carer.

Anxiety may be seen as a response to any threat, whether potential, actual or imagined. Some individuals experience a generalized feeling of apprehension and fear which they are unable to attribute to any specific focus. This is termed '*free-floating anxiety*'. However, where anxiety experienced is both disproportionate and produced in response to a threat recognized by the individual as not a genuine danger to wellbeing, the anxiety is termed *phobic*.

A lack of anxiety in some individuals may give rise to concern, for '*la belle indifference*' represents a markedly less than expected level of distress and concern exhibited by someone experiencing somatic symptomatology. Their apparent unconcern in relation to motor or sensory manifestations is a classical sign in the diagnostic category known as 'conversion disorders'. The physiological symptomatology occurs in the absence of a physical disorder. Instead, symptoms are a symbolic representation of psychic conflicts, for example, an individual who has difficulty acknowledging the traumas associated with an event witnessed, may express this conflict in the form of 'blindness', which exists for the individual and yet has no physical basis. The somatic problem may present less trauma to the individual than that associated with acknowledging the psychic conflict.

Guilt may be problematical where it is misplaced; for example, the survivor of a traumatic event who feels guilt because of his survival when others have died, or where it becomes excessive, creating incapacitating tensions that interfere with life and living. Equally problematical is the inability to feel guilt or remorse following anti-social activities or conduct, which is characteristic of individuals who lack insight into reality and also of some personality limitations.

Apathy represents a loss of interest and drive, and may be seen in combination with many other problems. It may be associated with severely depressed mood for example, in post-traumatic stress responses and organic brain damage. When witnessed in conjunction with a lack of insight, thought and perceptual problems, diagnostic labels of 'schizophrenia' or 'schizo-affective disorder' may be applied.

Lability of mood has been referred to above in relation to somatic dysfunction as rapid changes of mood, either in the absence of an appropriate stimulus or in response to very minor stimulation. Moods are mobile and unpredictable, and this problem is commonly witnessed in the care of individuals experiencing organic impairment. When extreme, it may be referred to as *emotional incontinence* and that less rapid, more persistent mood swing which may be experienced is termed *cyclothymia*.

Blunted affect refers to emotional expression that appears in response to stimuli and yet which lacks 'body'. It is neutral, flat and shallow and the normal range of emotional expression is restricted and lacking. *Incongruity* or *inappropriacy of affect* describes emotional responses that are out of keeping with the prevailing events or circumstances. A commonly quoted example is that of giggling at a funeral. Both emotional blunting and incongruity are associated with a lack of insight, and thought and perceptual problems.

Psychoactive substance *abuse* and *dependence* tends to be associated with the extremes of mood. Depression and anhedonia are commonly associated with the use of alcohol, amphetamines (and similarly acting sympathomimetics), cannabis and cocaine. Euphoria tends to feature in the use and dependence associated with phencyclidine (and similarly acting arylcyclohexylamines) and with sedatives, hypnotics and anxiolytic preparations. Opioids are usually similarly euphoric in effect,

although on occasions supplemental substances may be added, either to enhance the 'high' or to counteract any depressive effect experienced.

Intoxication may elicit other problems of mood. Where alcohol is the causative substance euphoria, depression and emotional lability may be observed. In amphetamine intoxication, anxiety and apprehension may occur and with cannabis, euphoria, inappropriacy, anxiety and panic attacks may feature. Cocain intoxication may provoke euphoria and anxiety and hallucinogens often create anxiety and depression. All psychoactive substances will create some degree of mood problem. *Withdrawal* from use will create similar problems, depression, anxiety and irritability all being common. Delirium, a state of altered consciousness, disorientation and confusion, is characteristic of acute and subacute organic reaction and may be a feature of both use and withdrawal of psychoactive preparations. Alcohol, amphetamines, cocaine and phencyclidine are examples of potential causes of delirium states, and emotional disturbances are very common in such scenarios. Anxiety, fear, depression, irritability, anger euphoria and apathy may all occur.

Some substances, notably hallucinogens and phencyclidine are specifically associated with a mood disorder. In either instance it may be difficult to ascertain whether mood disorder precipitated substance utilization—that is, the substance was taken to elevate mood, but depression was only exacerbated by its use—or whether the mood disturbance is a direct result of preparation usage. Most commonly, depression and anxiety are the problems experienced, and only rarely elation.

There are other problems associated with emotion that are often overlooked because they have not acquired psychiatric terminology. These are frequently experienced by individuals who fall through the mental health safety net one way or another, either because they keep their emotions to themselves and on a very tight rein, or because their response to such emotions is considered within the parameters of 'normal' behaviours.

Whilst many may not be as cynical as George Bernard Shaw when he said 'Love is a gross exaggeration of the difference between one person and everybody else' or Benjamin Disraeli who believed 'The magic of first love is our ignorance that it can never end' it has to be admitted that love is a major preoccupation for many and an integral part of life for most. Romantic love is the stuff of films, novels and poetry, and yet it is not the only focus of love feelings experienced within life and living. Think of parental love and its problems, which may be many and varied. Loving children too much, and trying to shelter them from the world, and being unable to love children at all, and eliciting an almost blatant disregard for their health and wellbeing, are two extremes of a continuum, and a happy medium, somewhere in between may be hard for some to find. Neither overprotectiveness nor neglect are of benefit to the developing youngster, but the parent who vacillates between the two extremes is even worse for the child's mental health prognosis.

Problems may similarly arise in the situation where parental love replaces a previous love-based relationship with a partner. The child(ren) form the focus of existence for one or both parents, preventing care between equals and that symbiotic love represented by a partnership. Difficulties present for all involved in situations where parental love somehow becomes distorted and assumes a heterosexual basis. Sexual abuse is a subject increasingly explored and reported by the media and will no doubt elicit continuing study over the next decade and beyond. The problems of physical and emotional abuse, too, are areas of difficulty which are well publicized, as is filial violence, that is violence perpetrated by a child upon a parent. All evoke major biopsychosocial traumas.

There are problems, too, associated with the parent who cannot 'let go' of an adult child. This is the parent who is unable to make the transition from protector and provider to friend. It is the parent who is unable, or experiences great difficulty, in allowing the child to develop new, lasting relationships outside of the family of origin and who often provokes guilt in the offspring in relation to 'having no further use' for the parent, who is 'obviously in the way'. This is the parent who may resent any attention that is not directed towards self, or any activity in which he/she has not been included as an automatic right. The

'unreasonable' expectations of a parent may create significant problems for the child's relationships and adult roles.

Romantic love must be considered problematical for many—if not most—of the population at some time within the life span. There are those who find themselves sacrificing self, own needs and aspirations to 'please' a partner who has been elevated to 'god' status. In addition there are those who expect too much of a partner and can never find someone sufficiently selfless to suit, and individuals who really do not expect another to love them, because they are so 'worthless', that is, lacking in confidence. Some have problems exteriorizing their love for another, whilst others will 'fall in love' all the time. Many may in fact be 'in love with being in love', desperately seeking someone to fulfil the idealistic dreams and images promulgated regarding romantic love. Whether the rescued or the rescuer, romantic love is envisaged by most as an integral and expected part of life, hence the roaring trade in dating agencies and 'introduction' services.

Sibling love may, for some, be non-existent, creating severe family discord and occasionally intense guilt within the individual. There may conversely be a prolonged or excessive dependence upon siblings to meet one's own needs, which may continue into adult life. Responsibility for an individual's health, happiness and achievements in life may be firmly placed on another's shoulders rather than being assumed by oneself, and that someone may be anyone, parent, sibling, partner or child. It may be that a relationship within the family of origin *always* assumes a higher priority than those with a partner and one's own children and again may create significant discord and resentment.

Altruism—that love experienced towards fellow man—again may be non-existent at one extreme and excessive at the other. Individuals who demonstrate a total disregard or disinterest in the effects of their behaviour upon others, for example, businesspersons who will tread on anyone to get whatever it is they desire, joy-riders who steal cars without thought for either the owners or anyone who may happen to get in their way, gun-runners who arm one or both sides in a conflict, generating financial gain at the expense of lost lives and maimed bodies, have no care for their fellow man. The individual who sacrifices self, own needs and aspirations within a total absorption of assisting others, whilst profoundly altruistic, may be missing out on a great deal of personal growth and development inherent in a 'well-balanced' life of partnerships—some equal, others not so equal—of giving *and* receiving, of being valued, valuing others and self, and all of the other experiences available within the lifespan.

There are those whose love for a spiritual god, of whatever nature and characteristics, assumes obsessional proportions, whilst others 'worship' material goods, which acquire a value above that of people. There may be a love of animals and pets which, again, may supersede that awarded to humans, for all sorts of reasons. For many, love may provide an area of considerable difficulty.

It would be inconceivable to mention love without mentioning hate and hatred, which may so often cripple the emotional lives of individuals and prevent attainment towards reaching their potential of 'being', feeling and experiencing other emotions. The emotion itself is often a very understandable response—the possible hatred of the Jews for the Nazi concentration camps and gas-chambers, that of an innocent victim towards the perpetrator of a terrorist bombing or that of a parent towards the individual who molested or murdered his child—and one with which everyone would empathize. Such hatred has to be managed and dealt with, to prevent the individual from falling victim to the event or occurrence, or from continuing to be such a victim for the rest of his/her life. To be totally preoccupied with seeking revenge, asserting the 'truth' of a situation or hurting others to compensate for the hurt and pain experienced by self, is damaging to the mental health of the individual and those who come into contact with him or her. It alters the perspectives applied to life and living and prevents maximization of opportunities available, or potentially available, for life, living, personal happiness and peace of mind.

There are individuals whose fear of life and living inhibits their experiences, creating continual unease and distress. Such fears may relate to almost anything in life, for example, afraid to try,

afraid to fail or afraid to succeed. Some may be terrified of showing their true self, for fear of rejection and 'not suiting' individuals who have no real significance in their existence. Others are afraid to find out about themselves, their likes, dislikes, needs, drives, emotions, for fear of having to face what may be traumatic revelations. There are people who are physically or emotionally afraid of loved ones, or who conversely enjoy the terror that they are capable of evoking or instilling in others. This lack of self-esteem, worth and confidence, or conversely, that lack of value, or trust and faith, in others, in comparison to self, cripples the individual emotionally.

Guilt feelings may be similarly problematical for an individual. Shame and self-loathing as a result of some action or omission on one's own part, whether actual, inferred, imagined, potential or exaggerated, may be persistent or intermittent in nature. Such feelings may evoke avoidance of situations or relationships that characterized the original problem, or a continuous placing of oneself in similar positions, whether compensatory in nature or as a form of punishment. There are those whose skill in life appears to be evoking guilt in others, perhaps to detract from their own responsibility in a situation or just as a means of achieving one's own ends. Again, there is a need to explore the emotion, come to terms with issues and feelings, and move on in life.

We have almost avoided the mention of anger as a response within this section, mainly for the reason that anger would be a relatively 'normal' reaction in biopsychosocial traumas. However, problems do occur for many individuals who may never approach mental health care services, and these merit identification. Just as with hatred and guilt feelings, some individuals always carry anger around with them, preventing the full experience of life. It may be a reaction to many events and circumstances—feelings of not 'being good enough' as a child and hence spending a lifetime proving parents wrong in their beliefs, is one such example. Being angry at a loved one's desertion of self, or at one's treatment at the hands of society, or an employer, are others. Some individuals find anger to be their predominant reaction in many situations and this may represent the individual's defensiveness and anticipation of attack by others, or blame being apportioned to them in other spheres of life. Lack of verbal fluency may predispose to violence and aggressive acts where anger or frustration feature. Certainly, the prime focus of anger may be either self or some vulnerable loved one—a parent, a partner or a child—or society at large via antisocial acts.

SUMMARY

A brief analysis of problems that may be observed within both individuals and society in general has been presented. When not publicized too loudly or broadly, in the main, people are left alone with their emotional distress. However, where antisocial activities result from feelings—a parent shoots the driver responsible for an accident which killed his child, a deserted wife repeatedly drives over the body of her husband's mistress, or a battered wife sets fire to her husband while he sleeps—society, often in the form of legal action, pays attention to the problems which have long exerted their detrimental influence.

Problems of emotion may be seen in a variety of shades and degrees and like all mental health problems, do not exist in isolation from problems associated with cognition and behaviour. A problem experienced in one domain will, of necessity, infringe upon the others and Chapter 10 will be seen to demonstrate this interaction.

FURTHER READING

Brain, W.R. (1985) *Brain's Diseases of the Nervous System*. Oxford: University Press.

Brunner, L.S. & Suddarth, D.S. (1986) *The Lippincott Manual of Medical Surgical Nursing*. London: Harper & Row.

Evans, P. (1989) *Motivation and Emotion*. London: Routledge.

Hinchcliffe, S. & Montague, S. (1988) *Physiology for Nursing Practice*. London: Baillière Tindall.

Hinwood, B. (1993) *A Textbook of Science for the Health Professions*. 2nd ed. London: Chapman & Hall.

Lishman, W.A. (1978) *Organic Psychiatry: The Psychological Consequences of Cerebral Disorder*. Oxford: Blackwell Scientific.

Roth, I. (Ed.) (1990) *Introduction to Psychology*, Vols 1 and 2. Milton Keynes: Laurence Erlbaum Associates in conjunction with the Open University.

REFERENCES

Ax, A.F. (1953) The physiological differentiation between fear and anger in humans. *Psychomotor Medicine*, **15**, 433–442.

Beck, A.T. (1974) The development of depression: a cognitive model. In Friedman, R.J. & Katz, M.M. (Eds) *The Psychology of Depression*. Washington: Winston.

Blaney, P. (1986) Affect and memory: a review. *Psychological Bulletin*, **99**, (2), 229–246.

Bower, G.H. (1981) Mood and memory. *American Psychologist*, **36**, 129–148.

Campbell, R.J. (1989) *Psychiatric Dictionary*, 5th edn. Oxford: University Press.

Cannon, W.B. (1927) The James–Lange theory of emotion: a critical examination and an alternative theory. *American Journal of Psychology*, **39**, 106–124.

Ekman, P. (1982) *Emotion in the Human Face*, 2nd edn. Cambridge: University Press.

Ekman, P. & Oster, H. (1982) Review and prospect. In Ekman, P. (Ed.) *Emotion in the Human Face*, 2nd edn. Cambridge: University Press.

Ekman, P., Levenson, R.W. & Frierson, W.V. (1983) Autonomic nervous system activity distinguishes among emotions. *Science*, **221**, 1208–1210.

Erdman, G. & Janke, W. (1978) Interaction between physiological and cognitive determinants of emotions: experimental studies on Schachter's theory of emotions. *Biological Psychology*, **6**, 61–74.

Garcia, J. & Rusinak, K.W. (1980) What the nose learns from the mouth. In Muller-Schwarze, D. & Silverstein, R.M. (Eds) *Chemical Signals*. New York: Plenum.

Hebb, D.O. (1972) *Textbook of Psychology*, 3rd edn. Philadelphia: Saunders.

Hohmann, G.W. (1966) Some effects of spinal cord lesions on experienced emotional feelings. *Psychophysiology*, **3**, 143–156.

Izard, C.E. (1984) Emotion-cognition relationships and human development. In Izard, C.E., Kagan, J. & Zajonic, R.B. (Eds) *Emotions, Cognition and Behaviour*. Cambridge: University Press.

James, W. (1884) What is Emotion? *Mind*, **9**, 188–204.

Jasmos, T.M. & Hakmiller, K.L. (1975) Some effects of lesion level and emotional cues on affective expression in spinal cord patients. *Psychological Reports*, **37** 859–870.

Johnson, J.E., Petzel, T.P., Hartney, M.N. & Morgan, L.M. (1983) Recall and importance ratings of completed and uncompleted tasks as a function of depression. *Cognitive Therapy and Research*, **7**, 51–56.

Lowe, J. & Carroll, D. (1985) The effects of spinal injury on the intensity of emotional experience. *British Journal of Clinical Psychology*, **24**, 135–136.

Mandler, G. (1982) *Mind and Emotion*. New York: Norton.

Maranon, G. (1924) Contribution to the study of the role of adrenaline in emotion. *Revenue Francaise d'Endocrinologie*, **2**, 301–325.

Papez, J.W. (1937) A proposed mechanism of emotion. *Archives of Neurology & Psychiatry*, **38**, 725–744.

Plutchik, R. (1980) A general psychoevolutionary theory of emotion. In Plutchik, R. & Kellerman, H. (Eds) *Emotion: Theory Research & Experience*, Vol. 1. New York: Academic Press.

Roget, P. (1982) *Roget's Thesaurus of English Words and Phrases* (1982). Harlow: Longman.

Roseman, I. (1979) Cognitive aspects of emotion and emotional behaviour. *87th Annual Convention of the American Psychological Association*, New York, September 1979.

Schachter, S. (1971) Some extraordinary facts about obese humans and rats. *American Psychologist*, **26**, 129–144.

Schachter, S. & Singer, J.E. (1962) Cognitive, social and physiological determinants of emotional state. *Psychological Review*, **69**, 379–399.

Seyle, H. (1956) *The Stress of Life*. McGraw-Hill.

Sperling, G. (1960) The information available in brief visual presentations. *Psychological Monographs*, **74**, 11, No. 498.

Tortora, G.J. & Anagnostakos, N.P. (1984) *Principles of Anatomy and Psychology*. New York: Harper & Row.

Zajonc, R.B. (1984) On the primacy of affect. *American Psychologist*, **39**, (2), 117–123.

8

BEHAVIOUR

F.C. Johnson and L.D. Smith

AIMS

i) To explore the concept of behaviour and innate influencing factors

ii) To discuss selected aspects of behaviour; the norms, expectations and characteristics associated with:
   1 Movement
   2 Eating
   3 Sleeping

iii) To determine potential problems which may indicate mental health assistance is required

KEY ISSUES

Definitions
Innate body rhythms
Paralysis, paresis, rigidity
Overactivity/stereotyping, etc.
Starvation, bingeing, compensation
Insomnia, nightmares and terrors
Withdrawal, compensation

Identify, analyse and assess factors causing distress and illness	Promote health, provide direct care and make interventions	Manage care programmes and services
Be critical, analytical and accountable, continue professional development	Counter discrimination, inequality and individual and institutional racism	Work within and develop policies, laws and safeguards in all settings
Understand influences on mental health and the nature/causes of disorder and illness	Know the effects of distress, disorder, illness on individuals, groups, families	Understand the basis of treatments and interventions

BEHAVIOUR—NORMS AND PROBLEMS

INTRODUCTION

After man's emergence as truly man, the same sort of thing continued to happen, but with an important difference. Man's evolution is not biological but psychosocial: it operates by the mechanism of cultural tradition, which involves the cumulative self-reproduction and self-variation of mental activities and their products. Accordingly, major steps in the human phase of evolution are achieved by breakthroughs to new dominant patterns of mental organisation, of knowledge, ideas and beliefs—ideological instead of physiological or biological organization.

The words above are those of the twentieth-century biologist, Julian Huxley (1958). Having evolved to the degree whereby locomotion could be achieved on two legs, rather than four, where objects could be manipulated as tools and weapons, thereby providing an advantage over many other species of the animal kingdom, and language could be utilized to share 'innovations' and observations, human physiological transformation was completed. A by-product of the increased interaction and control over the environment was the gradual development of an enlarged and more advanced cerebral cortex, which became incorporated into genetic coding and which continued to be perpetuated via the 'survival of the fittest' and the destruction of lesser able competition. The effects of environmental stimuli on the basic brain provided at birth are explored in Chapter 9 on cognition. Learning and experiencing the environment may be seen to be of the utmost importance in achieving potential function and abilities. Certainly it may be that limitations on performance are merely self-imposed or socially induced, and that the potential is almost limitless where the environment is appropriate and conducive to learning. As society, its systems and structures, its rules and norms are made by people and 'ideological

instead of physiological or biological' (Huxley, 1958), we may be only part-way along the path towards full emancipation from our animal origins. How far along the path may be inferred from the following discussion.

HUMAN NATURE OR ANIMAL INSTINCT?

Today, in a world of advanced technology and increasingly sophisticated methods of investigation and analysis, it is possible to confirm that we are indeed basically animal plus a highly developed cortex. The remainder of the human brain and its structures show very little difference, in situation or function, to those of 'lesser species'. The subcortical centres of grey matter elicit remarkable similarities, particularly the thalamus and hypothalamus, which, whilst regulating the autonomic nervous system and, to some degree, metabolic and endocrine activities, also, and importantly in the following discussions, play the major role in emotional and instinctual life, adding the affective elements to feelings. The thalamus, for example, possesses nuclei within its internal core, and the projections from these nuclei extend through the medial and basal telencephalon. Stimulation of these structures, in animals, is seen to create disturbances of feeding, fighting, pain avoidance, mating and nurturing behaviours. The hypothalamus is associated with temperature regulation, cardiovascular and endocrine activities but, in addition, appears to accommodate the mechanisms relating to certain drives, for example, hunger and thirst. The role of the hypothalamus within the exteriorization of behaviours associated with the docility–rage continuum, and within sleep, is similarly demonstrable and the relevance of thalamic and hypothalamic activity within each behaviour will be discussed in more detail within the appropriate sections of this chapter. Limbic influences are similarly brought to bear upon motor activity via connections between the basal ganglia and the areas generating emotion. The roles and effects of various neuro-transmitters, discussed by Farine in Chapter 20, provide an integral aspect of the study of behaviour and its influences: there is little difference at this point between the human brain and that of other animals.

Role of the cerebral cortex

In turning attention towards the cerebral cortex, it may be remembered that it is, essentially, the ultimate destination of data collected via the sensory receptors and organs. Its continual interaction with subcortical centres is elicited via the phenomena of perception arousing emotion, and, conversely, emotion focusing attention and therefore perception. Cortical regions are linked via association pathways and by this process, crude and raw perceptual experiences are transformed into meaningful information, with the addition of memories of previous experiences and learning. At the point at which all relevant data have been evoked, including that which relate to the current degree of angularity of joints and the relative tension of body muscles, the sensorimotor cortex activates the specific motor changes necessary to achieve rapid motor responses to information received. It is the cortex which discriminates between the perceptions emanating from internal and external environments, initiating and supporting responses to some stimuli, whilst concurrently inhibiting potential activities and reactions to others. With a highly developed cortex comes the potential to demonstrate a greater ability to discriminate between a wider range of somatosensory stimuli and their increased associations, plus an increased number of possible reactions are available from which to select an appropriate response. Thus our advantage over competitors within the remainder of the animal kingdom is, in theory, tremendous.

The evolutionary development of the frontal lobe of the cerebral cortex must, however, be our greatest advantage. Its role and value within social behaviour is well demonstrated within the following story:

In 1848, Phineas Gage was a hardworking, dependable and well-liked, 25-year-old foreman on a railway construction. An explosion at the site blew a thirteen pound metal rod through the front of his skull, causing extensive bifrontal lobe damage. Although surviving this horrendous accident, Phineas demonstrated a marked change in behaviour and personality. He was described as 'fitful, irreverent, indulging at times in the greatest profanity ... manifesting little deference for his fellows, impatient of restraint or advice when it conflicts with his desires, at times pertinaciously obstinate, yet capricious and vacillatory, devising many plans of future operations, which are no sooner arranged than they are abandoned'.

Phineas experienced no pain in relation to the accident and indeed spent some time with P.T. Barnum's circus, exhibiting himself as a freak along with the offending rod.
Harlow, 1848

There are direct neural projections from the thalamus to the frontal lobe and therefore a connection between emotion and innate behaviour and the higher functions related to judgement, reasoning, the development of intellectual resources and the pursuit of long-term goals. The frontal lobe assists in the demonstration of socially aware behaviour, tact, sensitivity and self-control—it is the 'policeman' moderating animal instincts.

From the above, it may be seen that the 'model' is that of 'animal' with the significant additions of judgement, the ability to plan ahead and work towards deferred gratification, and an emphasis on behaviour conducive to group acceptance.

AN INFLUENTIAL HERITAGE

Though basically animal, we have the higher cognitive powers necessary to interact to our advantage with the environment and control—within reason—our behaviour. It is observed, for example, that we may override some of our defence-orientated reflex actions when perceived to be beneficial to us:

Imagine, that knowing the pantry is bare, you

stop off on the way home from work to pick up fish and chips, or a take-away. By the time home is in sight, the meal is not feeling too warm and so, you put the meal on a plate in the oven to heat it up. Ten minutes later and presumably warm enough to eat with enjoyment, the meal is taken out of the oven, and despite the use of a cloth, the heat of the plate burns your fingers. Do you drop the plate? Not if it can be helped—it represents the only food in the house and the thought of scraping it off the floor into the bin would be more than a hungry stomach could condone. The instinct to release the plate and let it smash, food and all, is countermanded as evinced by the 'juggling act' undertaken in order to transfer the hot plate to a suitable surface. The pain in the fingers and hands is reduced to the greatest extent possible by the intermittent grasp of the plate achieved by the juggling act, but it remains the overwhelming priority of the moment to deposit the meal safely.

You will be aware, however, of situations and events when you were unable to control your own innate behaviours, which may have evoked feelings ranging in intensity from mild disappointment to intense anger directed at self. Wanting specifically to stay up late to watch a particular TV film and waking up only to find the credits rolling may be a 'mild' example. Losing control in a situation in which it is deemed important to maintain it, whether in the form of shedding tears or inflicting pain on someone, either verbally or physically, may provide another instance.

We need to be aware of the fact that there are biological influences which exert so subtle an effect upon general functioning, and hence behaviour, that the individual may not appreciate their existence. These influences may, in part, account for fluctuations in performance and are, in effect, rhythms adapted to the earth's cycles, and nature's norms. If we look at a garden, the rhythms of plants and flowers may be observable. The snowdrop *knows* when it is time for it to raise itself from the confines of the earth, as does every other bulb, shrub and tree in the garden. Daffodils are not evident in the long summer days and

delphiniums are not naturally seen in the border in the depths of winter or early springtime. It is known that some species of birds migrate to warmer climates for the winter and in the forest, some animals hibernate at that time. Salmon will find their way back to their birthplace in time to lay their eggs and then immediately die. How do frogs know when to spawn and tortoises to wake up from hibernation? The answer is that all possess in-built, genetically coded rhythms, which, whilst influenced by environmental conditions, are evoked automatically and at around the same time of the year and reflect a long evolutionary patterning of behaviour, designed to prevent disruption by weather vagaries.

There are three observable and natural rhythms that influence activities. Some garden flowers open their flowers in the day and close them at night, synchronized with the day/night—light/dark cycle of the day. Removed from the garden environment and placed in a dark cupboard, plants such as the heliotrope will continue to open and close their leaves in tune with the day/night cycle outside. It is not, therefore, stimulated directly by the amount of light and its pattern of opening and closing must be integral to plant structure. This is an example of a *circadian rhythm*, named from two Latin words, *circa* = about and *dies* = a day; rhythms that occur on an approximately daily basis.

In the human being, the sleep–wake cycle is the most visible of the circadian rhythms, but there are a hundred or so such cycles, many of which appear to be co-ordinated with sleep and wakefulness. Temperature, for example, is seen to rise and fall over the 24-hour period, with its peak in the afternoon and its low—about 1 to 1.5 °C lower—between 2.00 a.m. and 5.00 a.m. Urinary output is also governed by a circadian rhythm, as the antidiuretic hormone, produced by the posterior pituitary lobe, demonstrates a rise and fall in blood concentration levels, being lowest during the night. Cortisol, secreted by the adrenal cortex, peaks in humans just before dawn to prepare for the day's energy expenditure, whilst in nocturnal animals, that peak is seen in the early evening.

Infradian rhythms (*infra* = below, *dies* = day) occur at a rate lower than once a day, that is, are seen in a cycle of longer than a day's duration.

Animal hibernation is an example as, once each year, there is a prolonged inactive period, during which the body temperature of the animal drops significantly. The annual migration of birds follows an infradian rhythm, as does the return of the salmon to its birthing grounds. The stag grows antlers in the spring and summer for use as weapons of horn in the fight with other stags for possession of the does of the herd in the rutting season. The antler growth signifies the rising levels of the testosterone cycle and once rutting is over and hormone levels drop, the horns are lost to be replaced in the spring.

Within humans, the female menstrual cycle follows an infradian rhythm. Neurons within the pre-optic portion of the hypothalamus initiate the cycle via the release of gonadotrophin releasing hormone (GRH) which acts directly upon the anterior pituitary, stimulating it to produce two hormones in a precise pattern of secretion. Initially, follicle stimulating hormone (FSH) is released and acts upon the hollow ball, or follicle, within the ovary that contains the ovum. Development of this follicle is accompanied by its release of oestrogen in increasing amounts, which reduces further secretion of the follicle stimulating hormone by the pituitary gland, and prompts it, instead, to release high levels of luteinizing hormone (LH). Luteinizing hormone provokes a rupture in the follicle wall and release of the mature ovum. The process of *ovulation* is complete within a period of 10–14 days, and, during this period of the cycle, the lining of the uterus regenerates, beginning the gradual development of the endometrium.

The remainder of the follicle is transformed into the corpus luteum which secretes progesterone under the influence of LH. Progesterone has two effects, for it increases the blood supply to the uterus, facilitating further development of the endometrium, in preparation for implantation of the fertilized ovum, and also signals the pituitary gland to reduce production of luteinizing hormone. Where the egg remains unfertilized, levels of progesterone fall as the corpus luteum begins to degenerate, and this loss of hormonal support causes a reduction in blood supply to the endometrium, which ultimately leads to its death and evacuation as menstrual flow. Following fertiliz-

ation, the corpus luteum continues to produce oestrogen and progesterone for approximately three months, when the placenta takes over the function.

Seasonal affective disorder is of interest here, for whilst most individuals feel a little less energetic and enthusiastic as winter months approach, this is usually a subtle change accompanied by a similar slight lowering of mood. However, it has been noted that, in areas near or above the Arctic Circle in Scandinavia, there is a higher rate of suicide in winter than in summer. The phenomenon is not solely restricted to Scandinavia, for some individuals find that a significant depressed mood coincides with the onset of winter, only to lift with the arrival of spring. Wehr and his colleagues (1979) reasoned that provision of artificial sunlight during the dark winter days may relieve lowered mood and therefore experimented with full spectrum fluorescent lamps. By bathing the individual in bright white light for a few hours each day to supplement exposure to natural light, depressed mood was relieved quite dramatically for some within a couple of days of treatment commencing. Perhaps this is indicative of a period within the human evolutionary history when the species hibernated in winter!

There is a third type of rhythm demonstrable, that is, one that occurs more frequently than once each day. *Ultradian rhythms* (*ultra* = beyond, *dies* = day) are most easily discussed within the context of the human for several hormones are secreted into circulation episodically and over the 24-hour period evince an ultradian rhythm. The problems experienced by Mitch Heller provide a useful example:

An American engineer, avid hockey player and all-round sports enthusiast, Mitch was involved in a road traffic accident in August 1978, and sustained a minor blow to the head. Within a month of the bump, Mitch noticed that his desire for sexual intercourse was waning and that his body and facial hair seemed to be disappearing. His general practitioner suspected damage to the hypothalamus and referred him to William Crowley an expert in the area (Crowley *et al.*, 1980).

A defect in hypothalamic secretion of gonado-trophin releasing hormone (GRH), which in men, in exactly the same mechanism as women, prompts the pituitary gland to release sex hormones. These hormones act upon the testes, facilitating both sperm manufacture and secretion of testosterone, which provides male characteristics including the sex urge. GRH had been successfully produced artificially and was therefore available for treatment.

Ernst Knobil and his team (1988) at the University of Pittsburgh had discovered, in studies of monkeys, that the hypothalamus releases GRH rhythmically, in short sharp bursts. This knowledge was utilized by Crowley in Mitch's treatment, for a needle was permanently inserted into Mitch's abdomen, attached to an automatic syringe and pump worn on his belt. A timing device made it possible to deliver injections of GRH at two-hourly intervals throughout the day and night, in exactly the same way as nature would have organized it, or as Crowley himself stated, 'Only by administering the hypothalamic message in a pulsatile fashion could the normal physiology and normal endocrine conversation of the hypothalamus, pituitary and gonads be mimicked'.

Whilst initially hating the injections and associated paraphernalia, by the end of the first week, Mitch hardly noticed them. His desire for sex quickly returned, along with the hair on his chest, and within six months of the treatment commencing, Mitch and his wife, Debbie, were expecting their first baby.

Another similarly subtle ultradian rhythm is occuring in approximately 90-minute cycles in the human throughout the day and night, as demonstrated by electroencephalographic recordings of brain activity. Human alertness and cognitive performance appear to follow this same cycle, with verbal and spatial matching tasks eliciting differing levels of competency and accuracy at different points of the cycle (Lavie and Kripke, 1975). As we will discuss later within this chapter, this 90-minute cycle has long been known in relation to

the sleep hours, but largely was unrecognized in relation to day-time activity.

MOTIVATION

Campbell (1989) in his excellent definition of the term 'behaviour' includes the phrases:

—the manner in which anything acts or operates. With regard to the human being, usually regards to the action of the individual as a unit. He may be, and ordinarily is, acting in response to some given organ or impulse, but it is his general reaction that give rise to the concept of behaviour.

People are driven towards particular behaviours because of a desire or need and as such are motivated. But what motivates us? We believe that the basic initiators of behaviour may be divided into two main categories—*personal survival* and *progenitive* (or perpetuating the species).

For personal survival, people need internal homeostasis and a degree of environmental control. We need a constant amount of water to operate normal functions and, as those functions include respiration, micturition, defaecation and perspiration as methods of waste product removal, fluid intake is a necessary drive. Growth, repair and general activities of living utilize energy and this is only sourced by continual food intake of appropriate materials. The body's machinery and processes are designed to work within a particular narrow range of temperatures and therefore control of body heat is an important drive to behaviour. To actively achieve homeostasis, movement is a necessity. People must similarly protect themselves from the hazards of the environment and the power of movement is again an essential characteristic for this. During evolution humans have discovered the values of affiliation with others of our kind, for there is not only a greater degree of safety from predators by this, but also a valuable pool of sexual partners, to facilitate dissemination of superior genes, and in addition assistance is available to gather and produce food. Humans are at their most vulnerable in the dark, when there is no artificial light available. As sleep fulfils necessary functions apart from merely resting organs, the ideal time to use was the hours of darkness, and therefore humans are by nature, nocturnally inactive. Similarly aggression is an instinct that motivates behaviour, for via such actions, the individual is able to defend self—and dependents—from harm and ensure a reliable supply of food.

This brings us to progenitor instincts. There is little value in achieving survival of one generation, if there is no second generation to ensure the continuation of the species. Sexual reproduction is the method through which that further generation is ensured and sexual behaviour is therefore an instinct, designed to maintain the race. It is likewise necessary to protect and nurture offspring until sufficiently mature to function as a self-sufficient unit, and therefore humans possess the drive towards nurturing behaviour.

MOVEMENT

Although a detailed analysis of motor functioning is not within the remit of this chapter, a brief reminder of its basic characteristics is necessary.

Basically, the system comprises of an information 'originator' within the motor cortex of the brain, a series of pathways, formed by motor nerves, and action 'effectors', in the form of muscles. Simplistically, an impulse arises in the motor cortex, as a response to a sensory input, which then tavels to the appropriate muscle causing contraction of that muscle and therefore movement.

With exceptions such as those provided by the eyeball and the tongue, the majority of the muscles in the body link two bones across a common joint, and, when activated by a motor nerve, contraction causes shortening and bulking of the muscle and movement of the end of the bone, farthest away from the body, towards the body. Each muscle that moves a bone in one direction, like this, has an opposing muscle, that pulls in the opposite direction, thus facilitating standing erect and steady, against the effects of gravity and also graduation of the degree of contraction required to effect the desired movement.

A motor nerve, when activated, releases a neurotransmitter, acetylcholine, into specialized receptor sites at the junction with the muscle tissue, thus facilitating passage of the impulse to that tissue. Any one muscle fibre is controlled by only one motor neuron, but one motor neuron may control numerous muscle fibres via branches in the axon depending on the fine or coarse nature of movements necessary. The muscle fibres of the thigh, for example, may have one neuron for every hundred or so fibres, whereas the movements of the eye are evinced by one neuron for every three muscle fibres. The larger the axon branch serving an area, the larger the muscle served, so for example those controlling the fine muscle movements of the fingers are proportionally smaller than those controlling the biceps of the forearm. The motor neurons, axons and muscles which they control are referred to as *motor units*. The fact that such muscles usually move on volition renders this type of movement *voluntary* in nature, thus differentiating between this and *reflex movement*. Motor neurons which originate in the motor cortex and terminate at a synapse, with a short connecting neuron in the spinal cord, or at cranial nerve nuclei are termed *upper motor neurons*. Those that actually terminate in the skeletal muscle are referred to as *lower motor neurons*.

Reflex movement is involuntary and protective in function. Humans have the ability to override such reflexes at times. Reflex activities are achieved via spinal cord command, in conjunction with assistance from local sensory receptors. *Proprioceptors*, tiny sensors within muscle and tendon tissue, monitor the position and tension evident within these tissues and relay that information via the spinal cord to higher, cortical motor centres. Thus the cortex is always aware of the precise current degree of angularity, muscle and tendon tension relating to body joints, and has a knowledge therefore of the degree of movement necessary in order to achieve new positioning. In reflex movement, activity is generated via the spinal cord and the higher centres are informed with some slight delay of the need for action, thus it may be observed that the painful finger has already been removed from the hot plate before cognitive awareness has occurred. Pain activates sensory fibres which carry the impulse to the spinal cord. In turn spinal motor neurons are activated directly and impulses for movement are evoked. Muscle activity occurs and flexion of the joint removes the painful area away from the stimulus provoking the response. To maintain equilibrium, a counter-balancing manoeuvre is evoked, so that, for example, if you should firmly plant a foot on a pin during walking, as the injured foot is removed by flexion of muscles, the muscles of the opposite leg—which was up in the air, in the process of taking the next step—extend to compensate for the imbalance. *Crossed extension*, or this opposing movement of the limbs, is achieved as the sensory fibre of the injured limb interacts with the spinal motor neuron which controls the opposite limb, as well as its own effector. Therefore cross-innervation within the spinal cord provides for reciprocal muscle control, and balance is achieved during both normal and emergency muscular activity, with synchronized arm and leg movements made automatically.

The motor cortex is, of course, the originator of voluntary movement, and this is arranged as a strip in each cerebral hemisphere, adjacent to those relating to somatosensory function. The neurons in both the motor and sensory areas are organized in patterns of column-like, vertical structures and form a *functional column*. You may recall the disproportionate amount of space devoted to different surfaces of the body in relation to the somatosensory cortex and the mis-shapen little person, or *homunculus*, which represents this allocation of sensory neurons. The motor cortex is entirely different in its organization, with motor columns required to achieve specific joint positions rather than actually activate muscles. The knowledge of the *status quo*, that is, the current joint, muscle and tendon positions, is already available to the motor cortex via proprioceptor communication. The motor column is thought to be responsible for all muscles acting upon a particular joint and that an impulse to move is actually a command to assume a specific joint position, which all related muscles effect, rather than being an instruction to the various individual muscles to assume different degrees of contraction.

Some cortical motor neurons, the *Betz cells*, communicate directly with motor cells of the spinal cord and their axons amalgamate to form a large bundle of nerve fibres, termed the *pyramidal tract*. On the descending path towards the spinal cord, the pyramidal tract arising from the right motor cortex and that from the left, cross over each other, the *decussation of the pyramids*, so that the right pyramidal tract is seen to control movement of the left side of the body and vice versa. Also on this downward journey to the spinal cord, many axons produce spurs, or collaterals, to connect with other brain structures, for example the red nucleus of the reticular formation, the basal ganglia and thalamus.

Extrapyramidal motor control is the term generally utilized to describe the influences upon motor activity of other brain structures, the most important of which are the *basal ganglia* (Fig. 8.1).

---

1   The basal ganglia are paired masses of grey matter in each cerebral hemisphere.

2   The largest of these is formed by the corpus striatum.

3   The corpus striatum may be anatomically divided into:
    (a) The caudate nucleus, thought to control large, subconscious movements, for example, swinging the arms whilst walking.
    In conjunction with:
    (b) The putamen (and the cortex) controlled patterns of movement are attained.
    (c) The globus pallidus, controls muscle tone and hence positioning of the body for complex movement. (The putamen and globus pallidus together form the lentiform nucleus.)

4   The claustrum, a thin sliver of grey matter, lateral to the putamen, and the amygdaloid nucleus are, on occasion, considered to be a part of the basal ganglia.

5   The subthalamic nucleus is thought to

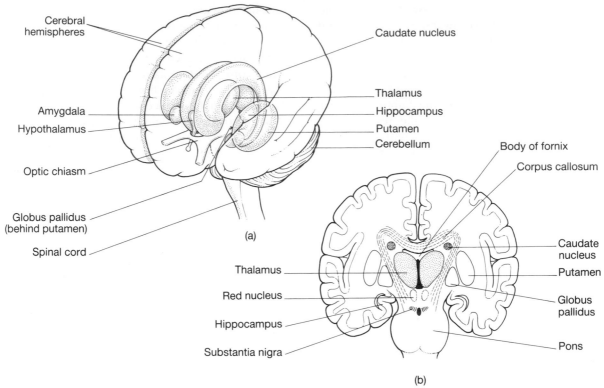

Fig. 8.1 *Basal ganglia of the brain (a) position of basal ganglia in the brain, (b) basal ganglia viewed in a coronal cross-section of the brain (from Hinchliffe and Montague, 1988).*

control walking and perhaps rhythmic movements.

6 The substantia nigra, comprising of dopa-mine-transmitting neurons which provide its colour, is necessary for smooth operation of the motor system, including the cortex, spinal cord and subcortical motivational control.

7 Potential functions of the basal ganglia are moderated, and therefore held in check, by the cerebrum.

The final area of significance for review in this section is that provided by the cerebellum, the large portion of tissue tucked underneath the cerebrum at the rear of the brain. It is attached to the brainstem by three pairs of fibre bundles, called the *cerebellar peduncles*, the *inferior* connecting it with the medulla, the *medial* with the pons and the *superior* to the midbrain. The grey matter on the surface of the cerebellum falls into fine, paral-lel ridges called *folia*, which, whilst increasing the surface area to accommodate an increased number of neurons, in the same manner as the convolutions or gyri of the cerebrum, are far less prominent. The white matter of the nerve fibres beneath the cerebellar cortex, resembles the branches of a tree and hence are termed *arbor vitae*. The *cerebellar nuclei* are small masses of neuronal tissue positioned deep within the white matter, just as the basal ganglia are subcortical to the cerebrum, and again like the cerebrum, the gross appearance of the cerebellum is of two hemispheres.

You may recall that, via proprioception, the motor cortex is made aware of the position of one joint in relation to all others and therefore is aware of changes necessary for continuing volun-tary movement. Impulses generated by the motor cortex pass to the pons and midbrain and thence via the middle and superior peduncles to the cerebellum. Subconscious impulses generated in response by the cerebellum pass via the inferior cerebellar peduncles to the medulla and spinal cord, and out to the muscles which will effect the voluntary movement desired. By inhibiting contraction of the opposing muscles, and stimulating the effector muscle to contract, smooth co-ordinated movement is achieved.

The cerebellum has connections with the inner ear and therefore is called into action when equilibrium is disturbed by the body leaning to the left or right. Impulses are initiated as a response by the cerebellum, causing contraction of appropriate muscles and restoration of balance. The area similarly controls postural muscles and therefore maintains muscle tone.

All areas are required to be fully functioning for voluntary movement and the defensive reflex activities to be performed. Proprioception is necessary for current knowledge of position, and therefore passage of impulses to the somatosensory cortex and an intact somatosensory cortex are a must. Transfer to the motor cortex plus the desire for particular movement activities provoke new instructions being sent via healthy motor neurones to skeletal muscles. Parallel and integrated modification via the basal ganglia and cerebellum provide smooth, co-ordinated, balanced and polished movement (Hinchliffe and Montague, 1988).

Of course, movement is influenced by so many factors, for example, by cognitive appraisal of a situation, by the emotional component of experiencing events within the environment, including interactions with others, and current motivation. Movement should, however, be goal directed, and therefore purposeful, synchronized and flowing.

PROBLEMS OF MOVEMENT

It is appropriate to start this section with an analysis of the degree of movement exhibited, ranging on a continuum of no movement to hyperactivity and you may be able to identify those aspects which might fall within healthy behaviour.

Many have experienced the phenomenon of being 'unable to move a muscle' and of remaining totally immobile for a period extending from a brief moment of time to several minutes. Conscious and aware but unable to move, perhaps because of shock, surprise or fear, such immobility is a well-known feature. You will no doubt be aware, however, of individuals who, whilst also conscious and aware, and despite a cognitive desire or intention to move are quite unable to achieve this because of some degree of *paralysis* being evident.

Paralysis

Paralysis simply infers a loss of power over muscle contraction and is a common manifestation of neurological problems. It may be exhibited as a total loss, or by a weakness, a *paresis*, and may be classified according to the extent of the affected area, for example, as *monoplegia*, a paralysis of one limb, *hemiplegia*, a loss of power to one side of the body, *paraplegia*, a loss of function in both lower limbs, or *quadriplegia*, where all four limbs are affected. Problems related to a paralysis of one side of the face plus paralysis of the opposite side of the body are occasionally seen and termed *alternate hemiplegia*, but all are indicative of a lesion within the central nervous system, the level of paralysis observable being indicative of the site of damage. You may have first-hand personal or professional knowledge of individuals experiencing hemiplegia associated with *cardiovascular accidents* (or strokes) or of individuals who have sustained damage to the cervical cord during a road traffic accident and are sadly paralysed from this point down. Both are unfortunately a common enough occurrence, and as paralysis is usually accompanied by loss of sensation to that area, the sequelae are obviously profound for the individual and their carers. Damage does not have to be of a central nervous system source, for a *peripheral nerve injury* may be sustained, resulting in the loss of contractile ability of one muscle of a group. This is an important distinguishing characteristic of the injury in regard to those paralyses seen within mental health care as will be demonstrated.

Some individuals may be predisposed to paralysis of skeletal muscle and a concomitant disturbance in the functioning of the body's smooth muscles, for example, cardiac and gut muscles, due to *hypokalaemia*, a depletion of potassium, necessary, amongst other functions, for the regulation of neuromuscular excitability and stimulation, and for nerve impulse transmission. Individuals who exteriorize a deficiency of potassium intake or an excessive loss, via prolonged vomiting and diarrhoea (including the individual experiencing problems of anorexia nervosa and bulimia), or use of diuretics or corticosteriod preparations are at risk. Muscle weakness, loss of tone and reflexes, and numbness gradually progresses to paralysis of arms, legs and respiratory muscles if untreated. Simultaneously, diminished peristalsis within the gastro-intestinal tract (a paralytic ileus) is demonstrated, with nausea, vomiting, abdominal distension and loss of bowel sounds and activity, and cardiac arrhythmias and increased sensitivity to digitalis may be seen.

Earlier we indicated that the *extent* of the paralysis is indicative of the site of the causative lesion, but the *type* of paralysis is also of significance. It may, for example, demonstrate retained reflex movements, exaggerated reflexes and hypertonicity (spasticity). This type of paralysis shows that damage is to the area of the cerebral cortex or pyramidal tracts and is termed therefore an *upper motor neuron lesion* or *spastic paralysis*. Injury lower down the pathway, in either the nuclei of cranial nerves, in the anterior columns of the spinal cord or the subsequent axons to the periphery, results in flaccidity because the reflex arc has been interrupted and therefore there is no reflex innervation or response. This represents a *lower motor neuron lesion* or *flaccid paralysis*.

All of the above is of great significance not only to the individuals experiencing the paralysis, who, it must be remembered, will have added problems to contend with besides the paralysis which result from the nature of the specific problem, but also for his carers and the professional within mental health services. Paralysis may be a feature of presentation where a deviation in mental health status is suspected and therefore differentiation between organic and psychogenic causation is necessary. Paralysis may be, for example, the major problem for an individual who has recently experienced one or more profound life stressors, such as unemployment, divorce or retirement. It

may be seen to develop within a three-month period of the event and is usually resolved within six months, and may be one of many features which become diagnosed as an *adjustment disorder*, causing impairment of social or occupational functioning and demonstrating an excessive reaction, above that considered expected or 'acceptable'. Similarly paralysis may be a problem where the diagnosis is one of *conversion disorder*, when the symptom is said to represent an expression or psychological conflict or need, and is associated with two elements of advantage. The first, or *primary gain*, keeps the conflict away from conscious awareness as, for example, a 'paralysed arm' will preclude the need for concern regarding a potential exteriorization of anger and damage to a loved one. The *secondary gain* may facilitate avoidance of an unpleasant activity and may evoke support from a previously or potentially hostile environment, and, again, an example may be provided by an individual who develops paraplegia, and whose wife therefore decides not to leave him for another man because of his inability to care for himself. The relative lack of concern regarding the problem—la belle indifference—may be suggestive of the nature of the symptom, but may also be exhibited by the stoic, but seriously ill, individual. Paralysis may also be seen in *somatization disorders*, where there is a persistent belief that one is 'sick' or has a specific physical complaint, and yet where medical opinion finds no evidence in support of this.

Since the 'paralyses' seen within mental health care correspond with the individual's subconscious ideas regarding the way the body works and performs, there are usually discrepancies in the area of distribution of the paralysis in comparison to that caused by an organic lesion, and symptomatology described is often physiologically impossible. Often when the individual attempts to move the 'affected' limb, as well as a strong prime mover-muscle contraction, a simultaneous contraction of the antagonistic muscle may be exhibited, thereby preventing any movement taking place. Such antagonistic contraction would not be evident when a 'true' paralysis exists and effort evokes little contraction of the prime mover at all. The 'hysterical paralysis' sufferer may exhibit a great expenditure of effort in his or her attempt to move the offending limb but with little result. The paralysis may appear flaccid or spastic, or there may be no disturbance of tone. Reflexes may be difficult to elicit but, when demonstrated, may be exaggerated or inconsistent, and are never diminished. Contractures and muscle wasting are rarely evident, except in situations where the problem has been exhibited for months or years. Even then, however, improvement may be achieved by electrical stimulation of antagonistic muscles, or under the influence of anaesthetic drugs.

You will no doubt recognize situations and circumstances where movement is possible but where individuals remain motionless and probably the best examples to be offered here are those that evince a total disregard or disinterest in the environment and that may occur for a variety of reasons. Deep thought and reflection is the commonest cause elicited for such behaviour within the general population, there being an intense concentration on some particular aspect of life and living which represents a challenge, problem or area of curiosity.

A reduced motor activity level is observable in those individuals experiencing a *mal-function of the thyroid gland* which results in insufficient secretion of its hormone, thyroxine. In the child, it is associated with a failure to achieve physical and cognitive milestones and a characteristic presentation of a limp, inactive, puffy and coarse-featured infant, the tongue often appearing too large for the mouth. The adult shows apathy, fatigue and the sequelae of decreased cellular metabolism, in addition to severely reduced activity levels. The latter may be considered as depressed or demonstrating the prodromal signs of organic impairment, on occasions, rather than somatically dysfunctioning.

Similarly, a reduced level of activity is associated with *Addison's disease* (primary adrenal insufficiency) and with the exteriorization of a lowered ability to cope with everyday stressors, tearfulness at the least cause, and the extreme fatigue and listlessness experienced, again may provoke thoughts of psychosocial rather somatic health problems. Irritability, impaired cognitive performance, and anorexia may compound the picture but the bronze/brown pigmented areas that develop on skin exposed to sunlight or friction is classically indicative of Addison's disease.

In mental health care, some individuals may experience extreme motor retardation, despite an intact motor system. The individual, for example, whose mood is *severely depressed* may appear as mute and motionless or, alternatively, exhibit a much reduced level of motor activity. *Catatonic stupor*, eliciting an almost total lack of reactivity to the environment, and a drastic reduction in spontaneous movement or activity, is a characteristic associated with a specific variation of the 'schizophrenia' group of syndromes. It may include features of *negativism*, in a passive resistance to being moved, *rigidity*, *posturing*, where an often bizarre position is voluntarily assumed and maintained for prolonged periods, and *waxy flexibility*, where limbs may be moulded into any position by an observer which will then be held by the individual for an indeterminable length of time. It appears that the individual's muscles do not feel fatigue in these postures assumed, or that such fatigue does not intrude upon conscious awareness. In many 'diagnostic classifications', where depressed mood is a feature, for example, *organic mood syndrome, phencyclidine mood disorder* and *primary dementia* of the *Alzheimer type with depression*, such catatonic behaviour may be evidenced in various degrees and shades.

Agitation

Accelerated motor activity may indicate that the mentally healthy individual is happy and optimistic, or terribly pressurized and rushed to achieve a goal. Sometimes a person may have so many priorities and stressors that this accelerated level of activity is unproductive, as there is a flitting to and from different targets with little being achieved. The anxiety levels may concomitantly rise, with the consistent failure to attain goals. Again, agitated behaviour may accompany both anxious and depressed moods, the individual finding difficulty in sitting still and settling to a specific task, needing to be mobile, active and occupied. Whether anticipating a pleasant or dreaded event, agitation may be a feature, and motor acceleration, a possibility.

A similar picture of agitation may be exhibited

by those individuals who have a neoplastic mass of the adrenal medulla—a *pheochromocytoma*. Its production of excessive amounts of epinephrine and norepinephrine causes hypertension, hyperglycaemia and hypermetabolism and therefore symptoms such as nausea, vomiting, air hunger, palpitations, nervousness, tremor and weakness are prominent. A severe and pounding headache, sweating, pallor, pupil dilation and tachycardia, complete a picture which could be that of anxiety. It is, however, a gradually increasing phenomenon, initially lasting for minutes, at most for hours. It is rarely of a continual nature. It is a problem, though relatively rare, that needs to be borne in mind by professionals.

Similarly *hyperthyroidism*, an excessive production of the thyroid hormone, may elicit agitated and hyperactive movement levels. The increased metabolic rate evoked by hypersecretion again provides a picture of nervousness, apprehension, irritability and restlessness, and may be indicative of an anxiety-type reaction. Gastro-intestinal symptoms, palpitations and shortness of breath are frequent features too, but an elevated sleeping pulse rate may be the observation that rings an alarm bell. The protrusion of the eyeballs (exopthalmos) and enlargement of the thyroid gland shown within textbook pictures may not always be evident or dramatic enough for a stranger to notice, and may have been so insidious in onset as to go relatively unnoticed by the family.

Within mental heatlh care, the prime example of hyperactivity must be that experienced by the individual labelled as '*bipolar mood disorder—manic episode*. The accelerated motor activity reflects the concomitant acceleration of cognitive processes, thought being rapid and transient, attention span severely limited, speech incoherent and circumstantial, and perceptions heightened. Social inhibitions are lost, and therefore there is a lack of insight into the implications of, what may be considered, grossly antisocial or meddling behaviour. Those individuals previously referred to as potentially experiencing catatonic stupor, its associated posture-related problems and negativisitic demonstrations, may similarly experience a *catatonic excitement* (or frenzy), where motor activity is highly accelerated, pur-

poseless and apparently not influenced by external stimuli. The transition from a stuporosed state to one of excitement, and vice versa, may be rapid and without warning, and may therefore evoke safety concerns in relation to the individual, other clients and carers. Whilst a potential problem in regards to any client evincing a lack of insight and accompanying hallucinatory and delusional experiences, it is more common in those where an organic aetiology is absent.

Agitation, in the form of pacing activities, a continual wringing of hands, pulling of clothes or playing with hair, is associated with individuals who feel tense and 'on edge'. You may hear the term utilized to describe varying degrees of restlessness accompanied by an excessive or increased motor activity, in a wide variety of individuals seeking mental health or assistance. The depressed or anxious person, those expressing phobic or intrusive thoughts, individuals experiencing problems associated with psychoactive substance use and those exhibiting problems provoked by organic impairment may all elicit such a problem.

MOVEMENT AND MENTAL DISORDERS

We mentioned within the last section the *rigidity* associated with catatonic behaviours and it may therefore be appropriate to consider other examples of the phenomenon, which may again provoke thought in regard to 'differential diagnosis'.

George was in his late 60s and had been an inpatient for many years. The various 'treatment' regimes utilized over those years, in efforts to ameliorate or eradicate mental health symptoms displayed, had achieved very little, for George continued to exhibit bizarre delusions and hallucinations, stereotyped and excited behaviour and the most dramatic catatonic posturing and posing features imaginable. Everyone in the hospital knew George, for, during medical and nurse education programmes, he would be identified as a valuable example of the various phenomena.

When, one morning, George 'refused' to bend in the middle and sit up for breakfast, no-one really thought it significant. Similarly when George vomited some dark brown granular fluid it was put down to his regular excursions into the ward bins and to eating cigarette tobacco. George did, however, not seem quite himself—the pallor of his skin was nothing so unusual but the cold, clammy sweating was and, whilst he didn't groan or appear to be in discomfort, his features seemed pinched and taut.

The morning saw no improvement and the doctor, doing his daily visits, was asked to see him. George was promptly diagnosed as suffering from peritonitis, and sent to the general hospital following commencement of intravenous fluid administration and nasogastric intubation. Laparotomy revealed a perforated duodenal ulcer, and, though seriously ill for some days, George made a full recovery.

People receiving mental health care may become somatically ill just like anyone else and yet, at times, symptomatology exhibited is assumed to be a 'part of the mental condition'. In George's instance—and many others—objective analysis and reflection of problems observed may just be a life-saver. The *board-like rigidity of abdominal muscles*, accompanied by 'coffee ground' vomit (*haematemesis*), clinical shock and pain are classical signs of irritation of the contents of the abdomen by some foreign substance and is usually indicative of a 'leak' from some part of the gastrointestinal tract. Observation by carers becomes even more important when an individual's ability to communicate and insight into reality is impaired by mental health problems.

Spasms

Painful spasms (*trismus*) leading to rigidity of the jaw and the distortion of facial muscles are the initial indicator of *tetanus*, the invasion of the nervous system by *Clostridium tetani*, a bacillus that gains entry through an open wound, and which is found in soil and the faecal material of both animals and humans. Whilst less commonly seen in this country in these days of prophylactic immunization, the all-encompassing and progressive muscle rigidity that results in cessation of respiratory function and the back arching off the bed (*opisthotonos*) is one of those experiences never to be forgotten. The spasms increase in frequency and severity for about 10 days but may be controlled with tranquillizers/sedatives and muscle relaxants. Human tetanus immunoglobulin and antibiotics are also administered and tracheostomy may be necessary. The spasms are associated with any sort of stimulation—noise, touch, movement—and therefore gentle handling and good communication prior to any attention given is the order of the day.

Rigidity

The *decerebrate*, or *decorticate rigidity* seen following the rupture of a cerebral aneurysm and severe haemorrhage into the subarachnoid space also provides a classical picture. The person is moribund and unresponsive. The adduction of the arms, flexion of arms, wrists and fingers, extension and internal rotation of lower limbs and plantar flexion exhibited is the result of interruption of the corticospinal tract, usually in the midbrain or poris. Such aneurysms are frequently asymptomatic until rupture occurs, which is often associated with psychological stress or physical strain and which produces sudden severe headache, nausea and vomiting and, in some instances, loss of consciousness. The decerebrate rigidity referred to signifies an extensive bleed and carries a poor prognosis, but many individuals with lesser bleeds will demonstrate *nuchal rigidity*, where the neck is stiff and attempts towards flexion provoke pain. A similar neck rigidity, to which flexion is resisted, is observable in individuals who suffer meningitis.

Hypoparathyroidism

Hypoparathyroidism, resulting in a fall in plasma calcium levels with a concomitant rise in phosphate concentration, will result in *tetany*, and demonstrate an increased excitability of nerves, pins and needle sensations (*paraesthesia*) and muscle spasm. *Carpopedal spasms*—flexion of the metacarpophalangeal joints and extension of the interphalangeal joints of the thumb and fingers— in adults and, more commonly, *laryngeal spasm* in children, are common findings. Hypoparathyroidism is fequently a complication of thyroidectomy, when parathyroid glands are removed along with a portion of an overactive thyroid. It may, however, be an idiopathic problem and a wide variety of mental health disturbances are associated with hypoparathyroidism. Robinson *et al.* (1954) reported the case of a 51-year-old woman who presented with status epilepticus, developed dementia-like symptoms and only 10 days after admission began to demonstrate signs of parathyroid deficiency. Fourman *et al.* (1967) studied 33 individuals, all of whom had previously undergone thyroidectomy, and whose mental health diagnoses were related to anxiety and panic attacks or depression. A quarter of the population studied showed calcium levels at the 'low end of normal' and yet no other indicators of parathormone problems were exhibited. Calcium citrate tablets were found to produce a significant amelioration in symptomatology, particularly in relation to lowered mood and poor appetite. Whilst more rare, schizophrenia and bipolar mood disorder, mixed, have also been presenting features of this endocrine problem and Denko and Kaelbling (1962) on discovering several clients similarly mislabelled as 'mentally retarded', suggest that serum calcium levels should be investigated as a routine on admission to facilities for those with learning disabilities. We repeat the plea in relation to individuals 'apparently' experiencing mental health problems.

Alkalosis/alkalaemia

The carpopedal spasms of tetany are a feature of any situation in which a rise in PH (the acid–alkaline continuum) of plasma is provoked, that is, an *alkalosis*, or *alkalaemia*. Severe vomiting, a depletion of potassium and burns may all be causative of a *metabolic alkalaemia*, whilst hyperventilation may engender *respiratory alkalaemia*. This is, of course, of great interest to those working within the sphere of mental health care, for the individual experiencing problems associated with generalized anxiety or panic attacks, or

indeed any diagnostic category in which anxiety presents as a major feature, may exhibit hyperventilation and therefore potentially may be prone to tetany and carpopedal spasms. Hyperthyroidism and fever may similarly provoke hyperventilation, as may certain central nervous system lesions—cerebrovacsular accidents, subarachnoid haemorrhage and meningitis.

Parkinsonism

The rigidity associated with Parkinsonism is again 'classical'. It affects both small and large muscles of the limbs, trunk and neck and agonists and antagonists equally. It may be unilateral, is unaffected by emotion and is found to persist during sleep. Limbs resist passive extension, the so-called *lead pipe rigidity*, and the combination of rigidity plus tremor demonstrates the *cogwheel rigidity*, best elicited by grasping the individual's hand, as in a hand shake, and alternately pronating and supinating the hand. As Parkinsonism is evoked by a variety of problems including neuroleptic drug administration, it may be valuable to shake hands with that individual on a regular basis, in an attempt to elicit minor changes in function. Parkinsonism tends to creep up on carers, who see the individual regularly and hence may not notice prodromal indicators of a problem.

Mannerisms

Voluntary movement is, by design, purposeful, smooth and co-ordinated but yet again there are exceptions to the rule. Many, if not most, people exhibit habitual movements and characteristic mannerisms which are apparently purposeless— and perhaps an irritant—to an onlooker and yet which are utilized on a more or less regular and even predictable basis. The automatic adjustment of spectacles when one is expected to make some reply to a statement from another individual, pulling an earlobe or earring during conversation, clearing the throat on cue, or twiddling a piece of hair, may all be habits that have been acquired. In the past the movement may have provided great value—comfort as felt by the thumb-sucking child, a focus of attention in an awkward or uncomfortable situation, such as playing with a loose thread on a hem, or as a relief of inner tension or anxiety, by, for example, sorting, straightening, lining up or generally tidying the immediate environment. The habit may have been found to be a valuable preparation for ensuing activities, for by clearing the throat prior to speaking it may prevent the necessity during speech and hence becomes habitual. Similarly a mannerism may provide useful thinking time and have acceptably covered slight hesitations in communication and so become integral or automatic in certain situations. Many classes—and not just those of children and early adolescents—have a mimic, who will entertain his peers in the breaktimes, or behind teacher's back, by imitating that individual's mannerisms and some manage to earn a very successful living at it. Mannerisms tend to be an individual's 'trademark' and hence are integral to behaviour.

Stereotyped movement

Mannerisms may be seen in an exaggerated form in several situations, for example, when an individual becomes pressurized or hassled, but when the patterned responses become a monotonously and frequent performed aspect of behaviour, the term *stereotyped movement* may be applied. This may be seen in the form of a single, or group, of actions or in the assumption of an unusual posture or position which may be maintained long after muscle fatigue would normally have forced cessation of the activity.

Stereotypic blindism may be associated with people who are congenitally blind. Activities such as head rocking, pressing the eyeballs, directing the eyes towards strong lights and exaggerated 'smelling' of objects or people, may all be utilized by an individual to create or increase sensory stimulation. On occasions, individuals may, knowing their propensity to self-injury during such activities, assume self-restraining characteristics, for example, keeping hands in pockets or inside a shirt or other clothing, and thereby assume another stereotyped activity.

Non-functional and apparently purposeless activities such as headbanging, body rocking, slapping, biting or picking movements, may be exhibited by individuals who have serious learning difficulties and profound multiple handicaps. The diagnosis of *stereotypy/habit disorder* relates to a wide number and variety of intentional and repetitive movements which may include teethgrinding (bruxism), air swallowing (aerophagia), breath holding and hyperventilation, all in a rhythmic fashion. *Pervasive developmental disorders*, the best known being that of *autistic disorder*, are diagnostic categories utilized to describe children whose development within spheres of reciprocal social interaction, verbal and non-verbal communication skills and imaginative activity are severely and qualitively impaired. Children with such problems demonstrate motor and verbal stereotypies. Hand clapping and peculiar hand movements, such as flapping, body rocking, dipping and swaying actions and repetitious sniffing and smelling of objects or feeling of textures may all be examples of stereotypies seen.

On occasions, stereotype motor activities may be seen to enable individuals experiencing the sequelea of progressive organic impairment to cope with everyday life and living activities. *Overly-orderliness* may be utilized to compensate for perceived deficits in intellectual organization, emotional control or social awareness, as the individual demonstrates a rigid adherence to routine and repeated checking activities. *Perseveration*, the repetition of a recent movement, despite the individual's efforts towards production of a new movement and *literative* phenomena, as endless reptition of words or phrases (*echolalia*) may therefore be a feature in the presentation of many individuals seeking assistance.

Stereotyped movements of the mouth and tongue, and sorting and piling manoeuvres are seen in situations where amphetamines or cocaine intoxication is creating problems for the individual and repetitive motor activities and grimacing are similarly a feature of phencyclidine intoxication. The face pulling in 'catatonic-schizophrenia' may include the lips being thrust forwards like an animals's snout (schnauzkramp), and is accompanied by bizarre and excited stereotype movements. The shorter duration 'schizophreniform disorder' may elicit similar characteristics as may manic episodes of mood disorders, and, whilst all may begin as an expression of emotional tension, or have a special and complex, almost magical, significance, they tend to become habitual and be produced automatically. The *compulsive* element of obsessive–compulsive behaviour differs somewhat in that the continued performance of ritualistic, stereotyped behaviour relieves the tensions and anxieties experienced and is therefore purposeful and intentionally conducted or initiated.

Tremors

Tremors are also something that you may have personal, or previous professional, experience of.

Her hands trembled and her knees shook, her legs feeling weak and powerless as he approached her. She could almost hear her racing heart as it thumped, in an effort to escape the ribcage which confined it ….

The stuff that 'Mills and Boon' paperbacks are made of or an 'encounter in the Mummy's tomb'? Suffice to say, people experience a tremor when angry, afraid or anxious, or alternatively when excited or full of anticipation for a pleasurable event. Tremor may be an integral part of any emotion and, just to destroy completely the romantic associations which may have been provoked by the above example, we will reveal that a tremor represents a rhythmic and repetitive movement induced by alternating contractions of antagonistic muscle groups. Three variations of tremor are clearly distinguishable, the *rest tremor* is more pronounced at rest, the *intention tremor* worse on initiation of voluntary movement and the *postural tremor* is exaggerated, for example, when limbs are outstretched.

Rest tremor is a characteristic of *Parkinsonism*, with Parkinson's disease reflecting just one cause of the clinical picture demonstrated. Parkinsonism may be drug induced (neuropletics), a sequelae of encephalitis or arteriosclerotic changes, or may be the result of repeated head trauma, for example, as in boxing. It may be seen following anoxia and carbon monoxide poisoning, as well as

many other events. The rest tremor of Parkinsonism is *coarse*, and demonstrates a characteristic '*pill-rolling*' action as the thumb moves across the fingers. It is the result of interference with, or degeneration of, the dopaminergic neurons in the substantia nigra and is accompanied by *bradykinesia*, a slowness in initiating and executing movement, including facial muscles and those related to speech production, and *rigidity*. The tremor of Parkinsonism is more resistant to amelioration by medication than the bradykinesia and rigidity experienced.

Intention tremor is associated with cerebellar lesions—tumours, aneurysms, abscesses, etc.— and is therefore often accompanied by *ataxia*, *dysarthria*, *nystagmus* and *dysdiadokinesis* (poor, rapid alternating movements). Multiple sclerosis is one of the best examples of a 'discrete' somatic problem associated with such lesions, as the degeneration of the myelin sheath and resultant secondary destruction of axons, whilst scattered throughout the brain and spinal cord, are more common around the sites of the lateral ventricles and cerebellum. In response to destruction, glial cells proliferate and lymphocytes and macrophage cells infiltrate the tissues, the subsequent scar tissue being macroscopically visible in the affected brain by translucent plague distribution. The neurological manifestions associated with multiple sclerosis are multifocal and relapsing in nature, providing serially gained evidence of the lesions produced, rather than an immediately obvious, visible diagnosis.

Early symptoms of oculomotor function (diplopia or nystagmus), lesion of the long sensory and/or motor tracts of the cord (paraesthesia or spastic paraparesis) and cerebellar involvement (ataxia and intention tremor) may settle in weeks or months, leaving no or little residual disability. Further attacks may bring new symptoms or exacerbate pre-existing ones, with relapses and remissions demonstrating a variable course. Most frequently, a progressive and accumulatory picture develops and the individual experiences multiple handicaps. A slight intellectual impairment has been elicited in Surridge's study (1969) particularly in relation to memory for recent events when it is often accompanied by confabulation, perseveration and dysphasia. Non-verbal reasoning abilities seemed similarly impaired along with general intellectual efficiency. Mood disturbances are also a common problem, with both depressed and elevated affect seen. Often depression is an early, and understandable, feature, whilst euphoria is more common as the lesions progress. Koenig (1968) described seven individuals who had presented and were diagnosed as dementia, with relatively silent neurological manifestations. Careful neurological investigation had elicited the disseminated central nervous system lesions of multiple sclerosis and Koenig therefore suggested that silent MS may be a commoner cause of organic impairment than had previously been assumed or recognized. We will return to this point later.

Postural tremor is relatively more commonly seen than either rest or intention tremor, and may arise as a result of a variety of problems. Transmission, for example, of an autosomal dominant gene may elicit tremor of the arms and head in an individual of any age within an affected family. *Benign essential tremor* is rarely progressive, but may be suppressed by moderate amounts of alcohol or, in about one-third of individuals, by propranolol or primidone medication. Similarly, *Wilson's disease* or *hepatolenticular degeneration*, transmitted via an autosomal recessive gene, is a problem associated with metabolism of copper and may present as a hepatic dysfunction (40%), a neurological disorder (40%) or a mental health related behavioural disorder (20%) (Bearn, 1972). Jaundice, liver and spleen enlargement (hepatosplenomegaly), ascites and ankle oedema may all develop, and rupture of oesophageal varicies (dilated veins in collateral circulation at the oesophago-gastric junction, 'haemorrhoids' in the oesophagus) may result in haematemesis. Neurologically, tremor may be one of several manifestations—rigidity, athetoid writhing movements and dystonic postures of the limbs. The tremor may be seen as a 'flapping' movement of the wrists, or a 'wing-beating' motion when arms are abducted and elbows flexed. The facial expression is stiff and the mouth is open and bears a rigid smile. Seizures, paralyses and disturbances in consciousness are not uncommon. A severe change in personality characteristics, hallucinations, delusional ideation, euphoria and catato-

nia and fatuous silliness have all been noted in relation to Wilson's disease. Whilst a rare condition, Scheinberg *et al.* (1968) found that more than one-quarter of the 49 individuals studied demonstrated mental health related problems as the first indicator of a dysfunction. Walker (1969) identified that all 12 of the people he studied had similarly developed mental health status deviations primarily and had been treated with drugs, electroplexy and psychotherapy.

Some early cognitive impairment, minor speech difficulties or distractibility provided the only evidence of neurological dysfunction in these individuals who had been categorized as school phobic, behaviour problem, personality disorder, depression, hysteria, schizophrenia and mental retardation. Eye examination, utilizing a slit lamp, will reveal the *Kayser–Fleischer ring*, a brown or greyish-green circle at the margin of the cornea and which may be visible to the naked eye. No Kayser–Fleischer ring—no Wilson's disease, and as treatment may significantly improve the indvidual's health status, and as symptom-free siblings may respond well to prophylactic attention, slit-lamp examination would seem to be a sensible inclusion in client examination. Postural tremor may arise, therefore, from genetic transmission.

It may similarly be demonstrated due to metabolic dysfunctions, for example, where carbon dioxide retention (*hypercapnia*) is a problem, as in respiratory disease, respiratory muscle disease, left ventricular heart failure and brainstem lesions. Yet again the 'flapping tremor', previously described, is evident. Coarse tremor is a feature of other metabolic dysfunction, such as that associated with liver failure, when it may be referred to as *liver flap*.

Postural tremor may be exhibited as an exaggerated physiological mechanism associated with thyrotoxicosis, where as in anxious individuals, a *fine finger tremor* is witnessed. Perhaps attention may usefully be directed at this point to the indicators that may ring a warning bell and evoke concerns towards a diagnosis of thyroid problems rather than purely psychosocial aetiology. Any sensitivity to heat and an individual's expressed preference for cold conditions and environments should ring that bell. Similarly the appetite of the 'thyrotoxic' individual is characteristically increased and yet there is a concomitant steady weight loss evident. The individual experiencing anxiety, when complaining of weight loss, typically complains of a poor appetite and reduced intake of food to boot. Some people are equally likely to put on weight when anxious, via 'comfort eating' and in this instance, thyrotoxicosis is not a differential diagnosis which evokes concern. A simple blood test may ascertain certain diagnosis where suspicions are raised.

The fine finger tremor of anxiety is often accompanied by complaints of disordered sensation—numbness (*anaesthesia*) and pins and needles (*paraesthesia*)—and by muscle tension and restlessness. Similarly, tremors may find exteriorization within somatically orientated mental health problems, for example, in *conversion* and *somatoform disorders*, where motor symptomatology associated with anaesthesias, paraesthesias, paralyses and co-ordination disturbances are frequent foci of attention. Tremors are a common experience in psychoactive substance intoxication and withdrawal with, for example, those individuals withdrawing from alcohol and sedatives, hypnotics and anxiolytic substances demonstrating a coarse tremor of hands, eyelids and tongue, as well as, on occasions, myoclonic jerks. Intoxication frequently produces tremor, incoordination and an unsteady gait.

Tics

Tics are involuntary in nature, and may be described as sudden, rapid, recurrent though non-rhythmic, stereotyped movements, or vocalizations. Simple tics, such as eye-blinking, neck jerking, coughing and grunting may be seen in childhood, and are always exacerbated by stress and greatly diminished during sleep. Tics may appear and disappear almost overnight for some, although any recurrence is always associated with stress. On occasions, multiple tics are seen and whilst at times these may revolve around the facial area, whole head, torso and limb involvement may also be a problem. Where more than one tic is evident, these may appear simultaneously, sequentially or randomly, and whilst

some individuals may become adept at suppressing them for varying lengths of time, they are eventually irresistible. Children and young adolescents affected are frequently seen to be 'uncomfortable' with themselves and social situations, and this may obviously lead to depressed mood.

Tourette's disorder is probably the best known of the pathological categories seen and involves multiple motor and one, or more, vocal tics which may appear simultaneously or at different points along the course of development. They are manifest several times a day, most days, and whilst typically affecting the head area, may also involve the rest of the body too. The vocal tics may resemble barks, grunts, yelps, sniffs or words, and *coprolalia* (uttering obscene words) may be a problem for approximately one-third of all sufferers. Lesser extremes of the Tourette disorder may be seen in some who demonstrate motor or vocal tics but not both, which may be referred to as a *chronic motor* or *vocal tic*, and where the duration of the problem is seen to be of less than 12 months, a *transient tic disorder* may be diagnosed.

Myoclonus is an involuntary, unexpected and sudden jerk of a muscle, or part of a muscle, and you may have experience of the phenomenon when dropping off to sleep at night. However, as well as being an innocent and benign occurrence, myoclonus may be indicative of serious somatic health problems. It may be seen, for example, in childhood as *benign essential myoclonus*, when it is associated with an autosomal dominant genetic inheritance. Similarly it may be indicative of encephalopathy in response to a variety of metabolic disorders, for example, lysosomal storage enzyme deficits, and focal myoclonic jerks may herald viral myelitis. Both single and multiple myoclonic jerks are associated with epilepsy, and, as epilepsy should be regarded as a symptom rather than as a specific dysfunction or entity in its own right, myoclonus may be associated with somatic health problems ranging in aetiology from trauma to space-occupying lesions, encephalitis to syphilis, hypo- and hyperglycaemia to hypo/hypernatraemia, and from liver to renal disease. Drugs may precipitate seizures, phenothiazines, tricyclics and cocaine may all be culpable, and similarly withdrawal from alcohol, sedatives, hypnotics and anxiolytic preparation may provoke myoclonus and seizures. There is, however, a rare epilepsy that is associated with inheritance via autosomal recessive gene. The *myoclonic epilepsy of Unverricht* comprises of increasingly frequent myoclonic jerks and a severe and progressive dementia. The link between epilepsy and myoclonus is well recognized.

Creutzfeldt–Jakob disease has recently been brought to public attention via the problems of 'mad cow disease' or *bovine spongeiform encephalopathy* (BSE). A progressive organic deterioration in which the grey matter of the brain degenerates and assumes a spongy appearance, the aetiology is one of a slow viral nature. Survival usually appears to be of a period not exceeding two years' duration, the individual sinking into a coma for several weeks prior to death. Myoclonic jerks and epilepsy are frequent features, and may be accompanied by spasticity, progressive paralysis or choreoathetoid movements. Speech may be impaired, with dysarthria and dysphasia, and cortical degeneration may provoke blindness. Neurological features vary considerably and are dependent, of course, upon structures involved. Progressive intellectual and neurological deterioration, with, on occasions, auditory hallucinations and delusional ideation demonstrated, leads to a profound dementia, spastic paralysis and severe emaciation.

The similarities between Cruetzfeldt–Jakob's disease, Kuru and 'scrapie' have long since been linked. *Kuru* is a dementia, restricted to the Fore tribe of New Guinea and, again, the sequelae of a transmissible agent, although genetic predisposition and a 'taste', in the past, for cannibalism may also have a role in transmission. *Scrapie* is a degenerative brain disease of sheep and is also the agent discovered in some forms of Creutzfeldt–Jakob's disease. All result in this spongy appearance of the brain and therefore are, in the present climate, worthy of further investigation, via, for example, the work of Beck and his colleagues (Beck *et al.*, 1966, 1969a,b). Links between scrapie and BSE are already confirmed, with aetiology of the latter firmly laid on feeding affected cows with infected sheep offal. Concern for human health must be raised in this regard.

Of course tics and myoclonus must be differentiated from a wide number of involuntary and more complex patterns of movement, for example, *choreiform movements*, which tend to be irregular, random, non-repetitive dance-like movements. These are semi-purposive and involve muscle groups of the face, limbs or trunk and, as in Huntington's chorea, which is inherited via an autosomal dominant gene, may begin as small tics or mannerisms, which are easily disguised, but progress to involve the whole body. That associated with an inflammatory encephalitis, Sydenham's chorea (or St Vitus' dance), may be seen to resolve slowly over several months but may recur at a later date. *Athetosis*, a slow writhing movement of fingers, hands and arms, is associated with damage to the putamen and globus pallidus and *hemiballismus*, characterized by sudden, forceful, violent and flailing movements of one side of the body, and commonly affecting proximal muscles of the limbs, is associated with subthalamic nucleus damage. It is, on occasions, a feature following cerebrovascular accidents, particularly in elderly diabetic individuals and usually subsides within months of the lesion. *Dystonia* are distressing, painful and involuntary muscular contractions which may commonly be associated with the eye, facial, neck, lingual and spinal muscles and more rarely the limbs. *Dystonia musculorum deformans* describes a generalized torsion dystonia, of unknown aetiology and yet with an apparently genetic basis in some instances, which is severe and progressively crippling. Anoxia or jaundice at birth may create a similar problem, as may tumours and infarctions of the basal ganglia. Cerebral pathology is known therefore to cause such problems, and the *oculogyric crises* and *spasmodic torticollis* occasionally seen following neuroleptic administration would appear to support such a view. However, there continues to be some dispute as to the organic versus psychogenic causation of several dystonias, including spasmodic torticollis, writer's cramp and blepharospasm.

Akathisia is similarly a problem associated with involuntary movement and again with neuroleptic use. The individual complains of an inability to stand or sit still and rocks, paces, shifts from foot to foot or taps his feet continuously, feeling 'tightened up and out of control'. This purposeless limb movement may be accompanied by myoclonus and a coarse tremor.

Tardive or *oro-facial dyskinesia* represents another extrapyramidal side-effect of neuroleptic use. It occurs in 1–2% of individuals administered such preparations for a year or more, though this risk is seen to increase in a variety of situations, for example, with increasing age (elderly women are said to be most at risk), increasing dosage and administration period, where there is underlying cerebral pathology and with anti-cholinergic medication, which may exacerbate existing, or expose latent, symptomatology. It may be seen to be reversible in only one-third of presentations (Appleby and Forshaw, 1990). Problems experienced by the individual include involuntary chewing, mouth and jaw movements, and grimacing. Mild choreiform movements of the extremities, shoulder shrugging and rocking actions may also be evident. An early, prodromal, indicator of the problem is the individual's inability to stick out (extrude) his tongue and keep it there for a minute or two. On occasions, a *tardive dystonia* or *tardive Tourette's syndrome* have also been exhibited in relation to neuroleptic use.

Ataxia

You may recall the previously identified need for proprioceptive information via skeletal muscles and tendons to facilitate kinaesthetic knowledge, that is, where and in what position limbs are currently in relation to the rest of the body position. *Ataxia* is the term used to describe a loss of that proprioceptive sense, with the result that there is a lack of co-ordination of muscle action between the extremities and the head and trunk. The individual is not quite sure of his position and is unable therefore to judge or control skeletal movements. The cerebellum, which receives all information concerning this orientation and is therefore crucial in co-ordination of such activities, may be elicited as the site of a lesion which evokes ataxia. The 'finger to nose' test is failed and a characteristic gait of staggering, reeling, erratic steps, with perhaps a deviation to one side is seen. This *cerebellar gait* is also characterized by the vigorous projection of the legs forwards and the forceful slapping of the feet on to the

floor. If truncal ataxia is seen to be worse when the individual's eyes are closed, the lesion is in the dorsal columns, the spinocerebellar tracts, rather than the cerebellum. *Friedreich's ataxia*, one of the commonest hereditary diseases of the nervous system, is also one of the commonest spinocerebellar ataxias seen. It is inherited via an autosomal recessive or, rarely, sex-linked gene, and with an onset typically in childhood or the teenage years, it may be mistaken for the 'normal' clumsy, inco-ordinated motor behaviour of youth. Spinocerebellar tracts degenerate, so that the original unsteadiness of gait progresses to the broad-based, lurching action associated with cerebellar dysfunction. Dysarthria, nystagmus and dysdiadochokinesis are all accompanying features. Myocardial involvement and optic atrophy may occur and characteristic deformities of musculature as *kyphoscoliosis*, a forward and lateral curvature of the spine and *pes cava*, a shortened, inverted, high arched foot, with clawed toes may precede neurological symptomatology.

Wernicke–Korsakoff's syndrome, often incorrectly solely linked with alcohol abuse, is in fact the result of a thiamine (vitamin B_1) deficiency of a variety of causes—dietary deficiency, pernicious anaemia, carcinoma of the stomach as well as alcohol-related problems. The problems demonstrated are the sequelae of tiny haemorrhages, particularly in the area surrounding the ventricles of the brain, with cell loss and subsequent glial and vascular proliferation. The *staggering gait* is accompanied by ataxia, demonstrated as the inability to stand upright and steady without support and on occasions by an inability to walk heel to toe, as along a straight line. These tests are of course utilized to assess an individual's capability to drive in relation to alcohol ingestion, indicating that intoxication will elicit similar, though temporary, features. Wernicke's encephalopathy is considered as the acute reaction to the causative factor and an emergency situation, whilst Korsakoff's is considered to be the stage of permanent damage. They represent two points on the same continuum, and may both elicit, therefore, confusion, nystagmus and eye muscle weakness or paralysis (*ophthalmoplegia*). The latter, due to third nerve lesion, shows an outward deviation of the eyeball and a dilated pupil, which is unresponsive to light and accommodation. *Ptosis*, a drooping of the upper lids, is also evident.

The *high-stepping gait* indicative of the *sensory ataxia* of *tabes dorsalis*, due to neurosyphilis, demonstrates the effect on co-ordination of degeneration of the ascending fibres. The individual describes the sensation of 'walking on cotton wool', with extreme skin hypersensitivity, paraesthesia in the legs and feet and severe, sharp, episodic stabbing pains in the legs which may extend to the trunk as girdle pains.

Whilst mentioning the specific gaits associated with ataxia, it is worth noting the characteristic *small-stepped gait* of *multi-infarct dementia*, the shuffling, flexed trunk, *festinant gait* of Parkinsonism and the *scissor gait* associated with spasticity of the lower limbs, where one leg is placed directly in front of the other and where thighs and legs are abducted, the knees rubbing with each step. The amount of information available by mere observation of the manner in which an individual walks into a room can be astounding.

Apraxia

We feel obliged to refer to one more phenomenon prior to closure of this section on movement and its related problems, and this relates to *apraxia*, the inability to execute purposive co-ordinated movement despite intact sensory and motor function and the desire to perform that movement. The association cortex of the parietal lobes, and particularly that of the non-dominant hemisphere, is responsible for an awareness of the body and the relationship between objects in the environment. Lesions within the non-dominant hemisphere lead to *constructional apraxia*, a defect in assembling or drawing items and *dressing apraxia*, where the individual is unable to get limbs into garments or clothing over the head. *Ideomotor apraxia*, an inability to perform a series of co-ordinated movements despite an understanding of request preceding it, is a feature of dominant parietal lobe lesion. *Gait apraxia* may be the explanation for a gait disorder when each of the separate components required for walking are found to be intact. It is seen to be

a problem where lesions affect bilateral frontal lobes or posterior temporal lobe regions. *Ideational apraxia* finds the individual 'unaware' of the co-ordinated actions necessary to achieve a task, for example, taking a match from a closed box of matches and striking it. The concepts of the required acts and the planning of the act both appear disturbed. It is always bilateral, usually a lesion of the dominant hemisphere and most frequently of parietal or temporal lobe origin. Apraxias are more often evident where damage is diffuse rather than localized and therefore cognitive and intellectual functioning is frequently impaired.

SUMMARY

We have outlined some of the problems associated with movement and provided examples of these problems both within somatic and mental health care specialties. There are very fine dividing lines at times between the two fields and frequently incorrect diagnosis is a potential. Clients have been admitted to mental health and learning disability care facilities when somatic health care was necessary and examples of somatic care being offered or instigated where problems are of a predominantly psychosocial origin abound. It is, therefore, of vital importance that the health care worker, regardless of the specialty service provided, has an awareness of what is on the 'other side' of that fine dividing line and is therefore competent to ask appropriate questions of the client, based upon that knowledge and the observations made. It is imperative that entrance into mental health orientated services does not evoke an assumption that problems exteriorized or experienced are automatically psychogenic in origin. Investigation may prove a somatic basis for the symptomatology, which may be eradicated or ameliorated with appropriate care and treatment. Similarly the individual with a history of psychosocial problems and mental health care *can* become physically ill in the same way as any other member of society and that any alteration in functioning is worthy of further exploration. Remember George!

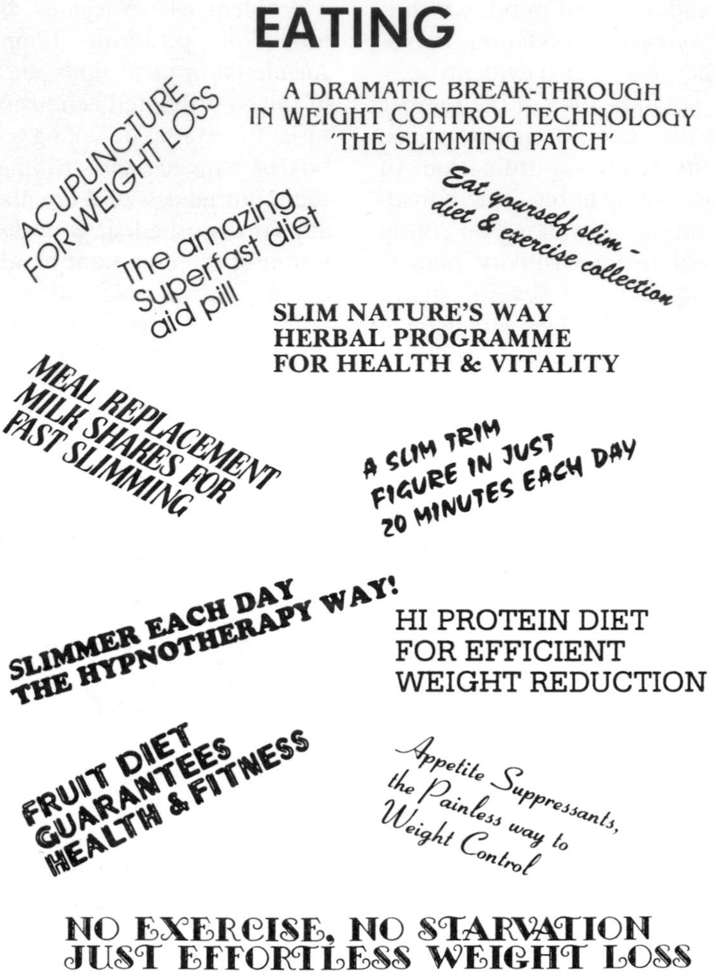

EATING

A DRAMATIC BREAK-THROUGH
IN WEIGHT CONTROL TECHNOLOGY
'THE SLIMMING PATCH'

ACUPUNCTURE FOR WEIGHT LOSS

The amazing Superfast diet aid pill

Eat yourself slim - diet & exercise collection

SLIM NATURE'S WAY
HERBAL PROGRAMME
FOR HEALTH & VITALITY

MEAL REPLACEMENT MILK SHAKES FOR FAST SLIMMING

A SLIM TRIM FIGURE IN JUST 20 MINUTES EACH DAY

SLIMMER EACH DAY THE HYPNOTHERAPY WAY!

HI PROTEIN DIET
FOR EFFICIENT
WEIGHT REDUCTION

FRUIT DIET GUARANTEES HEALTH & FITNESS

Appetite Suppressants, the Painless way to Weight Control

NO EXERCISE, NO STARVATION
JUST EFFORTLESS WEIGHT LOSS

Fig. 8.2 *Typical dieting slogans.*

INTRODUCTION

Millions of pounds every year are spent on slimming products and everywhere one looks, advertisements suggest products which will assist the individual, 'as part of a calorie controlled diet' to lose weight, more or less quickly, to have a 'fabulous physique in just 20 minutes a day' to produce a 'slimmer, more attractive youthful you' (Fig. 8.2). It is official, however, that some of the population *are* overweight and, if you were to secrete yourself in any large chemist store and note the number of slimming products purchased,

it would be assumed that the figure must be a high one. One of the targets included in *The Health of the Nation* (DH, 1992), indeed is the goal:

> To reduce the percentages of men and women aged 16–64 who are obese by at least 25% for men and at least 33% for women by the year 2005 …

So, it would seem that the diet-preparation manufacturers are set for a boom time over the next 10 years or so—or are they? The target continues by providing the actual figures of the 'obese' population as:

from 8% for men and 12% for women in 1986/87 to no more than 6% and 8% respectively.

Of course these percentages still represent a great many people, all of whom are 'at risk' in relation to a variety of somatic problems, but will the diets, slimming pills and exercises work and help in weight reduction, and will the slimmer, more healthy individual be able to maintain that loss? And, if so few—relatively speaking—within the population are overweight and remain overweight, then who is buying all of the diet aids? Perhaps if the dieter knew a little more about the body mechanisms involved, the individual would be in a more powerful position with regard to selection of 'regimes' and 'maintenance programmes' on offer. What does the evidence tell us?

INTAKE, UTILIZATION AND OUTPUT

Food taken into the body is converted, via processes of chemical, mechanical and bacterial breakdown in the gastro-intestinal tract, into substances suitable for absorption by the stomach and large intestine (10%) but mainly by the small intestine (90%). Glucose is derived from carbohydrates, amino acids from proteins ingested, and monoglycerides and fatty acids from fat intake, and in this form may be absorbed for utilization.

Material not required by the body for immediate use is converted to fat or to the insoluble glucose polymer, glycogen, and stored for future use. Glucose is the major energy source for all tissues, and, when necessary, the liver will convert the stored fat and amino acids into glucose for use.

Dieter's Tip No. 1
All food taken in excess of body requirements will be stored.

Dieter's Tip No. 2
All food *means* all food. Whether of a protein, fat or carbohydrate nature, excess will be stored.

Dieter's Tip No. 3
When energy requirements exceed circulating glucose availability, stored material will be brought into play to provide added fuel, thus depleting stores.

With the exception of the cells of the nervous system, insulin, manufactured by the beta cells of the pancreas, is necessary to facilitate cellular uptake of glucose from the circulating blood. It reduces blood sugar levels not only in this manner, but also by accelerating conversion of glucose into storable glycogen and stimulating conversion of glucose and any other excess nutrients into fatty acids. Insulin also increases the build up of proteins by cells.

HUNGER AND SATIATION

Despite the measures taken by any organism, no matter how simple or complex, to store available excesses of nutrients ingested, those stores require continual replenishment when normal activities are undertaken on a daily basis. Some animals, of course, overeat at the commencement of winter, storing as much fat as possible for both warmth and nutrition during hibernation. However, in order to survive that period of food abstinence, the animal must lower its metabolic rate and become inactive, merely ticking over in a state of suspended animation, until the spring, warmer climes and fresh vegetation appears to enable it to 'live' again. The fully awake, but store-depleted animal must now overeat until it reaches a weight at which it can match its energy requirements and yet still have a little 'put aside' for emergencies. This, as will be demonstrated below, is of great significance to the human 'dieter', but the fact is that the instinct for self-preservation in any organism initiates food-seeking behaviour, the feelings and sensations associated with which, we call 'hunger'.

The total mechanism for 'stock control and re-ordering of supplies' is less than completely understood but there would appear to be sufficient facts available to give an outline of the processes involved. Jean Mayer (1955), an American nutritionist, asserted that the body monitors glucose levels in the blood, via detectors called glucostats, specialized neurons which, it was proposed, fired at a higher rate when glucose levels were reduced, thus setting up the hunger drive and food-seeking behaviours. There is, indeed, monitoring of glucose levels in the lateral hypothalamus and also in the liver, which assesses nutrient absorption via the portal vein, sending information back to 'control' by way of the vagus nerve. However, experimentation in animals whereby the vagus nerve was severed (Tardoff *et al.*, 1982) demonstrated no effect on eating behaviour, indicating that hunger and glucose level fluctuation appeared only obscurely connected. Further studies demonstrated that glucose levels within the blood fluctuate very little, despite the amount, nature or timing of food intake, and again the assumption must be that efficient conversion and storage of superfluous nutrients facilitates immediate re-conversion and use when levels begin to signal a drop.

This is, of course, the point to reintroduce the example of the hibernating animal and his feeding patterns, pre- and post-sleep, for it has been found that an experimental animal, deliberately starved and exhibiting signs of weight loss, will, when given the opportunity to feed freely, overeat until it regains the fat it has lost. Conversely, the animal who has been force-fed until obese will, when in control of its own eating, undereat until the excess fat has been lost. There is a maintenance of total body fat at a reasonably constant level in adult animals and intake of food is regulated in relation to this. Somewhere within the brain there must be a representation of the amount of body fat necessary to the individual and his patterns of activity, in just the same way in which the brain is aware of joint and muscle position.

Role of the hypothalamus

Dieter's tip No. 4
Your brain 'knows' how fat you are supposed to be. No matter your weight loss on the diet, when you 'free-feed', you will adjust upwards to your normal body weight.

Two areas of the brain appear to be of significance here, for damage to the lateral hypothalamus of a rat results in a refusal to eat or drink. If not fed artificially, the rat dies, but where intravenous feeding is undertaken for several weeks, the rat begins to recover its appetite, initially for wet food but not for drink, and later for both food and drink. When feeding freely, the rat's weight is found to stabilize at a lower 'new' norm. Even in situations where the rat has been starved prior to the lesioning, when eating freely it will stabilize at a point of starved level (i.e. it will overeat for a time) but below that of its original weight. Lateral hypothalamic damage provokes a reduction and stabilization at a level below the previous norm (Mitchell and Keesey, 1974).

Conversely, where tissue of the ventromedial region of the hypothalamus is destroyed, the rat will initially overeat for a period of up to three months, but then reduce its intake by an amount sufficient to maintain the new obese 'normal' weight. Should the new 'obese' rat find that food is restricted, its body weight is found to reduce to its original level and then be maintained. However, when allowed to feed freely, the obese level is achieved and again maintained (Hoebel and Teitelbaum, 1966). It would appear, therefore, that both the lateral and ventromedial regions of the hypothalamus play a part in the set point for body weight, balancing each other to create the 'norm' to be expected and striven to be maintained, and indeed when precisely the same degree of damage is inflicted on both areas simultaneously, the animal exhibits no change in feeding behaviours, maintaining weight at its original, pre-operative level (Keesey and Powley, 1975).

However, omitted from the above is the fact that, in damaging these specific areas of the hypothalamus, nerve fibres in the area may also suffer damage and therefore may influence observations. Indeed, Friedman and Stricker (1976), point out that damage to the nigrostriatal bundle, nerve fibres associated with the initiation not only of feeding but other behaviours, inflicted at a point outside of the hypothalamus creates a variety of activation problems in the animal, including the refusal to eat and drink seen in the early stages of lateral hypothalamic lesioning. Similarly, branches of the parasympathetic nervous system pass through the area of the ventromedial hypothalamus, and, as these are seen to increase the rate at which nutrients are stored by the body at the expense of immediately available fuel, damage to these fibres will produce an animal constantly in need of circulating nutrients and therefore perpetually eating. The rat, therefore, behaves in the manner associated with that of a ventral medial hypothalamic lesioned animal.

There is, however, no doubt of the new weight level achieved by hypothalamic-damaged rats and it is possible that the specific regions of the hypothalamus and the named nerve pathways are synergistic, working together to achieve a balanced body weight, suitable to the animal's function on a long-term basis.

Other factors?

In addition to the long-term overview of a set point for optimum survival potential, a more immediately acting mechanism is necessary to facilitate adjustment of eating patterns and the rate of metabolism to meet those long-term goals for weight. The mechanism by which this appears to be achieved is via a circulating chemical substance, rather than by innervation, as demonstrated in the 'mouse experiments' conducted by Coleman and Hummer (1969). They surgically joined two mice, one obese and one normally lean, so that the animals shared a cardiovascular and extracellular fluid circulation, but had separate nervous systems. Therefore when the lean mouse began to undereat, just as if obese, this could not have been due to the influence of the obese mouse's nervous system, it had to have been achieved via a circulating messenger.

Insulin has been suggested as the regulator of body weight and therefore food intake and yet the cells of the nervous system utilize glucose directly and do not require insulin to achieve this uptake and indeed passage of insulin across the blood–brain barrier is achieved only with difficulty. Yet insulin is present within cerebrospinal fluid and there are receptor sites for this hormone within the brain, particularly in the olfactory lobe and hypothalamus. Indeed, micro-electrodes implanted in the hypothalami of animals elicit a decrease in neural activity within the region after glucose is given by injection and an increase in activity in the same area following administration of insulin, thereby demonstrating adequate and diminished levels of circulating glucose respectively (Stricker *et al.*, 1977). Further evidence to support insulin as an integral part of the initiation and termination of feeding behaviours is supplied by both Davis and Brief (1981) in their rat studies, and Woods *et al.* (1979) in their experiments on baboons. Continuous infusion of insulin into the cerebrospinal fluid, or persistent application directly on to the neurons of the ventral region of the hypothalamus, induces firing of the cells and heralds a reduction in eating behaviours and therefore weight loss. As a passing thought, this could account for the demonstration of insatiable appetite and yet continuing weight loss associated with the onset of diabetes mellitus. If insulin is deficient or absent, neuronal firing within the ventral area of the hypothalamus will not occur and feeding behaviour will continue.

Of course if you had to wait for depleted stores to be replenished before ceasing food intake, you would be eating for quite some time at each stretch, for it takes four to five hours or more for complete gastric emptying, approximately the same period of time to journey through the small intestine, where most nutrients are absorbed, and then storage activities must be undertaken. Most of the day would be spent in breakfasting! Instead, the reality is that you eat until you have 'had enough' or are 'full' and then push your plate away. How is it that you know that you have eaten sufficient to keep the brain happy and the stores replete? The ventromedial aspect of the hypothalamus requires absorption to have taken place before it can make adjustments based on the blood sugar level and the amount of insulin circulating and although valuable as a mechanism, insulin is not secreted until glucose and fats enter the duodenum which may again take some time, dependent upon the nature of the food taken.

Janowitz and Grossman (1949) looked to the upper portion of the tract—the mouth and throat—in their efforts to locate satiety sensors and severed the oesophagus of a dog from the stomach in an effort to assess the effects of food entering the mouth upon feeding patterns. The researchers found that, whilst the animal ate a larger than usual meal prior to ceasing activities, it soon recommenced eating. The assertion that satiation sensors exist within this area was therefore proven, for the animal did desist from feeding activities, but the more rapid than usual return to eating indicates the short-term nature of their effect. When redirecting attention to the stomach, it is obvious that satiety sensors are present within the area, for feeding via gastronomy satisfies hunger, and reduces food-seeking behaviours. Certainly stretch receptors in the stomach wall become activated when an animal risks injury by overfilling its stomach—the 'I just can't eat another bite' syndrome—and there is cessation of feeding. However, it would appear that the major satiation mechanism is mediated via the digestive hormones secreted by the gastro-intestinal system during food digestion. There are a number of such hormones and the exact ones secreted depend upon the nature of the meal taken. The intestinal mucosa secretes, for example, cholesystokinin (CCK) directly into the blood supply in response to protein- and fat-based foods entering the duodenum. Amongst other effects, CCK stimulates the pancreas to secrete its enzyme-rich secretion, provokes contraction of the gall bladder and therefore release of bile, and slows the rate by which gastric emptying occurs. There are other such hormones—secretin, vasoactive intestinal polypeptide (VIP), gastric inhibitory peptide (GIP) and somatostatin—all of which circulate in response to specific foodstuffs within the gastro-intestinal system and all of which appear to have a dual role. In their response to particular foods within the system, they achieve a tailoring of the appropriate digestive processes to match need. However, they also appear to interact with the nervous system to regulate intake. GIP, for example, is known to stimulate insulin production in response to glucose and fat entering the duodenum, and insulin is shown to influence feeding patterns. Injections of CCK have similarly been demonstrated as inhibiting eating (MacLean, 1977). Hungry rats when transfused with the blood of well-fed peers demonstrate reduced feeding activities (West *et al.*, 1982) thus indicating that these circulating satiety factors pass directly to the brain to influence the point at which eating should be terminated.

The link between the neurotransmitter *norepinephrine* is acknowledged but vague. It is known, however, that preparations such as amphetamines release stored norepinephrine from axon terminals or inhibit its re-uptake, and amphetamines can inhibit eating, hence their historical use as a diet aid. Passing through the lateral hypothalamus are several neural tracks that carry the transmitter and therefore it is present within the relevant locale. More about its specific role is not apparently forthcoming at this time but norepinephrine, and the similarly structured epinephrine, do play a substantial role in the sympathetic activity, mediated via the hypothalamus, during stress. A reduced rate of digestive action and increased blood sugar level in the body's preparation for 'fight or flight' are demonstrable and hence connections between feeding behaviours, the hypothalamus and the neurotransmitter appear strengthened.

One other point worthy of mention is that *endorphins* appear to increase the amount of food consumed during a meal. Endorphins are neuropeptides, the 'endogenous opiates', and are associated with suppression of pain, linked to memory and learning, regulation of body temperature, and sexual activity. There are connections, too, with the mental health problems diagnosed as 'schizophrenia' and 'depression'. Increased level of endorphins within the pituitary glands of genetically obese rats and mice suggest that there may be a relationship with feeding behaviours.

Metabolic rates

Metabolic rate influences intentional or naturally occurring diet reduction. The metabolic rate indicates the speed at which the synthesis and decomposition activities occur within the body, that is, the result of anabolic and catabolic reactions. An increase in the rate will elicit more rapid decomposition activities and foodstuffs broken down too quickly for the body to get the chance to do any storing activities. Unless the individual increases food intake, the inability to replenish utilized stores will result in weight reduction. A lowered metabolic rate will engender the converse, for food will be broken down more slowly and often incompletely and then stored. The individual gains weight easily. The sad truth for the dieter must be in the automatic response of the body to slow down metabolic activities when insufficient food is taken in to meet the brain's perceived needs. It is a protective mechanism designed to reduce energy expenditure and maintain store levels at the highest point possible for as long as is possible. The individual feels tired and energy-less, often complaining of feeling cold, as 'savings' are automatically made by the brain in whatever area possible, so that demands are reduced as far as possible in order to conserve those supplies. By this mechanism weight loss is reduced and it therefore falls to the higher cognitive powers of the human to initiate activities that will provoke a raise in metabolism, thus 'forcing' the brain to relinquish its hold on body stores, and facilitating weight loss acceleration.

Dieter's tip No. 5
Dieting, without a simultaneous increase in physical activity, may elicit disappointing weight loss. A combination of diet and exercise will be more likely to show results.

It would seem then that long-term regulation of food intake is controlled by the brain's representation of the fat stores of the body. Insulin would appear to provide indication of the current status of stores and hence signal the need for intake of food and therefore eating behaviours. Cessation of eating would appear to be the responsibility of the digestive hormones, or gut peptides, in conjunction with the hypothalamus. So where is the dieter in all of this? At the moment things do not look too optimistic in relation to intentional weight reduction. But if an individual wishes to maintain a body weight conducive to looking good, when the cerebral 'fat controller' deems differently, is it physiologically feasible?

PSYCHOSOCIAL INFLUENCES

Sometimes the wolf children would get there first and whether it was meat for the table or a dead animal or bird that they had found—they were particularly fond of rotten meat—they did not care to be obstructed ... it was a constant worry after witnessing their summary dealings with mice and cockroaches, that they would soon kill something larger.
MacLean, 1977

Amala and Kamala had been raised by wolves in their den until 'rescued' by the Reverend Singh, in 1920, and taken to his orphanage at Midnapore. At that time, aged approximately six and three years respectively, their diet, method of locomotion, communication strategies and sleep–wake cycle reflected their socialization by the she-wolf as her cubs. The Singhs tried hard to 'civilize' the children into a more acceptable lifestyle, but the older one survived only a year and Kamala, only nine years. The doctor in attendance believed their deaths to be due in part to the attempt to change their dietary intake radically by suppressing the availability of the accustomed raw meat diet and imposing cooked mixed food for which their gastro-intestinal tract was unprepared. This resulted in the generally weakened physical state and, in addition, gut irritability. Dysentery, fever and worm infestation further compounded the already lowered resistance and the exposure to human infections, for which sustenance by the she-wolf had given no immunity, found the children unprepared and unfit for human life and contact. Both children died of renal failure and even Kamala, an 'adolescent' 12-

year-old by the time of her demise, demonstrated a very limited degree of 'civilized' behaviour as the result of her nine years of human contact and 'assistance'.

We would probably find both our sensibilities and stomachs offended by the thought of killing dinner before eating it, or of being served with cockroach or mouse—raw or cooked—for this has not been a part of the socialization processes to which we have been exposed. Diet is one of the 'norms' of a culture, reflecting both traditional influences and the modifications concomitant in the changes of that society. In years past, an individual and family were reliant on what they themselves could produce, excess being exchanged or sold for other goods or services necessary. Today, few survive on the commodities that they home grow or rear and foodstuffs are mass-produced on a large, more efficient scale and sold to the rest of the population.

Socialization in regard to eating may be deemed as relatively unimportant and yet it provides the rules governing the individual's dietary and social behaviour. At a party, an individual will eat whether hungry or not, because everyone else is eating and food is an integral part of every major milestone in life—christenings, weddings and funerals being examples. Meals may be the only times that a family comes together because of the different daily occupations and as such may be considered as priority by the family, or at least, the adult members—the rule makers—of that family. It represents the continuing nurturing responsibilities of the adults towards their offspring and is governed by rules and hence provides socialization opportunities. Exclusion from the meal table or from a meal is a punishment used by adults to express disapproval of behaviour—'You don't deserve to join us, please eat in the kitchen' and 'No supper for you, go to your room', being typical admonishments. Similarly it is used as a weapon by the child, knowing that it will evoke parental concern and therefore increased, comforting-style attention. It provides a consolation when things go wrong or the child is hurt—a grazed knee evokes the offer of a 'sweetie' to take away the pain and coming second in a competition or race deserves a chocolate bar on the way home. Sugary, sweet things are seen as a reward and the principle may be instilled early. Sweetness is something special and desired, reflected in the offering of chocolates to say 'I'm sorry' or 'I love you', the Christmas tree chocolate novelties and the Easter eggs. Food, and especially sweet food, may be seen to represent much more to the individual than mere sustenance.

The importance of all of the above to the dieter is that, whilst the human and every other animal is born with a prescribed number of fat cells, genetics only prescribes the *minimum* number of fat cells and, though this minimum number cannot be lost, they can be increased in number by overeating both in childhood and adult years. As the overweight child frequently becomes an overweight adult (West *et al.*, 1982), both genetics and upbringing may play significant roles within weight control. Knittle and Hirsch (1968) demonstrated that rats with twice the normal number of fat cells are double the body weight of their control group peers and Faust (1984) found that by removing half of the normal size rat's fat cells, they developed to only half the size of their siblings. Obeser people similarly show larger fat cells than their normal weight counterparts, and Faust *et al.* (1978) suggest that it is the *volume* of these cells that provide the brain with its regulatory system. The assertion is that when fat cell volume decreases, the brain initiates food-seeking behaviours to restore the depleted volume to the set points discussed earlier.

The enzyme *lipoprotein lipase* is also of significance to the dieter for there is an increased level of this substance in the obese individual and animal alike. It is responsible for both the removal of fat from circulation and its storage in the adipocytes (fat cells), and when the obese restrict their food intake, the lipoprotein lipase level elevates further. It would appear that this higher level indicates continuing fat storage as a priority even where intake is restricted and may account for the periods of plateau experienced by dieters when they lose no further weight, or no weight at all, for often prolonged periods of time. It would certainly appear to be an integral part of the body's regulation of body fat and therefore weight control.

Upbringing and socialization processes may be

seen therefore to influence eating behaviours and weight control. An association between food—especially sweet sticky food—and comfort, ease and contentment, and the curer of all ills, pains and disappointments, is a coping mechanism of dubious value and potential detriment to the indvidual.

People, whether obese, normally or under-weighted, appear to fall naturally into two groups, those who show restraint in eating and those who do not. Studies (Herman and Polivy, 1980; Ruderman, 1986) consistently show the eating behaviours of the restrained eater are more similar to those of obese people than to the unrestrained eater. Restrained eaters consume more than their non-dieting counterparts, indicating their deprivation subsequently results in overeating, despite their original weight levels having been regained (Coscina and Dixon, 1983). This would account for the common phenomenon of dieters who initially successfully lose weight only to exceed their original level when restraints are relaxed. Similarly it may be responsible for the binge eating associated with anorexia nervosa, though of course weight increase is not seen because of induced vomiting and purging behaviours.

Obese people often demonstrate different attitudes and psychological responses to food, which may reflect the elevated lipoprotein lipase level and resultant chronic hunger associated with this enzyme. Similarities have been drawn (Schachter, 1971) between behaviours of obese individuals and those of the ventromedially hypothalamic damaged rat and yet no evidence of similar damage in these individuals has been demonstrated. However, overweight people are visibly more susceptible to food cues, such as the sight, aroma, texture and colour of foods than their normally weighted peers and tend to be more selective in their choice of food and drink. They will drink less of a nondescript tasting milk shake and more of a flavourful one than the normally weighted person, for example. Despite their interest in food, Schachter (1971) found overweight people less likely to make an effort to gain available food. In studies where obese and normal-weight individuals were left alone in a room with a bowl of nuts—still in their shells—

and a nutcracker, only 1 of 20 obese people used the nutcracker and ate a few of the nuts, in comparison to 10 of 20 normal weight subjects.

In our opinion, all of the above bodes poorly for the Government's weight-reducing target for the adult population. No matter how often an individual achieves a weight reduction, the brain will evoke its animalistic instincts and redress the balance, and indeed exceed the norm to ensure survival of the organism. The only way it would seem to us to achieve a reduction in obese adults is to educate parents into the necessity for sensible eating patterns in their children from birth and to inculcate the values of exercise for everyone.

PROBLEMS ASSOCIATED WITH EATING

There are a number of situations in which the individual is *unable* to control the intake of food and which may, therefore, produce a dependence upon others to ensure effective nutritional status. The most obvious of these is that of the young infant and the child and the previous identification of the reliance on parents' and carers' knowledge of how much food, how often provided and of what nature and balance is of value here. Education of nutritional needs and the advantages of exercise to the growing child are, however, not the only areas of importance for consideration here, as good food—low fat, high protein, low salt and sugar, and high in residue—is often more expensive than the 'stomach fillers' and therefore economics are a vital factor. The homeless, the unemployed, the one-parent families and the retired elderly people on no or low incomes to meet everyday needs at, what must be considered by anyone, a very basic level have little control over their diet.

We should also consider those at risk because of an actual physical limitation of movement, for example, the unconscious individual and those in whom the level of conscious awareness fluctuates, whether precipitated by injury, infection, metabolic disorder or tumour formation. Again these people are dependent for a varying period of time on the attention and support of others, as are those who, whilst conscious and aware, may not elicit a current appreciation of the need to eat. The *overactive individual* excessively preoccupied with his or her own thoughts and with responding to even the most minor environmental stimuli, has no interest in such mundane matters as eating, and therefore shows a drastic reduction in food intake and weight loss. The individual who, conversely, is experiencing the *psychomotor retardation* associated with *severely lowered mood*, or *apathy*, may again evince a disinterest in food, and diminished appetite, perhaps due to the overwhelming preoccupation with sad, distressing or negative ideation. Such depressed mood may indicate *organic impairment* or be a sequel to *psychoactive substance use*, in addition to representing the major problem in a *bipolar* or *depressive disorder*, or as seen in bereavement. Significant weight loss may be a feature of *dementia*, both Alzheimer and multi-infarct types. *Poor memory* may precipitate lack of awareness as to whether one has eaten or not, of the normal environmental cues that would suggest it is time for a meal, of the need to shop or prepare food for eating. Food that is prepared for, and presented to, the memory or intellectually impoverished individual may be hoarded, or used to feed the cat, rather than to fulfil nutritional needs, thus demonstrating poverty of judgement in addition to that of awareness and insight.

Within mental health care, individuals may be seen to refuse food and for a variety of reasons. 'Psychotic' individuals whose delusions include *persecutory beliefs* and fears related to being killed by some agency, may suspect all food and drink preparations as being poisoned or drugged and hence refuse them. Conversely they may believe that some vital part of their digestive system is missing, has been invaded or taken over by an alien being or animal, as with somatically orientated themes. Remember George's catatonia and ruptured duodenal ulcer (p. 130)?

When George was well on the road to recovery and therefore resident once again in familiar territory, he responded to any query after his health and all round attention by repeating the words 'rats, gnawing rats'! One or two members of staff recalled that a day or so prior

---

to his illness, George had given out the odd mutter about rats!

George would not be the only example from our repertoire of anecdotes in which investigation revealed a somatic problem in a body area which had been included in an individual's bizarre somatic delusions. It may at times represent the only way in which a client can communicate his physical sensations when the rest of his world is bizarre or unintelligible. Rats, mice and various insects 'gnawing' have all been indicated as causing problems and investigation has, on occasions revealed tumours, ulcers and strictures within the gastro-intestinal system. A thorough medical examination plus appropriate investigative procedures will exclude such problems. Similarly some will demonstrate *negativism*, refusing to accede to any request, whether in relation to food and eating, or any other behaviour. The individual may display an apparently motiveless resistance to any activity or perform the complete opposite of what is requested.

Some individuals may feel profound *guilt* in regard to a real or imagined act or omission in the past and consequently exteriorize thoughts and behaviours relating to their perceived current unworthiness to accept food, comfort or care. Others fear they are in reduced circumstances and, believing themselves needing to pay for services offered, will refuse food, drink and any other attention. Both are relatively common features demonstrated by the elderly who, accustomed and proud of their independence from 'national assistance' over many years, return to such long-ago held views when intellectual and memory impairments intercede and cause bewilderment. There is often little memory of the National Health Service, free at the point of demand, and if there is such an awareness, the individual may not recognize the environment as one of a hospital or other care facility. Of course, non-informed staff provide no clues to assist the individual, who therefore may believe themselves in a hotel, restaurant or paying facility. It is not unusual for any organically impaired individual to refuse to eat for those reasons.

Eating disorders

Anorexia nervosa provides a further example of food refusal or severe curtailment. Predominantly a problem of girls, aged 12–18 years of age, the theories put forward to account for the obsessive preoccupation with food and the pursuit of 'thinness' are numerous and inconclusive. Leibowitz (1983) suggests various brain structure/function abnormalities, for example, a norepinephrine-producing neuronal problem, to account for the behaviour of some anorexics, but there is little direct evidence to support this, and most clinicians believe it is a problem of a psychosocial nature. The Western image of the successful woman—the small breasts and narrow hips—as epitomized in adverts, films and the like is pressure to which all young women are exposed and therefore if it should be a strong influence on the anorexic, there must be some predisposition inherent in the youngster to achieve this influence. Crisp (1983) believes a fear of growing up, of achieving an independent identity and of adult responsibilities is translated into a fear of getting fat and yet other researchers suggest that eating may represent the only control over life and living that the youngster feels he or she may exert. Several studies have found high incidences of psychosocial problems within the families of anorexia, for example, psycho-active substance abuse, depression and psychosomatic disorders. Others point to the disordered body image perception as a key factor within development, though studies reveal that many women, particularly pregnant ones, demonstrate an overestimation of their own body size. Whatever the cause, the preoccupation with food and thinness is evident and may reach the point where 40%-plus of body weight is lost. It therefore presents a life-threatening situation in need of efficient and effective management.

In some situations intake is seen to be ineffective for a variety of reasons. In anorexia nervosa, for example, binges may be a feature, where vast amounts of food, and often thousands of calories, are ingested within a short period. The individual then induces vomiting, or utilizes laxatives and diuretics to prevent the absorption of those calories. This purge–binge behaviour is referred to as *bulimia*.

No aversion to food is seen in *pica*, where there is persistent ingestion of non-nutritious substances and these may range through materials such as plaster and paint, string and cloth, sand and pebbles, grass and leaves, insects and animal droppings. It is a problem associated with very young children, one to two years of age and most often remits in early childhood. On occasions the problem persists into adolescence and very rarely into adult life. It is frequently associated with those experiencing problems of learning disability and 'schizophrenia', but may also be seen in a 'mild' form within pregnant women.

The eating–bingeing–purging behaviours associated with anorexia nervosa and bulimia, combined with deliberate ingestion of large amounts of laxative preparations ensures no absorption of nutrients that have been eaten. Of course, the anorexic is not the only candidate for inappropriate use of laxatives, which, in essence, achieve their purpose by irritating the intestinal mucosa. Many individuals, whether labelled 'sick' or 'well' are obsessed with their evacuatory processes, demonstrating that laxatives may be another substance which is abused.

An increase in *metabolic rate* may obviously result in more frequent defaecation and perhaps diarrhoea and therefore the individual, for example, experiencing the effects of hyperthyroidism, may complain of the problem. Similarly *irritable bowel syndrome*, considered psychogenic in origin, reveals no organic disease in the intestine or elsewhere in the body, the individual often being described as 'nervous, sensitive and anxious'. *Generalized anxiety*, or a specific emotional conflict, generates increased peristalsis as an integral part of parasympathetic arousal, and therefore any situation in which the flight–fight mechanism is operational over a protracted period of time may see diarrhoea as a problem requiring attention.

The psychosocial sequelae of *diabetes mellitus* may be ignored and yet the individual has to monitor diet and physical health obsessively, administer insulin or other medication as prescribed and take full responsibility for judgement of the need to increase/decrease dosage in response to unusual daily events. This requires high levels of adjustment and readjustment in relation to daily activities initially and may, quite reasonably, become the focus of intense preoccupation. Overwhelming parental concern and anxiety may filter through to the young child and hence disturbances may ensue. Over-protective parental behaviour may smother a child, or food may be excessively valuable in parental manipulation. Wilful self-neglect may be a part of adolescent rebellion and sexual dysfunction—approximately half of diabetic men may experience impotence (Davis, 1978) and up to 35% of diabetic women may be inorgasmic (Kolodny, 1971; Ellenberg, 1977) for example—may contribute to relationship difficulties. Fear of the somatic sequelae of diabetes may result in *hypochondriasis* and episodes of hypoglycaemia and acidosis may damage brain tissue, both in those with early onset, that is before the age of five years (Ack *et al.*, 1961) and in adults (Ives, 1963) where cerebral atherosclerosis may be the predisposing problem. The diabetic may find a good mental health nurse a boon in adjusting to the changes and potential obstacles and problems which may be a necessary feature of living with insulin deficiency.

Obesity

Obesity indicates that calorie intake exceeds requirements and, rather than 'appearing overnight', tends to creep up on individuals. Whilst inherited fat cell numbers has to be a factor, obesity is either acquired via socialization processes or occurs as a direct result of changes in lifestyle that are not accompanied by a concomitant reduction in food intake. It is only occasionally that obesity is seen as a direct result of somatic health problems and where there is indication of physiological causation, it is symptoms other than the weight increase that provide the indicator of a problem. *Cushing's syndrome (adrenocortical hyperfunction)*, rare but more common in women, demonstrates as a decreased glucose tolerance, hyperglycaemia, muscle wasting (due to excessive protein catabolism) and weakness. The excessive production of cortisol similarly provides an abnormal distribution of fat and atrophy of lymphoid tissue, and hence the individual

presents with obesity of the head, neck and trunk (the classical symptom of *buffalo's hump*) on thin, wasted limbs. The oedematous, round bloated face—*moon-shaped face*—is again a classical sign.

Similarly *hypothyroidism* may be diagnosed on problems presenting, exclusive of increasing body weight. In congenital or childhood development, the limp, coarse-featured, thick-tongued appearance is unmistakable. The child looks 'puffy' and bloated, is pale, dry and cool skinned, and has problems in feeding and growth and development generally. Pulse is slow and temperature is subnormal, indicative of the reduced metabolic rate inherent in thyroid hormone deficiency. In adults, onset may be confused with depression or early organic impairment, but again, skin is dry, thickened and cold and the face is puffy with an enlarged tongue and lips. The individual feels weak, slow and lethargic, and there is a psychomotor retardation. Appetite is poor, despite the weight gain, and amenorrhoea is often a feature. Untreated, arteriosclerotic changes, cardiac insufficiency and coma may ensue and prompt treatment is therefore vital. One tip may be found within the hair distribution of the affected individual, as growth is reduced, head hair often becoming dry, coarse and sparse and eyebrows often disappearing or much reduced in quanity.

Lesions associated with the hypothalamus and its eating/appetite related structures, may create problems associated with obesity and therefore will present with client problems associated with that specific lesion.

Research indicates, however, that overweight individuals tend to eat more when anxious, whilst normal weight individuals eat more in low-anxiety situations (McKenna, 1972) and other studies have demonstrated that this increased consumption occurs in relation to any emotionally arousing situation encountered by the overweight person (White, 1977). Theories have been put forward to explain this increased eating both in anxiety-provoking situations and during emotional arousal in general. The scenario of food providing comfort during childhood, previously discussed, is important here and, where used as a panacea of all ills, it may be that differentiation between hunger and other feelings has never been attained. It follows, therefore, that obesity or significant weight increase may be a feature of *depressed* and *anxious individuals*.

SUMMARY

People eat to survive and therefore evolution has built in a system whereby a period of deprivation is automatically followed by overeating, thus maintaining optimum potential for species survival. The social functions of food and eating have been introduced by the 'civilizing effect' of the advanced cortex of the human and with this

'advancement' complications may be incurred in respect of a purely biological function. The dieting individual has to re-learn the habits of a lifetime to find continuing satisfaction with his/her shape and weight, introducing and maintaining new routines and schedules, until habitual in nature. In regard, however, to the targets within *The Health of the Nation* (DH, 1992), we would sincerely suggest that resources be applied towards parents and parents-in-waiting, and to the young generation who are likely to be the frustrated dieters of the future. Good habits learned early are the foundation for healthy lifetime eating.

SLEEP

INTRODUCTION

> Blessings on him that invented sleep! It covers a man, thoughts and all, like a cloak; it is meat for the hungry, drink for the thirsty, heat for the cold, and cold for the hot. It is the currency with which everything may be purchased, and the balance that sets even King and shepherd, simpleton and sage.
> *Andrews, 1987*

The words above are those of Miguel de Cervantes (1547–1616) and serve to illustrate the extent to which the sixteenth-century novelist, playwright and poet, creator of Don Quixote, was impressed by this simple, biological function. Of course, not everyone is quite so enamoured all of the time with sleep for, as with so many bodily functions, it may be taken for granted until it causes a problem. Whether it is an inappropriate 'nap', an ability to stay awake and alert at a point well past the normal bed-time, or sleep evading an individual, most people experience a difficulty on occasions. We will review the current knowledge relating to sleep, the manner in which it is mediated and the normal parameters associated

with the event, prior to exploring difficulties that may be experienced.

TO SLEEP ...

Sleep is an active physiological process, and not merely a failure of arousal. The most obvious of the human's circadian rhythms discussed earlier, it may be described as:

> A recurrent healthy state.
>
> A normal, periodic, physiological depression of function.
>
> A period of relative inertia and reduced environmental responsiveness.
>
> A circumstance where overt responses are absent, and covert responses diminished.
>
> A state clearly different to that of coma and stupor.

Were you to think about the overt signs of the onset of sleep, you may reflect upon the fact that an individual closes his eyes, that the normal breathing pattern changes, with respirations reducing the total flow of air breathed, and that the heart rate slows. Observations may also conclude that urinary output reduces sharply during the sleeping hours and that a stimulus of sufficient intensity—the ringing of the alarm clock or the sound of breaking glass—will provoke arousal.

However, more detailed reflection will elicit that you have far more knowledge than this about sleep and sleeping. For example, you will be aware that sleep is *species-specific*, each animal having its own pattern and time for sleeping and assuming a position conducive to the activity. Some sleep in the day, others at night; some lie down whilst others remain standing and a glance at a wildlife programme—or around the house and garden—will confirm this specificity of the sleep pattern. Observations of the pet, caged bird will, for example, elicit that it sleeps standing up at night and yet the owl likes to roam in search of food at night, and tends not to be active during daylight. The family dog may go through the routine of pawing and scratching at the carpet, circling several times and then settling himself off to sleep, whereas anyone with knowledge of bats will know that these are also night-time activists which hang upside down, wrapped in their wings to sleep through the day. The members of the monkey and ape genre lie on their bellies along the branch of a tree and human beings, all things being equal, take themselves off to a special room in the late evening hours, lie down and cover themselves.

Sleeping positions

Every individual exhibits a routine which prepares them physically and emotionally for relaxation and sleep, and deviation from that routine may provoke a feeling of unease or discomfort. On nights when the individual is excessively tired some bits of the routine may safely be omitted without detrimental effects, indeed the whole set of activities may go to the wall, without even a notice!

Besides this routine, there are other comforts that may be necessary to attain the desired goal. Position in bed, for example, may be central to going off to sleep. The right arrangement of pillows and blankets or duvet evokes that feeling of familiarity and hence safety and relaxation. Many people find great difficulty in sleeping in a 'strange' bed and room—they cannot quite get comfortable. Body position assumed in preparation for sleep is similarly an individual preference—are you a 'diagonal' sleeper, corner-to-corner, a runner in mid-stride sort of sleeper, a hanger-on-to-the-edge of the mattress sleeper, or do you assume a foetal position? There is one position that each person feels comfortable in and it may not necessarily be any of the four identified above. If forced to move into a different position, for example, because of a plaster cast applied to a limb or an ache or pain, an individual may find that sleep eludes them, because they just 'can't get comfortable'.

A partner's sleeping habits may be significant. If you have spent many years occupying a bed alone, it may take a considerable degree of adjustment to accommodate a second person in the same bed, particularly if it is discovered that this individual is a teeth grinder and a snorer who likes to sleep diagonally across the bed, wrapped in the entire duvet! As an interesting and passing thought, animals seem to curl up when sleeping, perhaps to reduce exposure to predators of their soft unprotected underbellies. Do humans curl up for similar, evolutionary reasons? Similarly the positioning of animals' bodies against something flat, maybe even another animal, where possible, has been noted and could this be to prevent any enemy attacking them from behind, so to speak, and out of eyeline? Many people prefer to sleep facing the bedroom door, rather than away from it. Is this, too, an evolutionary 'throwback'?

How much sleep?

It is known, for example, that the number of hours of sleep needed varies, not only with age but between individuals of comparable age and lifestyle. The newborn baby sleeps for most of the day, waking only for sustenance and comfort measures. As the days go by, the infant sleeps less, so that by six months of age, approximately 13 hours each day is spent in sleep, in two short 'naps' and a longer sleep at night. As a toddler, the two naps reduce to one and so on until in adulthood, the average period spent in sleep is about seven and a half hours. Again, however, the adult 'norm' must take account of those who seem to function best on less—as little as three hours a night for some—and those for whom eight hours or more is a must. It is a very individual need. As people age, there is evidence to suggest that there is a tendency to sleep less at night and to awaken earlier in the morning, often before 5.00 a.m. (McGhie and Russell, 1962). This may be of significance when looking towards problems associated with sleep. Most of us will have an acquaintance who is a 'night owl' who becomes active at night and also a 'morning lark'—the individual who is actually awake and fully alert and functioning before the first verse of the dawn chorus (Webb, 1975). The particular rhythm in operation is as individual as a fingerprint.

You may also have experienced more or less successful attempts to change the sleeping time or pattern away from the norm. Night duty will require you to be awake and fully alert throughout the night-time hours, when you would normally be tucked up and alseep. You will therefore need to sleep during the hours when the vast majority of people are awake, moving about and generally making a noise. Night duty patterns rarely provide you with sufficient time to adjust to the change required, internal rotation often demonstrating three or four nights on and then the rest of the week off, or vice versa. Worse still for adjustment are split nights off duty—the sort of two on, two off, two on, one off pattern—requiring adjustment to differing cycles several times a week. Of course many nurses working predominantly on nights do accommodate well, having grown accustomed to the alterations required in order to function well in both situations. Humans also have the ability to accelerate and retard the sleep period while travelling across different time zones and the hour on/hour off game that is played with British Summer Time. Whilst more or less 'jet lagged' by both, people do adjust where necessary within a few days.

What happens during sleep?

You need to be relaxed at bedtime to succumb to sleep and once you lie back in that darkened room and close your eyes, the passage from wakefulness into sleep is actually an instantaneous one. William Dement (1976) demonstrated this fact exceptionally well in experiments in which recumbent and sleep-ready people, whose eyes had been taped open, were asked to respond by pressing a button each time a light was flashed. The light was flashed every second or two, and the 'guinea pigs' showed no slowing of reaction, just an abrupt cessation of activity, indicating that, even with eyes taped open, they were fast asleep. The eyeballs deviate upwards, pupils constrict, but will respond slowly to light and a number of changed patterns of activity commence. The activity of the brain, demonstrable via electro-encephalographic recordings, elicits a recurring ultradian rhythm of differing patterns of electrical impulses (Fig. 8.3).

The awake but relaxed brain shows activity at 8–12 vibrations per second (referred to as Hz or Hertz) at the rear of the head, and is described as *alpha rhythm*. This is transformed into the low voltage disorganized *theta activity* as drowsiness ensues, interpreted by some researchers as a sort of random neuronal firing—a running down—prior to passage to *stage three*, characterizing light sleep. Within stage three, the activity moves predominantly to the front of the head. *Sleep spindles*, sudden bursts of impulses which last for less than one second at a time but which are synchronized at between 12 and 16 Hz, intersperse and interrupt low voltage slow activity. A series of *vertex sharp waves* and *K complexes* heralds the onset of *delta wave* activity and deep sleep. Activity is at 0.5–2 Hz and sleepers are harder to awaken at this point, although something familiar—their name being called, for example—will cause arousal. This is the stage of *orthodox* or *non-rapid eye movement sleep*, to be followed by a sudden descent into *rapid eye movement sleep*. Here the EEG resembles that of an awake and alert individual, hence the term *paradoxical sleep* is often applied. It shows a faster, low-amplitude activity which is punctuated by bursts of phasic events during which eye muscles show rapid movement, hence the term rapid-eye movement or *REM* sleep. The term 'paradoxical' is appropriate for, despite the brain's apparently alert activity, muscle tone in general across the body

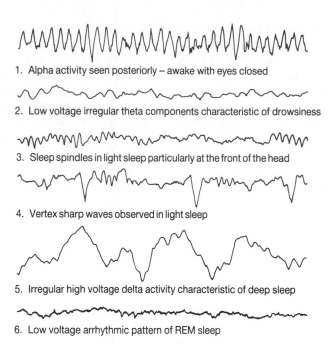

1. Alpha activity seen posteriorly – awake with eyes closed

2. Low voltage irregular theta components characteristic of drowsiness

3. Sleep spindles in light sleep particularly at the front of the head

4. Vertex sharp waves observed in light sleep

5. Irregular high voltage delta activity characteristic of deep sleep

6. Low voltage arrhythmic pattern of REM sleep

Fig. 8.3 *The EEG in sleep.*

shows a marked decrease and therefore complete relaxation of skeletal muscle, almost to the point of paralysis. The exact pattern of REM sleep varies from individual to individual and with age. The newborn infant spends approximately half of the sleeping time in REM sleep, and by the age of five years this has reduced to about a quarter or a fifth of total sleep. It then remains fairly constant through life at about 18% until old age. It is of interest to find that the premature baby spends about 75% of sleep time in REM as will become obvious during the later discussion on dreams and dreaming, for it is during this REM period that dreaming occurs.

REM sleep

The adult who spends seven and a half hours asleep each night will experience between one and a half and two hours of REM sleep. The first period is relatively short, lasting only 10 minutes or so, and occurs approximately 50–90 minutes after falling asleep. As the night wears on, REM periods become longer, interrupted only by return to stage 2. The length of the deeper stages of sleep, characterized by the delta waves, tends to reduce throughout the night and therefore the indvidual's sleep becomes lighter after the first few hours. Strenous physical activity increases the period of time spent in delta (slow) wave sleep and yet does not affect REM time. It has also been noted that REM sleep is increased in hospital patients who demonstrate psychosocial problems and also by women in the premenstrual phase of the monthly cycle, which may be a time characterized by mild psychosocial symptomatology, such as depression, anxiety and irritability (Hartmann, 1984).

During REM sleep, the rapid eye movements occur 40–60 times per minute and respiration and heart rate become rapid and irregular, in comparison to the almost absent eye movements and slow, regular breathing and heartbeat of non-REM sleep. There appear to be two distinct stages in REM sleep; one which is termed the *tonic phase* in which muscle tone is reduced and yet where, in men, an erection of the penis and, in women, increased vaginal blood flow is seen: the other is the *phasic period*, demonstrating the changes in heart and respiratory—and therefore blood pressure—rates mentioned plus an increase in cerebral blood flow, occasional myoclonic jerks and the conjugate eye movements. It has been suggested that REM sleep facilitates neural growth in the young (Roffware *et al.*, 1968), which would account for the higher proportion of REM sleep in children than in adults. The finding that protein synthesis rate is at its highest level during REM sleep would also support this hypothesis.

Physiological responses

There are other important features known in regard to sleep, for example, *cell division* is seen at various phases throughout the night but maximally during slow wave sleep. Similarly *growth hormone* concentrations are seen to rise with the onset of deep sleep and where sleep is delayed, so is the rise in growth hormone, thus indicating that its release is related to sleep *per se* rather than a 24-hour clock timing. This is helpful where investigating a possible deficiency of growth hormone for a sample of blood taken an hour after the onset of sleep would provide an indication of the capacity of the hormone. In adults, the *plasma prolactin concentration* is seen to rise about 90 minutes after the onset of sleep, and then shows a series of increasingly large secretory bursts, to reach a peak between the hours of 5.00 a.m. and 7.00 a.m. A rapid fall follows and the daytime low is seen to be achieved by about 10.00 a.m. Again it is sleep-related in onset, for if sleep is delayed, rises in prolactin levels are also delayed. However, it is not seen to be related to any one sleep-wave pattern. The circadian rhythm of adrenocorticotrophin hormone (ACTH) and cortisol shows a series of secretory episodes which cluster between 3.00 a.m. and 9.00 a.m., and yet little is produced between 11.00 p.m. and 3.00 a.m. This boost so late in the sleep period is obviously designed to prepare the individual for the energy expenditure needed upon rising. It is interesting that abnormalities in the 24-hour concentrations of plasma cortisol have been noted in those who have severe depressed mood, with return to normal levels noted following 'treatment'. In pre-pubertal children, luteinizing hormone levels are low and show no rise during sleep. However, at puberty there is an increasingly strong episodic release of luteinizing hormone during sleep and this is seen with a corresponding increase in testosterone levels. By the time sexual maturity is attained, daytime waking and night-time sleeping patterns of the hormone's release are the same. The release of *renin* from the kidney is seen to be abruptly halted at the initiation of rapid eye movement and levels of vasopressin, the antidiuretic hormone, are also rhythmic in function, thereby reducing fluid loss during the night-time hours by limiting urinary output at a period of reduced intake.

We have mentioned the increased protein synthesis associated with REM sleep, and must also identify, therefore, that the body's energy and fat stores are replenished during sleep.

MEDIATORS OF SLEEP

The *reticular formation*, or *reticular activating system*, is composed of the structures which facilitate sleep and wakeful states. The *mesencephalic portion*, comprising of areas of grey matter in the pons and midbrain, when stimulated, prompts impulses to spread upwards to the thalamus and onwards to generally stimulate the cerebral cortex, thus creating *wakefulness* and *consciousness*. The *thalamic portion* of the reticular activating system, which is made up of grey matter in the thalamus, appears to have a slightly different role, for stimulation of specific parts of the thalamus activates particular areas of the cerebral cortex and thus provokes *arousal* from sleep. Arousal requires sensory input, which stimulates the reticular activating system, and this input may be in the form of proprioceptive stimuli, pain or physical discomfort, bright light and loud noises. The cortex is then activated. Conversely, however, the cerebral cortex may be the originator of impulses which activate the arousal process, via somatosensory, motor or limbic system signals, and this reciprocal energizing effect is evident throughout the conscious part of the day, through a multi-circuit feedback loop. A similar arrangement is seen to be operating between the reticular activating system and the spinal cord, with impulses passing down through the cord to the skeletal muscles. The latter generate proprioceptive stimuli, which pass back via the cord and serve not only to sustain the activity of the reticular activating system, but also that of the cerebral cortex.

When it comes to sleep, several areas have been of interest to researchers. The *nucleus locus coerulus* is a group of neurons which contain *norepinephrine*, and the *dorsal raphe nucleus* comprises of *serotonin* enriched neurons. Both lie within the pons and recordings of the 'behaviour' of single cells within both areas demonstrate their maximum activity to occur during wakefulness. There is a progressive slowing of activity during the initial stages of slow wave sleep and a major depression of that activity prior to the end of the slow wave sleep phase. During REM sleep these cells are silent. Other pontine cells show a dramatic rise in activity prior to the EEG shift from slow wave to REM sleep patterns, indicating a responsibility in the transition from one stage to the other. It is clear, however, that this increase in activity is seen to be of a level 50–100 times that seen during wakefulness. These three groups of cells are thought to be connected to each other by various pathways and innervation, and it would appear that their activity is antagonistic. As activity increases in the REM-associated cells, a concomitant reduction in those related to consciousness and slow wave sleep is seen. Other substances produced within the area, for example, dopamine and acetylcholine, are known to be of importance within the wake–sleep cycle, though their exact role is obscure as yet. It is also possible that other pontine neurons are influential and have yet to be found. However, what does appear certain is that:

---

1 Fatigue + Withdrawal of afferent impulses → Reduction in the alerting system → Deactivation of cerebral cortex → Sleep.

---

and

---

2 Sleep + Afferent impulses → Stimulus to alerting system → Activation of cerebral cortex → Consciousness.

Early in the century, the French physiologist Henri Pieron (1913) demonstrated that the transfusion of cerebrospinal fluid from a sleepy dog to an alert one provoked the latter to fall asleep. In the 1970s, John Pappenheimer (1976) and his colleagues succeeded in isolating seven millionths of a gram of a substance—Factor S—from 3,000 litres of human urine, which they believed to be a sleep-producing substance. It was discovered to be a tiny, five amino acid peptide and since this time, studies from as far afield as Japan, Mexico and Romania have elicited substances which appear to be produced by the brain and which appear to trigger different stages of sleep (Krueger and Karnovsky, 1982). One such study demonstrated that a mere 600 molecules of the peptide *arginine vasotocin* induces sleep in a normal and alert cat. Sleep remains, to a large part, a continuing mystery.

Role of the pineal gland

We cannot ignore the role of the *pineal gland* in the cycles, including that of sleep, of animals, for, whilst no one can yet be sure, it may be that human physiological rhythms may be similarly influenced. The pineal gland converts the transmitter *serotonin* into the hormone *melatonin* and pours it directly into the bloodstream. Melatonin appears to have several functions in relation to both time and light, for example, it appears to cause a lightening in the colour of skin in certain lizards during the darkness hours and when injected into sparrows, they fall asleep. This conversion of serotonin to melatonin is acheved via the action of two enzymes produced within the pineal gland. One—N-*acetyltransferase*—determines the quantity of melatonin circulating and hence regulates cycles, for example, related to temperature changes and the sleep–wake cycle. It is a fact that, in many species of both nocturnal and diurnally active animals, the levels of N-acetyltransferase are always highest at night. This level may be 10 times that recorded in daylight hours and, for example, provokes chickens to roost and lowers their temperature. The mechanism by which melatonin levels are adjusted to match the normal variations of hours of light and darkness seen within the seasonal clock, is seen to be mediated via the pineal gland's sensitivity to light. Binckley's (1979) experiments with chicks kept in constant darkness elicited the normal *N*-acetyltransferase rhythm to continue. Those kept in constant lightness demonstrated a reduction in the levels of *N*-acetyltransferase circulating, whilst those exposed to alternating 12-hour periods of light and dark and which were then suddenly exposed to bright light during a dark spell, evinced a rapid drop in enzyme activity. It would appear therefore that the gland is sensitive to light, but it would also appear that there are certain times of the day when this sensitivity disappears and the rhythm is unalterable by environmental manipulation. The major influencing point appears to be related to light during dark periods and it may be, therefore, that the varying time of the early morning light is the re-setter of the biological clock. Light reaching the pineal reduces the activity of *N*-acetyltransferase, thereby reducing the amount of melatonin produced and circulated. The chick's body temperature begins to rise and its daily activities ensue. Different species sense these light alterations in differing ways. The rat, for example, has a branch of the optic nerve, unnecessary for vision, which conducts light inputs to the pineal gland, whilst birds monitor the light levels directly through the bony skull in addition to the eyes. In the rat, the sympathetic nerves release norepinephrine which activates the pineal gland and hence the enzyme, and yet, in chickens, the same norepinephrine release inhibits pineal gland activity (Binkley, 1979).

The human pineal gland, a small reddish-grey structure on the dorsal surface of the midbrain, which is attached to the roof of the third ventricle in the midline, also contains serotonin, melatonin and other active amines. However, its function is rather unclear, other than having an implication in the sexual development of the child at puberty. It does seem that there may be some similarities between the human function and that of the animals previously discussed. Man, for example, may be seen to demonstrate a similar body temperature cycle to the chicken. An approximate 1 to 1.5 °C difference is seen on the 24-hour cycle, with the lowest point between 2.00 a.m. and 5.00 a.m., and a peak in the afternoon. Body temperature is seen to influence the length of human sleep for those individuals on time-free schedules, and where no clock or environmental cues are provided to indicate bed-time is approaching. An individual retiring when his body temperature is at its lowest point sleeps for only eight hours. In contrast, retiring when the body temperature is peaking, demonstrates a sleep period of up to 14 hours. Most individuals have no perception of this temperature change and yet when still awake in the early hours of the morning notice how cold and chilled they have become. Similarly an extra long sleep is attributed to being extra tired, overfull with late-night dining habits or due to an extra glass of an alcoholic beverage, when it may simply be due to falling asleep when the body temperature is high.

Sleep–wake cycles

Many studies such as that of Michel Siffre (1963), a French cave explorer, have been conducted into the effects of living for a prolonged period of time without environmental cues to assist the body clock in timing of activities. Siffre, for example, lived in a carefully prepared cave, where no light could enter, for six months in Texas, USA. He ate and slept at will, wearing electrodes on his scalp to monitor his sleep cycles and passing specimens of urine up to the surface for analysis. When desirous of sleep, Siffre would contact the surface and artificial light sources would be extinguished. Each sleep–wake cycle constituted 'a day' and the length of Siffre's days were seen to extend gradually, to the point that Siffre's believed 151-day stay was in reality 179 days long. You may recall that the hostage, Jackie Mann, similarly miscalculated the number of days of his confinement because of reduction/absence of environmental cues. Mann 'lost' only a very few days, but Siffre 'lost' a whole month.

It was noted with Siffre that, whilst his days lengthened to approximately 33 hours, his temperature cycle remained in a 24.8-hour cycle so that, at times, he experienced both the temperature peak and trough within his 'daytime' activity and indeed on his twelfth day experienced two highs and two lows during one 'day'. It's not at all surprising that at the end of his cave sojourn he was confused:

Sullenly, mechanically, I stumble through my battery of tests. Just as I finish my laps on the hated bicycle, the telephone rings. Gerard tells me that it is August 10th, a stormy day, and the experiment has concluded; I am confused; I believe it to be mid-July. Then, as the truth sinks in, comes a flood of relief.

David Lafferty, however, who spent 127 days in a cave (Moore-Ede *et al.*, 1982), found that, whilst initially his cycles were erratic, they did readjust. Some 'days' were 19 hours long—10 hours awake and 9 hours asleep—and others were 53 hours long—18 hours awake and 35 hours asleep—but eventually, towards the end of his investigation, he settled to a 25-hour day.

In support of the role of melatonin in the human sleep–wake cycle, Arendt *et al.*, 1987) at the University of Surrey, conducted experiments with potentially 'jet-lagged' individuals. You may have personal experience of the fatigue, insomnia and disorientation which may spoil the first few days of a holiday abroad, and it is a fact that individuals suffer less of a problem when travelling in a westerly rather than easterly direction. The 23–25-hour inbuilt clock is actually extending the hours of its day during this westward travel and this would appear easier to accommodate than the daylength reduction inherent in travelling eastward. After a long flight, the day–night cycle of home remains 'locked into' the system and it is the attempts to override the norm by assuming a new holiday clock that creates the symptoms of jet-leg. Arendt *et al.* believed it to be the cyclical release of melatonin which maintains the inbuilt clock and therefore administered melatonin to jet-lagged volunteers during the evening when normally they would be sleepy. Far fewer of the volunteers complained of the ill-effects of jet-lag than the control group who had been given a placebo.

A more gentle movement of the biological clock has been seen to be of value in shift work situations. A one week of each day shift–night shift–evening shift system of working requires an individual to constantly turn back his clock by eight hours each week and provokes insomnia, digestive problems, fatigue and irritability. Labratory studies elicit the fact that animals exposed to such a rotating schedule have shorter life spans and an increased level of heart disease, so it is an important factor in health. Czeisler *et al.* (1981) utilized the natural preferences of the body for a forward adjustment rather than a backward orientated one, and also suggested that shifts should rotate on a three-weekly rather than a one-weekly basis to facilitate an adjustment to the adjustment in 'time zone'. The workforce were happy and healthier and productivity rose by 22%. The men found that a slight adjustment to their sleeping time, by going to bed a little later each week, made the transition even easier, in effect by gradually moving the inner clock forwards.

Perchance to dream?

It is not possible to leave the subject of sleep without a mention of dreams, and you may recall that REM sleep is the phase of the sleep cycle generally associated with the phenomenon. The studies of Aserinsky and Kleitman (1953) elicited the REM patterning of sleep and Dement and Kleitman's (1975) further investigations demonstrated that arousal immediately after the conjugate eye movements was more likely to evoke the report of a vivid dream, than arousal at any other part of the cycle. When Dement deprived individuals of REM sleep, by awaking them prior to its onset, subjects would show the signs of a sleepless night the following day and yet when woken the same number of times during other stages of sleep, a lesser degree of impairment was seen to follow. REM-deprived subjects similarly spent an increased amount of time in REM sleep the following night, as if to make up for the loss. Studies since the 1950s have pointed out that dreaming also occurs in slow wave sleep, for the subject awakened after only one hour of sleep and prior to the onset of the first REM period, often reports a dream. However, the more vivid and memorable dreams do appear to take place within the REM phase.

Of course it is a long time since Freud's *Interpretation of Dreams* (Freud, 1954) and, though we would recommend it as reading of interest, a great deal of scientific knowledge has been accrued since then. It is of some amusement to think of dreams being symbolic, acceptable representations of the wicked, pleasure-seeking 'id', and yet many still adhere to the theory. Stranger still, in this regard, is the knowledge that the newborn baby spends half its sleeping time in REM cycle and that the dog, cat and rat indulge in REM sleep and therefore presumably some variety of dreaming. Dogs definitely dream during REM sleep, with paws twitching and little yelping noises! Without Man's higher cortex and therefore 'conscience', do they need to disguise their basic impulses, especially when one considers how little control they exhibit over instinctual behaviour when awake!

Crick and Mitchison (1983) suggested that without the ability to dream, the cortex would be 'filled up' with out of date, uncorrected and superfluous information and that the organism would therefore require a very large cortex to continually absorb new information. Indeed, this appears to be supported by studies of the Australian spiny ant-eater (a marsupial) and the dolphin, both of which have an extraordinarily large cortex and neither of which demonstrate REM sleep ability. Crick believes the large cortex necessary because of the inability to unlearn material or re-vamp old learning in the light of further experience.

Sleep deprivation for three or more nights has been seen to produce both visual and auditory hallucinations, in addition to misperceptions. There are consistent reports of solid objects 'trembling', faces appearing from thin air and walls covered in insects and other items. Auditory hallucinations in the form of voices, talking about the subject, are similarly a regular complaint. Sounds familiar? It could be the clinical picture associated with a diagnosis of 'schizophrenia' and yet depressed mood has been successfully elevated via intentional sleep deprivation (Wehr *et al.*, 1979). The suggestion that dreaming is the brain's mechanism for removing old and incorporating new learning seems a sensible one when one views the mixed up nature of many dreams.

Events or information of the day appear often to be linked up with yesterday's activities and memories of many years ago, during sleep, in an apparently logicless sequence and certainly cause either amusement or bewilderment on the part of the subject. The new learning being incorporated, or replacing old memories, would appear a safe bet. However, the current state of physiological knowledge has many gaps with regard to sleep.

The evolutionary protective mechanism of sleep as the basis for all subsequent sleep-related activities also seems a realistic purport. Remaining tucked away from marauding predators during the night-time hours of darkness, when visual acuity has to be less effective, is an eminently sensible idea. The fact, too, that a period of inactivity and sensory deprivation is necessary to stock up on depleted food stores, provide a period of rest, recuperation, growth and repair of organs and to amend stored memories in the light of continuing inputs, would support the value of a prolonged and regular reduced awareness and response. Sleep is a necessary part therefore of the optimum potential for survival of any organism and thence should be viewed as valuable in its own right.

PROBLEMS OF SLEEP

Many of the everyday problems associated with sleep may be attributed to the adoption of a lifestyle which is not conducive—and may, indeed, be preclusive—to regular, restful sleep patterns. Children may never acquire the sleep hygiene measures necessary to ensure a lifetime of efficient sleeping, and sleep may be viewed as a waste of a third of the valuable waking time.

Sometimes people are less than helpful to their body rhythms, because of their attitudes to sleep, as one of something to do when there is nothing better on offer and not really of sufficient value to warrant specific attention. Whilst most people will not be happy to go past lunchtime without eating, and would certainly be really put out if their monthly/weekly income was unavailable on the correct day, the importance of *regular sleep hours* is often overlooked. Of course, there are many distractions to divert the individual's attention away from bedtime. Late and all-night television broadcasting, with all the best films screened during the bedtime hours, seems far more enthralling a proposition than bed at 10.30 p.m., especially if there is no deadline for getting up in the morning, as with the unemployed person, the afternoon shift worker or the college student. Entertainment, and leisure services in general, are encroaching more and more on the hours traditionally viewed as those for sleep, with midnight cinema shows, late-night restaurant and sports facilities all extending their opening hours to provide services for the more demanding population needs. There is more leisure time available and, in relative terms, the vast majority of the population have money to spend in excess of that needed for pure survival needs. Time and money are only two of three criteria necessary to enable the individual to go out and play; one needs the energy to spare in such activities and again, in comparison with our ancestors, today's generation expends far less physical exertion in their jobs and in general leads a far more sedentary lifestyle. *Daily exercise* promotes an increased blood circulation, raises the metabolic rate and assists in ridding the body of its toxins, as well as assisting in respiratory function and healthy bone and muscle maintenance. Steady daily exercise helps to promote sleep. No one would suggest a return to the days of 16–18 hours of hard graft, but the new found freedom from such major time constraints and commitments must be used to the human advantage and not detriment. Regular sleeping hours and daily exercise are two important sleep enhancers.

A third important factor again relates to the same general theme, for the individual needs to put aside *sufficient time* for sleep. There appears little point in spending a mere three or four hours in sleeping when the individual's biological activities undertaken during the period are programmed to personal requirements and require six or eight hours each night to complete. How can a person expect to feel refreshed and alert with so much unfinished business still to be attended to, which can only build up like an in-tray of unanswered mail? The duration of sleep which provokes this 'alert and refreshed' state is the amount needed to be set aside nightly to maintain health and wellbeing.

The environment is yet another area of importance when promoting sleep hygiene measures, for it used to be the case that a bedroom was solely, or almost solely, used for sleeping, but this is often no longer the case. Children often utilize a bedroom as a play area and hence it is filled to the brim with bright, attractive and stimulating material. It is an area associated now with socialization, friends being invited into the room and it being used as an entertaining area, rather than of peace, quiet and rest. For some, this valuable personal space may become inextricably linked with feelings of discomfort, isolation, punishment or physical and/or emotional pain. The child continually excluded from adult or family interactions and 'sent to his room' is more likely to resent the facility and associate it with negative, tumultuous emotions rather than the placid, peaceful, contented feelings which need to be engendered within a sleeping area. The physically and/or sexually abused child may feel fear and terror in regard to the environment where the injuries have been perpetrated. Such feelings are not conducive to restful sleep.

Of course, it is not only the child who may experience an environment unconducive to sleep. The student who lives in a hall of residence, with just one room available for all activities, may find similarly new and different associations being acquired in regard to what should be, in essence, sleeping quarters. Whilst communal cooking, eating and lounge facilities may be provided, the 'bed-sit' may become the centre for studying, socializing and sleeping. Adults who have access to a lounge in which to watch television may still insist on watching it in bed and hence again dilute the association with a sleeping area. The bedroom needs to be as free from distractions as possible and engender feelings of tranquillity, comfort and safety. Decor, too, needs to be restful rather than stimulating.

The individual gets used to the general sounds within the external environment too, and again changes may cause disturbances to sleep:

Mother's home is situated on the outskirts of a busy little town, whilst I live in the heart of the country and recently, when I'd got an overnight trip away, she came to 'dog-sit'. On my return, I was astounded to hear that she 'hadn't slept a wink all night for the noise'. The 'resident' owl, the cows and other farm animals in the locale had kept her awake when the passing—and often quite heavy—traffic outside her own home never disturbs her!

Whilst the problems identified above may provoke consistently *ineffective and inefficient sleeping routines*, the term *sleep disorders* is reserved for sleep problems of more than one month's duration, rather than transient sleeplessness or other disturbance associated with a short-lived psychosocial stressor or poor sleep habits. Sleep disturbance may be the initiator of other bio-psychosocial problems or may be a sequelae of mental health or somatic health difficulties, and therefore may represent a frequent complaint of the client or his significant others in many and varied care situations. Nurses will often wonder whether such problems represent a primary or secondary health deviation and it is therefore essential to ask the questions appropriate to elicit as much information as is possible, in order that relevant assistance may be provided.

THE DYSSOMNIAS

Dyssomnia is the generic term applied to problems associated with the *amount*, *quality* or *timing* of sleep. The group includes *insomnia*, where the duration or quality of sleep is insufficient for normal and expected levels of daytime functioning, *hypersomnias*, where despite an adequate night's sleep, the individual complains of excessive daytime drowsiness, and *sleep–wake schedule disorders*, where the individual's pattern of sleeping and waking is seen to be out of synchronization with what is considered to be the norm of the environment. A second generic group of problems, the *parasomnias*, are associated with the occurrence of abnormal events, either during sleep itself or in the twilight stage between sleep and wakefulness. These include problems related to dreaming, that is *nightmares and terrors*, and those relating to *sleep-walking* (*somnambulism*). Whilst all occur as a primary problem in the absence of any biopsychosocial health deviation, many may be seen as a secondary exteriorization to some other problem of health.

Insomnia may be diagnosed in response to client—or family—complaints related to:

1   A difficulty in initiating sleep

2   Difficulty in maintaining sleep

or

3   Non-restorative, though normal duration, sleep.

McGhic and Russell (1962) described insomnia as being reported with increasing frequency in older age groups, from less than 10% in the 15–24-year age group, to around 18% in the 45–54-year band and approximately 40% of 65+ year olds. They also note that 'symptoms' change with advancing age, as the younger group tend to complain of non-restorative sleep, whilst the older age groups complain of initiation–maintenance problems. Women appear to experience problems at twice the rate of their age-matched male peers—14% as opposed to 6% (Kripke and Gillin, 1985). The frequency of insomnia in men, whilst consistently lower than women, shows a sudden increase in the 65–74-year-old age group, and this may be related to the changes in general routines and exercise levels brought about by retirement. Researchers have discovered that individuals tend to overestimate the amount of sleep lost. One such study (Carskadon *et al.*, 1974) found that less than half of a group, who complained of protracted and severe sleep loss, were actually awake for 30 minutes during the night, and it has been suggested this overestimation may be due to one of two factors. It may be, for example, that, because there is no memory of having slept, the 'insomniac' remembers only the wakeful period, or that perhaps restless or light sleep may be interpreted as wakefulness and hence a miscalculation occurs.

In *primary insomnia*, sleep often becomes a major preoccupation with the individual anxious for the entire waking hours in relation to the difficulties experienced. The person tries hard to fall asleep, but this merely increases the prevailing tension and therefore sleep continues to be evasive. Often subjects report being able to sleep when not trying, for example, they may fall asleep easily in front of the television or in the cinema. Similarly, the individual may describe an improvement in the problem when sleeping in an unfamiliar environment. Often the individual reports a life-long sleep difficulty, although others may be able to pinpoint some event or psychosocial stressor in adult life which coincided with the onset of sleep disturbance. On occasions primary insomnia may be a complication of an insomnia which occurs as an integral part of a mental health or organic health problem. The client may 'get into the habit' of sleep disturbance during this time so that even when there is a resolution to the original problem, the sleep disorder remains.

Insomnia and mental disorders

Insomnia related to another, non-organic, mental health problem is frequently encountered, for many individuals experiencing lowered or elevated mood, or anxiety, will describe such disturbances. Where the diagnosis, for example, is one of *dysthymia*, a lowered mood, not associated with hallucinatory experiences or delusional ideation, there may be difficulties expressed with regard to initiation of sleep, but once asleep, the individual may be undisturbed for the rest of the night. In contrast, the individual experiencing a *major depressive episode*, with its concomitant absence of insight into reality, may initiate sleep relatively easily but exteriorize wakening in the early hours of the morning. The 'dysthymic' client experiences his lowest mood 'trough' of the day late in the evening just prior to bedtime, whilst the individual diagnosed as suffering a 'major' depressed mood awakens at his lowest mood point. Both may be of significance when nursing a client who has expressed or may be considering suicidal thoughts, for it is when mood is at its lowest point that such thoughts may find ex-

pression in enactment, and whilst close observation of this client is a priority 24 hours of the day, intense scrutiny during the quiet hours, when the client is expected to be asleep, and yet may not be, is of prime importance. You should be aware, however, that it is not only clients with a label of 'depression' who may experience a profound lowering of mood as an integral or concomitant feature of their total mental health problems and therefore any individual exteriorizing such mood deviation—for no matter how fleeting a period—may suffer severe sleep disturbance (and also ideas of self-harm).

Preoccupation with mental activities and imagery quite naturally will provoke unease, restlessness, agitation and perhaps motor acceleration and therefore any individual experiencing such problems is likely to find sleeping problematical. Clients exteriorizing elevated mood—as in diagnoses such as *cyclothymia* and *bipolar mood disorder* of a *mixed or manic nature*—may exhibit no inclination or desire to sleep, being unable to relax the body and quieten the mind for a sufficient period to allow sleep to encroach. Anxiety or fear for one's own health or safety and well-being may provoke a similar high level of mental alertness and a concomitant bodily tension and therefore preclude sleep initiation. This would encompass a wide number of individuals within care provision and not only those traditionally associated with anxiety. The individual, for example, who demonstrates obsessive ideation and compulsive, ritualistic behaviours may be too tense to sleep easily, whilst the person who is utterly convinced of the fact that someone is either intent on killing him or on 'interfering' with his or her mind or body during sleep, may be understandably unwilling to drop their guard to allow sleep. The young person experiencing anorexia nervosa and its associated problems may appear to have no sleep disturbance at all, for they seem to initiate sleep with no trouble and may still be fast off when approached next morning to get up, and yet the total sleep duration is often considerably reduced. How? The individual is frequently awake during the very early hours of the morning and may, within that wakeful period, exercise vigorously with no carer to observe the phenomenon. Bingeing and purging activities may similarly be quietly performed without other people's awareness.

Insomnia and organic disorders

It would be unreasonable, too, to assume that problems associated with somatic health during the day would miraculously disappear just because it is time for bed, and it is, therefore, a relatively common event to see *insomnia* which is *related to a known organic factor*. For example, the pain, stiffness or general discomfort associated with a broken bone, arthritic joints or the rigidity of Parkinson's disease may, indeed, be perceived as increasing at night, during the protracted period of enforced immobility and when environmental distractors and comforters are reduced in both quality and quantity. Some individuals may experience horror at the thought of lying down in bed, and people experiencing the effects of a left-sided heart failure are amongst this number. The difficulty in breathing (*dyspnoea*) which they experience is significantly exacerbated when lying flat (*orthopnoea*) due to the pulmonary oedema which 'clogs up' the alveoli and reduces the oxygen-filling capability of lung tissue. The individual may awaken suddenly during the night, often understandably panicked by inability to breathe easily—*paroxysmal nocturnal dyspnoea*. *Asthma* may also awaken the individual at night and cause early morning wheezing and dyspnoea, and, in fact, some paroxysmal disorders may be seen to begin with the REM sleep phases of the sleep cycle, for example, *duodenal ulcer pain* and *migraine*, causing disturbance in the early hours. Angina and cardiac arrhythmias occur more frequently in REM sleep, too, as do deaths from myocardial infarction. Whilst it is not clear during which phase of sleep infarcts occur, they usually happen between 5.00 a.m. and 6.00 a.m., when REM sleep predominates. Some people may experience *seizures* on a regular basis during sleep and the characteristic electroencephalographic 'epileptic discharges' may be seen to be activated in either REM or slow wave sleep, depending on the type of disorder. You are probably only too well aware of the disturbed sleep associated with a persistent cough in a short duration respiratory tract infec-

tion, but such a problem may be a long-term feature in a variety of respiratory problems and may be the result of both intrinsic stimuli (neoplasia, inflammation, foreign bodies and scar tissue formation are examples) and extrinsic stimuli (pleurisy, oesophageal growths, mediastinal lymphadenopathy) in addition to a psychogenic or attention-seeking origin. Sleep disturbance may serve to weaken the individual further and this type of intermittent night-time wakening may be a common feature in a variety of somatic health problems. The *pruritus* of jaundice and the *nocturia* (voiding during the night hours) associated with impaired renal function provide two such instances.

Within mental health care provision, individuals experiencing organic *impairment* may likewise exteriorize sleep problems. *Delirium* may be seen to provoke problems of both the insomnia-type and disturbances in the sleep–wake cycle later elucidated. The individual may be hypervigilant or hypersomnolent, and vivid dreams and nightmares may be seen to blend imperceptibly for the client into hallucinatory experiences during waking. There may be crying, moaning, muttering and calls for help during the night hours, thus disturbing the sleep of others within the environment. Delirium may be an integral feature experienced during a variety of somatic as well as mental health orientated problems—systemic infections, metabolic disorders, renal and hepatic disease and head injury to name but a few—and colleagues within all specialties of care should be aware of such sleep problems.

Psychoactive substance use and abuse is a frequent cause of delirium within the sphere of psychosocial health care and therefore this insomnia–hypersomnia pattern may be problematical. Withdrawal from substance use may elicit similar symptomatology and those experiencing the effects of a psychoactive-substance related organic mood disorder may have difficulty initiating sleep. However, it is not only the 'illicit' drugs that may provoke a sleeping problem, for steroids, bronchodilators and central adrenergic blocking agents given 'therapeutically' over prolonged periods may engender an insomnia disorder.

Insomnia, whether primary or secondary in

nature, is bound to result in excessive day-time fatigue, impaired day-time functioning and general irritability. Some may experience disturbances in mood, in memory and concentration and attention spans, and social and occupational functioning may become seriously disrupted if problems are protracted.

Hypersomnia

Hypersomnia on the other hand may engender disruption from day one, for, despite night-time sleep of an adequate amount, there are complaints of either excessive day-time sleepiness, sleep attacks or a prolonged transition from sleep to wakefulness, often referred to as *sleep drunkenness* (Roth *et al.*, 1972). That hypersomnia may be associated with other, *non-organic, mental health problems* has already been mentioned in passing. It may be a feature of *depressed mood*, in *bipolar disorders*, and in some other mood disorders, such as *major depression* or *dysthymia*. Similarly, hypersomnia may be a feature in the sleep of those diagnosed as '*schizophrenic*' and where '*somatoform disorders*' exist, but in the majority of instances the individual asserts that this excessive sleepiness is the result of non-restorative sleep. We have also made previous mention of hypersomnia in relation to a *known organic factor*, as in delirium and illicit and prescribed drugs, and other abused substance use/withdrawal.

Hypersomnolence may be a *secondary* phenomenon to a wide number of cerebral problems (trauma, tumour, vascular accident, inflammation and infection), in endocrinological dysfunction, for example hypothyroidism, and in respiratory, renal and hepatic failure (Guilleminault *et al.*, 1983). They may also be secondary to primary sleep disorders of which the subject is totally unaware. *Sleep apnoea syndrome*, for example, may result in day-time sleepiness because of persistent, short duration periods of respiratory cessation throughout the night. An individual may stop breathing in this way for one of two reasons; there may be a hyposensitivity of the respiratory centre to carbon dioxide or an upper airway obstruction to respiration, although mixed aetiology has been demonstrated. The com-

monest causes of obstruction would appear to be tonsillar hypertrophy, obesity or a sleep-induced hypotonia of the pharyngeal muscles, although deformity of the mandible has also been indicated as a predisposing factor (Lugaresi *et al.*, 1973).

The 'Pickwickian Syndrome', named by Burwell *et al.* (1956) after the fat boy in Dickens' novel, is, as the name suggests, seen in grossly overweight children. Some experience only mild headaches in addition to the sleep apnoea, but day-time somnolence does, of course, result in poor school performance. Other children may exhibit *cyanosis, right-sided heart failure* and *polycythaemia* (an increase in the number of erythrocytes and therefore an increase in the concentration of haemoglobin) in addition to the night-time periodic respiration and day-time sleepiness. There continues to be a dispute in regard to the specific aetiology of the problem (Passouant *et al.*, 1967; Schwartz *et al.* 1967).

Whatever the cause, each episode of apnoea may last from 10 to 80 seconds or more, and there may be anywhere in the region of 30 to several hundred such episodes each night. The individual must partially or fully arouse in order to breathe, although he or she is oblivious to the fact. There is a period of loud snoring and snorting, followed by a resumption in respiration. Gross movement of the extremities, sleep walking and enuresis (involuntary voiding of urine) may all be exhibited. If awakened at night, the individual may demonstrate automatic behaviour, amnesia, temporal disorientation, poor judgement and hypnagogic hallucinations. Day-time performance may be interspersed within micro-sleeps, or a generalized excessive sleepiness. Complaints may be made regarding decreased sexual drive and potency, personality changes and headaches and on examination hypertension and sinus tachycardia may be evident. Whilst it has been asserted that up to 10% of the population suffer from this syndrome, 'normal' sleepers may experience occasional apnoeic episodes too.

Primary hypersomnias may occur in short or long periods and, amongst the former, '*sleep drunkenness*' is by far the most common example. Subjects complain of not being able to wake up 'properly' for some considerable period after actually getting out of bed, which may extend to up to four hours. This half-awake/half-asleep period is accompanied by confusion, disorientation, retarded and inco-ordinated motor activity and a desire to go back to bed. Subjects will sleep, if left undisturbed, for up to 20 hours with no spontaneous waking and yet still experience daytime somnolence. Night-time sleep is rapidly initiated, often within seconds of putting the head on the pillow, and is extremely deep. Headaches, depressed mood and personality changes have frequently been reported, and occurrence is seen to be slightly higher in men. Whilst it may be seen to follow a period of sleep deprivation, in Roth and his colleagues' detailed study (Roth *et al.*, 1972), one-third of presenting individuals had a family history of such problems and most people demonstrated a life-long tendency towards sleep drunkenness symptomatology. It presented as a relatively common experience within this particular study of hypersomnia sufferers, with an approximate incidence of 30% of problems seen.

Kleine–Levin syndrome

In contrast Kleine (1925) and Levin (1936) described a much rarer type of hypersomnia which now bears their names. This syndrome is characterized by periods when the appetite is excessive (*bulimia*) and the individual will eat ravenously, and often anything in sight, yet if food is not available, neither complains of hunger nor demands food. The eating behaviour is compulsive, greedy and wolfish in nature and this is followed by a period of profound sleepiness, where the individual will sleep day and night, rousing only to eat, drink or perform evacuatory functions. During this period the individual is as easily awoken as any normal sleeper, but is irritable, bad tempered and may be physically aggressive. When awake, too, the individual demonstrates marked cognitive impairment—confusion, disorientation, muddled and de-personalized thinking and speech, and memory disturbances—and perceptions may be littered with vivid imagery which the individual finds difficult to differentiate from dreams. Auditory hallucinations and delusional ideation may also be exteriorized. Emotional and motor agitation and unrest are also a feature, with fidgety movements and gener-

alized unease. Abnormal—for the individual—levels of sexual behaviour have been reported (Critchley, 1962; Garland *et al.*, 1965) with frequent masturbation and hypersexuality.

The Kleine–Levin syndrome is seen to affect adolescent boys predominantly, though atypical cases have been documented where onset has been seen in an adolescent girl (Duffy and Davison, 1968), in women (Gilbert, 1964) and in middle age (Gallinek, 1954). An 'attack' may last for days or weeks, but typically are infrequent, the average being two per year though as many as 12 have been described. The onset is usually spontaneous, although it may be seen that a period of stress or flu-like condition may precede its onset. Indeed, whilst death during an attack is rare, a post-mortem examination of one fatality indicated the possibility of a viral aetiology (Carpenter *et al.*, 1982) though this has not been confirmed. In between attacks, the individual reverts to 'normal' characteristics and behavioural patterns, although mental health problems may exist for a short time before and after the episode. Onset and cessation of an attack may be gradual or abrupt in nature, and the individual may have only partial, or a complete lack of, awareness of the episode. The episodic problems of bingeing and somnolence appear to reduce in both frequency and duration with time, and ultimately cease completely (Gallinek, 1954).

Diencephalic abnormality has been suggested to account for the eating–sleeping behaviours of the syndrome, but no abnormalities within biochemistry, electroencephalography or physiology have been elicited during attacks. The problem for the client, and the professional must be in the syndrome's rarity and the apparently 'psychotic' symptomatology which may predominate within the clinical picture, for as Critchley (1962) and others observe (Robinson and McQuillan, 1951), the client may present with distinct schizophrenia-like symptomatology. The need for a comprehensive and accurate analysis of actual problems experienced by the individual, regardless of the symptomatology to be expected in a specific diagnosis applied, and the willingness to consider alternative explanations for behaviours exhibited, is therefore a necessary characteristic for all carers within mental health service provision.

Narcolepsy

Probably first described by Westphal (1877) but named by Gelineau (1880), narcolepsy is, by contrast, much easier to recognize. The individual experiences an irresistible desire to sleep during the day-time, and awakes easily enough from such naps, feeling refreshed and alert, experiencing no more episodes for several hours. The nap usually lasts for a period of 10–15 minutes and if the individual is prevented from napping, or awakened during the sleep, he or she may be extremely irritable. Naps most frequently occur at junctures of the day when events or activities are more conducive to drowsiness, for example, after meals and where environmental stimuli are reduced or monotonous, but some individuals experience the problem when talking, eating, dancing—even when making love—and attacks may lead to life-threatening situations if they occur during periods of driving, swimming or operating machinery.

In 75% of individuals presenting, there is evidence of other, additional features. *Cataplexy*, a sudden loss of emotional tone, appears to be evident in 70% of narcolepsy sufferers, and tends to occur following an emotion-provoking event, for example, after laughter or tears are evoked. Where all muscle groups are involved, the individual will fall to the floor, unable to move or speak, and possibly sustaining injury. Often the individual will remain standing, however, and reaction is appropriate to a limited muscular involvement, as the individual may drop something he was previously holding, or elicit a jaw- or head-dropping movement. Such attacks rarely extend beyond a minute's duration and the individual is always alert and fully aware of what is happening. Cataplectic attacks rarely occur more than once a day, and subjects may learn to avoid precipitating situations. Cataplexy has been described within one family, where 11 children were affected and attacks were laughter induced (Gelardi and Brown, 1967). The researchers believed it to be transmitted via an autosomal dominant gene and described only three of the children as evincing any—even if dubious—signs of narcolepsy, though *sleep paralysis* was occasionally demonstrated. Whilst rare, such an account is of value when attempting to discover aetiology of such problems.

Sleep paralysis, mentioned above, is again a relatively common accompaniment to narcolepsy, with an estimated 30% of narcoleptic individuals exhibiting the problem. There is a sudden inability to move either just before sleeping or immediately upon waking, which may occur in relation to both nocturnal and diurnal sleep periods. Abrupt in onset, there is a *flaccid paralysis* which is usually seen to encompass all muscles, although on occasions the individual may find some degree of eye movement possible. Duration does not usually exceed one minute, though one case has been reported where the paralysis exceeded an hour, and the experience may be dispelled by touch or by calling the individual's name. In a similar manner to cataplectic attacks, some rare instances of sleep paralysis occurring without narcolepsy have been described (Bowling and Richards, 1961) which affected 10 people from two families.

Hypnagogic hallucinations are reported by a slightly smaller percentage of narcolepsy sufferers than is sleep paralysis, and are commonly experienced via the auditory modality, though visual, tactile and multimodal perceptual disorders are also seen. They predominantly arise as the individual passes into sleep, but on occasions may occur during the transition from sleep to wakefulness, when they are referred to as *hypnopompic hallucinations*. You may have experienced similar bed-time experiences and both hypnagogic and hypnopompic hallucinations are 'normal' phenomena. The difference between the 'normal' and the 'narcoleptic' is that in the former, the perceptual experiences are often of a word or a brief image that has little emotional meaning to the individual, whilst the latter experiences vivid, intense and complex visions, often bizarre and sometimes unpleasant in content. They may be difficult to distinguish from a dream, because of these characteristics and are always accompanied by strong emotional reactions, and, whilst the subject may respond to his experience whilst it operates, there is the recognition, once awake, of the true nature of the hallucinatory experience (Zarcone, 1973).

Narcolepsy has its onset predominantly in the

10–20-year-old age group and it is rare to see a new subject of the 40-year-old-plus age group. Again it appears more common in boys and there is, in one-third of subjects, a family history evident. As has been identified, narcoleptic attacks as a sole problem presenting is less frequently seen—only 30% of instances, but to see all potentially associated features, that is cataplectic attacks, sleep paralysis and hypnagogic hallucinations, is much more rare at only 10% of all subjects with narcolepsy. The disturbed nocturnal sleep associated with narcolepsy demonstrates rapid initiation of sleep but subsequent restlessness and frequent wakeful periods. Many individuals, some 60% of those subject to both narcolepsy and cataplexy, experience vivid dreams, of an unpleasant and often terrifying nature, whilst where narcolepsy is a sole feature, the incidence is approximately 20% (Gelardi and Brown, 1967). Day-time sleep is not, however, associated with dreaming.

Whilst no such disturbance has been demonstrated in those experiencing narcolepsy alone, those individuals who exhibit one or more of the other accompanying features of sleep paralysis, hypnagogic hallucinations or cataplectic attacks, show REM sleep occurring out of the normal sequence during nocturnal sleep, with REM occurring immediately or very quickly after the onset of sleep, and also during the day-time 'catnaps'. The features of hallucinations and sleep paralysis both occur during this early REM phase, as do cataplectic attacks. In addition, or perhaps because of, this out-of-synchronization of the REM phase, the other stages of nocturnal sleep are disturbed accounting for the restlessness and frequent awakenings. It has been suggested (Rechtschaffen *et al.*, 1963), in the light of these EEG findings, that narcolepsy assumes a midpoint on a continuum that extends from hypersomnia at one extreme and narcolepsy plus cataplepsy at the other.

You will recall the emphasis we laid on the basic circadian rhythms, of which sleep is one example, and of the importance of environmental cues in the individual's awareness of when it is time to eat and sleep. Problems related to the *sleep–wake cycle* are seen to occur because of a mismatch between environmental norms and the individual's circadian rhythm, and again you may recall the 'jet-lag' and 'shift work' examples previously offered within the introductory discussion on sleep and its norms.

Sleep–wake schedules may be seen to be *advanced* or *delayed* in relation to the societal norms. Where an advance is seen, the individual is really desirous of sleep early in the evening, perhaps as early as 6.00 or 7.00 p.m. and is awake around 2.00 or 3.00 a.m., happy and alert. In delayed schedules, the reverse is seen with the individual actually wanting to sleep at around 3.00 or 4.00 a.m. and, if allowed, will sleep until perhaps 10.00 or 11.00 a.m., therefore finding great difficulty if needing to be at work or seeing the children to school at 8.30 a.m. An advanced sleep pattern is often a feature of older people and hence the nurse must be aware of this as a normal routine for an individual rather than merely assuming that is indicative of depressed mood, especially when one recalls that the need for sleep appears to reduce as age advances. The delayed sleep pattern is more likely to be a problem for the younger age group individuals and particularly those who have no rigid occupational or social commitments.

A third variation of the problem may be seen when there is no real 24-hour routine to life, and the individual is able to nap at will throughout the day, thus disrupting the circadian cycle of one major period of inactivity per day. The elderly and the bedridden individual may form part of this group of subjects, as may those individuals who fit their sleep into the voids created between work and socialization activities, thus demonstrating a *disorganized sleep–wake schedule*.

A *frequently changing pattern* of sleep–wake cycles may be seen to occur, yet again, as a result of lifestyle, in those jet-setters and shift workers, for example, who continually interfere with the normal routines of the body. You may recall that changes in 'time zone' require a period of adaptation to synchronize internal rhythms and environmental needs, and often an individual may try to mix the old and the new requirements, thus creating problems. The shift worker on night duty for a three-week period organized thus by his employer in order to ease the transition from one time zone functioning level to another, may attempt at the weekends when off duty to revert to a pattern of day-time wakefulness and night-time sleeping, thereby throwing the cycle's stability yet again. Having previously referred to the health problems associated with frequently changing schedules, it may be recognized as a detrimental practice.

For many of the individuals who experience sleep–wake schedule problems, the answers lie in their own hands in the need to assume a daily routine conducive to environmental norms and circadian cycles, for in a preponderance of instances day-time naps and night-time revelling interfere with normal sleep requirements. For shift workers and jet-setters, the answer is predominantly in maintenance of new 'time zones' until another change is on the horizon and then a gradual adjustment towards the new requirements, to prevent a total derangement of the cycle and an easier transition phase. Gradual sleep-time advance or retard may be of a similar value to those individuals experiencing an innate cyclical problem, and may be a far more advantageous option than medication-induced conventional sleep patterns or being tired for large parts of the morning.

Within mental health care, problems of the sleep–wake schedule may be associated with a variety of situations in which there is a lack of awareness of environmental reality or an inability to recognize, or accede to, the demands of the body for sleep and rest. Clients experiencing problems associated with organic deterioration and hallucinatory experiences and delusional ideation are therefore prime candidates, and may need intensive night hour assistance and support.

THE PARASOMNIAS

The parasomnias, the second category associated with problems of sleep experienced, are characterized by 'abnormal' events that occur either during sleep or in the transition from wakefulness to sleep. Whilst disturbing the quality or quantity of sleep attained, as, in the dyssomnia group, the individual's complaint is not related either to that disturbance or sleep loss as such—the person, or his partner or family, centre concerns upon the event(s) experienced, and thus a differentiation is immediately possible and necessary. Are clients having problems in initiating or maintaining sleep, or are they experiencing some 'happening' within the night-time sleep period which engenders fear to sleep or which wakens them and precludes a return to rest?

Who has not had the experience of a bad dream and awoken in the darkness, heart thumping and momentarily panicked that fantasy may indeed be reality, only to find that the bed and surroundings are safe and familiar, and breathe a sigh of relief? On the majority of occasions, having assured the security of the environment and of self within it, the individual will settle back to sleep, and it is only on rare occasions that the sleeper will remain disturbed and awake for the rest of the night. The REM phase of sleep is that commonly associated with dreaming and certainly this is the period when the vivid, bizarre and seemingly illogical visual images, which are labelled by individuals as 'dreams', occur. The individual 'running' or 'seeing' in his dream is actually experiencing the brain activity associated with these activities, and if it was not for the fact that his brain and skeletal muscles were 'disconnected' at this point via the loss of muscle tone, the individual would be running or seeing in actuality at that moment. In contrast, the dreams occurring in non-REM sleep are far less visual in nature, more logical and related to events occurring in waking life and are not as emotionally intense as REM dreams. Muscle tone is relaxed but 'connected' and available for use if necessary, as slow wave sleep predominates. The distinction is important when considering the potential events of sleep.

Dream anxiety, or *nightmare, disorder* occur during periods of REM sleep, which whilst occurring throughout sleep on a cyclical basis, occurs in longer phases as the night wears on, the longest period occurring prior to waking. Nightmares may then occur at any of these REM phases but become more frequent at the end of the night, when the period is more abundant. The observer will, of course, note very little physical indication of the sleeper's turmoil because of the lack of muscle tone and therefore no large movements are possible, although as the individual arouses from his sleep, movement is regained.

Nightmare content may be recalled in detail on waking, and typically relates to a threat to the individual's biopsychosocial integrity—to physical survival, to personal security, whether of a social or material nature, or to self-esteem. The nightmare theme may be a recurring one, is ultra-detailed, vivid and appears, to the sleeper, to be of a prolonged duration, and is often able to be recalled in the morning as efficiently as immediately upon waking after the experience. The nightmare content is extremely distressing and frightening and the individual, whilst gaining a rapid grasp of the reality of the situation, is often loath, or has great difficulty, in regaining sleep.

The years associated with childhood and the teens are most frequently those of the onset of the problem, and children tend to 'grow out' of the disorder. Where beginning in adults, it does tend to be rather more persistent and often continues for years. Nightmares are reported to occur as frequently as four or more times a week and therefore may provoke considerable disruption of the sleep pattern, regardless of the degree of fear or anxiety associated with the potential for the event. Many sufferers (about 60%) will describe the onset as related to some major life stressor that has occurred and indeed the frequency of nightmares is seen to increase at times of stress. In some instances, a change in the sleeping environment may engender a significant reduction in episodes experienced, as may physical fatigue.

Nightmares may be an integral problem, though not the primary problem, for many individuals seeking mental health assistance. Children, for example, who are experiencing a separation from a loved one, may describe nightmares comprising of people or monsters trying to hurt them, or people they love. Typically, too, they are afraid of the dark and unhappy to sleep alone, frequently finding protection and security by crawling into the bed of a sibling, parent or other significant adult. The child is little different to the adult, who may respond to estrangement, feelings of alienation or distrust, in a similar fashion.

Individuals experiencing the problems associated with organic cerebral impairment may find that their nightmares merge with hallucinatory events and may signify just one aspect of a disturbed sleep pattern which may also include insomnia and day-time hypersomnolence. Certain drugs have nightmares as a potential side-effect, for example, beta blocking agents and thioridazine, and withdrawal from REM-suppressing substances, for instance, alcohol or tricyclic preparations, will generally create a 'rebound' or compensatory increase in REM sleep and thus increase the likelihood of vivid dreams and nightmares.

In contrast, *sleep terror disorder* occurs during the slow wave, stage 3 and 4 delta rhythm activity and tends to occur during the first third of nocturnal sleep. Otherwise termed *parvor nocturnus*, the individual frequently sits up in bed with a scream (remember, there is full muscle tone in non-REM sleep), eyes open, pupils dilated and breathing rapidly. The picture is one of pure terror, the skin is pale, the individual is cold and sweating profusely, the hairs on his or her arms stand erect (*piloerection*) and pulse is accelerated. The individual's facial expression tells it all. At that moment the individual is totally unaware of the presence of any other person and is unresponsive to any attempt of comfort. The episode lasts for a period of up to 10 minutes, and when it subsides, the individual may recount a very fragmented nightmare scene and recall feeling the terror associated with it. They will, however, settle back to sleep and have no recall in the morning of the incident.

Where onset is in children, it appears to stand alone as a problem, with no apparent other psychosocial symptomatology. On occasions onset, which tends towards the 4–12-year-old age group, may be seen to follow a febrile illness, and the frequency of episodes may be variable, occurring on consecutive nights or with several days or weeks in between. Again the child tends to 'grow out' of the problem during adolescence. However, the adult does not tend to be so lucky, for where onset is in the 20–40-year-old age group—and it rarely occurs later than this—the course is often a chronic and persistent one, and is often associated with general feelings of anxiety towards life and living. Yet again, sleep terrors tend to occur more frequently in boys/men than their female peers and there would appear to be a higher incidence in first-degree biological relatives than within the remainder of the population.

Cerebral pathology should always be excluded at the outside, via an efficient and comprehensive neurological examination to ensure no underlying pathology is provoking the problem.

Sleep-walking (*somnambulism*) may damage health; many, including Scott (1981), have described children within care who have fractured limbs as a result of their nightly wanderings. Sleep-walking, too, occurs within slow wave sleep and may actually be initiated by lifting a child to his feet during this phase of the cycle, demonstrating the fact, amply, that the child is not responding to a dream. Again, more common in children, and boys rather than girls, it makes only a rare appearance in adulthood. Usually the activity witnessed is a gentle-paced aimless meandering, although, on occasions, running, jumping or searching behaviours may be seen. Sometimes the pattern of behaviour is very stereotyped and repetitive, totally purposeless in nature. The child will often reply to questions posed monosyllabically and some children will perform simple commands whilst experiencing this state. The episode may last half an hour or more, with the child then returning to bed and if awoken, contrary to popular belief, the child will display confusion and disorientation, but will gradually return to full awareness and have no recall of the incident. The problem tends to disappear as the child ages and matures into adolescence. There would appear again to be an increased familial prevalence of the problem, and an association with both *sleep-talking* (*somniloquy*) and *bed-wetting behaviour* (*nocturnal enuresis*).

Where sleep-walking is seen during adulthood, both onset (usually around the time of puberty) and episodes (about four or five a year) are associated with psychosocially traumatic events. These include separation from a parent, for a variety of reasons, the birth of a sibling or school change and the investigations of Sours *et al.* (1963) highlighted disturbed and difficult family situations and interactions as a common feature within the group they studied. Similarly, the majority of subjects had displayed antisocial behaviours—'theft, delinquency and acting out'—and demonstrated high levels of anxiety and depressed mood. Some of the group (9 of the 14) were diagnosed as 'schizophrenic' or of a 'schizoid personality', whilst others were considered to demonstrate symptomatology consistent with 'hysterical conversion disorders'.

Very seldomly, sleep-walking may be associated with an organic focus, for example, temporal lobe epilepsy, but, in general, it appears to be due to a partial arousal out of slow-wave sleep due to an abnormality—perhaps a lack of mature development—of the sleep-associated mechanisms.

Sleep-talking (*somniloquy*) is the production of speech, or other meaningful sounds, during sleep, of which the subject is totally unaware. Again more common in boys and seen within the slow-wave phase of sleep, it is often associated with sleep-walking children. *Bruxism* (*teeth grinding*) tends to occur in stages 1 and 2 of sleep and may lead to erosion and wearing down of the teeth. Aetiology and incidence is relatively vague.

Whilst not a 'sleep disorder', as such, *nocturnal enuresis* is an abnormal event which may punctuate sleep and hence warrants a fleeting mention. A behavioural problem, believed to occur in 10% of seven-year-old and 3% of 12-year-old boys, it may occur during any sleep stage but is more common in slow-wave sleep. It is less common in girls (3% and 2% for the respective age groups).

Micturition (the passage of urine) is heralded by a burst of EEG activity with stage 4 or 1 and 2, though when it does occur during REM sleep, the child may recall a dream in which he or she was urinating. However, in the majority of instances, the child awakes with no memory either of the dream or of voiding. Sufferers do outgrow the problem, with only 1% of 18-year-old young men still experiencing a problem, and almost a nonexistent incidence in young women of this age group.

The problem does tend to show a familial link, and developmental delay in bladder musculature and physiology that results in a low bladder threshold, and therefore involuntary voiding, may predispose the difficulty. Lax, inconsistent and delayed toilet training and psychosocial stress, for example sibling rivalry in response to a new baby, may also precipitate such involuntary voiding. Whilst not usually seen in relation to a co-existing mental health problem, more psychosocial problems are seen to exist within these children than in the general population.

Conclusions

Sleep is fascinating, and although an activity that everyone participates in, there are still many gaps in knowledge relating to the subject. Problems of sleep may indicate a significant biopsychosocial health status deviation or merely poor habits and a lack of understanding in relation to the great value of regular efficient sleeping within daily functioning. We assert the importance of a comprehensive, objective assessment of the individual's health needs and problems to ensure effective assistance is provided. The role of education, in regard to all aspects of sleeping patterns and routines, is important in the promotion of optimum psychosocial and somatic health.

SUMMARY

We have explored only some of the themes associated with the personal motivation resulting in exhibited behaviour and space precludes a more detailed and extensive analysis of both this area and that of social motivation. It is our hope that there is sufficient here to provoke both observation and reflection and to encourage you to look for similarities, as well as differences (or modifications) in behaviours exhibited by human beings and animals alike. To achieve the real degree of civilization desired rather than the superficial veneer so far attained requires more individual and societal attention, reflection and debate.

FURTHER READING

Abraham, S. & Llewellyn-Jones, D. (1987) *Eating Disorders: The Facts*. Oxford: University Press.

Allen Hobson, J. (1989) *Sleep*. New York: Scientific American Library.

Borbely, A. (1986) *Secrets of Sleep*. London: Penguin.

Brain, W.R. (1985) *Brain's Diseases of the Nervous System*. Oxford: University Press.

Brunner, L.S. & Suddarth, D.S. (1986) *The Lippincott Manual of Medical Surgical Nursing*. London: Harper & Row.

Duker, M. & Slade, R. (1988) *Anorexia Nervosa and Bulimia: How to Help*. Milton Keynes: Open University Press.

Hinchcliffe, S. & Montague, S. (1988) *Physiology for Nursing Practice*. London: Baillière Tindall.

Hinwood, B. (1993) *A Textbook of Science for the Health Professions*, 2nd ed. London: Chapman & Hall.

Lishman, W.A. (1978) *Organic Psychiatry: The Psychological Consequences of Cerebral Disorder*. Oxford: Blackwell Scientific.

Roth, I. (Ed.) (1990) *Introduction to Psychology*, Vols 1 and 2. Milton Keynes: Laurence Erlbaum Associates in conjunction with the Open University.

REFERENCES

Ack, M., Miller, I. & Weil, W.B. (1961) Intelligence of children with diabetes mellitus. *Paediatrics*, **28**, 764–770.

Andrews, R. (1987) *Routledge Dictionary of Quotations*. London: Routledge & Kegan Paul.

Appleby, L. & Forshaw, D. (1990) *Postgraduate Psychiatry: Clinical and Scientific Foundations*. Oxford: Heinemann Medical.

Arendt, J., Aldous, M., English, J., Marks, V. and Arendt, J. H. (1987) Some effects of jet lag and their alleviation by melatonin. *Ergonomics*, **30**(9), 1379–1393.

Aserinski, E. & Kleitman, N. (1953) Regularly occurring periods of eye motility and concurrent phenomena during sleep. *Science*, **118**, 273–274.

Bearn, A.G. (1972) Wilson's disease. In Stanbury, J.B., Wyngaarden, J.B. & Fredrickson, D.S. (Eds) *The Metabolic Basis of Inherited Disease*. New York: McGraw-Hill.

Beck, E., Daniel, P.M., Alpers, M., Gajdusek, D.C. & Gibbs, C.J. (1966) Experimental 'Kuru' in chimpanzees. A pathological report. *Lancet*, **2**, 1056–1059.

Beck, E., Daniel, P.M., Gajdusek, D.C. & Gibbs, D.J. (1969a) Similarities and differences in the pattern of the pathological changes in scrapie, Kuru, experimental Kuru and subacute presenile polioencephalopathy. In Whitty, C.W.M., Hughes, J.T. & MacCallum, F.O. (Eds) *Virus Diseases and the Nervous System*. Oxford: Blackwell Scientific.

Beck, E., Daniel, P.M., Matthews, W.B., Stevens, D.L., Alpers, M.P., Asher, D.M., Gajdusek, D.C. & Gibbs, C.J. (1969b) Creuzfeldt–Jakob disease: the neuropathology of a transmission experiment. *Brain* **92**, 699–716.

Binkley, S. (1979) A timekeeping enzyme in the pineal gland. *Scientific American*, **240**, 66–71.

Bowling, G. & Richards, N.G. (1961) Diagnosis and treatment of the narcolepsy syndrome. *Cleveland Clinic Quarterly*, **28**, 38–45.

Burwell, C.S., Robin, E.D., Whaley, R.D. & Bickelmann, A.G. (1956) Extreme obesity associated with alveolar hypoventilation—a Pickwickian syndrome. *American Journal of Medicine*, **21**, 811–818.

Campbell, R.J. (1989) *Psychiatric Dictionary*. Oxford University Press.

Carpenter, S., Yassa, R. & Ochs, R. (1982) A pathologic basis for Kleine–Levin syndrome. *Archives of Neurology*, **39**, 25.

Carskadon, M.A., Mitler, M.M. & Dement, W.C. (1974) A comparison of insomniacs and normals: total sleep time and sleep latency. *Sleep Research*, **3**, 130.

Coleman, D.L. & Hummel, K.P. (1969) Effects of parabiosis of normal with genetically diabetic mice. *American Journal of Physiology*, **217**, 1298–1304.

Coscina, D.V. & Dixon, L.M. (1983) Body weight regulation in anorexia nervosa: insights from an animal model. In Darby, P.L., Garfinkel, P.E., Garner, D.M. & Coscina, D.V. (Eds) *Anorexia Nervosa: Recent Developments*. New York: Allen R. Liss.

Crick, F. & Mitchison, G. (1983) The function of dream sleep. *Nature*, 304–311.

Crisp, A.H. (1983) Treatment of anorexia nervosa. What can be the role of psychopharmacological agents? In Pirke, K.M. & Ploog, D. (Eds) *The Psychobiology of Anorexia Nervosa*. New York: Springer.

Critchley, M. (1962) Periodic hypersomnia and megaphagia in adolescent males. *Brain*, **85**, 627.

Crowley, W.F. Jr, Beitins, I.Z., Vale, W. *et al.* (1980) The biologic activity of a potent analogue of gonadotrophin releasing hormone in normal and hypogonadotropic men. *New England Journal of Medicine*, **302**, 1052–1057.

Czeisler, C., Richardson, G.S., Coleman, R.M., Zimmerman, J.C., Moore-Ede, M.C., Dement, W.C. & Weitzman, E.D. (1981) Chronotherapy: resetting the arcadian clocks of patients with delayed sleep phase insomnia. *Sleep*, **4**, 1–21.

Davis, H. (1978) Sexual dysfunction in diabetes. *Medical Aspect of Human Sexuality*, **12**, 48.

Davis, J.D. & Brief, D.J. (1981) Chronic intraventricular insulin infusions reduce food intake and body weight in rats. *Social Neuroscience Abstract*, **7**, 655.

Dement, W.C. (1976) *Some Must Watch While Some Must Sleep*. New York: W.H. Freeman.

Dement, W.C. & Kleitman, N. (1975) The relation of eye movements during sleep to dream activity: an objective method for the study of dreaming. *Journal of Experimental Psychology*, **53**, 89–97.

Denko, J.D. & Kaelbling, R. (1962) The psychiatric aspects of hypoparathyroidism. *Acta Psychiatrica Scandinavica*, **164** (Suppl.) 1–70.

Department of Health (DH) (1992) *The Health of the Nation*. London: HMSO.

Duffy, J.P. & Davison, K. (1968) A female case of Kleine–Levin syndrome. *British Journal of Psychiatry*, **114**, 77.

Ellenberg, M. (1977) Sex and the female diabetic. *Medical Aspect of Human Sexuality*, **11**, 30.

Faust, I.M. (1984) Role of the fat cell in energy balance physiology. In Stunkard, A.T. & Stellar, E. (Eds) *Eating and Its Disorders*. New York: Raven Press.

Faust, I.M., Johnson, P.R., Stern, J.S. & Hirsch, J. (1978) Diet induced adipocyte increase in adult rats: a new model of obesity. *American Journal of Physiology*, **235**, E279–E286.

Fourman, P., Rawnsley, K., David, R.H., Jones, K.H. & Morgan, D.B. (1967) Effect of calcium on mental symptoms in partial parathyroid insufficiency. *Lancet*, **2**, 914–915.

Freud, S. (1954) Translated by Strachey, J. *The Interpretation of Dreams*, London: George Allen & Unwin.

Friedman, M.I. & Stricker, E.M. (1976) The physiological psychology of hunger: a physiological perspective. *Psychological Review*, **83**, 401–431.

Gallinek, A. (1954) Syndrome of episodes of hypersomnia, bulimia and abnormal mental states. *Journal of American Medical Association*, **154**, 1081–1083.

Garland, H., Sumner, D. & Fourman, P. (1965) The Kleine–Levin syndrome. Some further observations. *Neurology*, **15**, 1161.

Gelardi, J.A.M. & Brown, J.W. (1967) Hereditary cataplexy. *Journal of Neurology, Neurosurgery & Psychiatry*, **30**, 455–457.

Gelineau, Dr. (1880) De La Narcolepsie. In: Brain, W.R. (1985) *Brain's Diseases of the Nervous System*. Oxford: Oxford University Press.

Gilbert, G.J. (1964) Periodic hypersomnia and bulimia: the Kleine–Levin syndrome. *Neurology*, **14**, 844–850.

Guilleminault, C., Faull, K.F., Miles, L. & Van den Hoed, J. (1983) Post-traumatic excessive daytime sleepiness: a review of 20 patients. *Neurology*, **33**, 1584.

Harlow, J.M. (1848) Passage of an iron rod through the head. *Boston Medical and Surgical Journal*, **39**, 389–393.

Hartmann, E. (1984) *The Nightmare*. New York: Basic Books.

Herman, C.P. & Polivy, J. (1980) Restrained eating. In Stunkard, A.J. (Ed) *Obesity*. Phildelphia: Saunders.

Hinchliff, S. & Montague, S. (1988) *Physiology for Nursing Practice*. London: Baillière Tindall.

Hoebel, B.G. & Teitelbaum, P. (1966) Effects of force-feeding and starvation on food intake and body weight on a rat with ventromedial hypothalamic lesions. *Journal of Comparative and Physiological Psychology*, **61**, 189–193.

Huxley, J. (1958). *Evolution*. London: Allen & Unwin.

Ives, E.R. (1963) Mental aberrations in diabetic patients. *Bulletin of the Los Angeles Neurological Society*, **28**, 279–285.

Janowitz, H.D. & Grossman, M.I. (1949) Some facts affecting the food intake of normal dogs and dogs with oesophagostomy and gastric fistula. *American Journal of Physiology*, **159**, 143–148.

Keesey, R.E. & Powley, T.K. (1975) Hypothalamic regulation of body weight. *American Scientist*, **63**, 558–565.

Kleine, W. (1925) Periodische schlatsucht. *Mschr Psychiat Neurol*, **57**, 285.

Knittle, J.L. & Hirsch, J. (1968). Effect of early nutrition on the development of rat epididymal fat pads: cellularity and metabolism. *Journal of Clinical Investigation*, **47**, 2091.

Knobil, E., Neill, J., Ewings, L.A. & Greenwald, G. (Eds) (1988) *The Physiology of Reproduction*. New York: Raven Press.

Koenig, H. (1968) Dementia associated with the benign form of multiple sclerosis. *Transactions of the American Neurological Association*, **93**, 227–231.

Kolodny, R. (1971) Sexual function in diabetic females. *Diabetes*, **20**, 557.

Kripke, D.F. & Gillin, J.C. (1985) Sleep disorders. In Klerman, G.L., Weissman, M.M., Applebaum, P.S. & Roth, L.N. (Eds) *Psychiatry*, Vol. 3. Lippincott.

Krueger, J.M.P. Jr & Karnovsky, M.L. (1982) The composition of sleep promoting factor isolated from human urine. *Journal of Biological Chemistry*, **257**, 1664–1669.

Lavie, P. & Kripke, D.F.G. (1975) Ultradian rhythms! The 90 minute clock inside us. *Psychology Today*, **8**, 54–65.

Leibowitz, S.F. (1983) Noradrenergic function in the medial hypothalamus: potential relation to anorexia nervosa and bulimia. In Pirke, K.M. & Ploog, D. (Eds) *The Psychobiology of Anorexia Nervosa*. New York: Springer.

Levin, M. (1936) Periodic somnolence and morbid hunger: a new syndrome. *Brain*, **59**, 494.

Lugaresi, E., Coccaena, G., Ontavani, M. & Brignanv, F. (1973) *Journal of Neurology, Neurosurgery and Psychiatry*, **36**, 15.

Mayer, J. (1955) Regulation of energy uptake and the body weight! The glucostatic theory and the lipostatic hypotheses. *Annals of the New York Academy of Science*, **63**, 15–42.

MacLean, C. (1977) *The Wolf Children*. London: Allen Lane.

McGhie, A. & Russell, S.M. (1962) The subjective assessment of normal sleep patterns. *Journal of Mental Science*, **108**, 456.

McKenna, R.J. (1972) Some effects of anxiety level and food crises on the eating behaviour of obese and normal subjects. *Journal of Personality and Social Psychology*, **22**, 311–319.

Mitchell, J.S. & Keesey, R.E. (1974) The effects of lateral hypothalamic lesions and castration upon the body weight of male rats. *Behavioural Biology*, **11**, 69–82.

Moore-Ede, M.C., Sulzman, F.Z. & Fuller, C.A. (1982) *The Clocks that Time Us*. Massachusetts: Harvard University Press.

Pappenheimer, J.R. (1976) The sleep factor. *Scientific American*, **235**, 24–29.

Passouant, P., Cadilhac, J. & Baldy-Moulinier, M. (1967) Physiopathologie des hypersomnies. *Revue Neurologique*, **116**, 585–629.

Pieron, H. (1913) *Le Probleme Physiologique du Sommeil*. Paris: Masson.

Rechtschaffen, A.R., Wolpert, E.A., Dement, W.C., Mitchell, S.A. & Fisher, C. (1963) Nocturnal sleep of narcoleptics. *Electroencephalography and Clinical Neurophysiology*, **15**, 599–609.

Robinson, J.T. & McQuillan, J. (1951) Schizophrenic reaction associated with the Kleine–Levin syndrome. *Journal of the Royal Army Medical Corps*, **96**, 377–381.

Robinson, K.C., Kallberg, M.H. & Crowley, M.F. (1954) Idiopathic hypoparathyroidism presenting as dementia. *British Medical Journal*, **21**, 1203–1206.

Roffware, H.P., Muzio, J.M. & Dement, W.C. (1968) Ontogenetic development of the human sleep–dream cycle. In Webb, W.B. (Ed) *Sleep—An Experimental Approach*. New York: Macmillan.

Roth, B., Nevsimalova, S. & Rechtschaffen, A. (1972)

Hypersomnia with sleep drunkenness. *Archives of General Psychiatry*, **26**, 456–462.

Ruderman, A.J. (1986) Dietary restraint: a theoretical and empirical review. *Psychological Bulletin*, **99**, 247–262.

Schachter, S. (1971) *Emotion, Obesity and Crime*. New York: Academic Press.

Scheinberg, I.H., Sternlieb, I. & Richman, I. (1968) Psychiatric manifestations in patients with Wilson's disease. In Bergsma, D. (Ed) *Wilson's Disease. Birth Defects Original Article Series*, **4**, No. 2. The National Foundation.

Schwartz, B.A., Seguy, M. & Escande, J.P. (1967) Correlations EEG, respiratoires, oculaires et myographiques dans le 'syndrome Pickwickien' et autre affections paraissant apparentees: proposition d'une hypothese. *Revue Neurologique*, **117**, 145–152.

Scott, D.F. (1981) What is sleep? *World Medicine*, June 27th 1981, 57–58.

Siffre, M. (1963) *Hors du temps*. Paris: Julliard.

Sours, J.A., Frumkin, P. & Indermill, R.R. (1963) Somnambulism: its clinical significance and dynamic meaning in late adolescence and adulthood. *Archives of General Psychiatry*, **9**, 400–413.

Stricker, E.M., Rowland, N., Saller, C.F. & Friedman, M.I. (1977) Homeostasis during hypoglycaemia: central control of adrenal secretion and peripheral control of feeding. *Science*, **196**, 79–81.

Surridge, D. (1969) An investigation into some psychiatric aspects of multiple sclerosis. *British Journal of Psychiatry*, **115**, 749–764.

Tardoff, M.G., Hoffenbeck, J. & Novin, D. (1982) Hepatic vagotomy (partial hepatic denervation) does not alter ingestive responses to metabolic changes. *Physiology and Behaviour*, **28**, 417–424.

Walker, S. (1969) The psychiatric presentation of Wilson's disease (hepatolenticular degeneration) with an aetiologic explanation. *Behavioural Neuropsychiatry*, **1**, 38–43.

Webb, W.B. (1975) *Sleep the Gentle Tyrant*. New Jersey: Prentice-Hall.

Wehr, T.A., Wirz-Justice, A., Goodwin, F.K., Duncan, W. & Gillin, J.C. (1979) Phase advance of the sleep–wake cycle as an antidepressant. *Science*, **206**, 710–713.

West, D.B., Williams, R.H., Braget, D.J. & Woods, S.C. (1982) Bombesin reduces food intake of normal and hypothalamically obese rats and lowers body weight when given chronically. *Peptides*, **3**, 61–67.

Westphal, K.F. (1877) Eigen Hiü mluche mit eimshaffen. Verbundene aufälle. *Arch. Psychnevenkrar. British Medical Journal*, **7**, 631–635.

White, C. (1977) Unpublished Ph.D. dissertation. Catholic University, Washington DC.

Woods, S.C., Lotter, E.C., McKay, L.D. & Porte, D. (1979) Chronic intracerebroventricular infusion reduces food intake and body weight in baboons. *Nature (London)*, **282**, 503–505.

Zarcone, V. (1973) Narcolepsy. *New England Journal of Medicine*, **288**, 1156–1166.

COGNITION

F.C. Johnson and L.D. Smith

AIMS

i) To review and consolidate previous learning in relation to cognition
ii) To explore the characteristics associated with:
   (a) perception
   (b) attention
   (c) thinking
   (d) memory
   (c) language in health
iii) To determine problems which may be experienced in relation to the above abilities and which may indicate deviation from health status

KEY ISSUES

Definitions
Explanations
Relevant biopsychosocial development
Relevant theoretical perspectives
Illusions and hallucinations
Problems of attention
Problems of the form, content and nature of thinking
Memory distortions and difficulties
Language and speech problems

Identify, analyse and assess factors causing distress and illness	Promote health, provide direct care and make interventions	Manage care programmes and services
Be critical, analytical and accountable, continue professional development	Counter discrimination, inequality and individual and institutional racism	Work within and develop policies, laws and safeguards in all settings
Understand influences on mental health and the nature/causes of disorder and illness	Know the effects of distress, disorder, illness on individuals, groups, families	Understand the basis of treatments and interventions

INTRODUCTION

Imagine:

... a young woman, sitting on a bench, in the park, waiting for a friend. During the first few minutes, she is busy compiling a mental list of all the information she wants to share with her friend, but then she begins to shiver and notices how cold it has become.[a] Looking around her, she notes that the wind has strengthened and is whipping the dry, scrunchy-sounding, orange-gold leaves around the paths and between the shrubs. They congregate around her feet, the base of the bench and in the closed doorway of the cricket pavilion behind her. The trees are beginning to sway, and the windows behind her are rattling. The wooden verandah begins to creak and moan and the wind starts to howl. It's getting dark too, and shadows are forming around the foliage in the vicinity of the bench.[b] Whilst not afraid, the young woman is not feeling particularly comfortable either, as she snuggles deeper into her coat, reflecting that this was a less than ideal location to meet.[c] Looking about, the place is desolate, although she can hear traffic on the nearby road. She looks at her watch—it's five past four—her friend will be here any minute. Even as she's thinking it, she hears the iron gate, at the park entrance nearby, clang shut, and looks expectantly in that direction. Even in the dim light and shadows, she knows the figure is not that of her friend, and settles back on the bench.[d] A few moments later, a stranger passes her seat, just as the metal gate resounds again. This time the young woman, sure of the identity of the silhouetted figure, leaves the bench and hurries forward to meet her friend. They leave the park.

Some days later, the two friends are discussing a future meeting and on this occasion decide that the coffee shop should be the venue to meet.[e]

The scenario utilized hopefully reminds us of the operations inherent within cognition, that is, the vehicles via which an individual gains knowledge and understanding of both external reality and physiological status, thereby preparing for management of the situation presenting.

An analysis of the scenario identifies five distinct processes which culminate in cognition, namely:

(a) *Perception*, that is, the organization and interpretation of stimuli received into meaningful knowledge.
Longman's Dictionary of Psychology and Psychiatry, 1984

Within the scenario, the young woman has not been sitting with her eyes closed, whilst compiling her agenda for the forthcoming meeting, but even so was able to focus her concentration upon it during the period of time that the environment matched her expectations or remained relatively unchanged. However, when a change in stimulus occurred—she began to feel cold—she becomes specifically aware of her environment and begins to *perceive* her surroundings rather than mechanically *observe* them.

(b) *Attention*, represents conscious awareness, sensory clarity and central nervous system readiness to respond to stimuli received. It is a focusing on specific aspects of the environment and is a selective process, influenced by a variety of factors.
Campbell, 1989

The fictitious woman on the bench moves her centre of concentration to her environment, to facilitate assessment of the situation, by absorbing cues and clues available to her. She now clearly *attends* to the aspects of her surroundings that may influence subsequent activities.

(c) *Thinking*, where images and ideas, representing objects and events experienced, are manipulated, utilizing previous know-

ledge and general understanding of the situation to arrive at strategies by which changes in status may be changed.
Campbell, 1989

The young woman has done this, for she has identified the unsuitability of the environment for her purpose. Indeed her thoughts generate further focusing upon her immediate situation as she searches for more data to assist in activity planning. She is not only exposed to the elements within the present circumstances but notes the potential hazards to continued well-being in relation to the relative isolation and loneliness of the location. Therefore, she seeks information with regard to the proximity of people—the road and gate of the park—and an estimation of when company, in the form of her friend, may be expected.

(d) *Memory*—the ability to register, retain, recognize and recall past experiences for utilization at a subsequent time.
Campbell, 1989

She has employed memory, in conjunction with thinking activities to come to conclusions about her current situation, but, in addition, possesses sufficient details within her store of knowledge, in regard to the size, shape and general appearance of her friend, to know that the indistinct figure at the gate is not the person expected. The results of this experience—the perceptions, thoughts and feelings—will be stored too, for future use and consideration.

(e) *Language* is the mode by which thought and activity is made available to conscious awareness. It is the basic vehicle utilized to structure experiences and, other than for those few aspects of conscious thought when mental images are utilized or objects are rotated in space, is therefore depended upon to achieve conscious awareness. It may be vocal or utilize other methods but in essence is the manner in which communication between parties also occurs.
Longman's Dictionary of Psychology and Psychiatry, 1984

The young woman awaiting her friend utilized language to assess mentally her circumstances and to label the stranger as too fat/thin/short/tall to be her companion, to be wearing the 'wrong' sort of clothes or walk differently to her friend. In addition she manages her disquietude in regard to the environment my making alternative arrangements for the next meeting. She may not verbalize the 'why' but she utilizes language to inform, or negotiate, the where.

Cognition is the result of perception, attention, thinking, memory and language. The individual experiencing mental health problems may exteriorize a variety of divergencies from expected characteristics and it may therefore be valuable to explore briefly the basis for each process and the parameters and characteristics associated with it, prior to analysis of specific problems that may be evinced and the strategies that may be employed to manage/ameliorate their existence.

PERCEPTION

WHAT IS PERCEIVED AND HOW

We defined the process of perception as that encompassing the organization and interpretation of stimuli received, into meaningful knowledge. Such stimuli are recorded via a variety of sources, and, whilst we may automatically refer, at this point, to those senses that monitor the external

Table 9.1 *Sensation and the pathway to interpretation*

Sensation	Receptor	Quality	Sensing system	Primary relay level	Secondary relay level	Tertiary relay level

Vision	Rods
	Cones
		Brightness
		Colour
		Size
		Motion
		Contrast
			Retina	Retina	Lateral geniculate
					Superior colliculus
					Hypothalamus
						Primary visual
						  cortex
						Secondary
						  visual cortex

Hearing	Hair cells	Pitch
		Tone
			Cochlear	Cochlear nuclei	Lemniscal, collicular
					  and medial
					  geniculate nuclei
						Primary auditory
						  cortex

Touch	Ruffini corpuscles	Pressure	Skin and
			  internal
			  organs
				Spinal cord or
				  brainstem
					Thalamus	Somatosensory
						  cortex

	Merkel discs Pacinian corpuscles	Temperature Vibration				

Smell	Olfactory
	  receptor
		Floral
		Fruity
		Musky
		Pungent
			Olfactory
			  nerves
				Olfactory bulb	Piriform cortex	Limbic system
						Hypothalamus

Taste	Taste buds at tip
	  of tongue
	Taste buds at
	  edge and base
	  of tongue
		Sweet
		Salt
		Bitter
		Sour
			Tongue	Medulla	Thalamus	Somatosensory
						  cortex

environment, that is, the visual, auditory, tactile, olfactory and gustatory senses (Table 9.1), there are others to be considered.

The maculae and cristae, for example, are sense organs positioned within the semi-circular ducts of the ear. These monitor the position of the head relative to the ground—*static equilibrium or gravity*—and sudden movements of the head, such as rotation, deceleration and acceleration—*dynamic equilibrium*—respectively. Impulses pass, via the vestibulocochlear (viii) nerve, to the vestibular nuclei of the medulla, the cerebellum, thalamus and somatosensory cortex of the brain. Fibres from the vestibular nuclei transmit information to the nerves that control eye movements (iii, iv, vi) and to the accessory (xi) nerve nucleus which helps control the head and neck. Other fibres from the lateral vestibular nucleus, forming the vestibulospinal tract, transmit impulses to skeletal muscles, regulating the response of body tone to head movement. Pathways between the vestibular nuclei, cerebellum and cerebrum enable the cerebellum, which is continuously receiving sensory updates, to exercise a key role within the maintenance of balance (Tortora and Anagnostakos, 1984).

There is, too, the *kinaesthetic sense*, which provides the individual with an awareness of the activities of muscles, tendons and joints, which muscles are contracted and the degree of tension resultant within tendons. It is via this sense that the individual is able to judge the movements and positions of limbs when he walks without the use of his eyes, or in the darkness, by recognizing the location and rate of movement of one part, in relation to the other parts, of the body. There are joint kinaesthetic (or proprioceptive) receptors located within the capsule, and around ligaments in the area of the joint, providing feedback on the changing degree of angularity of the joint. Muscle spindles, comprising of sensory neurons, are positioned within most skeletal muscles, and provide information in relation to the degree of stretch within muscles. Tendon organs provide similar information relating to tendon tension, from their situation at the junction of muscle and tendon. All three types of proprioreceptors pass impulses for conscious utilization, via ascending tracts in the spinal cord, to the thalamus and cerebral cortex, whilst those resulting in reflex action pass, via spinocerebellar tracts, to the cerebellum (Tortora and Anagnostakos, 1984).

The above provides just two examples of sources of data, other than the five senses often considered to comprise perception. There are others, for example, baroreceptors monitor blood pressure, thermoreceptors respond to temperature changes and chemoreceptors measure levels of oxygen, carbon dioxide and hydrogen ions within arterial blood (Hinchcliffe and Montague, 1988). In addition, the endocrine system assists by maintenance of blood chemical levels within activities designed to ensure internal optimum balance, or *homeostasis*. Perception involves the use of information from various origins, and is rarely dependent upon just one source of stimuli reception. It is considered, therefore, to be resultant from *cross-modal transfer*, utilizing and integrating a combination of material from several sources. Indeed, the young woman within the scenario provided utilized data from visual, auditory and tactile senses to gain an understanding of her environment.

Despite the source of data employed, perception is dependent upon a stimulus being received by a specialized receptor. The stimulus is, at this point, converted from its original, physical, form (e.g. light, heat or sound) into action potentials, or nerve impulses, which are a representation of the event in the form of an electrical message. In this form, the information is despatched to an initial receiving unit, which, again, is sensitive to that specific form of sensation. This unit monitors the frequency of the impulses and the total number of receptors transmitting the information, indicating the extent of the object/event perceived. An example may be advantageous, and that of the stimuli emanating from an orange may be suitable. The colour, size, shape, fragrance and the distance from the orange's position, would all be noted in a primary receiving unit and passed to a secondary processing centre, where further judgements about the stimuli are made. The next step in the chain is transfer to an integrating centre, where sensations available from other sources (e.g. in the case of the orange, olfactory and visual receptors) and information from past experiences is added to the original data, via links with other similar centres. Thus cross-modal transfer is facilitated. Neural connections with motor areas of the brain provide for motor activity as a potential response to stimulus awareness (Hinchcliff and Montague, 1988).

The qualities of a stimulus (e.g. the pitch, loudness and location of a sound) are processed in parallel, via the specialist receptors, and conducted to the appropriate area of the brain—in the instance of sound, to the primary auditory cortex (Kandel and Schwartz, 1981). Associated cells, within the immediate area of the primary centre, receive impulses from the area and will respond to certain aspects to produce an overall stimulus. A useful analogy may be that of an orchestra—each individual member playing an instrument contributes to the composite sound produced, and yet on its own is only capable of eliciting a tiny fraction of the proposed end result. It is only when these parallel processes are combined that the perception of the complete stimulus is achieved. Once the entire details of any specific stimulus have been 'learned', it only requires the detection of a small number of these details in the future to enable recognition to take place.

MAKING SENSE OF PERCEPTIONS

In the same way as the qualities or specific aspects of a stimulus may be perceived, so a complex experience, or percept, may be broken down into its two or more distinctive elements. You will no doubt be aware of the research of Gestalt psychologists (Kohler, 1952) in relation to the perceptual organization of these elements of the stimulus, namely that:

1 Where two or more distinct elements comprise a stimulus, a proportion of the stimulus is perceived as 'figure' and the rest as 'ground'. There are many visual examples of this—a girl (the figure) seated by a tree (background), a house (figure) within a landscape (background), a train (figure) standing at a platform of the railway station (background)—but also auditory ones, too, for example, the voice of the soloist against the background of the chorus, the sound of the river or a bird's song against the rest of the outdoor noise, or one voice amongst many others at a party.

2 There is a tendency to organize into ordered relationships, generated by the pattern of stimuli.

Similarity

There is a tendency to perceive three alternating groups of a two row/line pattern, even though the letters are consistently spaced apart (Fig. 9.1). Individuals incline towards uniting similarities within the percept.

aaaabbbbaaaabbbb
aaaabbbbaaaabbbb

Fig. 9.1 *Similarity.*

Continuity

Individuals perceive dots as straight lines rather than unconnected items and, in addition, 'see' two continuing lines rather than four short ones (Fig. 9.2). The overall perception is one of a letter 'x', a meaningful symbol, rather than a pattern of dots. There appears a natural opposition to breaking a continuous line, shape or design.

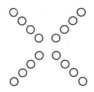

Fig. 9.2 *Continuity.*

Proximity

Individuals tend to 'see' three pairs of lines, plus one extra on the right-hand side of the figure (Fig. 9.3). It could be interpreted as seven lines, or one plus three pairs of lines—the 'one' being the first line on the left. However, the likelihood is that the perception is of three pairs plus one line.

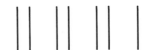

Fig. 9.3 *Proximity.*

Closure

Although incomplete, individuals tend to perceive complete geometrical shapes, in what appears to be a strong inclination to 'close' incomplete stimuli (Fig. 9.4).

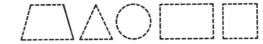

Fig. 9.4 *Closure.*

In addition, individuals perceive the elements within their environment as remaining relatively stable despite changing conditions or altering the position from which they are viewed, for example, the individual recognizes a pillar box, despite its cylindrical shape being distorted by bushes or a snow drift that is obscuring most of it. It is recognized when viewed from above and appears as a circular, one dimensional structure, and also from a two-dimensional sketch. Similarly it is 'known' to be red in colour, even when viewed in the darkness of late evening, and of an approximately constant size, the individual never having to lie face down on the ground to slip a letter into the box's opening!

Context

Individuals experience an element of a percept within a frame of reference provided by the context or setting in which it occurs. The perception of the size of an element is one aspect of this contextual setting. An example may assist here and, hence, a return to the example of the red pillar box may be valuable. When viewed from a distance the post box *appears* smaller than it actually is, and becomes progressively larger, the nearer an individual moves towards it. The individual recognizes the effect of distance on the apparent size of a structure, and does not consider for one moment that the real size of the object is actually changing. Similarly when both a building and the pillar box are viewed from a distance and appear to be of a similar size, the observer automatically accommodates the impression by inferring the house to be positioned at some considerable distance beyond the post box. The observer 'knows' that houses are much larger than pillar boxes and relates size to contextual setting.

Colour

Individuals are aware of the 'true' colour of a variety of objects and items within everyday life and will perceive that colour regardless of the wavelength of the light reaching the eye. Therefore, no matter the distance at which a tree is observed, the leaves are perceived as green, and, despite the dimness of an environment, an orange is 'seen' as orange in colour.

Location constancy

In regard to elements of a percept which do not generally move, despite the observer moving and the retinal image changing, objects are 'seen' to remain in the same place. Sometimes, indeed, individuals fail to recognize a familiar face or object because its contextual/location constancy changes. The bank manager may be a familiar and easily recognizable figure in the location of his usual environment (the office, the desk and its contents, filing cabinets, etc.) and dressed in pinstriped suit. However, meet him on the beach hundreds of miles from home, when he's wearing cut-off jeans, a tee-shirt, sporting a rude slogan and a three-day growth of beard and we may 'know he's familiar but can't place him'.

Shape constancy

The individual is aware of the 'real' shape of an article and perceives it to be that shape, no matter the angle from which it is viewed and despite the fact that a substantial portion may be occluded from view. Searching for a comb, should we see the last 'tooth' of it projecting from underneath a book, we will recognize just that one tiny aspect as the whole comb, and stop searching.

PROBLEMS OF RECOGNITION

Physiologically speaking, the systems involved in perception must be intact. The appropriately sensitive receptors must be available to monitor stimuli available within the environment and sensory pathways are required to transmit data to the responsible primary and association areas of the cortex for interpretation. However, despite the fully functioning physiological processes, on occasions individuals fail to *recognize* the stimuli perceived.

Agnosia is a term utilized to describe an inability to recognize an object despite intact sensation, and may take numerous forms. All are characterized by a lack of awareness and feeling of familiarity when encountering people, places, events or objects that have been encountered before and often 'known' on a daily basis. *Tactile agnosia*, or *astereognosis*, follows lesions in the dominant parietal cortex, especially the posterior aspects of the area and demonstrates a lack of ability to perceive, and identify, an object by touching and manipulating it alone. Whilst no defects are found within the sensory tract, a problem is identifiable within the processes of higher level correlation of proprioceptive sensation. *Finger agnosia* is an inability to interpret which finger has been touched by an examiner, and is commonly seen in childhood schizophrenia and also in children experiencing minimal brain dysfunction. *Anosognosia* is a denial of disability, particularly a part of the body evidencing disease of paralysis and *autotopagnosia* (or *somatotopagnosia*) is an inability to identify or orientate the body or the relationship of its individual parts.

Neuropsychologists working in Marseilles described the problems of a 19-year-old male patient who suffered the effects of bilateral temporal lobe lesions (Sirigu *et al.*, 1991). Intellectually, linguistically and perceptually, he experienced no significant impairment and yet his ability to recognize visually a wide variety of objects was quite profoundly deficient. The individual knew how to manipulate the objects and yet was unable to define either their function or the context in which they were utilized. The problems experienced by Paulette V., who had suffered a cerebrovascular accident some years previous, were described by Sergent and Poncet (1990). Since the stroke, Paulette had been unable to recognize faces as familiar or known to her (prosopagnosia) although able to match pictures of faces, even utilizing differing views of the same faces. Paulette was unable to recognize a slide showing the face of Dr Poncet, even though he sat next to the screen, and yet she could describe the facial features and approximate age of the doctor's face upon the screen. They concluded that there was a disturbance in the interaction between pertinent memories and facial representations, thus the latter remained meaningless.

The above are merely a few of the problems associated with *recognition* of objects via perceptual experiences when the sensory system remains intact. Physiological deficits are often readily identifiable—visual and auditory impairment are relatively easy to elicit during an efficient neurological examination, as is paresis or paralysis. However, when the client describes his world as colourless and perceived as shades of grey, it may be useful to discuss the matter with him further. Whilst rare, there is a problem associated with total colour blindness, termed *achromatopsia* (Zeki, 1991), where congenital absence of retinal cone cells, injury, inflammation or exposure to lead, or other toxic substances, render the individual unable to distinguish colour. Similarly, lesions outside of the striate cortex have been shown to cause cerebral akinetopsia—visual motion blindness—and again whilst rare, these

do occur. The two examples provided are obscure but hopefully serve to emphasize that it is unwise to accept clients' complaints, no matter how vague or 'florid', as automatic indicators of mental health status. Neurological disorders and dysfunctions may provoke seemingly bizarre symptomatology and present as deviation in mental health.

PROBLEMS OF PERCEPTION

We are aware that, at times, perceptions may mislead or confuse the individual with ambiguities, via illusions. An illusion may be described as a 'distorted perception or memory; a misinterpretation of sensory stimuli' (Campbell, 1989) and you may have seen examples of such illusions before (Figs 9.5–9.10). We may also have seen instances of 'reversible figures' in the past, where two differing images may be perceived but not simultaneously (Figs 9.11–9.13). However, illusions are not merely the result of either the artist's or psychologist's contrivance of an interesting possibility. They occur both within health, and disturbances of somatic and psychosocial equilibrium in a variety of situations and circumstances.

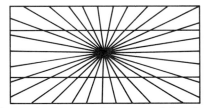

Fig. 9.5 *Are the horizontal lines parallel, or bent?*

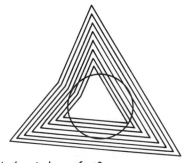

Fig. 9.6 *Is the circle perfect?*

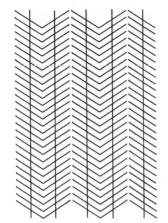

Fig. 9.7 *Zoller's illusion of direction.*

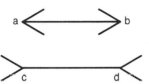

Fig. 9.8 *The Mueller–Lyer illusion of length.*

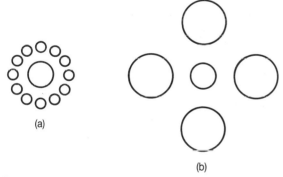

Fig. 9.9 *Which of the centre circles is larger?*

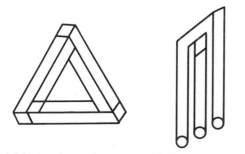

Fig. 9.10 *Are these objects possible?*

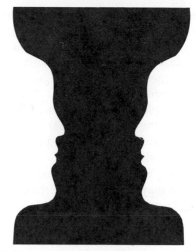

Fig. 9.11 *Rubin's vase. Face profiles or a vase?*

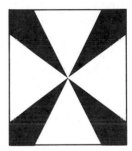

Fig. 9.12 *The Köhler Cross. A black or a white cross?*

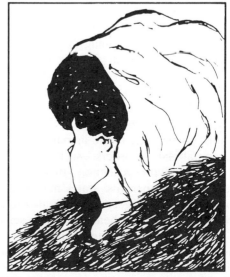

Fig. 9.13 *The Beauty or The Hag? (after Boring, 1930).*

Pareidolic images are one example of *sensory deception* which we may have experienced. A pareidolic image is a vivid perception of visual images in response to an indistinct stimulus. The image and the percept co-exist, and the image is usually recognized as 'unreal'. The commonly quoted example is that of objects, faces or scenes 'seen' within the flames of a coal fire. The individual sees the coal, the flames and the image—fantasy within reality.

An *eidetic* image, is vivid and usually visual although it may be auditory in nature. It closely resembles actual perception and is very detailed in composition. It occurs mainly in children—10% show a strong inclination and some 50% demonstrate a tendency (Leask *et al.*, 1969)—and may extend beyond adolescence in those who display an artistic ability or photographic memory. It may be referred to as primary mental image and the individual is able to scan a visual display even after the display has been removed. The image, whilst at times interfering with consequent stimuli, may be recalled with photographic accuracy long after the event or experience. Gardner and Roylance (1982) believe that the increasing ability of adolescents and adults to classify and re-label items weakens this figurative preciseness of memory and hence explains virtual absence from the older person's repertoire.

Pareidolic and eidetic images are examples of an illusion, that is, the *misinterpretation* of existing *stimuli*, and a relatively 'normal' phenomena. A similar form of eidetic imagery may be seen to occur in individuals with somatic disorder, for example, tetany (calcium deficiency due to hypoparathyroidism) and Basedow's disease (hyperparathyroidism causing demineralization of bone) (*Professional Guide to Diseases*, 1989). Systemic infections, particularly in the immature or ageing brain, metabolic disorders, such as hypoxia, hypercarbia, hypoglycaemia, thiamine deficiences, and postoperative states may also elicit the experience of imagery. Individuals regaining consciousness following head injury, or seizures, may similarly demonstrate illusions (Green, 1982), and within mental health care, those experiencing withdrawal from alcohol and those experiencing hallucinogen-induced organic prob-

lems provide examples of the exteriorization of illusions (Applyby and Forshaw, 1990).

Lyttle (1986) utilizes an example to facilitate differentiation between an illusion and a hallucination:

The alcoholic in delirium tremens (alcohol withdrawal delirium) may be startled by the pattern on the wallpaper as it resembles snakes to his fevered eye (illusion)—the snakes may then proceed to slide down the wall and climb up the counterpane (hallucination).

Hallucinations represent another example of sensory deception and may be defined as 'a false perception occurring in the absence of an external sensory stimulus' (Lyttle, 1986). They occur simultaneously alongside 'real' perceptions of the environment, and may be described as *elementary* or *complex* in nature. Elementary, or simple, hallucinations may take the form of a discrete noise, for example, as in a buzzing, banging or shuffling sound, whilst complex hallucinations may be a combination of sounds heard, as in voices or music. They are classified according to the sensory mode via which they are perceived.

Visual hallucinations may be clearly defined people, objects or animals, geometrical patterns, symbols or flashes of light. *Lilliputian (microptic) hallucinations* are those visual images that are seen as much reduced in size, for example, little people. They appear as a feature in typhoid, cholera and scarlet fever, temporal or temperosphenoidal tumour presence and are reported by some individuals experiencing petit mal epilepsy. Intoxication via alcohol, chloral, ether and trichlorethylene may also provoke Lilliputian hallucinations.

Auditory hallucinations may be of noises, but are commonly experienced as voices. They may be friendly or intimidating, clear or unintelligible, recognized as belonging to someone known or considered to be that of a stranger. Both *second-* and *third person* auditory hallucinations are reported, and the latter often involve voices keeping a 'running commentary' on the individual's actions, or arguing or discussing the individual and his activities. A *thought echo*, a repetition of a thought, is frequently considered as an auditory hallucination because the individual reports 'hearing' the echo.

Gustatory hallucinations are unpleasant tastes which often lead the individual to believe that his food is poisoned, and may occur in conjunction with *olfactory hallucinations*, again often of an unpleasant nature, and frequently perceived as being of poisonous gases, introduced to kill the individual.

Tactile (or haptic) hallucinations are often experienced as fingers touching the individual's skin, of sexually orientated sensations, pain or extremes of temperature. The term *formication* describes tactile hallucinations relating to bugs or vermin crawling in or under the skin, often associated with the experience of cocaine delusional disorders.

Kinaesthetic hallucinations are false sensations related to body movement, and one of the most common problems seen relates to a phantom limb. The individual feels that a lost limb is really present, finding great difficulty in correlating the absent limb and perceptions of body image. It is a 'healthy' response, that is, an expected one, and in time, as the amputee adjusts to reorganized body image, will disappear. Sometimes, however, individuals retain an 'extended phantom'—of the same length as the missing limb—for years, whilst others experience a 'retracted phantom' (a shortened missing limb) or a 'telescoped phantom', where toes are felt to be protruding from the stump.

Other hallucinations may be experienced, for example, *reflex hallucinations* occur when a stimulus in one sensory mode provokes an hallucination via a different sensing system. Such a reflex may relate to, for example, experiencing an auditory sensation in response to a tactile stimulus.

Functional hallucinations are experienced in conjunction with a real background stimulus, for instance, hearing water and perceiving voices in responses to the sound. *Extracampine hallucinations* occur when the individual experiences stimuli that are located out of range of the sensory field. The individual 'hearing' another person talking in Moscow, from his position in London,

without either the aid of a telephone or other 'eavesdropping' type of device, provides an example of this type of sensory deception.

Dissociative hallucinations, commonly elicited in individuals experiencing bereavement or grief, are feelings associated with the presence, or closeness of someone or something, to the degree where they can *almost* see, hear and feel the 'intruder'. Sometimes the term refers to bimodal hallucinations, where the image 'seen', 'speaks'. *Autoscopic hallucinations* may be dissociative in nature and relate to seeing self, that is, 'standing' outside of the body and watching one's own activities from a distance. Again these are commonly experienced by individuals following bereavement. *Pseudo-hallucinations* is the term utilized to describe those images that occur in the mind of the individual rather than within the external environment, or to those sensations and experiences which are perceived as unreal and yet where there is no ability to exert voluntary control over the image.

Mention has been made elsewhere (Chapter 8) of the 'normality' of hypnogogic and hypnopompic hallucinations—those visual or auditory perceptions occurring when falling asleep and waking up—and of those associated with febrile conditions, exhaustion and fatigue, and oxygen lack.

Indeed hallucinations may be induced experimentally by electrical stimulation of the temporal lobe, amygdala and hippocampus, plus other areas of the brain. They may occur as a feature of the aura of epileptic seizures, when they may be of the visual, olfactory or gustatory mode. Irritation of the vestibular apparatus of the ear may provoke false sensory perceptions, mainly visual and tactile in nature. Multiplication and diminution of the image, loss of colour and sometimes of half of the image, are evoked when the subject is subjected to a passive rotating movement. Similar *vestibular* hallucinations may be seen with those false perceptions experienced within alcohol-related mental health problems and in psychosis, vestibular hallucinations may be portrayed in sensations of the body's lightness or heaviness. In severe hypothyroidism (myxoedema) and a small proportion of individuals experiencing vitamin B_{12} deficiency they are vivid. Neoplasia and injury to the temporal lobe also exteriorized the hallucinatory experience. Within the sphere of psychosocial health, many individuals experience such a problem—those who are severely depressed in mood, often those who demonstrate psychomotor acceleration, as in 'hypomania', the 'schizophrenic' and the individual utilizing psychoactive substances or experiencing the sequelae of their use.

Illusions and hallucinations are sensory deceptions but, in addition, some individuals may show problems associated with *sensory distortion*. The intensity of perceptions may be heightened by alterations in physiological thresholds—for example, the individual utilizing lysergic acid diethylamide (LSD) may perceive vivid and intense colours. Similarly emotional status may affect perception, for the individual experiencing depressed mood may encounter a colourless, grey or drab world, whilst the hyperactive and over optimistic person may perceive a bright, exaggerated and florid environment. *Dysmegalopsia* may be experienced as the spatial form of objects alters. An example would be *micropsia* where objects are perceived to be smaller than they actually are and which may be a feature of temporal lobe epilepsy and psychoactive substance utilization. Distortion of the size perception accuracy—part of the 'physical appearance' construct—is seen within the diagnostic category of anorexia nervosa, where individuals perceive

themselves 'fat' despite actual emaciation. *Depersonalization and derealization* are sensory distortions, occurring where anxiety, depressed mood, schizophrenia, or temporal lobe epilepsy are featured, as well as in 'normal folk'. Depersonalization is the term utilized to describe the individual's feelings of lost personal identity, of being 'different', changed or strange and unreal. Derealization relates to similar feelings about one's environment, and the two may frequently be seen to co-exist.

CONCLUSIONS

We have provided examples of sensory deception and distortion and, not by any means, an exhaustive list. Whilst providing an overview of the problems of perception that may be encountered by the nurse because of an individual client's experience, we have also attempted to reinforce the fact that such problems are not solely encountered within mental health related care. The nurse in the adult, somatic-care orientated ward, the nurse within child care services and carers within facilities for those experiencing learning disability, may all witness such problems. There is therefore a requirement for all care workers to be able to recognize perceptual problems and employ strategies and interventions to manage the presenting situation.

ATTENTION

Our definition of attention was that attention represents conscious awareness, sensory clarity and central nervous system readiness to respond to stimuli received (Campbell, 1989). We also stated that attention is influenced by a variety of factors and that it is selective in nature.

Returning to the scenario at the beginning of the chapter, the young women's initial concentration was focused upon compiling the mental agenda of discussion topics for her meeting, and that it was only when she *perceived* a change in

her bodily status that she deliberately and consciously 'tuned in' to her surroundings and situation. People are constantly assailed with stimuli from competing sources and any sensory system that attempted to process every minute fragment of information available would quickly be overwhelmed with data and yet impotent to construct anything meaningful or valuable to the individual.

Imagine . . .

. . . just one instance from the past when, above

a cacophony of noise, a voice has emanated forth. 'Be quiet, I can't hear myself think!' ... and then, observe and register the composition of the room/environment in which you are currently seated. Look at the walls and decoration, the floor and its covering, the windows and the curtains. Take in the furniture detail—are there chairs, what type, how many and what colours? What about a table—is there one, what shape and size is it and what is it composed of? Is there a television, music centre or a video player? Are there books, pictures, photographs and ornaments—how many and what are the detailed features of each? How is the room heated and illuminated and who is sitting there within the environment other than you.

It is a myriad of different shapes, colours, sizes, textures and materials and the light and shade of the room is not static but ever subtly changing. Now imagine that every aspect of the room is communicating its detail to you simultaneously and continuously—a little like a speaking clock telephone service—repeating its vital statistics, current status, temperature, state of repair—and every particle of dust that settles upon it! A constant recorded message emanating from each element of the room, registering every fractional change in image would rapidly overwhelm you. There would be no time to register or record details provided and no opportunity to concentrate on one piece of furniture or other environmental feature, because of the equally demanding competition from the rest of the room. Chaos!

Attention is therefore of necessity a selective process. Physiologically speaking, some sensory receptor cells respond intensely to a novel stimulus, but as the stimulus continues, the response fades. This process is termed *adaptation*, and the speed and degree of adaptation occurring is seen to vary both in relation to the sensory modality involved and the prevailing circumstances or conditions. In this way, changes in environment or the status of self are incorporated into existing knowledge, to maintain the individual's mental construct—his or her current perception of the world or environment. Without adaptation, the imagery utilized to introduce this section would be the reality.

THEORIES OF SELECTION

Having decided that individuals are selective in their attention to the environment, how is this limited attention achieved? Broadbent (1958), utilizing *dichotic listening* tasks (i.e. sending one message to a person's left ear and a different one to his right ear simultaneously), found that the individuals participating made fewer errors when repeating messages back from 'one ear at a time' rather than trying to combine data from both ears and repeat material as it was presented (Fig. 9.14).

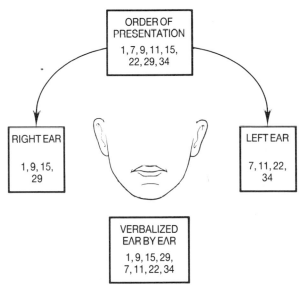

Fig. 9.14 *Dichotic listening I (Broadbent, 1958)*

Broadbent found that people tested, tended to repeat information back in this way which led him to theorize that individuals were only able to attend to one channel—in the above example, one ear—at a time, and that, furthermore, individuals found it difficult to change from one sensory channel to another at a rate of more than twice a second. His model suggests that information to the unattended ear is predominantly lost, though some elements may be held in the short-term memory store for a reduced period of time. Broadbent's *single channel model* asserts that it is the physical characteristics of the input (e.g. the source of the impulse, its strength and the number of times it is repeated) rather than the meaning of it which engenders attention and that understanding of the input occurs at a later stage after the filtering process. The model is limited, for it provides no explanation for those occasions when individuals are attending to one aspect of their environment but are distracted by, perhaps, overhearing a familiar name, or voice. Broadbent's theory would suggest that if attention is not being paid to the channel, material incoming via that channel is all but lost, and yet we know that such distractions are frequently experienced.

Gray and Wedderburn (1960) found, utilizing similar experiments of dichotic listening, that material could be combined from both ears and sorted to make sense, in a category by category response by participants, thus reducing the validity of the Broadbent model (Fig. 9.15).

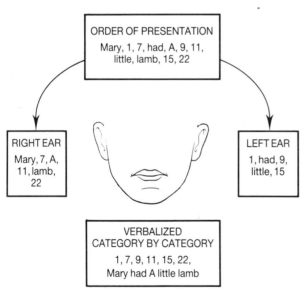

Fig. 9.15 *Dichotic listening II (Gray and Wedderburn, 1960)*

Speech shadowing, utilized by Treisman (1964) required the participant to repeat aloud material simultaneously being played into one ear, whilst an unconnected message was being played in the non-attending ear. Treisman found that individ-

uals could shadow the attending ear's material, but could also follow the information accurately when, unexpectedly within the duration of the experiment, the inputs to both ears were changed over. The non-attending ear became the attending ear often without the participant even noticing the change in channel. In addition, she discovered that bilingual participants were aware that the passage of French language being played into the non-attending ear, was a direct translation of the passage of English prose being played into the attending ear. Treisman and Gelade's *attenuation model* (1990), whilst agreeing with Broadbent with regard to the physical qualities of a stimulus being the attention-grabbing factor, asserts that the material inputting from non-attended channels is attenuated, or modified rather than lost. We would liken the process to turning down the television volume prior to answering a phone call—the background noise is still there but reduced. This model suggests, too, that both attended and relevant unattended (attenuated) stimuli pass through a second filtering system to ascertain their value for attention. Treisman and Gelade stated that a *threshold value* was required to be reached by stimuli in order that they pass through the second filter for attention, and that all attended stimuli would automatically reach this threshold. In addition, they suggested that some stimuli within the environment, for example, an individual's own name or those of other significant individuals, and words such as 'help' and 'fire', or screams, may have a permanently low threshold to facilitate passage through the filter. Temporary low thresholds, they asserted, were awarded to environmental features or other stimuli which had a relevancy of the moment.

The attenuation model, whilst more effective than Broadbent's single channel model, does not explain how information is processed to provide understanding. Deutsch and Deutsch (1963) tried a different analysis. The *late selection model* proposed that information is not selected until its meaning has been evaluated, and that filtering occurs only therefore after data have been recognized and its relevance or worth has been determined. Within this hypothesis, *all* inputs are screened at a high level and items selected as important are passed upwards for conscious attention. Research has provided some support for the late selection model via conditioning experiments, and those utilizing shadowing of ambiguous sentences. However, Dawson and Schell (1982) found that conditioned responses were only evident when the word stimulus was fed into the left ear of the subject, and Wexler (1988) found that such a conditioned response depended not only upon which ear was used but also on the personality of the subject.

The late selection model would appear to an extreme hypothesis, occupying the furthest end of a continuum that begins with Broadbent. From processing only attended material to processing *all* data appears too much of a quantum leap. Atkinson *et al.* (1987) propose a simplified theory, which draws upon elements of many and which they term a '*contemporary theory*'. The theory postulates that conscious perception and recognition of a stimulus may only occur when the *recognition* threshold of a specific neuron is reached and is dependent upon three factors. *Stimulus input* of a sufficient intensity and of an appropriate sensitivity will activate the specific neuron towards the recognition threshold, whilst an *attentional set* adds an internal input to the neuron relating the current context or relevancy, and the individual's motives and expectations. This added attentional set results in partial activation or inhibition of the neuron, with *selective attention* achieved via active neurons suppressing the activity of others. Reciprocal inhibition is suggested as the process by which less active neurons are suppressed and most active neurons are boosted towards the recognition threshold. The theory continues that the processing of stimuli is parallel to a point but that where attention is required, serial processing must take over to accommodate the fact that attention is limited to a small number of items at a time.

There is certainly little doubt regarding the features and characteristics of stimuli that attract attention and these may be viewed daily in the work of advertisers. A loud noise attracts where a soft one would not and repeated loud noises will attract attention even more effectively. Bright colours, changes in, or flashes of, colour have been utilized in neon-lighting adverts to good

effect, but any novel or incongruous feature will do the trick and you may find it is a valuable exercise to spend a few moments analysing the features of adverts that draw attention to a product.

'Attention set' is certainly of importance too, for, just as the dieting individual may constantly, and almost to the exclusion of all else, perceive food-related stimuli, and the person who is attempting to give up smoking may be able to smell cigarette smoke within a half a mile radius, so current interests and basic needs will influence attention. Similarly an activity already in progress may significantly influence attention. The athlete awaiting the starting pistol hears no background noise for example, and, similarly, the individual engrossed in a good book will attend to little else within the environment.

SUSTAINED ATTENTION

Sometimes, in situations where prolonged duration vigilance tasks are needed to be performed, attention suffers. Mackworth (1950) studied *sustained vigilance* in response to problems encountered within military operations during World War II, where the operator's task was beyond his control and his responsibilities centred around watching a radar screen for activity (particularly enemy activity), and lapse in concentration or attention could prove dangerous for a large number of individuals. Mackworth's findings in relation to performances similar in nature to those undertaken by military personnel elicited a rapid reduction in attention within the first 30-minute phase of the test, as accuracy of reporting stimuli dropped to 85%. Within the second and third 30-minute periods of testing, the decline noted was more gradual—74 and 70% accuracy in reporting respectively. Mackworth elicited the results of decline in arousal by stimuli presented and therefore reduced attention levels. Oswald (1960) demonstrated that prolonged exposure to repetitive and monotonous stimuli evoked electroencephalogram (EEG) patterns characteristic of sleep in subjects. Indeed, prior to sleep, subjects experienced short lapses of consciousness, of which they were totally unaware.

Wilkinson (1963) compared subjects' performance under 'normal' circumstances with that produced following sleep deprivation and with that exteriorized during exposure to noise. Within both of the 'abnormal' situations, performance was seen to decline and yet when combined (i.e. the subject was both sleep deprived and attempting to perform in a noisy environment), levels of performance were representative of those evoked under 'normal' circumstances. It may be logical to assume that poor performance following sleep deprivation may be the result of under-arousal, and that witnessed during exposure to high levels of noise, the result of over-arousal. The two combined may therefore cancel each other out to facilitate 'normal' performance supporting a theory of an inverted 'U'-shaped performance curve (Fig. 9.16).

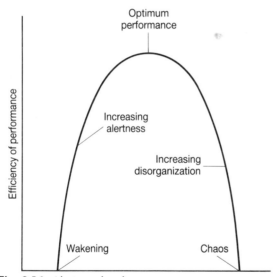

Fig. 9.16 *Alertness levels*

There are, according to this theory, optimum levels of arousal—not too little and not too much stimulation—required to evoke optimum levels of performance. Certainly Wilkinson's work would support such a theory, and therefore manipulation of the environment may be a realistic method of increasing attention thereby improving performance. You may have noted that prolonged periods of study are ineffective—attention wanders and no matter how frequently the passage has been read, it still is not absorbed or

understood. A change of activity—not more of the same, by reading a different passage—will restore attention at this point. For example, stopping reading after each couple of pages and jotting down notes of points required to be remembered or taking a complete break for five minutes and *doing* something different within the period, rather than dwelling on one's tardiness over a cup of coffee, will relieve the monotony of presenting stimuli.

PROBLEMS OF ATTENTION

Everyone is at times inattentive. The woman on the bench in the park exhibited inattentiveness whilst preoccupied with making her mental list of subjects to be discussed with her friend, and most individuals will be able to identify with this phenomenon. Short mental activities such as this are an integral part of daily function, and for those periods of time attention is turned inwards. In a similar fashion, most individuals have experienced a situation where too many issues are prevailing and consequently they cannot attend to one because of interference from another or others. These are problems encountered fairly frequently and most people learn to manage such situations more or less effectively. Temporary lapses in outward attention may, of course, be detrimental to health, should they occur, for example, whilst crossing a busy road or driving in heavy traffic. Many everyday activities may be performed almost by an 'automatic pilot', facilitating thinking about other things rather than the activity itself. Driving is one area where perhaps individuals do not always attend to the degree necessary to perform safely.

Problems associated with inattention are more common than you may think. In childhood, for example, attention deficits may be seen in combination with impulsiveness and hyperactivity, and this creates varying levels of difficulty within all settings. Some impairment in social and school functioning is always evident and follow-up studies show that in approximately one-third of such children, problems persist in later life. Attention deficit may be seen in children, without the added hyperactivity, but little is known about this, and more investigation is required.

An inability to attend or concentrate is a common problem experienced by those individuals experiencing maladaptive reactions to identifiable psychosocial stressors, termed adjustment disorders. These are evidenced within three months of the onset of stressor(s) and may take many forms, but will remit soon after the stressor ceases or when adaptation is achieved. Similarly inattention is a feature associated with depressed mood or hyperactivity in adults with anxiety, and those individuals experiencing the effects of psychoactive substance use. Poor attention levels may be responsible for complaints regarding 'poor memory', and differentiation of the actual difficulties experienced must therefore be employed.

The withdrawal from, and inattentiveness to, the environment described within discussions relating to schizophrenia were once thought, too, to be due to an excessive preoccupation with mental imagery and one's own thoughts and feelings. However, studies have demonstrated that, at least within the early stages of the experience, there is an inability to attend selectively to the environment and that therefore withdrawal is used as a defence against the bombardment of senses by the multitude of stimuli which compete for attention. The continuous distraction by the environment precludes adequate or effective general performance, by inability to exclude any aspect of surroundings. It may be that complete withdrawal may be the only alternative to the chaos of attempting to interact with the environment.

To be able to attend, of course, one has to be conscious and this area of function is the responsibility of the mesencephalic portions of the *reticulo-activating system* (RAS). When asleep, for example, inputs via sensory receptors stimulate the RAS into *general consciousness*, then pass upwards to the *thalamus*, causing the widespread cortical activity, termed *arousal* (Tortora and Anagnostakos, 1984). The RAS acts as 'the brain's chief watchguard', monitoring stimuli and forwarding only essential material to the conscious mind. Consciousness may be altered by various factors, from meditation to medication, and from somatic disorder to mental health problems. Hence problems associated with attention again may be encountered within all fields of health care, not solely that related to psychosocial service provision.

THINKING

The following definition of 'thinking' was used in the introduction to the chapter:

... the process by which images and ideas, representing objects and events experienced, are manipulated, using previous knowledge and understanding of the situation, to arrive at strategies by which changes in status may be managed.
Campbell, 1989

Thinking is something 'automatic' in nature, something that individuals take for granted. It represents a process that is continuous, from the time of awakening until the moment of drifting back off to sleep, and yet it is an area which most individuals never dream to analyse in relation to self. However, thinking is an area that has attracted the attention of philosophers, scientists and physicians for hundreds of years.

SOME THOUGHTS ON THINKING

Aristotle addressed the subject of thinking from his general philosophical framework and generated three primary laws to explain the *continuity*

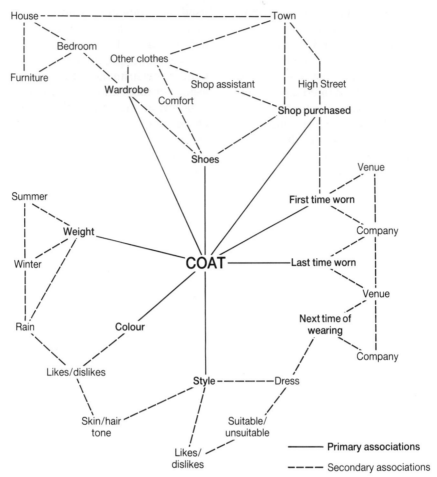

Fig. 9.17 *Potential associations.*

of thought and to elucidate the principles of memory.

1   Ideas are combined or *associated* because they are *similar* in some way, for example, bread and rolls have a similar *taste and function* within the eating process. Similarity of *location* provides another relevant association, therefore shoes and socks, table and chair, and garden and flowers are ideas that are associated.

2   The second law of association relates to the *contrast* between concepts, and therefore the association between up and down, in and out, black and white, and yes and no, are explainable.

3   The principle of *contiguity* suggests an association via concepts which have a relationship in *time or space*. Therefore an association exists between schools and learning, churches and worship, pens and writing, beds and sleeping and the like.

Aristotle and the early *philosophical associationists* (Warren, 1921) maintained that any specific concept may be accounted for by one of the primary laws, but that, in addition, one concept may generate several associations (Fig. 9.17).

Later associationists attempted to trace the construction of complex ideas, though it was generally accepted by all that the process involved a combination of all elements involved in some way. James Mill maintained that any idea, no matter how complex, was composed of discrete elements, each of which maintained its own identity, and which amalgamated with others to form a group. However, Hartley and Brown asserted that a complex idea involved a fusion of the properties of each individual element, and that such fusion evoked characteristics of properties in the whole which were not evident in the separate elements. Eventually Hartley and Brown's theory was accepted by the associationists and the view generally held became that related to the coalescence of elements to form a different, whole, and complex, idea.

Brown attempted to account for the *specific selection* of associations by providing a series of secondary laws. He asserted that concepts *most frequently* associated in the past were likely to remain so in the future—for example, school would continue to be associated with learning rather than a one-off visit to the seaside, which occurred at the age of five years. Where two associations had been made with almost equal frequency in the past, say school and learning and school and friends, Brown believed that the *most recent* association would take precedence, and that where a conflict occurred between the frequency or recency of an association, the one evoking the *most vivid* or *emotionally significant* association would predominate.

Herbart theorized regarding the manner by which conscious experience was *organized*, thus providing another set of principles for the combination of ideas and thoughts. He suggested that some concepts attract each other, that is, are *congruent*, whilst others repel or inhibit each other and are termed *incongruent*. Herbart believed that congruent material combined to make up the *apperceptive mass*—the existing body of knowledge and experience—which became the centre for the organization of conscious experience. Incongruent material, which is irrelevant or which does not 'fit' into the overall scheme, Herbart believed to be either rejected, and excluded from conscious experience, or 'made to fit in', according to its importance to the individual (Warren, 1921).

Wundt (cited in Watson, 1963) became known as the 'father of psychology' in respect of his activities, which separated the work of philosophers from that of 'scientists', who wished to conduct a more objective study of the mind. Wundt declared that the scientific methodology available was not applicable to the study of higher mental processes, such as thinking. However, observations of social phenomena, for example, language, and studies of reaction time, particularly those related to the focusing aspects of consciousness, provided Wundt with insight into the complexity of the subject, and, in addition, some objective information concerning thought. He asserted that thought and association were two different entities, and that thinking followed some logical sequence whilst association did not. He believed that associations did not, of necessity, make sense, for example, the individual who, when buying a book, gets soaking wet in a sudden downpour of rain, may associate the two events and yet there is no logical connection between them. The situation of needing the book for a specific purpose and the event of purchasing it, provide a logical consideration and, therefore, a logical connection. According to Wundt, cognitive connections are made upon logical considerations, relevancy and appropriacy.

Titchener (1909) also a structuralist like Wundt, arrived at his conclusions regarding thought and thinking via studies of the process of attention. For Titchener, the conscious content of an individual's mind comprised of various elements, or ingredients, and that any one element could be explained or described through the patterning of the others present. Much like a kaleidoscope may produce various images from a set number of different coloured pieces of glass, by adjustment of the pattern into which they fall, so any one element of conscious content depended upon the configuration of the others. Titchener believed that cognitive activities, such as thinking and attention, were composed of *images*, somewhat similar to those of sensation, in that they possessed characteristics such as quality, intensity, clarity and duration, and yet dissimilar, in regard to their 'transparency'. By this, he was referring to the images' characteristics of being less objective, appearing less realistic and being more easily destroyed than those of sensation. By equating thought with variations in the conscious content, he provided facility for the particular meaning of an image to be determined, not only by the appearance of the salient stimulus at a specific time, but also by the conscious content of the mind within the prevailing circumstances.

Titchener's European colleagues, however, objected to such a peremptory dismissal of the area of cognitive function, and with reference to this discussion of thought, whilst agreeing that images could occur within thinking processes, asserted that *imageless thought* was the typical component comprising the processes of thinking.

William James (1890) considered the processes of thinking, reasoning and believing were biological in essence and resultant from the elaboration of sensory processes within the central nervous system. He believed these processes to be dynamic in nature and that, therefore, any attempt to break down the overall processes into sub-units of 'ideas' or 'images' was both pedantic and artificial, engendering a rigidity where, in his view, the essence was of fluidity and flexibility. He believed thinking to be the vehicle via which biological needs were met by the individual, facilitating adjustment to the environment, goal-directed behaviours to achieve basic needs, and the anticipation of difficulties, and generation of solutions to problems encountered on the way. According to James, it is an irrational process, directed by biological need. He did not differentiate between the roles of thinking and memory within this process. He believed both to be dependent upon two separate and differing sequences. The first of these he referred to as *sagacity* or *insight*, and described this as a creative ability, combining the capacity for perspective, with the ability to select the relevant features of the problem from the accompanying minutiae. Thus a 'sagaciously structured' problem is one that has been clearly identified with regard to its detailed nature, and which has been examined from a variety of points of view. Having achieved this sequence, the second one begins operation, with an arousal of previously learned associations and the application of these to the decision, or choice of solution, to arrive at a reasonable course of action within the circumstances.

Whilst not differentiating between thinking and remembering, James did distinguish between thoughts and beliefs. The latter he asserted to be more closely related to emotion than to thought and reasoning, because of their *coercive* nature. He considered that beliefs determined an individual's psychological reality, by exerting pressure upon the person to perceive the world in accordance with those beliefs. Beliefs were, he asserted, established on the basis of biological need or instinct and their continued existence served only to gratify that need. Hence beliefs were irrefutable.

Tolman (1932) developed his theory relating to *cognitive maps* from his work with rats. He had observed that rats *learned* about a maze during his experiments, rather than merely utilizing a series of responses to deal with it. He discovered that, given the opportunity, the rats would select the shortest pathway between two points even if they had no previous experience of that specific path and were on unfamiliar territory. He believed that the rats had constructed a 'map' which represented the salient features of the maze and the spatial relationships involved. In addition, Tolman considered the rats not only to be aware of the relationships among stimuli, but also to have generated expectancies about their meanings and a readiness to respond in appropriate ways. It was as if the rats had 'visualized' the journey from A to B and the activities necessary to complete the journey successfully and in the shortest period of time.

Tolman asserted that human beings create cognitive maps, too, and in their instance, such maps are not solely related to locations. People exhibit 'maps and expectancies' relating to what self and others should, or would do within a number of different situations, and he concluded that individuals possess a symbolic representation of all biopsychosocial aspects of their environment, plus their potential reactions to them. These anticipations, maps and the ability to mentally 'try out' scenarios presenting held no meaning in themselves, for he asserted that they were derived from, and relevant to, whatever purpose was influencing behaviour.

It was Tolman's belief that consciousness (*awareness*) and thinking occurred only within situations where behaviour could not be automatically evoked, for example, in novel situations where anticipations and predictions could not be inferred with any certainty. The absence of knowledge was not considered to be the cause of consciousness or thinking, but merely provided an *opportunity* for their utilization. Where new relationships emerge from productive thought, engendering new anticipations and novel responses, he coined the term *inventive ideation*, to indicate an especially creative process. In general, however, Tolman believed that once the novelty had diminished within a situation, conscious awareness and thinking were also reduced, allowing automatic processes and habitual responses to assume responsibility for continuation of activities at the earliest appropriate opportunity.

To understand the beliefs of Sigmund Freud (1922) and psychoanalytical theory in relation to thought and thinking, a brief review of his considerations of consciousness and personality is required. You may recall that Freud characterized *conscious activity* as that encompassing an awareness of events occuring both within the individual and his external environment. In addition, however, he believed that there were other occurrences of which the individual was unaware, situated within the *unconscious*, and again material which, whilst the individual had no current awareness of it, could be recalled into consciousness at will, within the *preconscious*.

With regard to personality, Freud delineated three regions—the *id*, *ego* and *superego*. The id he described as a composition of primitive and unsocialized biological urges and drives, guided by the *pleasure principle*, and maximizing the pleasure of the moment, uncaring of eventual consequences. The ego assumed the role of mediator between the id and the real world, seeking realistic outlets for id impulses whilst simultaneously keeping within expectations of the environment and avoiding painful experiences of injury, rejection and punishment on behalf of the id. The guiding feature of the ego was referred to as the *reality principle*. The superego provided the region of the personality that included the person's moral values and ethics—the conscience—which often influences behaviour without the individual's awareness, via social learning taking place prior to the child's ability to understand or verbalize such material. The superego

basically interacts with reality and the external world and is, therefore, like the ego, necessarily conscious in nature.

To recap, Freud believed the mind to be influenced by animal drives (id), moderated by the demands imposed by reality (ego) and censored by moral values (superego). Of necessity, the individual is aware (conscious) of the demands of the ego (reality) and of some of the material of the superego (moral values and ethics). However, the individual is totally oblivious (unconscious) of the true nature of his animal urges, because awareness would create distress. Awareness constituted only the salient stimuli, impulses and memories necessary to performance, with the preconscious providing a reservoir for the additional resources necessary.

Freud maintained that the infant, at the mercy of, and solely influenced by, the pleasure principle (the id), can neither perceive nor think, but reacts both impulsively, and automatically, to maximize satisfaction of biological urges and drives. Gradually, however, the child becomes aware of the need to adjust behaviour to the reality of the situation, because of the pain that may result from its disregard. To avoid such pain—rejection, punishment and injury—the individual evokes thoughtful behaviour, to analyse and respond appropriately to the demands of reality. Thoughtful behaviour represents a more mature stage of development and signals the influence of the ego. Freud asserted that once an individual exhibited sufficient maturity to maintain a realistic orientation, he was able to revert to the drives of pleasure principle only when the ego was rendered inactive—in sleep, fantasies, neurotic and psychotic symptomatology.

Freud believed thought to be a symbolic representation, rather than an entity in itself, and that these symbols, words and images are representative of objects, events and feelings and are mostly learned. The child is unable to think until such learning has taken place. In addition he believed thought to be symbolic in another way, being an expression of unconscious material, and therefore a mechanism via which primitive, repressed urges may be satisfied. This type of symbolism, he determined, was often a product of cultural and racial heritage and found expression within fantasy, day dreaming and aimless mental wanderings. His interpretation of dream symbolism is an extension of this element of the theoretical perspective. According to Freud, then, thought is a learned symbolism, relating to feelings, events and objects, which originates with the reality principle and which assists the ego to moderate the relationship between the id and the external reality.

We have identified just some of the many perspectives that have been applied to thought and thinking. There are many others, including those of Adler, Harry Stack Sullivan, Lewin, Hebb, Piaget and others, plus those attributed to Gestalt, phenomenological and cybernetic schools of study (Neel, 1969). Limitations of space alone preclude their outline within this section, though we would suggest their perusal to be valuable in relation to any detailed study of the area. In providing broad examples of 'thoughts about thinking', we have attempted to provide insight into the widely differing perspectives held and promulgated by philosophers and psychologists. However thinking arises and whatever influences are applied to the process, individuals do think, and in some recognizable ways.

TYPES OF THINKING

McKellar (1957) differentiated between two different types of thinking processes. The first— *autistic thinking*—related to that mental activity which is more or less subjective and removed from reality. It represents the narcissistic, egocentric material that day-dreams and fantasies are made of and the type of thinking experienced within dream states. The second category identified by McKellar is that of *realistic* or *imaginitive thinking* and in this he is referring to a more logical, rational, goal-directed thinking, in which words and symbols, representing objects and events, are manipulated mentally, rather than in reality. Realistic thinking is the process inherent within problem solving and scientific thinking, and any goal-directed activity requiring the ability to *reason*. McKellar believed realistic thinking to be influenced by learning and experience.

Experimental psychology has been, for the most part, concerned with realistic thinking, and yet there is evidence—if one looks for it—of autistic trends in the everyday thinking of adults, who would, no doubt, consider themselves objective and logical beings. Autistic thinking is, for example, a prerequisite for spiritual beliefs. 'In sure and certain hope' is reliant upon faith, not logical, objective evidence and yet millions of people world-wide believe in a God, of some specific name, of an after-life and of this existence being a preparation for another, better one. People either have faith or they do not believe. Individuals who are superstitious are similarly a little less than logical, for, whilst there was frequently a sensible basis for a superstition in the past, circumstances change and actions or beliefs are now no longer relevant. Whether one believes that the 'third light' from a match is unlucky, a broken mirror brings seven years' bad luck or walking under a ladder bodes badly, there is no longer a logic to underpin the beliefs held. Prejudices and stereotypes are irrational, as are the 'miracle' cures which promise to ameliorate everything from obesity to shyness. Anyone utilizing a sweeping generalization in a statement or accepting a 'quick fix' to solve a personality problem has got to believe in magic!

We believe that any relaxation of attention or redirection of thoughts from goal-orientated activities is an opportunity for autistic-orientated thought. Indeed mental health nurses encourage it—'For the next few moments I want you to close your eyes and relax. Imagine yourself walking along a beach ...' Everyone has fantasies and day-dreams. Many people 'relive' a particular incident within their minds, where they engender a more effective self—'I should have said that ... if only I'd have thought about saying ...'. On any continuum of thought where the autistic type provides one extreme and realistic thought the other, the vast majority of people will be seen to move somewhere between the two extremes at various times of the day.

Realistic thinking is goal-orientated and logical, being subject to the influence of learning and experience. You may find it valuable to undertake a small analysis of the day's events in regard to the number and type of activities that required a deliberate effort of thought. A day at home may include, for example:

Switched off alarm clock ... got up, washed and dressed ... listened/watched news ... made and ate breakfast ... jobs around the house ... an hour in the garden ... shopping ... more food ... reading ... listened to music/TV ... got showered and changed ... out with friends ... home ... bed ... slept.

Who has such a simple, selfish and wonderful day? You, will, no doubt, have to include activities related to a partner, children and relatives. Walking the dogs, cleaning the car and arguing with a salesperson in a shop may also figure, but of your list, how many of the day's activities were 'routine' and undertaken with habitual action or reaction, and how many really required thinking about? Whilst constantly thinking, many of your daily activities *will* be undertaken on automatic pilot and those that require 'thinking about' *are* those in which an obstacle of some nature prevents goal achievement. They are those situations that require the individual to utilize the reasoning process to effect a removal of the impediment and facilitate goal success. If the individual applied logic to the situation, the answer to a new problem is to be found externally, within the nature of the problem and internally, via the stored memories of previous learning experience. Inhibition of the irrelevancies of a situation facilitates organization of the information available in a way that will lead to solution. That would be logical and rational. The question to ask, of course, is do individuals do this within the reasoning process?

Unless prevented from acting freely, the individual will randomly apply various responses when faced with a novel problem to achieve a solution. One has only to think of completing a jigsaw to see our meaning. The individual will try to fit a piece of the jigsaw into a specific place even though the colour shading is inaccurate, the shape is wrong and the part picture upon the piece is totally out of tune with the area. The individual will even turn the piece of puzzle around to try to fit it in, perhaps two or three times before deciding it is the wrong piece. People are most likely to attempt a solution via trial and error when faced with unfamiliar tasks which can be physically manipulated. Many people prefer to utilize trial and error thinking—even Edison tried hundreds of substances, one by one, rather than reasoning through the qualities necessary in a substance to render it an effective filament for his incandescent light bulbs. His response to critics of his trial and error methods was, 'Now I know hundreds of things that won't work!'

In some situations trial and error thinking may be the most practical solution. Ruger (1910) set up experiments with people who had to solve a wire puzzle. He found that an analysis of the solution *followed after* the solution was reached and not before, and that understanding was achieved in two distinct stages. Firstly the subject would analyse which bit of the puzzle he had successfully manipulated and then retrace the movements utilized to attain that success. After several attempts, the subject would finally experience an abrupt understanding and perform speedily and successfully from this point onwards. 'The penny dropping' and suddenly 'seeing the light' are phrases used to describe *insight*.

We are certain that there is no need to recount the classic tale of Archimedes, his bath and running naked down the streets of Syracuse, but the anecdote reinforces the abruptness of the understanding associated with insight. The mental restructuring of the situation that is required to attain insight may occur *prior* to solving the problem and will result in a reduced period of time taken to achieve the desired outcomes. The Gestalt school of psychology—particularly Wolfgang Kohler (1925)—was responsible for extensive investigation in this area.

Harlow (1949), in his experiments with monkeys found that, after several exposures to tests where the animals were required to 'select the odd one out', the monkeys seemed to understand the concept of 'oddness' and became very adept at choosing the correct—that is the odd—object from the group offered. He argued that the monkeys were not simply learning to respond to a specific stimulus, because they would select the appropriate object in one test, where its selection in a previous test had proved incorrect, and hence the monkeys had failed on that occasion to gain a record. Harlow argued that the monkeys had developed a 'learning set', a state of mental preparedness to solve this particular type of problem.

Luchins (1959) asserted that humans develop such a readiness, too, and that, with sufficient experience, in any one particular method of problem-solving activity, individuals would tend to choose that method, above easier and quicker ways of solving the problem. He discovered that such *mental sets* may be both a hindrance and a help, for though they may assist an individual to find a solution quickly in some situations, they may also prevent alternative possibilities being looked for and used. Glucksberg (1962) found that the use of mental sets precluded an ability to think of using objects outside their normal function—something he termed *functional fixedness*—and that, because of this, solutions to some problems were unavailable to the individual. The Gestalt psychologists believed that, partly because of this tendency to adopt mental sets and partly due to the nature of thinking itself, individuals could be reluctant to accept new modes of activity and alternative ways of problem solving.

LOGICAL REASONING

'Logic' is the branch of philosophy that is concerned with analysis of *inferences* and *arguments* (Salmon, 1973). An 'inference' is the formation of a conclusion based upon available evidence, whilst an 'argument' is that conclusion plus the evidence. Such evidence used to support this conclusion may involve one or more theoretical statements, called *premises*, and the strategies of logic facilitate an analysis of the reasoning involved from premises to conclusion.

Pierce (in Steiner, 1978) asserted that the major stages of inquiry comprise of three kinds of reasoning: *deduction*, *induction* and *retroduction*. Deduction is reasoning which commences with the 'general' and proceeds to the 'particular', as

specific conclusions are drawn from more general premises or principles. An example may assist:

---

1   If A were true, then B would be true

2   A is true

3   B must be true

Some arguments are *deductively valid*, that is, it is impossible for the argument (conclusion) to be false if the premises (the statements which build the conclusion) are true (Skyrms, 1986):

To be a registered nurse, you must pass the appropriate examinations

Jayne works as a registered nurse

Therefore, Jayne passed the examinations

This sort of argument may be evaluated in two ways: the first requires an analysis as to whether the conclusion follows logically from the premises: the second requires an assessment of the truth—or otherwise—of the statements used. Deductive arguments may comprise of all true statements, as with the above example, or they may contain one or more incorrect or false statements. When the latter applies, the argument is referred to as *deductively invalid*, for example:

All hawthorn berries are red

This berry is red

Therefore this is a hawthorn berry

The conclusion reached is not supported by the evidence of the premises. The information provided within the premises is neither implicit or explicit enough to arrive at such a conclusion. Now if *only* hawthorn berries are red, that would be a different matter.

Inductive reasoning describes the exact opposite process to the above, for a generalization is arrived at from a number of specific observed instances. It is less well developed than deductive reasoning (Pospesel, 1974) and is based on the assumption that what is true of randomly selected members of a group or classification, is true for all members of the group:

Susan's husband drank too much and always became violent

Margaret, Josie, Pam and Ann were also married to men who drank to excess and then became violent

All married men are alcoholic, wife-beaters

The conclusion reached is generalized well beyond the small number of instances observed, to the whole group or class of 'married men'. Similar assumptions may be seen to be applied by pollsters in election campaigns:

56% of the survey stated that they will vote for Party A

Therefore 56% of the population will vote for Party A

Excluding for the purposes of this analysis, the fact that some of those surveyed in the poll (a) may have deliberately lied, (b) may change their mind before actually voting, (c) may not actually make it to the polling station, (d) may spoil their ballot paper by placing a tick rather than a cross against the candidate's name, or (e) may not be entitled to vote, this conclusion is based on limited evidence and therefore can clearly be erroneous. The population sample may, for example, have been only 25 people, 14 of whom may have been approached as they came out of Party A's election headquarters! The survey may have been limited in any number of ways—the age group selected, sex, occupational group, area of domicile, etc.—and hence the conclusion would be disputable. However, the valid–invalid assessment utilized in relation to deductive arguments is not applied to those of inductive arguments. An inductive argument is viewed in terms of the *probability* of the premises leading to a given conclusion, therefore degrees of high,

medium and low probability may be applied to any inductive argument. An appropriately sized, representative sample used in the survey, or several such surveys used in combination to achieve a premise, may be awarded a higher level of probability than the one provided as an example.

The third type of reasoning identified by Pierce (in Steiner, 1978) was that of retroduction, which he viewed as the first stage in the analysis of a 'surprising phenomenon', to generate a potential explanation. Once an explanation of some description was available, he believed deductive reasoning could be employed to develop it and that, finally, inductive reasoning could be used to assess the degree of probability of the hypothesis in practice. Retroductive reasoning does not seek to establish a 'truth', but merely to originate ideas about a phenomenon, which may then be evaluated. It is therefore of value in areas where little is known about a subject and innovation is required to advance current knowledge and understanding. An idea or conjecture related to a new area of study or observation may be devised from previous knowledge in a different field, for example, explaining brain activity and function via the workings of a telephone switchboard, as an analogy. In relation to human activities of an everyday nature:

In situation 'A', behaviour 'X' was successful

Situation 'B', whilst relating to a different problem, has some similarities

Perhaps the principles of behaviour 'X' could be modified to produce behaviour 'Y' and achieve the goals desired

---

Applying Pierce's theory the individual may then deduce the conclusions of the activity—"if I do 'this', then 'that' will follow" and later use inductive reasoning, to analyse the probability of the conclusion actually being the outcome—"but, if I do 'this', then 'that' may not necessarily follow; the result may actually be ... or ..."—and, therefore, the potential value of any specific activity undertaken.

The question begs 'Do human beings use

logical reasoning?' Hudson (1966), in an extensive study of school children, analysed the cognitive patterns that characterized those who selected 'arts' or 'science' subjects. He discovered two distinctly varying *cognitive styles*, which he termed *convergent* and *divergent* thinking. Convergent thinkers tended to choose science subjects, and exhibited an extremely logical and linear focused style of reasoning. Those considered as divergent thinkers exhibited more intuitive and impulsive thinking, would utilize a range of potential options in problem-solving activities than their convergent peers, and tended towards the art-type subjects at school. Discrete convergent and divergent thinkers each represented approximately 30% of the population tested, whilst the remaining 40% of the sample tended to mix the characteristics of the two, emphasizing different styles in different situations. Hudson's study found support in that conducted by Pask and Scott (1992) and therefore it may be that some individuals are more 'logical' in cognitive styles than others.

Those then, who may be more logical in their reasoning—how logical are they? Wason and Johnson-Laird (1970) discovered that, despite two statements being 'logically equivalent', individuals take longer to process a negative statement than a positive one, for example:

Statement 1
If the carpet is blue, the curtains will be red

Statement 2
If the carpet is not green, the curtains will not be yellow

Individuals took more time and found it more difficult to process the information presented in a negative form, as in Statement 2, than in a positive form, as in Statement 1. In addition, Wason and Johnson-Laird asserted that humans utilize a less than formal logic, for they utilize their broader knowledge to analyse what is *likely* or *probable* to occur within problem-solving activities, rather than what is *definite* or *certain* in the situation, as logic would dictate. Rips (1986) demonstrated that people tend to use 'short-cuts'—*heuristics*—by applying previous experi-

ences and learning to a situation or problem requiring a solution. Such previous experience facilitates ease of application of the problem-solving strategy—it is already in the individual's repertoire—and may be successful in its outcome. Johnson-Laird (1983) suggested that, rather than reasoning a problem through, individuals showed evidence of applying a concrete example to the situation presenting, so that instead of mentally manipulating concepts or language, images representing the problem are utilized. The image content, he believed, of the concrete representation would be selected by the nature and content of the problem to be addressed. Again the evidence suggests people to be less logical than philosophers would have us believe.

Tversky and Kahnemann (1973) demonstrated that, in tests to ascertain how individuals arrive at a judgement regarding probability and the degree to which something is likely, people frequently ignore—or at least fail to take into account—evidence available to assist in determining probability. Despite the fact, for instance, that subjects were presented with a neutral character description which related to one or other of a group of 70 lawyers or 30 engineers, the subjects assessed the probability of the description being that of an engineer as '50–50'!

Individuals are not necessarily logical in reasoning and problem-solving activities and, whilst this may be viewed in some quarters, particularly by philosophers and purists, as detrimental to functioning, it would appear to others to be far more sophisticated and of a higher cognitive order than logic. Human reasoning encompasses more than mere logic, for it uses previous knowledge of past experiences and learning, of social context and meanings, and personal choices to come to a conclusion. The human being does far more than 'compute' information to arrive at an answer to a problem—people 'think' about problems.

PROBLEMS OF THOUGHT AND THINKING

Minor 'aberrations' of thought content and thinking patterns are relatively common within the mentally healthy individual and you may not only be able to identify with some of the examples provided here, but also be able to proffer one or two of your own. Discussions within preceding pages of this section identified the frequently illogical basis for thoughts and beliefs, for example, the shades of autistic thinking evident within superstition and religious, or spiritual, beliefs. It is relatively easy to recognize elements of *magical thinking* within the above examples, that belief or certainty that, somehow, specific thoughts, words or actions may precipitate or prevent a particular outcome, thus thwarting the laws of cause and effect. Children commonly exteriorize such thinking patterns in activities like refusing to step on the cracks in the paving of a street and it represents an integral part of development and growing up. Adults, too, may rely on charms and rituals to provide a sense of security, safety or continued wellbeing. People talk about 'tempting fate', believing that to think about or verbalize the possibility of an event or occurrence, may be sufficient to provoke its happening. Others speak of lucky charms or significant items—footballers may believe their skill increased by wearing a specific pair of boots, golfers have favoured putters that they are unable to hole a ball without and gamblers may have 'lucky dice', with which they 'just can't lose'.

Frequently such talismen and amulets provide the wearer with a sense of increased confidence, optimism and self-esteem, thus facilitating enhanced performance. The individual feels good and therefore functions well—the self-fulfilling prophecy. Such a reliance on an external object, however, detracts from the individual's ability to recognize and value the power, skill and personality characteristics which essentially generate the successful, or otherwise, outcome and which are built in and readily accessible to the person. You may recall the Walt Disney film of 'Dumbo the Elephant'. Dumbo was able to fly, he believed, because of the influence and power of a magic feather. He was confident until he dropped the feather and then panicked, believing himself incapable without it. His mouse-friend and mentor convinced him otherwise just in time to prevent Dumbo's sad demise from a great height. You may wonder why we recount this tale, but it

would seem very clear to us, that a token may initially be a boon in promoting confidence in one's own abilities, but the sooner the individual realizes that this is exactly what it is and that he or she alone is in control of 'fate' and the hand that is dealt, the more effective the efforts made towards reaching optimum development will be.

Many people experience a transitory *blocking of thought* processes, where a train of speech is interrupted before a thought or idea has been completed. Often it happens to the individual who is uncomfortable or anxious within a situation, in an interview, at the end of a driving test or in the middle of a soliloquy or speech of some kind. You have no doubt—at least once in a lifetime—experienced that dreaded pause, when you find it impossible to recall what you were saying or meant to say, and therefore are unable to continue. That dreaded 'drying up' of the actor, on stage and in mid-flow, which requires one, or several, prompts from off-stage, happens to everyone at some time and is provoked by some feeling of 'threat' to one's own psychosocial integrity and wellbeing. Such an elevated level of anxiety is inhibitory to performance and the individual whose confidence levels are sufficiently poised to facilitate the view of 'what is the worst case scenario, resultant from my failing to achieve the desired outcome?' is one who will perform more effectively, for there is the realization that life will not come to an end because of a 'negative' event. There will be a great deal of learning achieved, just by the experience, and hence there is a potential value to the individual which may far exceed that of actually achieving the desired ends. There will be another opportunity and all is not lost.

Many have experienced differences in the speed of their thought processes, as they accelerate or retard. An increased *pressure of thought*, as ideas move more rapidly through the mind, may be more noticeable in two distinctly different situations. The first occurs when the individual is overjoyed or excitedly anticipating some event. The individual finds great difficulty in concentrating or attending as the thoughts that preoccupy flit through the mind, one often leading to another via association. Similar patterns of acceleration may be experienced in those who feel anxious or overwhelmed, as thoughts flow in rapid succession regarding things that have to be done. Conversely, when a person is severely fatigued or stressed, thought processes may *retard*, and a great effort of will may be necessary to accomplish reasoning activities. Those who are sad and distressed, or somatically discomforted, may find their thought processes slow and stultified, heavy, cumbersome and difficult to achieve. Boredom and insufficient stimulation may evoke retardation of thought in a similar way.

We mentioned elsewhere the relative normality of *obsessional thoughts*, those persistent, recurrent and intrusive ideas that many people experience. You may recall individuals who are compulsive 'picture straighteners', 'precise folders' of paper or linen, 'centre-ists', who need one article to be positioned symmetrically on top of another or other precise activities. To resist the desire to respond to the thoughts that generate such activities may create discomfort and unease, though the recognition exists that the action is meaningless and futile. These small obsessional thoughts provide the individual with feelings of 'same-ness' and stability, and hence security, plus feelings of control over the environment, which again promotes ease and confidence.

Thought aberration, particularly *delusional ideation*, may accompany a number of primarily somatic health problems. A delusion may be defined as a false belief, which cannot be shared by others of the same culture, or social standing, and which cannot be altered by logical argument or contrary experiences. The central nervous system of 75% of individuals suffering from systemic lupus erythematosus—a multisystem disease, characterized by inflammation and biochemical and structural changes in collagen fibres of connective tissues, throughout the body—and delusions, accompanied by problems of perception, may be a feature requiring attention for some. Similarly, individuals experiencing the cerebral infective process, termed encephalitis, may present within mental health facilities because of bizarre thoughts and odd behavioural changes. Cerebral neoplasia and perceptual disturbances (temporal) may present with delusions, the individual experiencing the effects of an overactive thyroid may complain of thought acceler-

ation and the person whose thyroid is underproductive, may demonstrate slow, sluggish, dull thinking or conversely delusional thoughts. Vitamin B_{12} deficiency may provoke significant thought disorder in approximately 10% of individuals concerned, whilst drug preparations, for example, steroids and cardiac glycosides, may also affect the quality and speed of thought processes. Preoccupation of thoughts with distressing facts and fears may, of course, be a problem for anyone experiencing somatic ill health, its treatment or sequelae.

Within mental health care, problems of thought and thinking may, for ease of description, be subdivided into those relating to:

1 Thought content

2 Form of thought

3 Thought possession

4 Stream of thought

5 Judgement and decision making

We have referred previously, within this section, to the delusional ideation that may be associated with somatic ill-health, and, in particular, neurological disease and dysfunction. At that juncture, meaning was given to the term '*delusion*'—that is, a false belief, which cannot be shared by others of the same culture, or social standing, and which cannot be altered by logical argument or contrary experiences. One may assume, then, that all false beliefs may be delusional and indicative, therefore, of deviation in psychosocial or somatic health. However, that assumption would be erroneous, for many individuals may demonstrate *over-valued ideas*, which whilst indicative of eccentricity, may not be considered as evidence of a deviation in mental health status. An overvalued idea assumes an integral and important role in the individual's life because of its associated emotions and personal significance. These, too, are immune to rational argument, but differ from delusions in that they become comprehensible in the light of the individual's previous experience or in relation to the beliefs of his family or his subculture. Commonly quoted examples of the phenomenon include a brief that the world is flat; that a daily purgative is essential to health and that modern-day wet summertimes are due to space exploration.

Delusions represent problems of *thought content*, and, as such, are associated with those who lack insight or contact with reality, that is the individual ascribed the label of '*psychotic*'. A delusion may be referred to as *primary*, or *autochthonous*, in nature, when it arises fully formed and without any identifiable precursors. There may be no apparent relationship with the subject's prevailing mood (though on occasions and in reprospect, mood may be considered aberrant) or with any recent event. The subject *suddenly knows* that he or she is God, that the two hemispheres of his brain have been transposed or that he or she has a personal and profound mission in the world. Jaspers (1963) suggests that this *sudden delusion idea* provides one example of a *primary delusional experience*, and that this, plus the second example of a *delusional perception*, may both arise from a *delusional mood*. He described a delusional perception as that event which occurs when a full delusional meaning is ascribed to a normal, innocuous perception that is totally unrelated—for example, running water evoking the subject's belief that he or she is God. Subjects believe that their environment has dramatically and inexplicably changed; it is usually unpleasant and self-referential. They are convinced—or at least strongly suspect—that mundane events are of tremendous significance, but they remain perplexed and apprehensive, as they attempt to make sense of their environment. Grandiosed or paranoid ideas (see later discussion) may be entertained and quickly discarded, and the problem resolution is seen either in the form of recovery or development of a stable delusional system. Delusional mood may be diagnosed retrospectively, following the emergence of a sudden delusional idea or perception. Sometimes, however, the term is used loosely by practitioners, who may attribute little diagnostic importance or specificity to its presence.

Individuals may present with the problem of a persistent delusion and very few other, associated problems. Behaviour does not appear 'odd' or bizarre, and, whilst on occasions, the delusion may be accompanied by perceptual problems—notably visual or auditory hallucinations—these are neither distressing nor prominent for the individual and his or her daily performance. When present in this, almost isolated form, the label of *delusional disorder* may be assigned to differentiate between this and more complex problem experience. You may observe that an individual's delusions tend to follow one or more distinct themes of content. *Somatic type* delusions may be exteriorized by a belief that certain parts of the body are malfunctioning, harbouring a parasite or emitting a foul smell. Subjects may believe that insects inhabit their skin or have burrowed beneath it, causing an infestation, or perhaps that organs, or body parts, have become distorted in size, shape or appearance. All available evidence refutes the individual's beliefs, but he or she will frequently present to somatically orientated health care facilities with his apparent problems.

Jealousy may similarly assume a delusional theme, with the subject certain that his or her partner is unfaithful and yet there being no just cause for this belief. The subject may prevent the partner from leaving the house alone, may initiate a surveillance upon the individual's every move and collect 'evidence'—in the form of creased clothing or use of a new perfume—to support this belief. The subject may actually confront the partner with the supposed infidelity, as, indeed, he or she may accuse a 'lover' of these activities, and violence may ensue.

The belief that one possesses a great, and, hitherto, unrecognized skill, talent or knowledge, for which there is no apparent basis or evidence, is characteristic of the *grandiose type* of delusion. Beliefs that one has a special relationship with a well-known personality—a film star, politician, footballer and so on—whilst less common, similarly occur and where this is exhibited, the well-known personality is often accused of being an imposter, and not the 'real' individual at all. Where grandiose delusions have a religious content, subjects may assume elevated, it not leading, positions within cult movements.

In *erotomanic-type* delusions, individuals believe themselves romantically and spiritually united with someone—often a public figure, sometimes a complete and utter stranger—whom they will avidly pursue, whether by telephone, letter, via sending gifts and cards, or by following the individual in daily life or through the person's publicity. The 'erotic' connotation of the descriptor would suggest a sexual desire as the basis of the fantasy relationship, but this may not be so, the beliefs and desires being 'pure and unsullied', idealistic and loving rather than lusting in nature. Sometimes, people experiencing this delusional theme may come to the notice of the police because of the harassment, stalking or attempts to 'rescue' their loved one from some imagined threatening individual or situation. Often, however, the subject maintains a secrecy around their beliefs and desires and is unwilling to discuss or share them with anyone, even their closest relatives or peers.

The *persecutory theme* is one of the most commonly encountered, and may be simple or complex, and single, or multiple and intertwined, delusional ideas. Most revolve around an injustice of some sort—the individual is being cheated, mistreated, excluded from events or being drugged or poisoned—and the subject feels 'hard-done-by', often angry and sometimes is overtly violent towards the believed perpetrators of his problem. On occasions, the subject may persistently attempt to gain legal redress for the imagined injustices—*querulous paranoia*—and initiate proceedings via the courts, repeatedly and determinedly using all channels and avenues available to him.

The above themes—somatic, jealous, grandiose, erotomanic and persecutory—may be viewed as embellishments, expansions and explanations of a primary delusional idea or perception and hence may be referred to as *secondary delusions*. They may feature in association with other characteristic problems within a variety of discrete diagnostic 'psychotic' categories utilized by medical colleagues including schizophrenia, bipolar affective disorders, psychoactive substance use and misuse, and organically precipitated problems.

Delusions of control—passivity—may be seen when the individuals believe that their thoughts, feelings, actions or will are being determined, influenced or controlled by an external or alien power. When related to movement, it may be referred to as *motor passivity* or *made acts*, to sensation as *somatic passivity* or *made sensations*, and to emotions as *emotional passivity* or *made emotions*. Individuals believe themselves to be the passive recipient of some external influence and in essence, have an experience that simultaneously acquires a delusional interpretation or explanation. Passivity phenomena are characteristic of the multiple problems categorized as 'schizophrenia'.

Delusions of reference are characterized by the subject's belief that events, objects, overheard conversation and similar mundane occurrences not in reality relating to the individual, have great personal significance, are self-referential, and may have been deliberately arranged to influence or affect him or her personally. Any event may be misconstrued by the individual and ascribed as an important indicator of his or her beliefs regarding the situation. The specific manner in which a pint of beer is pulled, the method used to fold a table cloth, or the particular direction in which a shopper fills his trolley may all be highly significant to the individual experiencing this problem. *Ideas of reference* is the term applied to a similar phenomenon but of lesser intensity and therefore not reaching delusional proportions. These may be exteriorized by the mentally healthy individual as well as many individuals experiencing a deviation in mental health status.

Problems associated with the *form of thought*, or *formal thought disorders*, are those that relate to the *process* of thinking and the consequent expression of those thoughts. They include the difficulties associated with conceptual or abstract thinking, particularly experienced by those individuals diagnosed as suffering from schizophrenia and organic impairment, and, whilst several authorities have described the various problems associated with form of thought, differing terminology has been utilized in describing those problems.

Bleuler (1950), for example, identified a distinct lack of connection between the individual's ideas, and termed this *loosening of association*. As a result of this loosening, Bleuler believed that the subject's use of concepts becomes imprecise and fluctuates, and he identified three Freud-orientated factors which he believed contributed to the problem. The first he termed *condensation*, describing the merger of two or more associated ideas to form a false concept; the second he related as *displacement*, where a correct idea was replaced by an incorrect, but associated one; the third he named *misuse of symbols*, and this described the concreteness of interpretation of a symbol, rather than its abstract, more 'symbolic' meaning.

Cameron (1938) similarly noted this lack of connection of ideas, and termed it *asyndesis*, and, in addition, the imprecise, idiomatic and shifting conceptual expression, which he labelled as *metonyms*. He described the subject's confusion by other themes when attempting to consider one subject, and called this *interpretation of thoughts*, and the lack of organized thinking, the inability to set parameters to a topic or to differentiate between central themes and peripheral, unimportant, details as *overinclusivity*.

Schneider (1959) considered that healthy thinking exhibited characteristics of *constancy*, *organization* and *continuity* and that, in 'formal thought disorder', these were disrupted to produce *transitory*, *drivelling*—the mixing of the elements of a complex thought—and *desultory* thoughts. He similarly identified problems of *fusion*, *omission*, *derailment* and *substitution* as occurring. He regarded fusion as the enmeshing and weaving together of separate thoughts in a confusing manner; omission refers to the exclusion of major parts of a thought; derailment is the term used to describe the individual's penchant of moving from one train of thought to another, without logical connection; substitution was the term used to describe the replacement of one thought by another, unconnected, one.

Certainly the term '*knight's move thinking*', which illustrates the peculiar 'angled' thought pattern demonstrated by the individual experiencing the multiplicity of problems categorized as schizophrenia (as illustrated by the 'L' shaped movement of the knight piece on a chess board) would approximate to both Schneider's terms of derailment and substitution. In addition, problems of over inclusivity and concrete thinking are commonly encountered within the individual's exteriorization of his mechanism or form of thinking.

Further discussion on problems associated with derailment, incoherence and poverty of content are undertaken within the final section of this chapter and relate more easily to language.

Problems associated with *thought possession* are relatively easy and quickly related. In 'normal, healthy' individuals, their thoughts are their own, and remain inside their head unless they choose to verbalize and hence share them with others. Whilst they may be persuaded, or manipulated, to think in a particular way, individuals are in ultimate control of that thinking, which occurs in response or reaction to their environment and experiences. Individuals may demonstrate problems within aspects of the above, for, as an example, they may believe their thoughts to be foreign or alien to themselves and that they have been placed there by others—*thought insertion*. Similarly, individuals may experience, what they believe to be, a sudden removal of thoughts by an outside individual, agency or authority—*thought withdrawal*—or that one's own thoughts are available to others, that they are being *broadcasted* and that others speak with those thoughts.

The above are commonly verbalized by individuals who are diagnosed as 'schizophrenic' and, whilst not delusions but experiences, may acquire embellishment and stability via additional delusional ideation.

Problems related to the *stream of thought* are, again, frequently exteriorized. We have already mentioned *thought blocking* as a common experience accompanying anxiety but for some individuals there is a sudden cessation of the train of thought, which leaves a vacant expanse within the cognitive function without evidence of anxiety. The subject finds that when his or her thoughts resume, they follow a totally unrelated train and will continue in that new vein unperturbed. The anxious individual will frantically search their mind for the lost thread and desperately try to remember what he or she was thinking or verbalizing, not so with the person whose mental health status is significantly altered. *Perseveration* is similarly indicative of a major mental health disruption, as a thought—it may also be a word or phrase—is repeated persistently, long after it has become irrelevant. Both thought blocking and perseveration may be exhibited by the individual categorized as schizophrenic, and thought perseveration may also be a problem for the individual experiencing temporal lobe epilepsy.

The speed of the stream of thought may similarly create difficulties for both the individual and others. We previously mentioned the minimal levels of acceleration and retardation which the mentally healthy individual may experience on occasions. However, the degree of the problems that may be experienced by the individual may be prolonged, extensive and create severe disruption to life and living. *Retardation of thought* is a common problem for those who are intensely depressed, and may form part of an overall psychomotor retardation, with poor concentration, attention, memory and motor activity reduction. *Pressure of thought* describes an increased speed of flow of thoughts and ideas through the individual's mind, whilst *flight of ideas* relates to a more accelerated thought pattern, in which ideas are linked or associated and continue to flow without respite. Both pressure of thought and flight of ideas are associated with the generalized psychomotor acceleration and increased rate of activities and functions indicative of elevated mood problems. They are, therefore, a problem in situations where mood and affect is aberrant—that is in those using psychoactive substances, for example, hallucinogens, phencyclidine, or similar preparations, those experiencing organic impairment and deterioration, of various aetiological factors, and those experiencing a primary mood disturbance, often categorized as 'affective' or 'bipolar disorder', of elevated or mixed mood.

Circumstantiality may also serve to slow down or retard thought processes and this occurs when trivial details are persistently included within thinking processes. The individual then has so many items to consider within any reflective period or decision-making process that a conclusion is well nigh impossible to achieve. The normal speed of thought may similarly be reduced if other, recurring, and intrusive thoughts persistently interrupt thinking. We have previously mentioned obsessions, that is, those repetitive thoughts—or perhaps actions—which one feels compelled to resist and yet is unable to do so successfully. When excessive, the individual may experience a life that is organized around such obsessional thoughts and their overt responses—compulsive, ritualistic activities. However, there are many examples of recurring, intrusive thoughts—perhaps relating to hopelessness, suicide, or a preoccupation with having been assigned the wrong gender role by society. Individuals may find themselves returning time and time again, and often unwillingly or without deliberate intention to a recurring often distressing theme, thus inhibiting thought processes related to daily living.

Judgement may be impaired within the cognitive functioning of those whose mental health is giving rise to concern. The ability to collate all available information, to weigh it, piece by piece and then make decisions in the light of projected value, anticipated outcomes and rationale within overall goals, may be disturbed within any state of intoxication, for example, and therefore there may be a problem in excessive utilization of alcohol, cannabis, opioids, inhalants and other psychoactive substances. Similarly, because of elevated mood and accelerated thought processes, individuals experiencing hyperactive functioning, those diagnosed as 'mood disorders—manic/mixed', and those whose cognitive abilities are deteriorating due to organic impairment from a variety of causes, may exhibit such uncertain judgement. Certainly any individual who demonstrates impulsive, antisocial or extremely dependent behaviour will exteriorize problems associated with judgement and decision-making, as will anyone who, for whatever reason, finds attention and concentration limited or easily disrupted.

Problems of thought and thinking may create significant disruption in the individual's life and total functioning and represent a considerable challenge to carers.

MEMORY

INTRODUCTION

'Memory is the diary we all carry around with us'.
Oscar Wilde, 1969

This observation, made by Miss Letitia Prism to her student, Cecily, in Oscar Wilde's comedy of manners *The Importance of Being Earnest*, could not be more succinct or accurate, and hence provides an effective analogy for use here.

The diary that many individuals rely on, and carry around in a handbag or pocket, has two distinct functions. It provides a record, and hence a reminder, of what an individual has spent time doing, when and where. In addition, however, it enables the individual to plan, predict and anticipate the future thereby assisting in the organization of current and continuing activities.

Memory is very similar in action, for where the diary is a written record of previous events and occurrences accessible via visual scanning, the memory provides a store of past learning, related to the experiences of life and living, that is able to be accessed in various formats, in a variety of different ways, for use in current activities. The value of memory is not appreciated by the individual until it does not provide the service that has come to be expected. Most people have 'forgotten' something, somewhere, sometime—that is, have failed to recall a name, an important date, the time of a meeting, and the like. Many have experienced 'losing' a piece of information—a word, perhaps, which elicits the exact meaning wished to be conveyed—and having to enter into a long drawn out explanation of material, associated with the 'lost' item, to compensate. Behaviours, learned in the past, are often automatically evoked by the adult who, if required to explain how an action is to be achieved, may now be unable to 'remember' exactly what processes are performed and in which order they are carried out. The experi-

enced driver trying to teach a novice is a prime example of this, driving having become so integral to the behaviour evoked by opening a car door and sitting in the driver's seat, that the individual no longer has to think about the series of activities or manoeuvres required. When one considers the traumas often associated with learning a complex set of inter-related movements for the first time, such as is involved in driving, it has to be a relief to realize that such activities do become an integral aspect of functioning. If one had to learn to dress and tie shoe laces every morning, no one would ever get out of the house! It is irritating enough to forget one item of vocabulary in a day, but imagine being unable to recall something done only a few minutes ago— not just once, but as a common regular occurrence of everyday life.

SURGICAL SEQUELAE—A CASE HISTORY

In 1953, a young man was referred to a hospital in Hartford, Connecticut, USA, for advice and assistance from the neurosurgeon, William Scoville. The young man, known to the world as HM, was, at that time, 27 years old and had, from the age of 16, suffered severe epileptic seizures, with terrible frequency. Neurological examination depicted the temporal lobe as the focus of the fits and both hemispheres appeared equally affected. Medication had failed to effect any relief and therefore surgical intervention, in a manner never previously attempted, was deemed appropriate. The surgeon removed parts of both temporal lobes, including the hippocampus and amygdala. Miraculously the seizures ceased, and the team were, of course, delighted, until, within a few hours of surgery, it became obvious that HM was experiencing difficulties in a different area of function. He was unable to recognize care staff, or even find his way back to his room in the hospital. It was soon discovered that HM was unable to remember any new fact or experience.

HM had good recall for the early part of his life

and for those elements learned during that time, so, for example, his linguistic abilities, and psychomotor skills of walking, dressing and eating remained intact. His level of intellect was unimpaired and, using standard intelligence tests, his IQ was, in fact, a little higher following surgery than preoperatively. However, HM lived entirely in the present, being able to recall objects, people or experiences only whilst they remain in his short-term memory. Brenda Milner, of the Neurological Institute of Montreal, who had known the individual for over 25 years, presented as a stranger every time they met. She reported (Milner, 1972) that 10 months after the operation, HM and his family moved to a new house not far away from their previous residence. A year later, HM was still unable to provide his new address to questioners and proved unable to go home alone, for he continually returned to his old address. Milner described his ability to repeat the same jigsaw puzzles, day after day, without showing any evidence of the practice effect, and to read repeatedly the same magazines without any evidence of familiarity with, or recognition of, their contents. An individual who chatted with HM and then left the room for a few minutes, returned as a stranger, for HM had no recollection of either the individual or the previous discussions held.

HM and his family moved to Boston in the late 1970s, and were supported by Massachusetts General Hospital. Material and events stored within his memory up to a period of three years before the operation were available to him. That stored within the year or two preceding surgery had suffered some impairment and he could remember little since surgery. As a result of the unforeseen sequelae, the procedure was never performed again, for whilst the well-meaning surgeon achieved his objectives in preventing further epileptic seizures, it was at a devastating cost to the individual and his family.

HM, sadly, became one of the best-known amnesiacs in the world, but from his experience, much was able to be deduced:

1 The hippocampus and the medial part of the temporal lobe play a role in the processes inherent in memory consolidation, that is, the physical and psychological changes that occur as the brain organizes material which may become part of permanent memory.

2 That the part played by these structures appears to be related to making memories, rather than their storage (his memory for up to three years pre-operation was intact) or recall.

3 That memory may continue to be consolidated for some considerable time after learning has taken place.

ACCIDENTAL EVIDENCE—A SECOND CASE STUDY

NA presents another saddening lesson in the search for the biological basis of memory, this time via injury (Squire, 1984). He was on army service in the Azores, in 1960, when during some friendly horseplay in the barracks with a room mate, a fencing foil penetrated his brain, via his left nostril. His recollections after the accident are that he really had no control over immediate activities or himself—'I really became someone outside of my body ... I didn't really care too much about it because I didn't think it was me'. NA recalls the details of the actual accident with clarity. He did not experience pain, but a sensation of 'shock' felt by his brain. He tried to remove the foil but found it to be stuck hard, so he persuaded his companion to try. The foil was withdrawn with relative ease, again with only a sensation of a shock felt by his brain. After a few seconds, a thick clear substance began to run from his nose, which would not stop flowing.

NA did eventually collapse after the accident but not for some minutes and not until after he had walked down some stairs. He spent months in hospital, often seeming to watch events that were happening to him from outside of himself, sometimes feeling that these things might be happening to him and on other occasions certain that they were. For much of this period he was unsure of who these events were happening to.

After the accident, NA went to live with his

mother, and, about a year following the accident, suddenly was able to pull the fragments of his identity together, to become a 'whole person', and yet remained amnesic. Computerized axia tomography (CAT scan) enabled Squire to identify the area damaged by the fencing foil. The area of damage proved to be that of the dorsal medial nucleus of the thalamus, that area of the limbic system that lies quite close to the hippocampus and amygdala. The damage was on the left-hand side of the brain structures, an element of importance when identifying the exact nature of memory loss experienced.

According to Squire, the fact that pre-1960 memory was intact whilst post-1960 memory demonstrated impairment, would indicate a 'difficulty in laying down new memories', that is, a disruption of the learning process itself rather than the retrieval process. This assertion is strongly contested by other scientists who believe the memory store to be the area damaged. Squire connects all three phases—learning, storage and recall—but asserts that the storage of memory probably functions in the larger, overlying areas of the brain, within the cortex. The thalamus, he believes, is part of the system that establishes and forms memories and that elaborates them over time.

The damage to NA's brain was on the left-hand side of the organ, where it is known that centres concerned with speech and language are situated. NA's visual memory was existing, as Squire demonstrated via a test utilizing cards with black and white line drawings upon them. All of the drawings were of everyday objects, and half an hour after being shown them, NA could recall that he had been shown the cards and that one was of a fork. He was unable to recall the reason for being shown the cards, but could at least remember being shown them. A second test, comprising of written words on cards, was followed 30 minutes later by Squire's posing a question as to whether NA remembered *either* of the tests. NA recalled the cards with drawings upon them, but had no recollection of the word-card test.

The inference would seem to be that there is a system for learning verbal material and a separate one for learning visual material.

DRINKING TO FORGET

Amnesia is also seen to occur in Korsakoff's syndrome, a result of vitamin B (thiamine) deficiency which is progressive in nature and a relatively common sequel to chronic alcohol misuse. Treatment, if the problem is discovered early enough, is with extensive doses of the deficient vitamin.

The problems associated with memory in Korsakoff's syndrome are not only related to forming new memories, but in addition, to pre-damage events. There are problems associated with thinking and problem solving, shown in tests requiring differing strategies to be utilized, to solve a puzzle. For example, a test may be conducted with a number of cards, each of which depicts a different geometrical shape. Given no information, the subject will pick up cards, one at a time, until he is told that one in particular is 'the right card' for example, the circle-card. In subsequent tests the individual selects that same card and is told that he is correct on each occasion. When on the next trial, the experimenter changes the solution to a different card, say a card depicting a square, the subject chooses the circle-card and is told he is incorrect. Instead of trying a different geometrical design, the individual experiencing the Korsakoff-related amnesia will continue to select the circle-bearing card and will do so despite being told on each occasion that this is the 'wrong card'. He will persevere with the strategy long after it has proved inadequate or incorrect in the problem-solving experience. The 'normal' subject—and indeed HM and NA—would try different cards until they selected the right card.

Proactive inhibition is the term used to describe the interference of old learning on new learning related to the same topic. For example, when learning successive groups of words all belonging to one category—say the names of birds—the content of earlier lists learned interferes with those learned later. The phenomenon disappears when later word groups to be learned relate to a different category, for example, types of dogs. The individual experiencing amnesia associated with Korsakoff's syndrome, demonstrates no improvement when categories are changed, continuing to display proactive inhibition.

The damage of Korsakoff's syndrome includes the same thalamic nucleus that NA damaged in his fencing accident, but, in addition, there is neuronal loss in both the cerebral cortex, particularly the frontal lobe, and in the cerebellum. The question to ask would seem to be 'Is the long-term-memory deficit of Korsakoff's syndrome due to cortical loss, or does cognitive dysfunction—problem solving and concept formation difficulties—prevent reconstruction of past memories?'

Studies by Moscovitch (1981) of individuals who do not demonstrate amnesia and yet who have sustained trauma to the frontal lobe, reveal that such people have similar problem-solving difficulties as those experiencing Korsakoff's syndrome. The answer to the question becomes more obscure at this point, because further questions related to the different degrees of damage that have been sustained, and exactly where such damage lies, may be significant. Plus, of course, damage may have been incurred in those alcohol-related Korsakoff's syndrome sufferers, through head traumas, that have not been accounted for.

MEMORY AND LEARNING

To conclude the valuable information gained from the unfortunate experiences of HM and NA, an identification of the continuing abilities of such individuals to learn is available. Whilst cognizant of the fact the individual would not remember the new learning, Cohen and Squire (1981) taught a group of amnesic individuals the skill of mirror reading. It took three days for the individuals to become adept at the task—about the same time as 'normal' subjects—though of course, they could not remember ever having worked on the skill before, and none could later remember the words he or she had read. The group retained a high level of skill for the entire period of testing, some three months. Indeed, Cohen (1981) found HM capable of learning to solve puzzles and repeat the successful solution, though he had no recall of working on the puzzle in the past and appeared not to know what was expected of him.

Cohen and Squire suggested that problems such as those experienced by HM were not related to retrieval of memory as many had suggested, but indicated a failure to store as much information as others do, to facilitate problem solving (Cohen and Squire, 1980). In the light of this, they advanced the theory that the brain handles and stores two kinds of information in different ways. *Procedural knowledge* is that related to how to do something, which probably developed early in the evolutionary period, and, at a later juncture, there will be an exploration of evidence which would support the existence of such a memory. However, in addition to procedural knowledge, they suggested the existence of an 'explicit, accessible record of individual previous experiences, a sense of familiarity about those experiences', which they termed *declarative knowledge*. It is this latter type of knowledge that they believe to be processed in the temporal region and parts of the thalamus, and which requires a remodelling and adjustment of neural circuitry in those areas, differing from that of procedural knowledge, in which only stuctures directly involved in the procedure being learned seem to be changed biochemically or biophysically.

It is of interest to note that, in relation to learning, the rates of forgetting shown by HM, NA and individuals experiencing Korsakoff's syndrome, show some differences. Where the primary injury site was the medial dorsal thalamic nucleus, as in the case of NA, and those with Korsakoff's syndrome, the individuals 'forgot' at a normal rate, as compared to that of a control group of 'normal' people. HM—and individuals receiving bilateral electroplexy by the way—demonstrated an abnormally rapid rate of forgetting. It would appear, therefore, that the hippocampus, amygdala and related structures are necessary in memory consolidation, that is, the transfer of declarative material to long-term memory. The thalamus, on the other hand, may be necessary to perform the initial coding of certain kinds of declarative information and material.

In the introduction to the chapter, we asked you to imagine being unable to recall something done only a few minutes before, on a consistent, everyday basis. Perhaps the words of NA may assist:

There are, I guess, many missing pieces but I don't remember that I miss them. I don't remember what it is I'm missing, so I don't pay much attention to it.

LEARNING AND THE BRAIN

A combination of the work of anatomists, psychologists and neuroscientists has, over the past century, provided a wealth of knowledge in relation to the effects of learning upon the brain.

The brain of a new-born baby is approximately a quarter of the size of that of the adult. At six months the brain has assumed almost half the size of that of the adult and at the age of two years, 75% of the final dimensions. The number, size, shape and function of neurons is decreed at conception via genetic inheritance and no new brain cells are created after birth. The increase in the size of the brain of the developing infant is accounted for in part by the increasing size of the neurons, their increasing number of connections via axon growth and dendrite branching, new glial cells and myelin sheath growth. However, the remainder of this growth would seem to be related to the interaction between the individual's genetic plan and the environment.

Animal experiments, in the main, have provided evidence that denial or reduction in sensory input will inhibit development. Woolsey and Wann (1976) found that each of a mouse's whiskers relays sensory data, via two synaptic relays, to a group of cells—a barrel—within the cerebral cortex. Removal of one row of whiskers, shortly after birth, shows a failure of the related cortical barrels to develop, with cells shrinking and losing their function. In addition, however, the barrels of adjoining rows of whiskers will be larger than normal, showing a compensatory mechanism in operation, to make up for the deficit experienced. This compensation is termed *plasticity*. Hubel and Wiesel (1977) demonstrated similar results in a kitten. One of the kitten's eyes

was covered shortly after birth and within a few months, the kitten was unable to see through that eye. The 'defect' was not in the eye or its structure, but due to a failure of the visual cortex to develop. Conversely, Rosenzweig (1984) showed that rats raised in an 'enriched environment' developed more extensive cerebral cortices than those 'deprived' and raised in isolation. A large cage, plenty of company, and objects to play with resulted in an improved learning ability within maze experiments. The 'pampered' rats could run faster and more reliably than their lonely rat counterparts, their learning in relation to the maze being swifter and more accurate. The cortical neurons evinced more spines in the enriched rats, these spines acting as extra receivers of impulses at synaptic relays (Globus *et al*, 1973). The size of these synaptic contacts was seen to be 50% larger than those of the deprived rat (Mollgaard *et al.*, 1971) and far more frequent in number (Greenough *et al.*, 1978).

The cortex of humans may be seen to be similarly affected. Freeman and Thibos (1973) found abnormal cortical development in the brains of adults who had an astigmatism at birth, which had gone untreated. An astigmatism is a refractive error, where horizontal and vertical curvatures of the cornea of the eye are uneven, producing differences in focusing of light rays. Whilst some may fall upon the retina, others may fall short and others may be carried beyond the retina, causing blurring of the image. Freeman and Thibos (1973) demonstrated a reduced cortical response from the area of the cortex related to the dimension that had always been blurred. Dennis (1960) demonstrated the effects of severe sensory deprivation in his study of infants in Iranian orphanages. Babies were handled, in essence, only once a day, for bathing, otherwise human contact was negligible. Feeding was achieved via bottles propped upon pillows and any physical attention required was performed in the cot, where babies lay all day. To prevent draughts, the cot sides were covered hence reducing potential stimuli even further. The study showed that many of these orphans were unable to sit up, unaided, at the age of 21 months, something usually achieved by nine months, and that less than 15% could walk at three years of age, where most children are walking well before the age of two years. The normal stimulation of the brain was absent and therefore infants failed to develop and learn the skills associated with normal milestones. The cortex failed to develop.

Curtiss (1977), a psycholinguist, described the sad account of Genie, a 13-year-old girl who came to the attention of Californian welfare authorities in 1970. Genie's father was severely mentally ill and her mother, almost blind. From the age of 20 months, Genie had been confined solely to one room, kept naked and tethered to a commode chair, by a harness designed by her father. Fed only baby food and milk throughout her short lifetime, the girl weighed 26.8 kilograms when discovered, and did not know how to chew food. She was unable to recognize words or speak—father had forbidden mother to talk to her throughout her incarceration—had no control over bowels and bladder, and was unable to straighten her arms or legs, having only experienced free movement of her hands and feet. Father committed suicide soon after the discovery of Genie, but mother asserted that Genie had been a normal, healthy baby. Father had apparently hated children, and had placed a previous baby, aged two months, in the garage because it cried. That baby died of pneumonia.

During the following six years, Genie was provided with a great deal of general and expert assistance. She made great advances in some areas—she learned to use tools, to draw and had some ability to orientate herself and find her way around, for example, in a supermarket. In simpler instances, Genie could relate cause and effect and yet her linguistic skills remained at a level similar to a two-year-old child. In 1977, her IQ, on non-verbal tests showed a low—normal score of 74 and EEG patterns indicated that Genie was utilizing the right hemisphere of her brain for both language and non-language functions. Normally the specialist skills relating to language would be sited in the left hemisphere.

Curtiss asserts that language acquisition provokes or facilitates the hemispheric specialization pattern that is normally seen and that failure to acquire language may engender cortical degeneration and atrophy of those areas relating to linguistic functions.

WHAT HAPPENS WHEN AN ORGANISM LEARNS?

Neuroscientists have investigated the simple learning that occurs in animals at an unconscious level—that is, that learning which occurs without the organism's awareness of a change in behaviour.

Habituation is said to occur when a stimulus, which initially provoked a response, is presented so frequently that the organism fails to respond to it any more. The organism becomes accustomed to the stimulus and its meaning to the environment and the organism's own survival, and simply ceases to react to its presence. Kandel and Schwartz (1982) studied a marine snail, *Aplysia californica*, and demonstrated that changes at a cellular level accompany habituation. *Aplysia* demonstrates a reflex action implicit in survival. It has a gill-withdrawal ability, which facilitates retraction of the gill and hence its protection in rough waters or when debris may cause damage. In quiet water, the gill is extended to allow the *Aplysia* to breathe. When conditions become adverse, retraction occurs, being controlled by one ganglion, containing six motor and 24 sensory neurons. Connections between the two are provided both directly, via excitatory synapses, and indirectly, via interneurons. Repeated stimulation in the laboratory, provoked initially a less-vigorous withdrawal and after 10 stimulations, no withdrawal was elicited at all. Less neurotransmitter substance was released by sensory neurons across the synapse to motor neurons, which, because they were in receipt of a lower level of activation, performed less intensely. A short-term habituation results because of decrease in excitation at the synapses of the existing neural pathway. The researchers discovered that after no further experimentation, the gill-withdrawal reflex returned to its usual vigorous activity within a few hours. This return is due to a change in the amount of transmitter substance released at the same synaptic junction. It is brought about by the release of another chemical transmitter substance, by other sensory fibres in response to stimulation of another part of the organism. This is termed *sensitization*, and reflects a second type of simple learning, in essence, a reversal of habituation. The animal learns to respond vigorously to a previously neutral stimulus.

The study has parallels in the behaviour of the newborn human infant who demonstrates a capability for habituation. A sensing device attached to the soother of a four-hour-old baby detected a cessation of sucking at the onset of a tone, loud enough for the infant to hear. After a few seconds—presumably of listening to the tone—sucking was recommenced, and it was only when a tone different from the first was played that the infant stopped sucking again to listen. The first tone had been habituated (Bronshtein and Petrova, 1967).

Pavlov's (1927) experiments with dogs and classical conditioning are well recorded and frequently cited. In Pavlov's experiments, a stimulus which naturally produces a particular reaction, is paired a number of times with another stimulus. The neutral stimulus becomes representative of, and elicits the same reaction as, the primary stimulus. To achieve conditioning, the two stimuli must be presented close together.

Alkon (1983) has demonstrated neural changes occurring in response to conditioning in another genus of marine snail, *Hermissenda crassicornis*. This particular snail naturally feeds in well-lit water near the surface of the sea and therefore instinctively moves towards light. Like *Aplysia*, it dislikes turbulence, as it tends to injure the delicate appendages of the organism, and therefore, in response to rough water, will contract its foot, reducing the speed of its movement towards light. Alkon and his colleagues paired turbulence with a preceding light, conditioning the snails to associate light with the onset of turbulence. The snails slowed their rate of movement towards light, their feet contracting when they saw light, and this response was maintained for several weeks. The researchers found the response had been mediated on three different levels.

Anatomically speaking, light generates impulses in two types of photoreceptors in the snail's eyes, which are in turn transmitted to interneurons, motor neurons and muscles. Water turbulence is detected via hair-like structures in, what are the equivalent of, the snail's ears. Impulses are similarly transmitted along an inter-neuron–motor neuron–muscle pathway, but some axons have synapses with the light sensitive, receptor axons, allowing the two systems to interact.

Of the photoreceptor cells in the eye, one is excitatory and one inhibitory. When the latter is activated, impulses along the neural path, which drive muscle contractions allowing movement towards light, are inhibited. The hair cells usually maintain these inhibitory receptors in a state of rest and during turbulence, that resting state is increased. When turbulence ceases—after the light has flashed—the hair cells release their effect on the inhibitory photoreceptor, allowing it to become excited, impulses to pass, and dampening down of the movement towards light. Following conditioning, the light alone will cause these inhibitory photoreceptor cells to exert their role.

In addition to the above, Alkon noted *biophysical* changes in the cell membrane. To recap on the physiology, you may recall that:

A neuron at rest is polarized, the inside of the cell being negative in respect to the outside environment. The potassium concentration is higher inside the cell than outside it. The concentration of sodium is higher outside than inside the cell

Na	K		Na	K	
		Na		Na	

K	Na	K		K	
	K			K	Na	K

	Na				
Na			Na		Na
	K			K	

Owing to the effects of a chemical transmitter or in response to a sensory stimulus, channels in the cell membrane open, allowing sodium (and calcium) ions to flood in, causing depolarization. Similarly potassium channels open, allowing potassium to move from an area of high concentration to an area of low concentration, outside of the cell membrane. When movement across the cell membrane is at an appropriate level, a wave of activity—the nerve impulse—is able to pass through the length of the axon.

When activity ceases, the reverse process occurs, and the cell membrane returns to a state of rest.

Before conditioning, the photoreceptor cell receives inhibitory messages from the hair cell and thus the photoreceptor cell is kept at rest and negatively charged by allowing potassium ions to pass out. When the light flashes, the photoreceptor becomes excited, and sodium ions, followed closely by calcium ions, pass into the cell. At this precise moment, the turbulence commences, prompting the hair cell to increase its inhibitory action on the photoreceptor cell, and upon cessation of the turbulence, the hair cell relaxes its influence. The photoreceptor cell assumes a more positive charge as further calcium channels open, allowing an increase in the concentration of calcium within the cell cytoplasm. Potassium channels close, preventing further loss of these ions, and the cell is depolarized. Passage of the impulse then inhibits the snail's movement towards the light. This excited state may last for days and within this time a flash of light alone will cause continuing cessation of movement.

Alkon (1983) demonstrated that the behaviour exhibited could persist for weeks, with the photoreceptor cell maintaining its excitability and inhibiting the muscle action which would move the snail towards the light. Levels of calcium had been seen to be elevated within the photoreceptor cell during training but these reduced to normal levels once training had been discontinued, and yet the learned response persisted. It had been noted that these previously high levels of calcium had activated enzymes that combine proteins and phosphate molecules. This *phosphorylation* was thought to both change the character of the protein and the ion channel specificity, which may directly reduce the outflow of potassium from the cell, and thus maintain the excited state. It seems, too, that once activated, these phosphorylating enzymes continue to function despite the return of calcium levels to normal.

Simple learning in lower-life organisms may be seen, therefore, to create changes in anatomical, biophysical and biochemical neural mechanisms, and remembering that human beings *evolved* to their current abilities, it is sensible to assume that such simple cellular learning has been preserved, even though the complex and complicated nervous system of vertebrates may have additional mechanisms and systems for memory storage.

Certainly Kandel and Schwartz (1982) point to the similarities between the signalling properties of the nerve cell of a snail, cat, monkey and human, stating that the kind of chemical substances used as transmitters and patterns of synaptic interactions closely resemble each other. They comment that '. . . one has reason from just the tradition of biology to feel that the basic processes like these are very likely to be similar in simple animals and complex ones'.

WHAT IS STORED AND WHERE?

Individuals who have sustained damage to the *cerebellum* report that they have lost the ability to move automatically and now have to consciously perform each step of a complex movement, for example, lifting a cup and actually stopping it at the right position before it 'hits' the mouth. McCormick *et al.* (1982) believe that a wide number of classically conditioned, learned responses may be stored in the cerebellum. Experiments with rabbits indicated that a memory trace, associated with eye-lid conditioning, developed in one particular area of the cerebellum called the deep cerebellar nuclei. Destruction of the region destroyed the memory trace and completely removed the conditioned response. With the area removed, the rabbit was unable to relearn the conditioned response, thus indicating the relative contribution of the cerbellum to the storage of memories of learned responses.

We have already mentioned the apparent role of the *hippocampus* in relation to memory, via the case study of HM's surgery and its sequelae. O'Keefe and Nadel (1978) in studies of the brains of rats, found some neurons within the hippocampus only respond when the animal is in a certain position within familiar territory. The rat may be moving about, and a specific cell be quiet until a particular location is reached, when the cell will fire vigorously. As the rat moves its position, the nerve cell activity ceases, only to re-fire when the rat returns to the precise position. O'Keefe and Nadel found that different cells scattered throughout the hippocampus fired in response to different regions of the rat's cage, thus prompting the researchers to suggest that the animals keep a mental map of their immediate environment 'in mind' in a sort of short-term memory facility. They believe that in simpler animals, the hippocampus may store information relating to environments previously encountered, helping the animal to plan continuing exploration of that environment. It has been demonstated that removal of the rat's hippocampus reduces the effectiveness of its ability to find its way around a maze, thus supporting the hypothesis.

Olton *et al.* (1980) found that, when foraging for food, 'normal' rats learned about their environment to the point where they would remember where they had already been and never retraced their steps to cover a path twice. However, when the hippocampus was removed the rat frequently retraced its path, apparently unable to remember where it had been before. It appears, therefore, that the hippocampus provides a short-term memory related to current activity.

Thompson *et al.* (1983) identified the role of the hippocampus in the conditioning of rabbits. With no hippocampus, conditioning was still possible, but with disruption of neuronal activity in the hippocampus, the rabbit was unable to learn a conditioned response. Thompson found that a slight delay between the presentation of conditioned and unconditioned stimuli provoked hippocampal neurons to commence firing activities as if the hippocampus was maintaining a state of readiness for the arrival of the unconditioned stimulus. Tasks of increasing complexity seemed to require increased neuronal activity within the hippocampus and evidence accumulates to demonstrate continuing firing long after stimulation has ceased. This *long-term potentiation* appears to evoke neuronal structural changes and hence may be indicative of learning (Swanson *et al.* 1982).

The *cortex* of the brain is the probable ultimate home of many memories but the actual way that these are spread out, or how this is achieved, is as yet unknown. It is possible that cerebral cortical cells have the ability to change the strength of their responses to incoming signals in a manner similar to that of the hippocampal cells, and that initial cortical activity is responsible for short-term conscious memory. This may then be transferred to the hippocampus for processes aimed at conversion to long-term storage and then returned to the cortex, where it results in permanent neuronal change, and long-term storage.

The role of transmitter substances has been implicated within learning and memory, particularly norepinephrine secreted by the adrenal medulla, at times of arousal. Whilst unable to cross the blood–brain barrier, norepinephrine is seen to consolidate memory formation. McGough (1982) demonstrated that animals given a small amount of the substance following the use of pain as a punishment showed a greater propensity and better memory for correct behaviour.

Increased protein synthesis is seen in animals during learning, as demonstrated by Rose *et al.* (1973) in their work with chicks. The imprinting behaviour exhibited by chicks as they become attached to, and follow, the first moving object they see—usually the mother—was shown to be associated with an increased production of protein in the chick's brain, within two hours of exposure to the stimulus being imprinted. It is suggested that the extra available protein may be transferred to the synapse to facilitate a temporary increase in its effectiveness and hence may provide the basis for learning.

Whilst researchers continue to uncover elements of the memory-learning processes, a great deal remains to be clarified to facilitate a complete understanding of the subject area.

PROBLEMS OF MEMORY

Most people forget something at some time, and there is usually a simple reason for this. On occasions, the individual has not attended effectively to the exposed stimulus and does not, therefore, absorb the data available. This inattention may be due to a variety of factors—disinterest or boredom, a lack of perceived relevance of information to self, excessive preoccupation with other data, or activities, are examples—but whatever the causation, the result is the same, for an individual may not expect to recall material which has not yet been learned and retained.

At times, too, an individual attempts to recall information which was only in temporary storage, long after it has disappeared. The telephone number which one expects to use on a single occasion only, would not be available within memory the following day, for example. Whether because of decay (Brown, 1964) or because new information disrupts or replaces previously stored data (Tulving and Madigan, 1970), the original memory has disappeared and is unavailable for recall. We have already mentioned retroactive inhibition, the process whereby new learning interferes with and influences previously learned material, which has not had time to consolidate and be transferred into permanent storage sites. This knowledge may infer that theories of disruption or replacement may provide a more reasonable hypothesis for the loss of transiently stored material than those of decay.

The process of forgetting material from remote memory storage may be due to similar processes, but, in addition, may be a problem associated with an ineffective retrieval process. It is noted, for example, that, utilizing computerized information retrieval systems, the 'correct' word or command—that is, a word already within the system—is needed to access the desired information. The computer is not capable of substituting a similar meaning word for the one entered; the operator must utilize the appropriate terminology. It may be that formal retrieval processes are used within the human brain in relation to memory recall and that some part of this process is disrupted.

Freud, of course, would have asserted that forgetting is 'motivated', and the means by which unacceptable, unpleasant or threatening scenarios or data is removed from conscious awareness. His original work, later embellished and expanded by Anna Freud, asserted that the defence mechanism of *repression* was the primary vehicle via which the elimination from consciousness was achieved and that under free association or hypnosis, recall was possible (Freud, 1986). However, Eysenck and Wilson (1973) declared there to be little experimental evidence available to support Freud's hypothesis.

You may be aware, from personal experience, of other factors which may influence recall abilities, for example, excessive tiredness and fatigue, the general malaise associated with colds and influenza, and the 'saturated solution' scenario, where your mind is so full of the events of the day, that you are just not able to give of your best. Any situation which has a detrimental effect on attention and concentration may affect recall abilities. Stress and anxiety may have quite opposite effects in that an individual experiencing longstanding and cumulative stressors may be so overwhelmed that he or she forgets a variety of aspects of life and living, and yet, given an 'acute' and threatening situation, the same individual may be able to recall the tiniest and most obscure detail of the event.

The case studies of HM and NA demonstrate that cerebral trauma, whether accidentally or surgically induced, may create memory problems, and, even a relatively 'innocuous' bump to the head, may evoke an amnesia that may persist for minutes or hours. Frequently an individual does not recall the incident that precipitated damage or bodily injury, for example, there may be no recollection of a road traffic accident or the few minutes preceding or following it. However, sometimes there may be a persistent and recurring memory or 'dream sequence', where the precise nature of the incident—the actual movement of impact, say—is re-lived, time and time again, as in *post-traumatic stress disorder*. Certainly where an individual exhibits memory disturbances that are accompanied by sensorimotor symptomatology—paraesthesias and/or hemiparesis—evidence of recent injury to the side of the head opposite to that showing the sensorimotor impairment should be excluded.

Previous examples of memory problems associated with temporal lobe damage have been provided, but any irritable focus of the cerebrum may evoke a disturbance. Temporal lobe seizures, for example, may disrupt memory for a period of minutes or hours. Where verbal memories show disturbance, the focal area of irritation is found within the left hemisphere, whilst graphic and verbal amnesia is due to right hemispheric dysfunction. Cerebral tumours within the temporal lobe may precipitate early cognitive deficits, as may cerebral abscesses and a subdural haematoma, the latter being more common in alcohol-dependent individuals (approximately 50%; Lishman, 1987) and the elderly, for obvious reasons of limitations or difficulties in mobility.

Cerebral hypoxia may similarly precipitate memory problems. Those associated with carbon monoxide poisoning, for example, may be accompanied by sensory disturbances—tingling and numbness—and be profound in nature. Vertebrobasilar circulatory disorders, whether caused by ischaemia, embolus, haemorrhage or infarct, may be abrupt in onset, last for some hours and then end as abruptly as they commenced. On occasions, there is a global loss of recent memory associated with feelings of bewilderment in an otherwise alert and responsible individual (transient global amnesia). For others, there is blurred, or double vision vertigo, dizziness, nausea and vomiting, and ataxia. Remaining symptomatology subside to a vast extent as the episode is resolved, but amnesia remains.

Individuals, recovering from the effects of Herpes simplex encephalitis, a viral disease affecting predominantly the medial temporal and orbital regions of the cortex, may demonstrate a residual amnesia and be associated with olfactory and gustatory hallucinations, and, similarly, those experiencing cerebral involvement due to syphilitic infection, may exteriorize problems associated with memory.

It has previously been noted that endocrine and metabolic problems may exteriorize as, or precipitate, deviations in mental health status and are significant, too, in relation to memory disturbances. Addison's disease (primary adrenal insufficiency), hypopituitarism, hypothyroidism, under or oversecretion of parathyroid glands and hypoglycaemia may all encompass problems associated with memory.

Within mental health care, one may hear several terms utilized to describe the particular 'shade' of memory problem experienced by the individual. One such term may be *psychogenic amnesia*, where there is an abrupt inability to recall personal details and information and yet no organic reason is elicited to explain the phenomenon. One such type of psychogenic amnesia has been identified in the example relating to the in-ability to remember the details surrounding a road traffic accident and on occasions, this amnesia may extend to the period of two days or so following the trauma. This is termed a *localized* (or *circumscribed*) *amnesia* and is characterized by this inability to recall the events occurring within a 'circumscribed' period of time. *Selective amnesia* is less common and is the failure to recall some—but not all—of the events of a circumscribed period. Utilizing the previous example of the road traffic accident, the victim may recall a passer-by assisting him from the car and, at some time within the episode, sitting at the side of the road, and yet nothing else of the event. *Generalized amnesia*, a total inability to recall any aspect of previous existence, and *continuous amnesia*, where amnesia extends from a specific event and includes present functioning, are more rarely seen. The psychogenic amnesias are associated with stress or an intolerable life event, for example in war situations and other life-threatening or psychosocially devastating experiences. It usually disappears abruptly, leaving the individual completely recovered.

Another, less common, absence of recall is again exhibited at times of great personal distress, and has been well documented in times of war and following natural disasters. *Psychogenic fugue* is the term used when an individual demonstrates a total lack of recall for his previous life, assumes a new identity and moves away from his home location, abruptly and unexpectedly. With the assumption of the new identity, the individual frequently assumes a new personality, which often tends to be more extroverted, disinhibited and socially gregarious than that hitherto displayed. The individual appears well integrated and competent within socially complex situations, and is therefore accepted by others as 'legitimate' and as presented. On occasions, the fugue state is less well developed and is incomplete. There may be little more than abrupt, purposeful travel which is of brief duration. Although a new identity may be taken, it may be less well systematized and patchy in development. In these situations, social contact may not be so extensive and may be avoided by the individual. Again, on occasions, psychogenic fugue may be associated with acts of violence, either related to person or property.

Such fugue states may last for hours, days or, occasionally, months. Recovery is usually abrupt and reoccurrences are rare; the problems which tend to be exteriorized are those related to the social implications of the abrupt disappearance and return, and because there is no recollection of events or experiences that took place during the fugue period. Differentiation needs to be made between such problems of a psychogenic nature, and those automatisms and fugues associated with typically temporal lobe epilepsy. Lishman (1987) makes the point that many experienced clinicians view all epileptic fugues as essentially psychogenic in nature, and asserts the inextricable link between organic and psychogenic factors. Despite this potential dispute between researchers regarding the aetiology of such experiences, the nurse's management of the individual, being tailor-made to the exteriorized and potential client needs, will differ due to the problems which may be concomitant in the experience of epilepsy *per se*.

Amnesia associated with Herpes simplex encephalitis, head injury, hypoxia and cerebral circulatory disorders has previously been mentioned in relation to the somatic aetiology of memory problems. In mental health care, such *amnestic syndrome* is relatively rare, but when demonstrated tends to be by those people exhibiting a chronic use of alcohol and the consequent thiamine deficiency. Recent memory shows impairment via the individual's inability to learn new material, and that which has been learned is quickly forgotten—termed *anterograde amnesia*. As a result of this the individual so affected demonstrates disorientation related to time, ordering of events and frequently place and person.

Retrograde amnesia may cover a period of months or years prior to the onset of the problem and may be patchy and incomplete. *Remote memory* related to learning beyond the retrograde gap is relatively unimpaired and therefore speaking, writing, calculation and other early learned skills remain intact. Some individuals lack the awareness or insight to appreciate the impairment of memory, whilst others will acknowledge it, but be unperturbed by it. The gaps in memory may be filled by *confabulation*, that is the recounting of 'imaginary' events, but this tends to

disappear with time. Individuals often demonstrate apathy, shallow affect and a distinct lack of initiative, though superficially they may appear gregarious and companionable. When related to alcohol utilization, the individual may be experiencing profound neurological deficits, for example, cerebellar ataxia, peripheral neuropathy and myopathy. Alcohol amnestic disorder is also referred to as *Korsakoff's syndrome*.

Memory impairment is commonly associated with any situation in which *delirium* is evident. Memory disturbance is related to recent events, and is associated with disorientation to time and place, though in relation to person, it is rare. Thinking is often disorganized and speech irrelevant, rambling and incoherent. Psychomotor activity may be severely aberrant, with restlessness and hyperactivity at one end of a continuum, and sluggishness and stupor at the other. Rapid fluctuations from one extreme to the other are common, and the individual may grope or strike out at non-existent objects. Misinterpretations, illusions and hallucinations are common, and frequently via the visual mode, although any sense may be involved. The sleep–wake cycle may be severely disturbed, with drowsiness, which may assume semicoma level, or hypervigilance and insomnia. Emotional disturbances may be exhibited, with lability, or a constant emotional tone displayed throughout. Physiologically, various autonomic symptoms—tachycardia, palpitations, elevated blood pressure, dilated pupils, etc.—are common. Psychoactive substance utilization may precipitate such problems, for example, it may be seen 24 hours after the use of amphetamines, cocaine, phencyclidine and similar-acting preparations. It is similarly evident during withdrawal from alcohol, sedative, hypnotic and anxiolytic preparations, and in the intoxication phase associated with opioid, sedative, anxiolytic and hypnotic substances.

Memory impairment associated with dementia is accompanied by problems of abstract thinking, impaired judgement and other higher cognitive deficits, plus changes within the personality characteristics demonstrated. The problems of memory may be moderate and predominantly relate to recent events, or be severe, showing marked anterograde and retrograde amnesia.

Thinking difficulties, of an abstract nature, are exhibited via difficulty in managing novel tasks and processing new or complex information. Problems associated with judgement are particularly evident where frontal lobe damage is a feature of the cerebral deterioration. Inappropriate, rude and coarse speech and behaviour may be exteriorized, with impulsive, reckless or antisocial activities—for example, sexual overtures to strangers, shoplifting, incautious gambling or risky business ventures—often being a problem. *Aphasia*, *agnosia* and *apraxia*, the failure to name articles, recognize them and carry out motor activities respectively, may all create difficulties for both the individual and his carers. Personality characteristics may demonstrate a profound alteration or accentuation, with, for example, the previously neat and tidy individual becoming either slovenly and unkempt, or obsessively, hyperattentive to the minutest detail of his appearance. Where some awareness of the extent of the deterioration is retained, fear or depression may be evident, and delusions, of a persecutory or jealous nature, may also be exteriorized. Dementia may be the unfortunate sequelae in a number of situations, for example, following:

1 Vascular disease, when it is termed multiinfarct dementia

2 Central nervous system infection—tertiary neurosyphilis, acquired immune deficiency syndrome (AIDS) related disorders, viral encephalitis, fungal and tuberculous meningitis and Creutzfeldt-Jakob disease.

3 Cerebral trauma

4 Toxic/metabolic disturbances—bromide intoxication, pernicious anaemia, folic acid deficiency, hyopthyroidism, posthypoglycaemic and post-anoxic states

5 Normal pressure hydrocephalus

6 Neurological disorders—Pick's disease, Parkinson's disease, Huntington's chorea, multiple sclerosis and cerebellar degeneration

Absence of memory is not the only problem that may be experienced, for there may be *distortions of recall* (*paramnesias*) exhibited by some. We have previously mentioned confabulation, where past fictitious events are described in some detail to 'fill in' the gaps evident in memory. Berlyne (1972) supports the earlier distinction, provided by Bonhoeffer (1909) between two distinct types of confabulation. One is brief in content, may often be related to a real event which has become misplaced in time or context, and has to be provoked. This may be referred to as the *momentary type* of confabulation. The second type, the *fantastic type* or *delusional confabulation*, is rarer to encounter, but relates to impossibly, far-fetched accounts of events or experiences which could never have taken place, for example, the detailed memories of being born. Often the content is grandiosed in theme, and the 'memories' are sustained and elaborated, with no stimulus required for their exteriorization.

Retrospective falsifications, are memories which are modified by the individual to be consistent with current thoughts, beliefs, experiences and mood. This may be exhibited by all individuals at one time or another 'Nothing ever goes right for me, I remember nothing but a catalogue of disasters and mistakes, just like this one'—it happens when the individual feels down and deflated. Where depressed mood is of a prolonged and severe nature however, such retrospective falsifications may be a common and persistent feature.

Retrospective delusion, on the other hand, is the term used to describe the individual's 'backdating' of his delusional ideation, to a point within his life history which is well before the actual origination of the false belief. An individual may claim, for example, that his recently acquired persecutory beliefs have been held for some years. *Delusional memories* are exhibited when a delusional interpretation is applied to a previous experience. Both problems may be exteriorized by individuals diagnosed as 'schizophrenic'.

Doppleganger or *reduplicative paramnesia*, are terms used to describe the belief that an exact replica of an individual or place exists somewhere, and this is associated with problems in the non-dominant parietal lobe.

Similarly, *distortions of recognition* may occur and create potential problems for an individual. People may, during a totally novel experience, event or situation, feel that they have seen this exact situation before. They do not know where or when, and yet there is an illusion of familiarity and recognition which they cannot eradicate or account for. This is referred to as *déjà vu*, and happens to most people and one time or another. Quite the opposite experience is encountered in *jamais vu*, for in a familiar and previously met event, place or situation, the individual feels a distinct lack of recognition, and strangeness and unfamiliarity. Again, *jamais vu* may be experienced very occasionally by the individual who has no problems related to mental health status as such, but both phenomena are a more common feature for those subject to temporal lobe seizures, and within mental health care situations. There are other distortions of recognition, for example:

Déjà entendu	the feeling that something has already been heard or perceived
Déjà eprouve	that something has already been tried out or tested
Déjà fait	that something has already been done, or has happened to the individual before
Déjà pense	that 'an idea' has previously been thought
Déjà reconte	that something has already been told or recounted
Déjà voulu	that feelings of wanting or desiring something are the same now as they have been in the past; something has already been desired

These feelings associated with false recollections are common occasional experiences within the general population, but may be far more frequently encountered within those requiring mental health care.

Positive or *negative misidentifications* may create problems for some. In the former, strangers are 'recognized' as friends or relatives and responded to as such. In the latter situation, friends and family members are not 'recognized' as in any way known or significant to the individual or his life, and are therefore treated as strangers. The *Capgras syndrome*, describes the individual's belief that either significant others, or himself, or both, have been replaced by identical doubles. It is also referred to as the *illusion of doubles*, and often follows changes in the quality of significant relationships. Negative feelings are directed towards someone previously loved, and it may be that the individual is unable to manage this dichotomy. The misidentification of the spouse having been replaced by an imposter may facilitate coping. It may be common in situations where persecutory ideation is a feature, or where mood is significantly depressed. The *Fregoli phenomenon* or *illusion*, named after an actor who was renowned for his ability to change his appearance, relates to the belief that a persecutor has assumed the guise of a variety of people who are encountered in everyday life. In the *Amphitryon illusion*, the individual believes his or her spouse alone to be a look-alike imposter, whilst in the *Soaias illusion*, friends, acquaintances and other relatives are considered to be such. All again relate to the persecutory type theme of thought problems.

Hypermnesia is the term used to describe an excessive retention of memories, which are recalled in very fine detail. You may have observed such abilities in show business personalities, who have made a career out of their enhanced abilities to remember. There is, for example, one individual able to remember 36 digits at a time and this he achieves by linking each number proffered with a consonant of the alphabet, which he then converts into words by adding vowels. The words provide an image within the individual's mind and hence enable him to recall the original numbers. Certainly there are references from a variety of sources to indicate that the eidetic imagery utilized in childhood (Leask *et al.*, 1969; Gardner and Roylance, 1982) (refer to section related to perception) may continue to be employed by adults. Cicero (1927) relates the story of the poet, Simonides, who attended a banquet thrown in honour of Scopas, a nobleman, in order to provide part of the evening's 'cabaret'. After Simonides left the stage, the roof of the building collapsed, killing, and mutilating beyond all recognition, Scopas and many of his guests. Simonides' 'photographic memory' facilitated the task of the relatives claiming the correct body of their loved one, for he could remember, precisely, the position of each individual seated within the auditorium.

Similarly, Luria (1987), a Russian neuropsychologist, in his book *The Mind of a Mnemonist*, recalls his studies of a Russian reporter, who worked for a newspaper in Moscow, in the 1920s. This individual was able to reproduce the most detailed reports of events and situations without ever taking a written note. Luria observed that this individual's memory apparently had no limits for capacity or durability, the reporter being able to store the required information quickly—in minutes—and yet recall it days and weeks later. Luria actually tested the individual 30 years after their original work together and was astounded to discover that the newspaper man still retained, in perfect detail, that information first learned during their initial experiments together, all those years before.

In relation to those experiencing such a deviation in mental health status, there is a wonderful book, initially published in 1909, which recounts the experiences of Clifford Whittingham Beers during his encounters within American institutions and asylums at the turn of the twentieth century (Beers, 1962). In it, he describes the thoughts, feelings and behaviours associated with his, initially, severely depressed mood and then his over optimistic, grandiosed and hyperactive state. He similarly identifies the 'care' and 'attention' he received during that time. The following is a selected abstract from that work:

'That one's memory may perform its function in the grip of Unreason itself is proved by the fact that my memory retains an impression, and an accurate one, of virtually everything that befell me, except when under the influence of an anaesthetic or in the unconscious hours of undisturbed sleep. Important events, trifling conversations, and more trifling thoughts of my own are now recalled with ease and accuracy: whereas prior to my illness ... mine was an ordinary memory when it was not noticeably poor'.
Beers, 1962

The recollections contained within the book would certainly appear to bear out the statement above, for the author goes on to elucidate the events fixed within his 'supersensitive memory'. The individual experiencing elevated mood and psychomotor acceleration frequently exhibits such a retentive memory for detailed events occurring to him, as may those individuals eliciting delusional ideation of a persecutory theme. Hypermnesia may be related to hypnosis, fever or cerebral trauma. In addition, it may be elicited during neurosurgical procedures, where the temporal lobe is stimulated, and where delirium is a feature.

We have continually mentioned *insight*, that is, the individual's awareness and understanding of the *status quo*, whether that relates to the specific nature of a puzzle or problem, the way forward within a situation, or his own biopsychosocial health and wellbeing in the current environment or circumstances. The problems experienced by those requiring mental health assistance may be seen to form a continuum on the scale of 'no problems recognized' to 'Help, I need assistance' (Fig. 9.18). At each stage of the continuum, the particular individual experiencing the problem will need specific assistance. This failure to be aware of the status of a situation may relate to any aspect of functioning, for it is just as likely that an individual will ignore or deny that a problem exists at work, within a current relationship or within somatic health status.

All require and will respond to the same principles of therapeutic intervention—time, assistance to ventilate problems, education and strategies designed to facilitate movement forwards. Warmth, emotional support and understanding is demonstrated in the approach utilized by the carer and is of importance regardless of the field of practice.

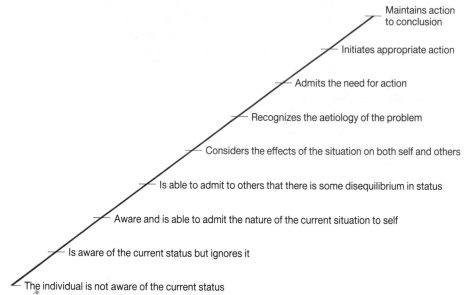

Fig. 9.18 *Degrees of insight.*

LANGUAGE

INTRODUCTION

The term language has previously been defined as:

> ... the mode by which thought and activity is made available to conscious awareness. It is the basic vehicle utilized to structure experiences and, other than for those few aspects of conscious thought when mental images are utilized or objects are rotated in space, is therefore depended upon to achieve conscious awareness. It may be vocal or utilize other methods but in essence is the manner in which communication between parties also occurs.
> *Longman, 1984*

Language is yet another skill that the individual takes for granted, only perhaps valuing it appropriately when unable to find the words necessary to express current thoughts and feelings—one becomes speechless—or perhaps when someone demonstrates eloquence, fluidity and versatility in respect of his or her native, or another, tongue.

Most of the time, little credit is given to the value of language in the evolutionary process and yet Julian Huxley, the eminent biologist, has asserted that:

> 'For their (our pre-human ape ancestors) transformation into man a series of steps were needed. Descent from the trees; erect posture; some enlargement of the brain; more carnivorous habits; the use and then the making of tools; further enlargement of the brain; the discovery of fire; true speech and language; elaboration of tools and rituals'.
> *Huxley, 1969*

Wendt, again in the attempt to differentiate between animals and humans goes so far as to say:

> 'Certainly we modern men are chiefly distinguished from all other living animals by the development of speech and our ability to think in abstract terms—but where word symbolism and the formation of abstract concepts began

in fossil hominids is of course something we cannot determine'.
Wendt, 1972

Language is a remarkable phenomenon. Directly as a result of it, the knowledge and wisdom accrued by humans over centuries, becomes accessible to the individual in the here and now situation. Individuals are then able, if they so desire, to learn via lessons of the past, to build on current knowledge and disseminate new information to others. By utilizing language, people are able to name, describe, explain and often predict the components of their worlds and experiences. Once a name, and characteristics or descriptors are applied to people, places, objects, situations and other environmental variations, information may then be filed away within the appropriate memory frameworks, to be recalled at a later date for use. What, then, does the term 'language' infer?

CHARACTERISTICS

Brown (1973) asserted that, before any system of communication could qualify as a language, three distinct criteria needed to be fulfilled. The first he termed *semanticity* and by this he meant that the symbolic representations utilized to convey meaning must denote the same thing to all users of that language. This is sensible, if you consider the point, for if our words are communicated with one meaning intended but, when received by you, are interpreted as something entirely different, the result may be that you may now believe that you have been instructed in the care of hardy annuals in the garden, rather than in the analysis of the problems associated with an individual's mental health! Secondly, Brown (1973) identified the need for communication to relate to past, present and future elements of life and living, and this he termed *displacement*. Again, this would appear eminently sensible when one considers the limitations imposed by verbalizing only about the present. There would be no 'had a nice day?'—it relates to the past—and no 'Where shall we go

tomorrow?'—it's all in the future! Reflection would be nigh impossible, as would planning or anticipating, for there would be no appropriate, meaningful terminology to apply to such situations. *Productivity* was the term applied to the third criterion, and in this, Brown was referring to the need for communication to facilitate the combination of a limited number of symbols into an unlimited number of varying uses. A simple example would be the way that, within the English language, it is possible to change a statement into a question by using the same words but altering the order or sequence of those words—'I shall get you a cup of coffee' easily becomes 'Shall I get you a cup of coffee?' The addition of the appropriate punctuation at the end of the sentence provides a visual clue to the intent of the words, whilst in verbalizing the sentence the individual's tone of voice would provide the added clue. However, without either, the offer of a cup of coffee would be inferred by the specific meaning of the words used.

Certainly the manner in which *concepts* are utilized within language would support Brown's criterion of productivity, for consider how many extra words would be needed within a vocabulary, for example, if every variation in an object's shape, size, colour, composition or location required it to be allocated a new name. Imagine the situation where only one, very specific shade, of red carpet was termed a carpet, and all of the other shades of red carpet were allocated individual names, as would be all shades of all other colours available. A 'carpet shop' would only be able to sell one particular shade of red carpet—if a vendor wanted to sell more than just examples of this one item, he or she would have to run a 'floor covering shop!' Now it would seem to us that this would be a very precise way of doing things, but remembering that colour is only one of the variations possible in carpet selection, the mind boggles when wandering in the direction of the number of words needed to describe each and every variation with an individual name! Think of the chaos of asking for a patterned, multicoloured carpet! Concepts, then, are a boon. They provide the individual with a mental impression of the properties commonly associated with an object, event, activity, etc. and therefore one word may encompass a significant number of variations on that one theme.

Rosch (1973, 1975) asserts that there are two distinct categories of concepts. The first she refers to as classical concepts, in which all characteristics are exhibited by every member of the group, for example:

Bachelors have to be unmarried adult men

Wives have to be married, female and, in our legal system, 16 years old plus

Nephews and nieces have to be the offspring of the individual's sibling(s)

Squares have to have four sides of equal length joined at 90° angles

Circles have to be plane figures, bounded by a single curved line, every point of which is equidistant from its centre

---

Classical concepts are less commonly encountered than the second type, which she identified as *probabilistic concepts*. The term describes those situations in which members do not always share the same properties or characteristics, or where, perhaps, there is not one common feature shared by all members of the group. All birds, for example, do not fly, all chairs do not have arms, all books may not be for reading. Despite this, one is aware that there are sufficient features in common, for an individual member to be assigned to a particular group, and that a penguin is, for instance, 'probably' a bird. Rosch suggested that most everyday concepts are of this type.

Labov (1973) believed that individuals are significantly influenced in their conceptualization of objects by the context of their surroundings, and that because of this there was a necessary vagueness, or *fuzziness*, regarding the boundaries of many concepts. A useful example may be that of the chamber pot, which, as we are sure you will be aware, used to sit under most people's beds prior to the introduction of 'plumbed in' water closets within house structures. Nowadays, where observed at all, they tend to be adorned with a plant. The concept is fuzzy, for, under a bed, or at first glance, it would be recognized and viewed as something to urinate into, whilst in the middle of the dining-room table, it is hopefully otherwise defined. Similarly a cup may only be conceptualized as such when used to drink from. When positioned upon a dresser or display unit, with its saucer placed behind it, it is more likely to be viewed as an ornament, or considered a financial investment and irreplaceable.

Rosch (1975) asserted that, in addition to recognizing and accumulating knowledge regarding the properties of concepts, individuals have insight into their relationships with other concepts. Fruit, for example, is a division, or *subset*, of food, and other subsets may include vegetables, meat, grains and fish. She believed that the properties of concepts and their relationships to each other, formed a *hierarchy*, thus creating finer, more detailed delineation of the overall concept:

Mother: What would you like for lunch?

Son: I don't know—what have we got?

Mother: (opens fridge door) Well, a sandwich, something on toast, meat and veg?—give me some idea.

Son: I don't know—what is there?

Mother: Well, there's ham, corned beef—

Son: I don't feel like meat.

Mother: (in addition, now opens cupboard door) There's tuna or sardines—

Son: Haven't we got something else?

Mother: How about beans or spaghetti on toast?

Son: No thanks, I don't want toast.

Mother: What about bacon and egg or fish and chips?

Son: There's never anything to eat in this house! I'll have a cheese and tomato sandwich please.

Concepts have to be learned and analysis of the

properties and relationships which link elements of the world are acquired over the years, but, in addition to concepts, other components of language have to be learned.

LINGUISTICS

It is highly probable that most individuals fail to recognize the complexities of language until, at some point following their initial mastery of their native language, they embark on trying to acquire a second one. It is at this point that the individual recalls a teacher, within the past, differentiating between nouns and verbs, or adjectives and pronouns, though these have, most likely, never *appeared* to influence one's speech since that period. It is often when one realizes the difference in the sounds of letters in the new language, compared to the old, or that verbs are conjugated to provide variation in tense and person that an individual is more likely to appreciate the task of the child as he masters his native language. For example, the child is required to learn the precise sounds each letter makes and that sometimes one letter may make more than one sound, depending upon its combination with other letters. There are more exceptions to learn, for example the differing sounds of pairs of letters—cough and about, please and lease, and chop and chaos—and that some words sound the same but are spelt differently and convey very different meanings—by and buy, sore and soar, sail and sale. The study of the specific sounds and how they function to indicate a change in meaning is termed *phonology* and Ladefoged (1975) defined the smallest sounds, which may be distinguished by their contrasts in words, as *phonemes*. The word apt, for instance, has three phonemes—a-p-t—whilst, by replacing the 't' with an 'e' to form the word 'ape' would only provide two phonemes, due to the long 'a' sound produced by the a–e combination. Of course, the child, unlike the majority of adult learners, absorbs and remembers the sounds of language long before those sounds are correlated with the appropriate symbolic letter. A child may have no problems learning and verbalizing his native language and yet encounter great difficulties in reading and writing, as may be seen later in

this section, and, of course, the child who is deaf, or reared in an environment of severe sensory deprivation, may never hear the sounds required to be amalgamated to form language.

Phonemes combine to create larger, more complex units of sound, termed *morphemes*, for example, the words 'turn' 'excite' and 'develop' are all morphemes. These cannot be reduced further and yet still have sensible meaning. They can, however, have other morphemes added to them. For instance turn + 'ed' = turned, or + 'ing' = turning, or + a single s = turns and this, in English, changes the *tense* of the verb, or in the case of 'turns' may convert the word to its *plural* form, as in 'We took turns on the swing'. Of course there are other ways in which added morphemes are utilized, for example to create *comparatives* and *absolutes*—tall, taller, tallest and dark, darker and darkest—and other contrasts— excite, exciting, unexciting, and develop, developed and undeveloped.

Having said all of the above, one has most surely heard the errors of childhood language, such as 'mummy, is it time we goed now?' or 'Do it be for me?'. It, again, takes time to learn *syntax*—the rules that govern the ways in which words may legitimately be combined, to form meaningful sentences in a language. Similarly, the child requires to understand the actual meaning of words utilized, and many parents have, no doubt, experienced great embarrassment as a youngster repeats a word that has been overheard, perhaps in 'adult' conversation, and yet has no idea of the meaning or nature of the term. This knowledge of word meaning is referred to as *lexical knowledge*, whilst *semantics* is the term utilized to convey that necessary understanding of combined sounds, as words, phrases or sentences. Certainly if language is to be utilized to the full and employed in both verbal and written form, it is necessary to understand that the symbols selected to form an alphabet represent words with meanings.

It is possible, of course, to have a detailed linguisitic knowledge and yet fail to be understood, and a useful example may be provided by the situation where a non-English speaking tourist detains a passer-by to ask directions to the nearest lavatory. His speech is, probably, grammatically perfect and yet he is unable to share the meaning of his communication. It appears a very simplistic observation to make, but it is vital that speaker and listener share enough common ground or knowledge, and have enough relevant information, to understand what is conveyed by the language used. We make the point to remind you that professional groups utilize a language which may not be completely or correctly understood by those who are not a part of that group. Therefore, it is necessary to be willing and able to discard the terminology and jargon associated with the professional tongue, to facilitate communication appropriate to the experiences and norms of the listener. Language is utilized to achieve an aim relevant to a specific social context and in this sense is a very self-referential activity. Whether an individual is seeking or conveying information, persuading, influencing, negotiating, demanding or instructing, the use of language is *pragmatic*, for it achieves the individual's aims and purposes.

Language is, it would seem, a complex skill, with regard to the elements which need to be mastered. However, having looked previously at thinking, and acknowledged that the vast majority of thinking is achieved via language, it seems appropriate to examine the relationship between the two cognitive functions.

LANGUAGE AND THINKING

There are three main perspectives with regard to the relationship between language and thought:

1 Thinking is dependent upon language

2 Language is dependent upon cognitive development

3 The two functions develop separately and amalgamate early in childhood

For many years, it was believed that all individuals think in similar ways, but in the second and third decade of this century, two individuals, working separately from each other, put forward theories in opposition to that commonly held view. An anthropologist and linguist, Edward Sapir (1949) and Benjamin Lee Whorf, an insurance company fire prevention officer and avid spare-time linguist, both asserted that people's languages confine and constrict methods of perception and thought, and hence, individuals in various parts of the world both perceive and think about their world in different ways. The *Sapir–Whorf*, or *linguistic relativity hypothesis*, proposes that the environment and way of life experienced within the different cultures of the world engender the development of a unique view of that world and its important features. This specificity evokes a vocabulary, concepts and grammar appropriate to the needs experienced and that, therefore, determines the parameters and nature of thinking. Thus, in learning the native language, children also learn the concomitant and implicit view of the world expressed via that language, for vocabulary is not available for, what are considered, culturally unimportant or irrelevant features. *Linguistic determinism* is, then, the hypothesis that language determines thinking. Whorf produced a great deal of evidence to support his beliefs, which included his work with the Hopi Indians, who, he pointed out, have no expressions or words relating to time—past, present and future—as European languages have, and who, often, have just one word to describe a whole performance:

'The light flashed', we say in English. Something has to be there to make the light flash; 'light' is the subject, 'flash' the predicate .... A Hopi Indian ... says Reh-pi—'flash'—one word for the whole performance, no subject, no predicate, no time element.
Stuart Chase (in Carroll, 1956)

The emphasis is placed on what actually happened—not the 'how, when, why, how or where' of it happening. These factors would appear unimportant to the Hopi and are therefore not delineated, thus, according to Whorf, altering the perception of the event and the thinking associated with it.

A second, commonly quoted, example used in support of the hypothesis relates the fact that the Eskimo people have more words to describe snow—27 in fact—than are available in English. There are specific names, for instance, for drifting snow, packed snow, fluffy snow and words for the snow suitable for igloo construction and for sledging on, indicating the importance of the feature within their way of life and not that of Europeans. Therefore, according to Whorf, each of the two cultures will adopt a unique view of their world, the paramaters of which, will be provided by language.

There has been evidence both to support and refute the Sapir–Whorf hypothesis in the years since its inception. As early as 1932, Carmichael *et al.* confirmed the fact that verbal labelling significantly *influences* perception and hence thinking. In their studies, two experimental groups were given the same neutral drawing. Each group, however, was given a different verbal label in association with the picture. When later requested to reproduce the previously viewed drawings, subjects were found to produce very different drawings, according to which verbal label had been offered.

Carroll and Casagrande (1958) studied the language of the Navaho Indians, and compared children of the same age, who spoke Navaho only, English only and both languages. The Navaho language places great emphasis on the form of objects, with separate verbs, for example, to describe the performance of handling an item, which is dependent upon the qualities of the object being manipulated. There is, therefore, a verb used in relation to handling long, flexible items, such as string, another for handling long rigid items, such as sticks, and yet another related to the handling of flat and flexible articles, such as pieces of cloth. American children, in contrast, learn object recognition first in relation to size, then colour and finally form or shape, so that some items will initially be recognized as big or little, then red or green and finally round or square. In their studies, Carroll and Casagrande discovered that children who spoke only Navaho were more aware of the form of an object than their English-only speaking peers, and were able to recognize items by their form. A surprising

second comparison, however, between the English-only speaking children and the English–Navaho speaking group of youngsters, revealed the former to be more adept in recognition of the form of objects than the latter, and this Carroll and Casagrande accounted for by the experience gained by the English-only speaking children within preschool nursery education.

Slobin (1979) maintains that the Sapir–Whorf hypothesis is too strong an assertion, for whilst he agrees that language may *influence* thought, he refutes its action as a *determinant*. He identifies points of emphasis in other languages—French and German—which do not appear in English, for example, the familiar and polite terms used for the second person pronoun. In English, the term 'you' is consistently used, with no differentiation made between a personal or formal reference. This is not so in French, where 'tu' and 'vous' are used, or in German, where 'du' and 'sie' are delineated. Slobin remarks that in all forms of speech, the French and German speakers are required to incorporate an assessment of the social relationships involved within communication, whilst English speakers are not so obliged. This does not mean, avers Slobin, that social relationships are not recognized, or that they are not considered within intercourse, it merely indicates that the English language does not emphasize the need to do so.

Berlim and Kay (1969) analysed the ways in which different languages label and differentiate colours and their variations in shade. Native speakers were presented with over 300 coloured squares and asked to name them in their own language. All languages had at least two terms for, what were described by the researchers as, *focal*, or *main colours*, whilst some languages identified as many as 11 words. The best example of a colour—the best example of red, yellow or green for instance—was identified as such regardless of the language used, but despite the lack of a specific word to name a shade of colour, shades were still recognized as being related to the appropriate focal colour. Heider (1972) similarly found that the Dani, of Indonesian New Guinea, had only terms to distinguish two main colour features. The word 'Mola' means light, and 'Mili' means dark, and yet native language speakers were able to perceive and recognize focal colours better than the non-focal examples. Language did not influence perception and thinking, but only items of sufficient relevance or significance to life had warranted a unique label. Perhaps language may influence thinking, but it certainly does not appear to determine it.

Piaget, of course, believed language depended on, and indicated the level of, cognitive development attained:

'… language and thought are linked in a genetic circle …. In the last analysis, both depend on intelligence itself, which antedates language and is independent of it'.
Piaget, 1968

Whilst he would acknowledge the important role of language in extending the range of symbolic thinking, Piaget asserted that language represented only one element of such symbolic function, which, in addition, included the rudimentary forms of symbolic play and imagery. Development of intelligence, he proposes, begins at birth and pre-dates the acquisition of language, and, therefore, Piaget believed that the initial thoughts of the child are expressed via images and activities, which he termed *autistic thought*. The child, he believed, was unable to understand the linguistic expression of a concept until competent to master the concept *per se*. Certainly, there is some everyday evidence to support that specific element of the theory:

When are we going to the park, mummy?

Tomorrow, dear.

When's tomorrow, Mummy?

It's the day after this day, dear.

When's this day over, Mummy?

When we've been to sleep tonight and then wake up in the morning, that will be tomorrow, dear.

The child ponders.

When are we going to the park, Mummy?

The child has no understanding of the concept of 'tomorrow', has no understanding of when he will be taken to the park, or when it will be his birthday or Christmas day, or can reference any other future element in time.

Piaget believed that babies develop impressions or outlines of their world via their experiences and that such outlines or schemas are embellished and new ones created as the world is explored. In the same way that a child is able to understand that he can 'pretend' that four dining-room chairs appropriately positioned are his car, that is, he has learned the one is a symbolic representation of a 'real' object in his life, so the child is able to understand that a word represents an object. The child's initial speech is, Piaget believes, merely an expression of his own thoughts—a sort of running commentary on his world and his activities within it—and that only at a later point in cognitive development, will the 'social aspects' of language be introduced, as he begins to incorporate the responses or interjections of a significant onlooker into account.

Again, direct observation would support Piaget's assertion of the egocentric and self-absorbed nature of early language displayed. One only has to watch children in a pre-school setting to note that whilst within the group, the younger children are actually playing alone, and that, whilst talking, they are not actually communicating with the child next to them. However, Piaget did not pay any credence to the fact that exposure to language itself may assist the child to absorb and understand new concepts. Returning to the example of the 'tomorrow' concept, the child does learn via explanations and experience when 'tomorrow' will arrive, that is, the concept of time.

Vygotsky (1962), a Russian psychologist, believed that thought and language initially develop as separate entities, and whilst continuing in this fashion to a greater or lesser extent into adulthood, also combine to form a third and major component of the thinking–language processes. Like Piaget, Vygotsky believed that:

---

1 Children think before they speak

2 They build up schemas related to their experiences of their world

3 Early thinking is comprised of images, perceptions and actions

4 Initially, speech is egocentric and basically a verbalization of thinking

5 Symbols begin to double for 'reality'—the four chairs standing for a car—at around the age of two years

---

Vygotsky referred to this early thinking as *pre-linguistic thought*. However, he diverged from the theory put forward by Piaget in his assertions that language develops simultaneously throughout this period, as the child practices the sounds that will amalgamate to form speech. This he refers to as *pre-intellectual language*.

The crux of the matter for Vygotsky was the differentiation he made between *inner speech*, which reflected personal thoughts, and *external speech*, which represented social communications with others. He proposed that early speech is thoughtless speech and purely social in nature, for the child's ability to reason and think about his environment, and experiences, has no language available to describe it. However, about the age of two years the thoughtless speech and language-less thought processes begin to merge, with words used as representative symbols for thoughts. Vygotsky believed that only at this merging point within cognitive development could individual social development begin, as children explore their world and that of others with the aid of language. Similarly, the child absorbs the socio-cultural norms that surround him, as thinking and language create two interlinking circles, and activity in one area generates a concomitant response in the other. Vygotsky believed that the egocentric speech of early childhood, rather than disappearing in the light of social speech, actually continues, but in the child's head. He found that both children and adults, when faced with a difficult or complex task, would verbalize their egocentric speech via thinking aloud. Certainly, individuals are aware of the continuation of languageless thought into adulthood, because of their ability to manipulate images, not just words, within their minds.

The theories of Sapir–Whorf, Piaget and Vygotsky seek to explain the relationship between thinking and language, and certainly you may consider elements of each to be feasible even if you cannot accept one perspective in its entirety. The next, seemingly logical, point requiring analysis would appear to be related to the methods via which the child masters his or her native language

ACQUISITION

Jakobson (1968) studying the language of babies and young children, concentrated his attention on the sounds and sound patterns (phonology) which were used regularly and which appeared to be employed by the child with distinctive meaning.

It may be a valuable exercise, at this point, for you to analyse the parts of the mouth and the way the tongue is utilized in making the sounds symbolized by the alphabet. Is there, for example, a significant difference in the way in which the sounds of vowels and consonants are produced, and are all consonants formed by the same movement?

Jakobson believed that the child initially differentiates between vowels and consonants in very broad terms, though these broad terms do not immediately include an ability to distinguish between the sounds within either group. Each group is then further embellished, for example, by a distinction between consonants produced nasally and non-nasally, and later between those that are produced in various sites of the mouth, to build up an extensive 'menu' of available sounds. He uses embryological development as a simili for the process, with an initially undifferentiated group of sounds, repeatedly subdividing until the sound system is fully differentiated. The original work by Jakobson was published in 1941, and, since this time, elements have been questioned by others researching the field. One example of dissonance is seen in relation to his proposals that the order of acquisition of contrasts was consistent for all children and all languages, for Menn (1985) amongst others, has refuted the actuality of such proposals. Jakobson was, however, a pioneer in the field, for previous studies in phonology had concentrated on the number and specific sounds available in a child's vocabulary at different ages.

Stampe (1969) asserted that the child's phonological development is determined by ease of articulation, and is best described in terms of simplifying functions that affect whole groups of phonemes, rather than single sounds. He maintains, for instance, that whilst able to perceive the difference between the 'k' or 'g' sounds (velar stops) and the 't' or 'd' sounds (alveolar stops), the latter are easier to articulate and therefore 'cup' is pronounced 'tup' and 'girl' becomes 'dirl'. One sound replaces another. Similarly one sound may be seen to influence the pronunciation of a second sound in the same word, for example 'kekkle' and 'goggie' for 'kettle' and 'doggie', despite the child's ability to make the sound of 't' and 'd' as in 'tap' or 'bed'. Others have shared Stampe's belief in the child's ability to differentiate between sounds, though the factors involved in the order of acquisition of speech sounds continue to be disputed. Dodd (1987) would assert that visual as well as auditory cues are utilized by the child to learn the required sound system for language development.

Early studies of grammar and its development in the child, concentrated on the quantity of material learned—the number of words used, how many different types of words are employed and how much of speech conformed to adult grammatical rules. Studies during this time, for example, by Gesell (1950) merely established the fact that the length of speech and the amount of that speech which complies with grammatical rules, increases with age. However, Brown (1973) asserted that, even in the earliest stages of speech production, there is order and regularity within

that speech, both in the type of words used and the way in which they are combined. This regularity could not be accounted for in grammatical terms alone, and Bloom (1970) asserted that meaning, too, was a vital element requiring consideration alongside grammar. Semantics, the meanings of words used, is discussed below, but one aspect of grammar is certain and that is, it is not produced by imitating adult speech alone. Rarely can it be considered that a child will hear and adult state 'I no go', 'I not want', 'I goed', 'I feeled it', or similar errors of speech, and yet these are terms used at a particular point in language development by all children. Children definitely learn rules, rather than merely imitating adults, for they recognize that, for example, adding an '-ed' to a verb will—in some situations—change present tense to past tense—for example, I wanted, I wished. The child applies the rule consistently across all verbs only later absorbing the exceptions observed. The grammatical complexity of a child's speech is seen to increase with his general maturity (Crystal, 1984), and a full set of sentence types is in use by the age of five years (Wells, 1985).

We have previously mentioned Bloom (1970) and his emphasis on meaning within early word combinations used by children. He asserted that the meaning of words uttered could be construed by the context in which they occurred, and used the example of 'mummy sock' to prove his point. When the child is offering mummy one of her own stockings, the child's meaning is inferred as 'there, mummy, this is one of your stockings', that is 'mummy's sock'. However, where the child is sitting barefoot, with a sock in his hand, his speech may be translated into, 'mummy please put my sock on'. Children consistently string more words together, adding common linking words (the, on, at) and those of relationships (my, your) until grammatical sentences are produced. First words produced are proper nouns—mummy and daddy—progressing to common nouns where differentiations have to be absorbed—dogs and cats (small), horse and cow (big)—and where full meaning of the noun is rarely understood despite the term being used. It is common to hear one term misused by an over-generalization, where, for example, all animals are dogs, which is termed *overextension*. Similarly, misuse of a word may occur as the child over-specifies, with only, for example, the family pet, or a particular breed of dog, labelled as an instance of the word. This is referred to an *under-extension*.

The linguist, Noam Chomsky (1959) believed that the capacity for human language is an innate element, as are the internal 'rules' that enable the individual to decide whether sentences both convey the meaning intended and are grammatically appropriate. Chomsky asserts that people do not use the same 'stock' sentences time and time again, but are constantly creating new ones. If an individual were only able to repeat sentences previously heard, speech and language would be severely limited, but he maintains that *because* humans are born with the rules of grammar, they are capable of inventing and understanding sentences never previously heard. Chomsky stated:

'One can only conclude that children do not build grammars primarily from the evidence they hear, but according to an inner design—a genetic program'.
Chomsky, 1980

He compares the development of grammar to the growth of the child's physical organs, with the environment providing both activation of the system and its support, in exactly the same way as oxygen and nutrients facilitate the growth of an embryonic heart. The fact that children learn a culturally specific language which reflects their native environment and therefore varies greatly between cultural groups does not deflect Chomsky (1986) from his proposals. He asserts that the inner rules relate to a *universal grammar*, which provides an automatic knowledge of the general form any language should take. Hyams (1986) raises objections to such a hypothesis on the grounds that all languages do not conform to the same grammatical rules, citing the norm of saying 'went' in Italian, whereas, in English, a subject is grammatically necessary, as in 'she went'. Chomsky replies to such criticisms by proposing that environmental influences will modify

such parameters as are necessary to meet cultural aberrations.

Chomsky is a prolific writer and his work is very valuable in any detailed study of linguistics. However, his theories suggest that individuals produce perfectly grammatical sentences which frequently they do not. A point of some interest, though, is the work of Werker and Tees (1985) who discovered that babies lose their initial potential to recognize all possible sounds in languages as they begin to assimilate a single dialect. Eight-month-old babies, immaterial of their nationality, immediately detect and react to changes in sounds which adults fail to recognize. By the time the child reaches 12 months, this ability to recognize such subtle shifts in sound is lost if exposure to them is not undertaken on a regular basis.

FACTORS IMPLICIT IN DEVELOPMENT OF LANGUAGE

You may recall the lack of verbal recognition and memory associated with Genie, the 13-year-old girl discovered after being confined to a small room under conditions of extreme physical restraint and sensory deprivation from the age of 20 months by her parents (Curtiss, 1977). You may recall, too, that Genie had failed to acquire language skills and despite intensive expert assistance, has not achieved linguistic competence to date. The cerebral hemisphere specialization that one would expect to occur had failed to develop and Genie's language-related cerebral structures had degenerated. Similarly in this area of memory and learning, we recalled the work of Dennis (1960) with children in Iranian orphanages and their slowness to develop, due to sensory deprivation. All spheres of growth were severely retarded and the children failed to reach any of the expected milestones of the early years.

It would be a relief to believe that these were isolated instances, but, unfortunately, this is not the case. There are many historical examples of children deliberately isolated in attempts to analyse the nature and development of language. The Egyptian pharaoh, Psammetichos, the Holy Roman Emperor, Frederik II and King James IV of Scotland are all alleged to have used such experiments (Curtiss, 1981) and within the twentieth century, alone, there are a number of instances of children isolated from human contact and interaction besides Genie:

Anna, a five-year-old girl, found tied to a chair in a store room of the family farm, where she had been since babyhood. Removed to a children's home and later to an institution for the elderly infirm, Anna was cachexic and frail physically, and expressionless and apathetic. She was thought to be deaf and probably blind. Once removed to a foster home and one-to-one attention, however, Anna began to acquire both cognitive and motor skills. Anna was, for some reason, transferred to a private home for 'retarded' children and after two years there, was reported to be uttering single words and attempting conversation. She died, aged approximately 10 years old, of jaundice.

Isabelle, as six year old, was kept isolated because of her illegitimacy. She and her mother, who was both deaf and mute, were housed in a darkened room, away from the remainder of the family, who had rejected them. After their escape, the child was admitted to a children's hospital for orthopaedic surgery and physiotherapy, necessary due to rickets and abnormal bone development. In hospital she was withdrawn and mute, showing extreme hostility to strangers, especially men. Her acquisition of language was quite remarkable, however, for within two months she was singing nursery rhymes, could read and write within a year, and after eighteen months possessed a vocabulary of some 2,000 words and could create stories.
Davis, 1967

Space precludes more examples than proffered above, but many more are documented—the Koluchova twins (1976), Mary and Louise (Skuse, 1984), Alice and Beth (Douglas and Sutton, 1978) and Adam (Thompson, 1986) are just a few. Similarly there are recorded examples of children being raised from babies, as 'Wolf children', Victor, the 'Wild boy of Aveyron'

(Itard, 1801) and Amala and Kamala of Midnapore (Singh and Zingg, 1942), who experienced isolation from humans, but adopted the animal parent's language and way of life. Other studies, too, of institutional care and its effects on the development of children, for example, Skeele's (1966) comparison between a group of children raised in an unstimulating orphanage and a second group who had been transferred from the home to an institution for 'retarded adults' at about 20 months of age, and Dennis' study of a poor foundling home in Beirut, Lebanon (Dennis, 1973), all direct attention to the importance of environmental stimulation in language development.

Bruner (1983) and others have stressed the importance of a stimulating environment in the prelinguistic period on the acquisition of speech. Certainly psychosocial deprivation at this point has been shown to impair preverbal vocalization and babble (Provence and Lipton, 1962) and Dennis (1941) discovered that, whilst babies still expressed preverbal sounds within situations of minimal verbal interaction, they did not progress to use any sound that corresponded with a 'real' word during the 61 weeks of his study.

Piaget (1967), of course, would assert that the lack of opportunity to play in such isolated and deprived circumstances would inhibit a child's progression to the level of cognitive function necessary for thought, and hence language, to develop. His belief in symbolic function, including mental imagery and symbolic play, as the precursor and facilitator of an appropriate level of sensorimotor behaviour to engender the representational skills necessary for thought and language, firmly places language in the primary role of personal communication strategy first, and social interaction strategy second in importance. Yet others (Tomasello and Farrar, 1984; Gopnik and Meltzoff, 1985) have asserted that the earliest words used usually relate to social relationships and are uttered in social contexts.

Certainly malnutrition was a common factor experienced by the isolated children referred to above, but many studies have indicated that this alone fails to produce permanent mental impairment. In conjunction with social and intellectual deprivation, cognitive development is depressed.

In many of the case histories provided which relate to 'wild' children, whilst linguistic abilities were poor on discovery, progress was rapid after rescue and the implementation of strategies to enhance psychosocial development, for example, play school attendance and speech therapy. Many of the children actually reached age-appropriate lanaguage skills within a few years of rescue, with little difference in acquisition between those removed at an earlier or relatively later age. Lenneberg (1967) suggested that to proceed normally, language must be acquired during the first 12 years of life and the story of 13-year-old Genie, who never achieved more than the single word speech associated with a toddler, may be used as evidence to support his proposals for this critical learning period.

Common sense would indicate that the child must be able to hear efficiently in order to identify and discriminate between the speech sounds of a lanaguage. Therefore any loss or distortion of auditory stimuli within the early years of language development may significantly impair its acquisition. The visually impaired child, too, may be disadvantaged during the preverbal period of speech development. In normally sighted children, the partner in an interaction will utilize the direction of the child's gaze as indicative of the focus of attention, and also his visually directed gestures, such as pointing to objects that stimulate him, to choose topics of interaction. These are absent or greatly reduced in the visually impaired infant and therefore cues to assist the partner are missing, engendering difficulties in understanding the child's desires or intentions. Rowland (1983) found that, in such situations, whilst affective states could be communicated successfully to an adult, sightless babies vocalized less than, and in different patterns to, sighted babies. Rowland suggests that listening becomes so important in the baby's assessment of the environment that perhaps his lack of vocalization is to prevent 'clutter' of the auditory cues. It must be difficult to relate the word 'tree' to something that is noiseless and out of reach, and to try to associate 'dog' with certain tactile, olfactory and auditory cues, and yet generate the concepts relevant. Structural abnormalities of the speech apparatus, such as cleft palate and lip, do not necessarily preclude normal speech production, for in most instances surgical repair is instigated before the child starts to talk. Articulatory abnormalities are higher for these children than the normal population; often the child exhibits a more nasal quality in verbalizing consonants. Some conductive hearing loss may also result from the impaired functioning of the Eustachian tube (auditory tube), with a concomitant phonological developmental difficulty. Motor speech impairments (*dysarthria*) result from problems within the central or peripheral nervous system. Children experiencing such problems as cerebral palsy may exhibit an ability to talk but verbalizations are often slow and distorted. In extreme situations, the child may be unable to speak at all, termed *anarthria*.

The examples provided above serve hopefully to remind us that language acquisition and speech production are complex biopsychosocial skills, involving processes which, as yet, are incompletely understood.

PROBLEMS ENCOUNTERED WITHIN MENTAL HEALTH CARE

Throughout we have attempted to emphasize the fact that problems encountered within mental health care are also encountered in other spheres of care delivery and those associated with language are no exception.

The cerebral hemispheres function asymmetrically, with one hemisphere, termed *dominant*, determining language, and the favoured, or *preferred*, hand, foot and eye use. People talk of being left or right handed, referring to the side of the body most favoured, and the vast majority of the population—90%—are right handed with the left hemisphere dominant. The remaining individuals, though left handed, may have a right hemisphere dominant (30%) or a left (70%). Various tests for dominance are available, for example, an electroencephalogram demonstrates greater alpha wave suppression in the dominant hemisphere during verbal thought. Language is mediated via different areas of the cortex of the dominant hemisphere, although they are interconnected. Any problem occurring within any of these areas, or along the interconnecting network of fibres associated with them, may affect the ability to speak, write or understand language.

Broca's area, associated with the mechanisms by which words are selected, articulated and constructed to form sentences. Damage in this area (frontal cortex) may produce *primary motor dysphasia*, otherwise termed cortical motor, expressive or Broca's dysphasia, and whilst comprehension remains relatively unaffected, speech is slow, sparse and hesitant. Its rhythm and intonation is disturbed and the individual experiences great difficulty in word-finding, with 'wrong' words being utilized and often being incorrectly pronounced. Individuals often recognize errors made and in attempting to correct them, become irritated and annoyed. They may compensate by miming words 'lost' or using gestures, but when offered the correct word, can recognize and select it. Sentences are abbreviated with words omitted, but are meaningful. Problems of writing reflect those of speech.

Wernicke's area, spanning the temporal and parietal cortex, posterior to the medial end of the Sylvian fissure, is associated with comprehension of language, both spoken and written, therefore lesions here reflect those functions. *Primary sensory dysphasia*, otherwise termed receptive or Wernick's dysphasia, demonstrates a defective appreciation of the meaning of words and grammatical constructions. The individual is less able to respond to instructions and has difficulty in repeating back phrases provided. The cortical system for analysing incoming speech are affected, and therefore speech is affected, with words used incorrectly, *neologisms* (new words, distortions or combinations of existing words) and errors of grammar and syntactical construction. Speech is fluent and easy, unlike Broca's dysphasia, with rhythm and inflexion preserved and no articulatory defects, though it may be pressurized. Individuals are unaware of linguistic errors, and are unable to recognize a 'correct' word when offered. They seem unable to discard words already used and speech is often *contaminated* by previously used words. Both these individuals and those experiencing Broca's dysphasia demonstrate *perseveration*, that is, repetition of a word or phrase long after its relevance is past. Whilst

the individual may be able to read a single word aloud with no problems, reading of longer sentences is jumbled and contaminated, with no comprehension and therefore an inability to carry out written instructions.

A lesion in the dominant temporal lobe, which is adjacent to the primary receptive area for hearing, is rare but, when occurring, produces an agnosia for spoken words which is interpreted as sounds, but not words. The individual hears because pathways in the non-dominant hemisphere are intact, but information related to speech cannot reach the receiving centre in the dominant hemisphere. Speech and writing are fluent and without error, and the term used for the problem is *subcortical auditory dysphasia* or pure word deafness. Similarly, lesions of the left visual cortex and the splenium of the corpus callosum evoke pure word blindness, or *subcortical visual aphasia*. Visual input is possible to the right hemisphere only and therefore access to the language systems of the left hemisphere is not available. The individual speaks normally and can understand the spoken word. Difficulties relate to comprehension of visually perceived language, that is, written words. Pure word dumbness, or *subcortical motor aphasia*, creates a picture of individuals able to comprehend both spoken and written language, and who are able to express themselves in writing, thus indicating that their inner speech is unaffected. Their problem relates to articulating speech, which may be complete or achieved with great difficulty (dysarthria). Where speech is achieved, it is slurred, and individuals cannot repeat words heard, or read alone, neither can they verbalize at will. *Agraphia*—an inability to write—may be seen to occur in any general dysphasia, or as a problem associated with movement difficulties termed *apraxias*. However, a pure motor agraphia is thought to be associated with an interruption of the pathway from the left angular gyrus to the hand area of the left motor cortex. Speech is unimpaired, as are understanding of written and spoken words. Spontaneous writing or that related to dictated material is disturbed, though individuals may be able to copy written words provided for them.

Nominal dysphasia (amnesic or anomic aphasia) is the term describing difficulty in evoking names at will. Individuals may be able to describe the object, its use and even recognize the name if offered to them, but its name eludes them. Speech is fluent, but at times word-finding pauses may be demonstrated, or individuals may have to go 'all around the houses' to make their point—*circumlocution*. Sometimes, individuals exhibit difficulty in comprehension or execution of oral or written commands, demonstrating that internal speech is affected. Nominal aphasia is associated with both diffuse cerebral dysfunction but also with lesions of the dominant temporo-parietal region.

There are other disturbances of language, for example, lesions which disrupt links between Broca's and Wernicke's areas—*conduction dysphasia*—and where it is thought that the links between these areas remain intact and yet the area is isolated from other parts of the cortex—*syndromes of isolated speech area*. However, sufficient examples have been provided here to provoke consideration of somatic aetiology for disturbances of speech exhibited by an individual rather than an automatic assumption that they are indicative of a primary deviation in mental health status.

Neologisms have previously been mentioned in relation to primary sensory dysphasia. New words are created, standard words may be given a new and highly idiosyncratic meaning or more than one word may be combined. Within mental health care, the use of such new words is indicative of a lack of contact with reality and is therefore observed in individuals who are subject to a 'psychosis'. It is always necessary to incorporate an assessment of the individual's cultural and educational experiences prior to labelling an aberration of speech, a neologism, for errors of speech, and meaning may, on occasions, be an integral, though incorrect, part of 'normal' speech.

Circumlocution, has also been mentioned, as indirect speech which is delayed in reaching the point, because of difficulty in word finding. *Circumstantiality* is a similar meandering of speech but on this occasion is due to the inclusion of unnecessary and tedious details, and parenthetical remarks. The latter are meaningful and connected clauses, related to the point of the speech, which the speaker never loses sight of. Circumstantiality is a feature frequently encountered within the mentally well, but may be a feature of those categorized as 'obsessive compulsive personality disorders' and schizophrenia. You may recall within the section on thinking, that *loosening of associations* was mentioned. Circumstantiality demonstrates connections between areas of speech whereas in the individual experiencing loosening of associations, the original point is lost, and thoughts and speech wander off in a new and unrelated direction. *Tangentiality*—statements either totally unrelated to each other, or only obliquely so, are juxtapositioned—may be the verbal evidence to support loosening of association, and is demonstrated where the individual exteriorizes the complex problems labelled as schizophrenia.

Perseveration, mentioned in relation to both primary sensory and motor dysphasias, may also be evidence of mental health difficulties. The persistent repetition of currently irrelevant words is associated with organically evoked mental health problems and also others which demonstrate a lack of contact with reality. *Echolalia*, however, is the term used to describe the constant repetition, or echoing, of words or phrases of others. The intonation of the individual's voice during this persistent repetition may be mocking or staccato, or conversely the individual may 'mumble'. This may be exhibited by those experiencing pervasive developmental disorders, such as autism, and again by those demonstrating the mental health related sequelae of organic impairment, and 'schizophrenia'. Words selected for use in speech may be seen at times to depend on their sound rather than their meaning. *Rhyming* and *punning* (the construction of poor quality jokes) are features associated with *clanging* or *clang association*, evident in those experiencing psychomotor acceleration problems and where contact with reality is disturbed. *Word salad* may be the term used to describe the jumbled, incomprehensive speech exhibited by some 'psychotic' individuals, particularly those experiencing the multiplicity of problems labelled together as 'schizophrenia'. Similarly '*talking past the point*' may be demonstrated by this individual, who provides an answer to a question posed which, whilst related to the topic itself, is inappropriate and incorrect.

Slurred speech, previously mentioned in relation to subcortical motor dysphasia, is associated with intoxication due to various psychoactive substances when seen within mental health care. Alcohol, opioids and inhalants may all evoke the problem. *Incoherence* is differentiated easily and quickly from slurring, for, whilst there is a lack of logical, or meaningful connections, between words or phrases, changes in subject matter and the inclusion of irrelevances, words emitted are not dragged or drawn out in articulation. Speech may be *pressurized*, reflecting the speed of thoughts experienced by the overactive individual, or may demonstrate the *interruptions* of flow associated with blocking of thoughts and ideas. Similarly, *mutism* or *elective mutism* may be features indicating a mental health problem. The severely depressed individual may initially show a slowing of the stream of speech which may dry up completely, but such silence may be the result of hallucinatory experiences, or delusional ideation, or extreme difficulty in thinking. Elective mutism, demonstrated by children, is a persistent refusal to talk though gestures and odd monosyllabic responses may be evoked. This is often situationally specific, occurring in a discrete social setting. Only rarely is total mutism seen, but the excessively shy, withdrawn or isolated child, or conversely the controlling, negativistic child, may exhibit the problem. On occasions, there may be delayed language development or articulatory problems, but in the main, such children will have normal language skills.

There are a myriad of problems associated with language and speech production, but a selection has been included to encourage further observation and reflection on the linguistic functions and abilities demonstrated by people within care. An efficient neurological examination may preclude an incorrect diagnosis of somatic problems which may require neuromedical or surgical intervention but the nurse's observations may be the prerequisite and provoking factor which results in more detailed investigation.

FURTHER READING

Brain, W.R. (1985) *Brain's Diseases of the Nervous System*. Oxford University Press.

Bruce, V. & Green, P. (1988) *Visual Perception, Physiology, Psychology and Ecology*. London: Lawrence Erlbaum.

Brunner, L.S. & Suddarth, D.S. (1986) *The Lippincott Manual of Medical Surgical Nursing*. London: Harper & Row.

Gellatly, A. (Ed.) (1986) *The Skilful Mind*. Milton Keynes: Open University Press.

Hinchcliffe, S. & Montague, S. (1988) *Physiology for Nursing Practice*. London: Baillière Tindall.

Hinwood, B. (1993) *A Textbook of Science for the Health Professions*, 2nd edn. London: Chapman & Hall.

Lishman, W.A. (1978) *Organic Psychiatry: The Psychological Consequences of Cerebral Disorder*. Oxford: Blackwell Scientific.

Loftus, G.R. & Loftus, E.F. (1976) *Human Memory: The Processing of Information*. Hillsdale, NJ: Lawrence Erlbaum.

Roth, I. (Ed.) (1990) *Introduction to Psychology*, Vols 1 and 2. Milton Keynes: Lawrence Erlbaum in conjunction with the Open University.

Thouless, R.H. (1974) *Straight and Crooked Thinking*. London: Pan.

REFERENCES

Alkon, D.L. (1983) Learning in a marine snail. *Scientific American*, **249**, 70–84.

Applyby, L. & Forshaw, D.M. (1990) *Postgraduate Psychiatry: Clinical and Scientific Foundations*. Oxford: Heinemann Medical.

Atkinson, R.L., Atkinson, R.C., Smith, E.E. & Hilgard, E.R. (1987) *Introduction to Psychology*, 9th edn. Florida: Harcourt Brace Jovanovich.

Beers, C.W. (1962) *A Mind that Found Itself*. New York: Doubleday.

Berlim, B. & Kay, P. (1969) *Basic Colour Terms: Their Universality and Evolution*. Los Angeles: University of California Press.

Berlyne, N. (1972) Confabulation. *British Journal of Psychiatry*, **120**, 285–292.

Bleuler, A. (1950). Translated by Zinkin, J. *Dementia Praecox or the Group of Schizophrenics*. New York: International University Press.

Bloom, L. (1970) *Language Development: Form and*

Function in Emerging Grammars. Cambridge, MA: MIT Press.

Bonhoeffer, K. (1909) Translated by Marshall, H. Exogenous psychoses. *Zentralblatt fur Nervenheilkunde*, **32**, 499–505. In Hirsch, S.R. & Shephard, M. (Eds) (1974) *Themes and Variations in European Psychiatry*. Bristol: John Wright.

Broadbent, D. (1958) *Perception and Communication*. Oxford: Pergamon.

Bronshtein, A.I. & Petrova, E.P. (1967) The auditory analyser in young infants. In Brackbill, Y. & Thompson, G. (Eds) *Behaviour in Infancy and Early Childhood*. New York: Free Press.

Brown, J. (1964) Short term memory. *British Medical Bulletin*, **20**, 8–11.

Brown, R. (1973) *A First Language: The Early Stages*. Cambridge, MA: Harvard University Press.

Bruner, J. (1983) *Child's Talk: Learning to Use Language*. New York: Norton.

Cameron, N. (1938) Reasoning, regression and communication in schizophrenics. *Psychological Monographs*, **50** (1).

Campbell, R.J. (1989) *Psychiatric Dictionary*, 5th edn. Oxford University Press.

Carmichael, L., Hogan, H.P. & Walter, A.A. (1932) An experimental study of the effect of language on the reproduction of visually perceived forms. *Journal of Experimental Psychology*, **15**, 73–86.

Carroll, J.B. (Ed.) (1956) *Language, Thought and Reality: Selected Writings of Benjamin Lee Whorf*. Cambridge, MA: MIT Press & Wiley.

Carroll, J.B. & Casagrande, J.B. (1958) The function of language classifications in behaviour. In Maccoby, E. *et al.* (Eds) *Readings in Social Psychology*, 3rd edn. New York: Holt.

Cicero, M.T. (1927) *Tusculan Disputations*, text and English translation. Cambridge, MA: Harvard University Press, Loeb Classical Library.

Chomsky, N. (1959) Review of Skinner (1957). *Language*, **35**, 26–58.

Chomsky, N. (1980) *Rules and Representations*. New York: Columbia University Press.

Chomsky, N. (1986) *Knowledge of Language: It's Nature, Origin and Use*. New York: Praeger.

Cohen, N.J. (1981) Neuropsychological evidence for a distinction between procedural and declarative knowledge in human memory and amnesia. Ph.D thesis, University of California.

Cohen, N.J. & Squire, L.R. (1980) Preserved learning and retention of pattern analysing skill in amnesia: dissociation of knowing how and knowing that. *Science*, **210**, 207–209.

Cohen, N.J. & Squire, L.R. (1981) Retrograde amnesia and remote memory impairment. *Neuropsychologia*, **19**, 337–356.

Crystal, D. (1984) *Who Cares about English Usage?* Harmondsworth: Penguin.

Curtiss, S. (1977) *Genie: A Psycholinguistic Study of a Modern-Day 'Wild Child'*. New York: Academic Press.

Curtiss, S. (1981) Feral children. In Wortis, J. (Ed.) *Mental Retardation and Developmental Disabilities*, Vol. xii. New York: Bruner/Mazel.

Davis, K. (1947) Final note on a case of extreme isolation. *American Journal of Sociology*, **45**, 554–565.

Dawson, M.E. & Schell, A.M. (1982) Electrodermal responses to attended and unattended significant stimuli during dichotic listening. *Journal of Experimental Psychology: Human Perception and Performance*, **8**, 82–86.

Dennis, W. (1941) Infant development under conditions of restricted practice and of minimal social stimulation. *Genetics of Psychology Monographs*, **23**, 143–189.

Dennis, W. (1960) Causes of retardation among institutional children: Iran. *Journal of Genetic Psychology*, **96**, 46–60.

Dennis, W. (1973) *Children of the Creche*. Englewood Cliffs, NJ: Appleton-Century-Crofts.

Deutsch, J.A. & Deutsch, D. (1963) Attention: some theoretical considerations. *Psychological Review*, **70**, 80–90.

Dodd, B. (1987) The acquisition of lip-reading skills by normally hearing children. In Dodd, B. & Campbell, R. (Eds) *Hearing by Eye: the Psychology of Lip-reading*. London: Erlbaum.

Douglas, J.E. & Sutton, A. (1978) The development of speech and mental processes in a pair of twins: a case study. *Journal of Child Psychology and Psychiatry*, **19**, 49–56.

Eysenck, H.J. & Wilson, G.D. (1973) *The Experimental Study of Freudian Theories*. London: Methuen.

Freeman, R.D. & Thibas, L.N. (1973) Electrophysiological evidence that abnormal early visual experience can modify the human brain. *Science*, **180**, 876–878.

Freud, S. (1922) *Introductory Lectures on Psycho-Analysis*, 10th impression. London: George Allen & Unwin.

Freud, S. (1986) *The Essentials of Psychoanalysis*. London: Pelican.

Gardner, H. & Roylance, P.J. (1982) *Developmental Psychology: An Introduction*. Boston: Little Brown.

Gesell, A. (1950) *The First Five Years of Life*. London: Methuen.

Globus, A., Rosenzweig, M.R., Bennett, E. &

Diamond, M.C. (1973) Effects of differential experience on dendritic spin counts in rat cerebral cortex. *Journal of Comparative Physiology and Psychology*, **82**, 175–181.

Glucksberg, S. (1962) The influence of strength of drive on functional fixedness and perceptual recognition. *Journal of Experimental Psychology*, **63**, 36–41.

Goldenson, R.M. & Barrows, H.S. (1984) *Longman's Dictionary of Psychology and Psychiatry*. New York: Longman.

Gopnik, A. & Meltzoff, A.N. (1985) From people, to plans, to objects. *Journal of Pragmatics*, **9**, 495–512.

Gray, J.A. & Wedderburn, A.A.I. (1960) Grouping strategies with simultaneous stimuli. *Quarterly Journal of Experimental Psychology*, **12**, 180–184.

Green, B. (1982) *Intensive Care for Neurological Trauma and Disease*. Orlando: Academic Press.

Greenough, W.T., West, R.W. & DeVoogd, T.J. (1978) Subsynaptic plate perforations: changes with age and experience in the rat. *Science*, **202**, 1096–1098.

Harlow, H.F. (1949) The formation of learning sets. *Psychological Review*, **56**, 51–65.

Heider, G.R. (1972) Universals in colour meaning and memory. *Experimental Psychology*, **93**, 10–20.

Hinchcliffe, S.M. & Montague, S.E. (1988) *Physiology for Nursing Practice*. London: Baillière Tindall.

Hubel, D.H. & Wiesel, T.N. (1979) Brain mechanisms of vision. *Scientific American*, **241**, 150–162.

Hudson, L. (1966) *Contrary Imaginations: A Psychological Study of English School Boys*. London: Metheun.

Huxley, J. (1969) *Evolution*. London: McDonald.

Hyams, N.M. (1986) *Language Acquisition and the Theory of Parameters*. Dordrecht: D. Reider.

Itard, J. (1801) In Maison, L. (Ed.) (1972) *The Wild Boy of Aveyron*. London: NLB.

Jakobson, R. (1968) Child language, aphasia and phonological universals. *Janua Lingaurum*, Series Minor, 72. The Hague: Mouton.

James, W. (1890) *The Principles of Psychology*. New York: Holt, Rinehart & Winston.

Jaspers, K. (1963) Translation by Hoenig, J. & Hamilton, M. *General Psychopathology*. Manchester: Manchester University Press.

Johnson-Laird, P.N. (1983) *Mental Models: Toward a Cognitive Science of Language, Inference, and Consciousness*. Cambridge, MA: Harvard University Press.

Kandel, E.R. & Schwartz, J.H. (1981) *Principles of Neural Science*. New York: Elsevier, North Holland.

Kandel, E.R. & Schwartz, J.H. (1982) Molecular biology of learning: modulation of transmitter release. *Science*, **218**, 433–442.

Kohler, W. (1925) *The Mentality of Apes*. New York: Harcourt Brace.

Kohler, W. (1952) *Gestalt Psychology*. London: Vision Press.

Koluchova, J. (1976) The further development of twins after severe and prolonged deprivation: a second report. *Journal of Child Psychology and Psychiatry*, **17**, 181–188.

Labov, W. (1973) The boundaries of words and their meanings. In Bailey, C.J.N. & Shuy, R.W. (Eds) *New Ways of Analysing Variations in English*. Washington, DC: Georgetown University Press.

Ladefoged, P. (1975) *A Course in Phonetics*. New York: Harcourt Brace Jovanovich.

Leask, J., Haber, R.N. & Haber, R.B. (1969) Eidetic imagery in children. *Psychonomic Monograph Supplements*, **3**, 25–48.

Lennenberg, E.H. (1967) *The Biological Foundations of Language*. New York: Wiley.

Lishman, W.A. (1987) *Organic Psychiatry: The Psychological Consequences of Cerebral Disorder*. Oxford: Blackwell.

Luchins, A.F. (1959) Primary–recency in impression formation. In Hovland, C.I. (Ed.) *The Order of Presentation in Persuasion*, New Haven: Yale University Press.

Luria, A. (1987) *The Mind of a Mnemonist: A Little Book about a Big Memory*. Cambridge, MA: Harvard.

Lyttle, J. (1986) *Mental Disorder: Its Care and Treatment*. London: Baillière Tindall.

Mackworth, N.H. (1950) Researches in the measurement of human performance. *MRC Special Report Series*, **268**. London: HMSO.

McCormick, D.A., Clark, G.A., Lavord, D.G. & Thompson, R.F. (1982) Initial localisation of the memory trace for a basic form of learning. *Proceedings of the National Academy of Science USA*, **79**, 2731–2735.

McGough, J.J. (1982) *Memory Consolidation*. Hillsdale, NJ: Lawrence Erlbaum.

McKellar, P. (1957) *Imagination and Thinking*. London: Cohen & West.

Menn, L. (1985) Phonological development: learning sounds and sound patterns. In Berko Gleason, J. (Ed.) *The Development of Language*. Columbus, OH: Merrill.

Milner, B. (1972) Disorders of learning and memory after temporal lobe lesions in Man. *Clinical Neurosurgery*, **19**, 421–446.

Mollgaard, K., Diamond, M.C., Bennett, E.K., Rosenweig, M.R. & Lindner, B. (1971) Quantitative synaptic changes with differential experience in rat brain. *International Journal of Neuroscience*, **2**, 113–128.

Moscovitch, M. (1981) Multiple dissociations in the amnesic syndrome. In Cermak, L.S. (Ed.) *Human Memory and Amnesia*. Hillsdale, NJ: Lawrence Erlbaum.

Neel, A.F. (1969) *Theories of Psychology*. London: University of London Press.

O'Keefe, J. & Nadel, L. (1978) *The Hippocampus as a Cognitive Map*. Oxford University Press.

Olton, D.S., Becker, J.T. & Handelman, G.R. (1980) Hippocampal function: working memory or cognitive mapping. *Physiological Psychology*, **8**, 239–246.

Oswald, I. (1960) Falling asleep open-eyed during intense rhythmic stimulation. *British Medical Journal*, **1**, 1450.

Pask, G. & Scott, B.C.E. (1972) Learning strategies and individual competence. *International Journal of Man Machines Studies*, **4** (3), 217–253.

Pavlov, I.P. (1927) *Conditioned Reflexes*. Oxford: Oxford University Press.

Piaget, J. (1967) *Play, Dreams and Limitation in Childhood*. New York: International University Press.

Piaget, J. (1968) Language and thought from the genetic point of view. In Piaget, J. (Ed.) *Six Psychological Studies*. London: University of London Press.

Pospesel, H. (1974) *Propositional Logic*. Englewood Cliffs, NJ: Prentice-Hall.

Professional Guide to Diseases (1989). Springhouse Corporation.

Provence, S. & Lipton, R.C. (1962) *Infants in Institutions: a Comparison of Their Development with Family Reared Infants During the First Year of Life*. New York: International University Press.

Rips, L.J. (1986) Deduction. In Sternberg, R.J. & Smith, E.E. (Eds) *The Psychology of Human Thought*. Cambridge: Cambridge University Press.

Rosch, E. (1973) On the internal structures of perceptual and semantic categories. In Moore, T.E. (Ed.) *Cognitive Development and the Acquisition of Language*. New York: Academic Press.

Rosch, E. (1975) Cognitive representations of semantic categories. *Journal of Experimental Psychology*, **104** (3), 192–233.

Rose, S.P.R., Bateson, P.P.G. & Horn, G. (1973) Experience and plasticity in the nervous system. *Science*, **181**, 506–514.

Rosenzweig, M.R. (1984) Experience, memory and the brain. *American Psychologist*, **49**, 150–162.

Rowland, C. (1983) Patterns of interaction between three blind infants and their mothers. In Mills, A.E. (Ed.) *Language Acquisition in the Blind Child: Normal and Deficient*. London: Croom Helm.

Ruger, H.A. (1910) The psychology of efficiency. *Archives of Psychology*, **19**, 15.

Sapir, E. (1949) *Language, Culture and Personality: Selected Essays*. Berkeley: University of California Press.

Salmon, W.C. (1973) *Logic*. Englewood Cliffs, NJ: Prentice-Hall.

Schneider, K. (1959) *Clinical Psychopathology*. New York: Grune.

Sergent, J. & Poncet, M. (1990) From covert to overt recognition of faces in a prosopagnosic patient. *Brain*, **113**, 989–1004.

Singh, J.A.L. & Zingg, R.M. (1942) *Wolf Children and Feral Man*. New York: Harper Bros.

Sirigu, A., Duhamel, J.R. & Poncet, M. (1991) The role of sensorimotor experience in object recognition. A case of multimodal agnosia. *Brain*, **114** (6), 2555–2573.

Skeels, H.M. (1966) Adult status of children with contrasting early life experiences: a follow up study. *Monographs of the Society for Research in Child Development*, **31**, 3.

Skuse, D. (1984) Extreme deprivation in early childhood 1. Diverse outcomes for three siblings from an extraordinary family. *Journal of Child Psychology and Psychiatry*, **25**, 523–541.

Skyrms, B. (1986) *Choice and Chance: An Introduction to Inductive Logic*. Belmont, CA: Dickenson.

Slobin, D. (1979) *Psycholinguistics*, 2nd edn. Glenview, IL: Foresman.

Squire, L.R. (1984) Memory and the brain. In Friedman, S. *et al.* (Eds) *Brain, Cognition and Education*. New York: Academic Press.

Stampe, D. (1969) The acquisition of phonemic representation. *Proceedings of the Vth Regional Meeting of the Chicago Linguistic Society*, 433–444.

Steiner, E. (1977) Criteria for theory of art education. Paper presented at the seminar for Research in Education, Philadelphia.

Steiner, E. (1978) *Logical and Conceptual Analytic Techniques for Educational Research*. Washington, DC: University Press.

Swanson, L.E., Teyler, T.J. & Thompson, R.F. (Eds) (1982) Hippocampal long-term potentiation: mechanisms and implications for memory. *Neurosciences Research Program Bulletin*, **20** (5). Cambridge, MA: MIT Press.

Thompson, A.M. (1986) Adam—a severely deprived Colombian orphan: a case report. *Journal of Child Psychology and Psychiatry*, **27**, 689–695.

Thompson, R.F., Berger, T. & Madden, J. (1983) Cellular processes of learning and memory in the mammalian CNS. *Annual Review of Neuroscience*, **6**, 447–491.

Titchener, E.B. (1909) *Lectures on Experimental Psychology of the Thought processes*. New York: MacMillan.

Tolman, E.B. (1932) *Purposive Behaviour in Animals and Men*. New York: Appleton Century.

Tomasello, M. & Farrar, M. (1984) Cognitive bases of lexical development: object permanence and relational words. *Journal of Child Language*, **11**, 477–495.

Tortora, G.J. & Anagnostakos, N.P. (1984) *Principles of Anatomy and Physiology*. New York: Harper & Row.

Treisman, A. (1964) Verbal cues, language and meaning in selective attention. *American Journal of Psychology*, **77**, 206–219.

Treisman, A. & Gelade, G. (1980) A feature integration theory of attention. *Cognitive Psychology*, **12**, 97–136.

Tulving, E. & Madigan, S.A. (1970) Memory and verbal memory. In Mussen, P.H. & Rosenzweig, M.R. (Eds) *Annual Review of Psychology*, **21**.

Tverskey, A. & Kahnemann, D. (1973) On the psychology of prediction. *Psychological Review*, **80**, 237–251.

Vygotsky, L.S. (1962) *Thought and Language*. Cambridge, MA: MIT Press.

Warren, H.C. (1921) *A History of the Association: Psychology*. New York: Scribners.

Wason, P.C. & Johnson-Laird, P.N. (1970) A conflict between selecting and evaluating information in an inferential task. *British Journal of Psychology*, **61**, 509–515.

Watson, R.I. (1963) *The Great Psychologists: From Aristotle to Freud*. Philadelphia: Lippincott.

Wells, G. (1985) *Language Development in the Preschool Years*. Cambridge: Cambridge University Press.

Wendt, H. (1972) *From Ape to Adam*. Thames & Hudson Ltd.

Werker, J.F. & Tees, R.C. (1985) Cross-language speech perception: evidence for perceptual reorganization during the first year of life. *Infant Behaviour and Development*, **7**, 49–63.

Wexler, B.E. (1988) Dichotic presentation as a method for single hemisphere stimulation studies. In Hugdahl, K. (Ed.) *Handbook of Dichotic Listening: Theory, Methods and Research*. Chichester: Wiley.

Wilde, O. (1969) *The Importance of Being Earnest*. In *Complete Plays*. London: Methuen.

Wilkinson, R.T. (1963) Interaction of noise with knowledge of results and sleep deprivation. *Journal of Experimental Psychology*, **66**, 332–337.

Woolsey, T.A. & Wann, J.R. (1976) Areal changes in mouse cortical barrels following vibrissal damage at different postnatal ages. *Journal of Comparative Neurology*, **170**, 53–66.

Zeki, S. (1991) Cerebral akinetopsia (visual motion blindness), a review. *Brain*, **114** (2), 811–824.

10

SHARING A COMMON LANGUAGE

F.C. Johnson and L.D. Smith

AIMS

i) To review the communication needs and norms of those significant in the care programme

ii) To interpret and give relevance to diagnostic categories utilized within psychiatry

iii) To explore the values and limitations of psychiatric diagnostic categories for all concerned

iv) To reaffirm the foci of client centred care in relation to each individual significant in care

KEY ISSUES

Individual and team perceptions of problems

Lay and professional communication and terminology

Labelling

ICD and DSM categories—a comparison

Common diagnostic categories

Treatment available

Identify, analyse and assess factors causing distress and illness	Promote health, provide direct care and make interventions	Manage care programmes and services
Be critical, analytical and accountable, continue professional development	Counter discrimination, inequality and individual and institutional racism	Work within and develop policies, laws and safeguards in all settings
Understand influences on mental health and the nature/causes of disorder and illness	Know the effects of distress, disorder, illness on individuals, groups, families	Understand the basis of treatments and interventions

INTRODUCTION

Perhaps the most valuable and effective manner to open a chapter such as this, is to use the words of an individual describing the care and treatment of a relative and the family's need for information during the period:

The consultant was, initially, very 'up front' and revealed the diagnosis to her and her husband straight away. He identified the need for surgery plus radiotherapy before any analysis was undertaken regarding the size or degree of invasion of the tumour. There were no options provided and no discussions relating to the merits or otherwise of the planned intervention. There were, therefore, no decisions to be made and the treatment went ahead.

I tried to prepare her for the potential side-effects of the radiotherapy, but the responsible medical officer informed her that she'd only be very sore, and that there would be no other detrimental effects. She didn't know who to believe, but preferred his version. Of course, when the first handful of hair lay on the pillow, she was devastated and by the time the nausea and vomiting was so severe that she was unable to tolerate even soda water, mistrust in the professionals began to creep in.

The mental health problems appeared almost overnight, immediately after the cessation of the radiotherapy. Hallucinations and delusional ideation were consistent with intense depression one moment and yet, intermittently, she demonstrated persecutory or grandiosed themes. She was agitated and confused, having no insight into the everyday dangers of the environment.

It seemed that there were several potential causative factors for the problems exhibited and the family really needed to know the 'culprit', to facilitate decision making and action planning for the future. If this was the original tumour, an extension or secondary growth from it, then this was an indicator of what the family could expect in the future, at best. We needed to be prepared for this and accept that she

would, perhaps, deteriorate further if the entire tumour had not been eradicated. We wondered if this was a more or less temporary phenomenon, created by the radiotherapy, or if, perhaps, she was experiencing the well-documented side-effects of the analgesia prescribed and again, should this be the case, this was a temporary problem and not indicative of a poor overall prognosis. This could, quite possibly, be a reaction to the news of the potential threat to life and living, in the form of diagnosis of malignant neoplasm, to the facial scarring and the loss of her feminine tresses. Whatever the cause, we needed to know, for no-one had offered any sort of indication as to the prognosis which could be expected. If it was to be grave in nature, we wanted to make the best of the time left and that included taking her home. She hated the hospital ward and was distressed to have to stay. The nurses were trained in the surgical specialty relevant to the ward, not mental health care, so there seemed little advantage in her remaining there, in regard to the latest sequelae. She didn't need somatic care as such.

In my opinion, the consultant was very hard on us. We had to ask very pointed questions and, whilst he eventually informed us of the very poor expected outcomes to the treatment, he only referred us to his associates—the other consultants involved, because of the nature of care—for the information we needed. He did inform us that at the time of surgery there was no apparent cerebral involvement, but felt unable to comment further.

The psychiatric opinion offered related to discontinuation of the potentially offending analgesia and commencement of a low dosage of a major tranquillizer, to ameliorate symptomatology presenting.

A lot more water has flowed under the bridge since that point, but, obviously cachexic, she's now at home, with the family none the wiser as to what is actually happening to her. The mental health problems are controlled with medication and so she's not distressed at all. The pain is relatively well controlled, so I suppose we can't hope for anymore.

I am disappointed in my health care colleagues. As a professional nurse, in addition to a relative, it seemed to be grossly unfair that I should be aware of the prognosis before she or her husband were, and merely because of my previous experiences. It was hard on me, because in knowing what I would be expecting within this situation, and then the actuality not meeting those expectations, I was in the position of either having to collude with the medical staff by staying silent, or risk them looking inept or dishonest in their dealings with my family by stating objections to the activities and mode of management employed. As it was, by trying to gain the best of both worlds, I achieved little bar upsetting doctors and instilling gross mistrust in the family, of all professionals.

I expected an analysis of the extent of the tumour initially and in the light of findings, sensible options put forward in regard to various treatments and their potential sequelae. With such a poor prognosis generally, as a professional, one would need to question the value to the client of extensive surgery when palliative interventions may be less distressing for the individual and of equal effect in prolonging life. Certainly the quality of life, and the individual's participation in making decisions related to that quality of life, should, in my view, be paramount in such situations. She and the family were at the mercy of the medical staff. She was 'treated' by the experts, who 'know best', there was no inclusion, no opportunity to control or influence proceedings. Having heard of similarly distressing mental health sequelae in others who had the same surgery performed, one must sincerely question the value of surgery to the individuals concerned.

I expected that she and her husband would be kept informed of what was happening and why it should be so, but I was disappointed. I certainly expected the several consultants involved in her care to hold a case conference and communicate with each other regarding specialist input given in the total care provided. It was more than obvious, however, that there was little collaboration except via formal letters. The 'left hand was rarely aware of what the right hand was doing', as one consultant would make a decision, completely contradictory to that of another of his colleagues.

I had expectations that any form of treatment or care provided would be evaluated in the light of results achieved, whether that be by medical, nursing, or any other professional group undertaking the activity, but that certainly didn't appear the case here. Where multidisciplinary care was being provided, one would have expected a multidisciplinary team approach to planning and evaluating total care, but the nurses on the ward asked us for information, not the other way around, in regard to the progress of the tumour. They had no more data than we did.

I suppose my greater knowledge and enhanced expectations engender the greater disillusionment I feel, in comparison to the rest of the family. Where they feel anger, I feel hurt and ashamed of the professions involved, I suppose, because of the vested interest and personal efforts made over the years, within professional activities.

Whilst the family have come to terms with the fact that someone who is very loved amongst them is dying, that is down to their own observations rather than to professional advice. There seems an unwillingness on the part of the doctors to admit the fact, though when pushed they will allude to death as an 'if the worst comes to the worst she'd be better off at home' sort of possibility. We're making the best of an awful situation, responding on a day-to-day basis in regard to problems encountered within her care.

I don't believe the family will ever really trust the health care professionals again, and that includes me. They have learned to demand answers and attempt to ask the appropriate questions in an area where they have no

knowledge or expertise. But, at what cost to the one we love?
Personal communication

The comments reproduced above represent one person's perceptions and views concerning a relative's care and management. They may be significantly biased and therefore reflect unjustly on the professionals concerned, for a variety of reasons. The reality of the situation, the degree of objectivity attained by the participant and the fairness or otherwise of the comments made are of little importance as we have no wish to validate or legitimize the particular and individual details of the experience recounted. We do wish, though, to use the above as an example of the perceptions and interpretations of events which *may* be made during care management. It is of great value in regard to many aspects of the ensuing discussion concerning the communication rights and needs of individuals significant with health care delivery and is hence utilized to guide the following text.

THE PATIENT'S RIGHTS

The central focus of all care delivery and management is necessarily upon the individuals who are experiencing the health related difficulties. It is of paramount importance that health care personnel remember that such health care difficulties 'belong' to the individuals concerned. They are their problems, their experiences and their symptoms. Individuals should be responsible for their own health and well-being. Health care personnel only provide services which may, or may not, be valuable in assisting the individual to restore the optimum level of health available, within prevailing circumstances. An analogy may be of use here to set an appropriate perspective of the client–professional relationship:

Individuals experiencing problems with a piece of household equipment will, if unable to effect a safe repair themselves and if they have any insight into the presence and potential repercussions of the malfunction, seek the services of

---

someone with a greater knowledge and expertise in the relevant area.

They have the right to expect a competent and skilled performance from individuals offering themselves up as advisers and service providers in this situation and may check that the providers are appropriately recognized as such by peers and relevant 'approving' bodies. The purchaser has the right to expect the service to be provided by competent practitioners, or those designated as equally skilled, and would, most likely, consider it unacceptable for the work to be undertaken by an inexperienced apprentice.

The purchaser similarly expects to be provided with an analysis of the extent of the mechanical problem, though this may, of necessity, be a provisional judgement and not exact in nature until the equipment has been stripped down and examined more closely. At that point, however, an estimate in the degree of work required to render the equipment fully functioning, options worth considering in relation to the work and a quotation regarding the projected cost to the individual would be expected.

Should the purchasers believe the cost of the work to be beyond that which they are willing to pay, that replacement of the equipment may be a more cost-effective option or that the charge is too high for the work involved, they have the right to review their options in the light of the skilled advice provided. They are not, however, obliged to purchase the service if it fails to meet their needs or expectations in any way, or if they consider the action too expensive. They have the right to make judgements regarding the relative value of advice offered, and take responsibility for those judgements.

The client–professional relationship should be based upon similar principles, for health care personnel only provide services in the same way as a plumber, electrician or heating engineer provides a service that is reliant on the consumer expressing a need for such a service. At times it is difficult to envisage the factors operating which have elevated one service provider so much above others in status, and whilst this may have been acceptable in the past, it can no longer be the case. Of course, we would admit that health is not a piece of machinery able to be replaced, and would, therefore, consider it too precious a commodity to be unconditionally relinquished into the hands of another, no matter how skilled or well meaning that individual may be. The right to be given 'a clear explanation of any treatment proposed, including any risks and alternatives, before you decide whether you will agree to the treatment' is identified within the Patient's Charter (DH, 1991) as one of seven 'well established rights' to which the Government was to add three more on 1 April 1992. Another of those seven rights relates to the individual's ability to choose to participate in medical research and medical student training and the remaining ones identify entitlements to access to health care services and to personal health records, with respect to which it is confirmed that NHS personnel 'are under a legal duty to keep their contents confidential'. This latter, and important point, will be returned to below but, for the present, we wish to concentrate upon the issues of rights to information relating to treatment and that of choosing to participate in research and training activities.

Whilst every household has received a copy of the Patient's Charter, this does not guarantee that everyone has read it, and that is, of course, the prerogative of each recipient. Of those who did peruse its contents, how many could be assumed to have internalized their rights to the extent that they would be able to evoke them automatically in a health crisis? It's hard to judge, but of those who are aware of their rights, how many *would* actually evoke them, and take the risk of casting doubts upon the quality of advice/instruction given by the all powerful and infallible, 'curer of all ills'. Whilst any fragment of such a perception remains within the general population, it may be unreasonable to expect the public to assert their rights, and demand relevant information. There is, of course, always a fear of the possibility of reprisals in the minds of those who do insist upon the fulfilment of their rights, and, in the situation where personal health and well-being, or that of someone close and loved, is at stake, it is a risk that for many is not worth contemplating. As pro-

fessionals, nurses and other health care providers would automatically defend colleagues as incapable of such behaviour and yet responses to the 'unco-operative' or 'non-compliant' individuals have long since been recognized and documented (Stockwell, 1984). Sad as it may seem, it may be a genuine fear experienced by the individual seeking care, which relates to the potential for a second class professional reaction to the assertion of rights.

A more effective way of facilitating communication and the sharing of all appropriate and relevant information may be achieved by awarding a joint responsibility to both partners within the interaction for the activity. Whether the client asks the 'right' questions to elicit necessary data or not, the professional should provide that information as an integral part of each consultation— it should reflect a professional, inescapable and unavoidable duty implicit in the contract with the client. We have noted in our travels, posters within hospital corridors and waiting rooms which identify the standards, both nationally and locally ascribed, relating to particular aspects of care management and organization. However it would be a brave, forthright and innovative care provider who handed a copy of those expectations to the client immediately prior to seeing the responsible medical officer, along with guidelines relating to examples of some of the questions which it may be prudent to ask the professional. Similarly, a large poster, positioned behind the consultant's head, in direct line of vision of the client, in every consulting and examination room, bearing the words:

You have the right to know:

1 The nature of your problem

2 Its cause and continuing effects on you

3 Treatments available and outcomes associated with each

4 My considered opinion of the best of those alternatives for you and why that is so

Please ask me if you are unclear about any of the above

---

may help to remind both parties of the appropriate client–professional relationship and prompt information passage. It would certainly boost the client's confidence within the situation, by provision of an implicit permission to ask and be given data.

Within the Patient's Charter, however, there is no right to know the diagnosis made by the consultant. There is currently only a requirement to explain 'any treatment proposed, risks and any alternatives', and if consultants should decide that there is no real option to the treatment proposed, they may see fit to exercise their professional judgement and provide information only relating to the treatment of their choice. Thus patients have a limited 'right' as it stands, and it relies too heavily upon the consultant's interpretation of a relatively vague statement.

This, of course, opens up the whole debate regarding 'what to tell the patient?', which is long running and vehemently argued. Professionals who make judgements regarding an individual's ability to 'cope' with negative or distressing information, may do that individual a grave disservice, if they consciously deprive him/her of the opportunity to take control of, and direct, activities that influence the quality of life and living. People will cope with the most horrendous news if they are prepared, supported and cared for during the process; the proof lies within the success of hospice care. Surely, if the worse-case scenario occurred, and the individual 'didn't cope', isn't the role of the professional to help them cope; to educate and assist, in the development and implementation of plans and strategies to optimize the management of life and living? To draw relatives into collusion activities seems even more controversial and places great pressure on those concerned, as indicated by the relative's account at the beginning of this chapter, and why should the relatives be able 'to cope' more appropriately and effectively than the individual? It may be considered immoral to introduce such deceit and dishonesty into a relationship, at a point when its days may be numbered.

Many doctors will admit to the paucity of education and training within the area of giving information and those who seek further experience are the wise ones. Whatever the factors influencing communication contents and the levels of skills employed within the process, they require addressing within both initial and continuing medical training. It is, of course, difficult when one is viewed as the 'curer of all ills' to admit impotence or inadequacy in regard to a specific client's care and treatment, when such admission may herald death or, worse in our view, a prolonged, painful and debilitated future. Sometimes one considers that there may be a fear of getting the diagnosis or prognosis wrong and of the repercussions of such an error. Perhaps it is just a lack of the appropriate skills to engender confidence in one's own abilities to be the bearer of bad tidings and manage the implications of such news to the benefit of the client. Maybe it is a defence to protect self. Certainly the nurse finds a potential dilemma, when charged by the code of professional conduct to engender partnerships in care and negotiate actions and outcomes, rather than dependency and compliance (UKCC, 1992). This is not possible when one party is in possession of information pertinent to care and influential in the decision-making processes that the other party is unaware of. This would be no partnership and any negotiation undertaken would be meaningless. Of course plumbers, electricians or mechanics, do not have such problems. They offer to do their best within the situation presenting but may be unable to guarantee to restore the equipment to its original status, particularly if the machinery is old, the problem unusual or the parts hard to come by. Sometimes, one has to admit that a problem is 'irreparable' but it would be a dishonest worker who asserted that the machinery had been repaired in that situation or refused to impart the status of the situation.

In regard to the 'right to know', great hope and optimism can be held out in the light of a private member's bill on this subject, laid before the House of Commons by the Stoke Central MP, Mark Fisher (Campaign for Freedom of Information, 1992). However, whilst there is much contained within it which will enhance information availability in regard to many areas of health and health care, on this specific issue of focus, there is only a requirement for accessibility to medical records predating November 1991, where current access is to material added since that date. Even then the proposed bill identifies exemptions to that availability and the one of particular reference here is that such information:

---

may be withheld, if disclosure would be likely to cause serious harm to the applicant's health.

Though in accordance with both the Access to Health Records Act 1990 (HMSO, 1990) and the Data Protection Act 1984, and whilst it would be possible to appeal against a decision to withhold that material, yet again someone—probably a member of the medical profession—other than the individual will be making a decision on what will or will not constitute 'serious harm' to health! The proposed bill would give individuals the right to access information that directly affects them and which relates to a variety of issues and activities of everyday life, and, as such, is laudable. However, if people are to be given the right to information regarding, say, the effects of certain Government policies, or the level of safety achieved by the local railway station, and be trusted to utilize such information to their advantage, why should they be deprived of the right to decide for themselves whether personal health details may 'damage their health'.

In regard to the right to 'opt out' of medical research and medical student training activities, the former would appear to be relatively well safeguarded by the invaluable work undertaken by ethical committees. They rely, of course, on being informed of proposed research, its nature and parameters, and the potential effects on the participating population. In addition, the committee requires to be convinced of the benefits to be accrued by such activities. However, in relation to the right to opt out of medical student training, several problems can be envisaged. The first of such problems relates to the recognition of the status of an individual who is involved within the environment, for anyone walking around toting a stethoscope and wearing a white coat is assumed, by the seeker of care, to be a doctor. Male nurses, wearing uniform, are frequently mistaken as such, despite the adornment of a badge, a couple of inches long, stating name and

'rank'. Perhaps an instantly recognizable differentiation by appearance, such as with nurse–students, would facilitate the individual perceiving a difference between those participating in care, and prompt inquiry as to the relative experience of the individual. Many clients will ask about the different uniforms worn by nurses, but to be absolutely certain, perhaps that brave and innovative health authority that we referred to earlier may see fit to issue information to attenders of the various facilities relating to that colour coding system used, and again display appropriate posters on service area walls. The practice of providing 'mug-shots' of the staff who may be encountered within an area is a laudable idea, but requires constant adjustment and renewal in the face of staff changes.

Of course, within mental health care, uniformed staff are more rare and therefore the badge system, the 'mug-shot' board and the willingness of personnel to inform clients of their identity and areas of competence, within the overall care delivery, is vital. The really brave authority may find it useful to indicate those individuals who are deemed competent and sufficiently experienced to deal with all aspects of, for example, medical, nursing or other specific care activities, and assert the clients' right to care by those individuals, or by personnel being directly and continuously supervised, in practice, by those individuals. Utopia? Perhaps, but every individual should have the right to health care delivery provided by skilled and experienced personnel who have been recognized as such by an appropriate authorizing body. Those who are in the process of acquiring such skills and competence require to practice under close and full tuition and support. No one has the right to inflict any member of the public with an apprentice-level, unsupervised service. It would not be acceptable with the household plumbing and should certainly not be acceptable within the health care provision.

Where does the onus of responsibility lie for notifying the client of the student's status and reaffirming the right to request him or her to be excluded from ensuing activities. Is it the responsibility of the student, prior to the commencement of the planned procedure or activity, or perhaps of the consultant at the same juncture? Or is there the expectation that the client will ask for the identity and relative status of each individual participating in care? Of course, for the client to make such a request, there must be an awareness of the potential for such to occur and, as previously stated, if someone is dressed like a doctor, why should he or she be assumed as less than so?

One wonders why other students within the health care professions have been excluded from this right of the patient to 'opt out'. Are student nurses, for example, less of a potential threat and less able to wreak havoc to health than the medical student? Are they less likely to do the client harm within the process of acquiring the skills inherent in professional practice, and, if that should be the case, why should it be so? Equally, student nurses could be considered to be a potential danger to clients, due to their close and prolonged daily contact and because of the hazards implicit in activities conducted during that time. Something so basic within nursing activities as lifting, moving and positioning a client, something performed maybe a dozen or more times a day on one individual alone, may potentially damage the client—and the nurse—for life. This is just one example of the potential damage to the health and wellbeing of the client. Errors in administration of diets and medication may have a profound effect on physical well-being, just as incorrect information and inadequate support may induce prolonged psychological distress and distrust.

Consider students of physiotherapy and the 'damage potential' during their acquisition of competency to practice. Similarly, students of clinical psychology, pharmacology, dietetics, radiography and the rest, may all engender risk to the client, so why should medical students be singled out as 'different'? Could it be that they are considered more 'important' than the others, or worthy of special consideration? Why should the vulnerable public not be protected from all unqualified personnel?

Of course, it is not solely unqualified staff who may influence the client's experience of health care provision, Should there not be the right to refuse to be treated by inexperienced, though qualified, personnel? The 'junior' doctor undertaking a six-month experience in one specialty or another cannot be considered competent to direct or undertake care without supervision from individuals appropriately qualified and experienced within that field. Similarly, the nurse with a basic qualification in adult, somatic care should not be considered competent to care for neonates or children, those primarily experiencing problems associated with learning disability or mental health, or any other specialty area. They have a basic education in the broad principles of one field and with one client group, and, whilst the skills acquired may be valuable in another specialty, they should not be assumed to imply competency within that field. The client should have the right to be cared for by an appropriately qualified, or approved, and experienced professional.

If we are serious in our assertions regarding patient's rights, partnerships and client-centred care provision, and our activity in this area is not just a superficial veneer of change to pacify activists, greater thought and appropriate, meaningful action is required to facilitate sensible, logical and consistent planning and implementation of appropriate activities to prompt and support that change. Clients need to know and no one should have the power to deprive them of health-related information.

CARERS' NEEDS FOR INFORMATION

What then do relatives need to know regarding a family member's health status and action to be taken? The answer must come back as 'the same' and yet they have no right to such information unless permission has been sought of the client and has been granted. The exception, of course, relates to the legal parent of the minor or the designated guardian, in various other circumstances. The client is entitled, by law, to confidentiality regarding his or her personal health details, and this is similarly a requirement of the code of professional conduct for nurses (UKCC, 1992). Yet again this right is taken lightly for, unless a client specifically states otherwise, health care personnel automatically involve relatives in care management, revealing details or problems experienced and/or action to be initiated, and sometimes to a greater extent or depth than has been provided to the client himself. The situation whereby the consultant and relatives collude in keeping information from a client has already been discussed, but where, within such a situation, do the client's rights to confidentiality of information figure? It is the right and responsibility of the client, with assistance and support, education and facilitation by professionals where necessary, to impart information to his family members to the degree considered appropriate. The presence of the professional may be valuable during such information sharing and personal disclosure and indeed the client may choose to pass the responsibility for this to the professional. The latter, however, may not be the most therapeutic way of managing the situation, for repeating information and discussing it with others may assist the client greatly in managing the reality of the situation and hence accepting it. Avoidance of reality is not valuable to the client and whilst professional assistance may be necessary initially to facilitate accommodation and acceptance prior to disclosure, again this is what the professionals should be doing, rather than removing unpleasant responsibilities from the client. Professionals should be asking permission from the client prior to disclosure of any specific details of health status, but wherever possible, because these problems 'belong' to the clients, they should be the primary source for information required by relatives.

Client care should be delivered within a multidisciplinary, co-ordinated and focused framework and whilst every member of the team may not be inputting into a client's care, the observations, reflections and objective analysis which those professionals are able to offer may be invaluable to those personnel directly involved in care delivery. Without an overall insight into the problems experienced by the client, a professional is unable to analyse the values to the client of the skills and resources that are implicit or associated with his specialist role and function in health care delivery. Thus beneficial or advantageous services may be unavailable within total client care directly due to ineffective communication amongst pro-

fessionals. The days should be long since past when the consultant referred a client to another 'team player' for treatment of a specialist nature, though, of course, investigative procedures are still requested mainly by this method. The physiotherapist, occupational and speech therapist, clinical psychologist and similar care team members need to make their own assessment of client needs within their specific parameters of knowledge and expertise, following a general problem identification within the multidisciplinary team setting. This then facilitates action planning to meet needs, in collaboration and negotiation with the client by the responsible practitioner, and subsequent implementation of that action. The team's general and broad discussions may be seen then to generate specific and relevant attention from those with the necessary skills to assist the client. Feedback to the team ensures an awareness of the nature of interventions and resources utilized by all team members, and not just each care provider, thus facilitating cohesion of plans and actions and preventing omissions or duplications in service delivery. The 'right hand knows what the left hand is doing'—a need identified by the relative at the commencement of the chapter. Where a true multidisciplinary framework of care provision is utilized, with all professionals assuming an equal status within the group because of their specific roles, skills and functions, effective communication between professionals is built in, and should not be a cause for concern or dispute.

ENGENDERING UNDERSTANDING

If all of the above had been standard practice, would the relative, whose words opened this chapter, have perceived care management as more effective and able to meet both client and family's needs? One has to presume so, according to the expectations expressed. However, we would add a rider, in the form of the *terminology* used within care settings and delivery. Brown (1973) asserts that, to qualify as a language, any system of communication needs to fulfil three criteria:

1 *Semanticity*—symbolic representations used to convey meaning must denote the same meaning to all users of the language

2 *Displacement*—that the mode of communication used includes the facility to relate to past, present and future tenses

3 *Productivity*—a facility for combination of a limited number of words, or symbols, in an unlimited number of ways, or uses

Terminology used by medical personnel, and absorbed into the language of other professional carers, is, in most cases, unintelligible and meaningless to the rest of society. Exceptions to this are those words that are used by both professional and lay sections of society, but with each group applying a different interpretation or meaning to the term.

Within somatic care, the word 'tumour' automatically is called to mind. If mentioned within a medical consultation as a 'diagnosis', health professionals and others with knowledge of the field would, probably, wait to panic until they had heard the word 'malignant' or until they had been informed of the degree of accessibility attributed to a benign overgrowth of tissue. This, however, is solely dependent upon the fact that those involved have a basic insight into the area under discussion, which enables them to make such judgements relating to 'when to panic'. To the average person, a 'tumour' is synonymous with 'cancer' and death, and they are unable to differentiate between the harmful and relatively harmless examples encountered. The word 'growth' or phrase 'new growth' conjures up similar associations.

The term 'abortion', to the average person, is an alternative to continuing with a pregnancy. It is construed as a deliberate and intentional cessation of foetal life and is often accompanied by high emotion and perceptions of 'criminal activity'. Clients refer to their experiences of 'miscarriages', to infer a natural, unintentional interruption of pregnancy and the public response to 'miscarriage' is entirely different to that of abortion. There's a great deal of hand-patting or squeezing, expressed sympathy and profound sorrow at the event, and, whilst it may represent as unwanted a pregnancy as many of those therapeutically terminated, affected individuals are wished 'better luck next time'. Even the term 'termination' is very negative when applied to the interruption of a pregnancy. The word 'abortion' is still frequently used by professionals, and, whilst other terminology may be added to clarify the 'type' of abortion, such as 'incomplete', 'missed', 'therapeutic' or 'threatened', it creates an opportunity for misinterpretation and potential distress and unhappiness for many, who may feel wrongly accused of disposing of a baby.

The terminology used within the mental health care specialty is probably more, rather than less, open to such misinterpretation. Mention the word 'schizophrenia' to many within the general population and they will respond with explanations of 'split personality' or 'Jekyll and Hyde' behaviours. Similarly, lay individuals use the term 'hysterical' to describe the weeping, wailing, over-emotional and over-reacting acquaintance, and the word 'senile', as a derogatory descriptor applied to anyone over the age of 65 years, who does not behave in a manner desired by the younger observer. The words 'obsessive' and 'neurotic' are often levelled as accusations to those who are particular or pedantic in habits, whilst the term 'psychopath' is retained for any passing murderer, paedophile or rapist.

With such obvious a mismatch in terminology utilized by professionals and the meanings ascribed by society in general, one wonders as to the continuing value of medical terminology. Certainly within mental health care, there are difficulties not only within professional–lay communications, for the Mental Health Act 1983 evokes similar difficulties for professionals (Gostin, 1983). Although operational for only a decade, the Act maintains definitions for terms such as 'mental disorder', 'mental illness' and 'psychopathic disorder', words that many professionals would refuse to use. The debate continues, for example, as to the existence of this thing 'mental illness', which will find further discussion later within this chapter, and, perhaps because of the connotations inferred within general language, the term 'psychopath' has long since found replacement with the equally derogatory term 'personality disorder' and an appropriate descriptor, for example, hystrionic, dependent or sadistic.

The intra-professional dispute continues within mental health care, as exposed by studies such as that by Dean *et al.* (1983) which compared research diagnostic systems and the results generated by their use. It would appear that, even where diagnostic categories are accepted and agreed between professionals, there may be disagreement with regard to which individuals, within a sample, are 'ill' and the way in which they are 'ill'. Dean and his colleagues demonstrated the fact that, whilst two commonly used methods of assessment yield prevalence rates, for anxiety and depression, which were not too dissimilar from each other, the degree of a 'match' attained in the selection of the same individuals as 'cases' or 'non-cases', and, in the assignment of a similar diagnostic label, was poor. Whilst the period of time allocated to the task of data collection varied with each assessment technique utilized and hence may account for some of the discrepancy seen in the labelling of symptomatology observed or elicited, it is of great concern that the same individuals were not identified by both systems as in need of assistance.

Thus, according to which system of diagnostic labelling is in use by the psychiatrist, a single client may, or may not, be viewed as in need of 'treatment'. There are two diagnostic categorization systems available to the practitioner. The first, published by the World Health Organization, is the *International Classification of Disease*, now in its tenth edition and hence referred to as *ICD 10* (WHO, 1988). The second, compiled by the American Psychiatric Association is termed the *Diagnostic and Statistical Manual*, which is now in its third edition and a revised form, referred to as *DSM IIIR* (American Psychiatric Association, 1987). In *ICD 10*, for example, an individual must have experienced the 'menu' of appropriate symptomatology for 'several weeks' before the application of the label 'generalized anxiety disorder', The *DSM IIIR* categorization system requires the presence of a similar 'menu' of symptoms for six months before the label is awarded. Such a basic discrepancy between the point at which an individual is considered to become 'ill', is common when comparing the two systems. Whilst the major categories of each system correspond, the *ICD 10* has subdivisions within each major category which describe the varying features that may be viewed by the observing psychiatrist. These varying features include additional symptomatology and the severity and course of problems experienced. An analogy that comes to mind is that of a plain omelette equating with the major category, with the addition of cheese, or mushrooms, or ham being recognized as such on the menu, that is an omelette with cheese, etc. The *DSM IIIR* system, on the contrary, would be very prescriptive in its definition of an 'omelette' and where much was added to its definition would insist on it being recognized as a separate major category—within the menu offered, for example, that it is a cheese omelette.

ICD 10 Menu

1 Omelettes—plain, cheese, ham, mushroom

2 Potatoes—boiled,   chipped,   sautéed, mashed

DSM IIIR Menu
1 Omelette

2 Cheese omelette

3 Ham omelette

4 Mushroom omelette

5 Potatoes—boiled

6 Chipped potatoes

7 Sautéed potatoes

8 Mashed potatoes

In such a situation, *DSM IIIR* would assert that two categories of 'illness' are present simultaneously, for example, 'a major depressive episode' and an 'undifferentiated somatoform disorder', though the severity of both sets of symptoms would need to meet the appropriate criteria to be labelled as such. However, *ICD 10* would assert the client to be experiencing 'moderate depression with somatic symptoms'. *DSM IIIR* was published in 1987, and a fourth edition is now awaited, whilst *ICD 10* was published in 1988. The former is less unwieldy—and daunting—and hence is easier to use. Perhaps this, in part, explains its increasing popularity with clinicians.

The same difficulties within the terminology and diagnoses used by medical practitioners are not as prevalent within somatic care. The diagnostic labels of 'thyrotoxicosis', 'myocardial infarction' and 'cerebral haemorrhage', for example, would rarely represent a fertile area for dispute. The organs and systems of the body are relatively well-known territory, in that the 'normal parameters' associated with size, shape, position, function and interaction with other systems within health have been investigated and documented over many years, and with the continuing benefit of advancing technology. The science has moved on considerably since the second century, Greek physician, Galen asserted that physical function and illness were dependent upon the distribution of the 'four humours', though his beliefs went relatively unquestioned for 1500 years. Whilst 'total' knowledge in somatic care may have to await further technological advances, because, for example, the liver's functions are known, their dysfunction is easily recognized. There may be dispute regarding aetiology of a problem or its most effective treatment, but the actual malfunction is usually comparatively obvious.

A ROSE BY ANY OTHER NAME ...?

All individuals use at least one form of 'linguistic shorthand' in their incorporation of concepts into communication. Words such as 'plants', 'animals', 'cars' and 'clothes' form an integral aspect of language, and, as long as the individual is conversing with another English speaker, there is usually no problem, for most people will possess a common understanding of the parameters of such words. Individuals also acquire other forms of 'linguistic shorthand' relevant only to the specific subcultures of which they are a part. The term

'albatross'' would mean the name of a large seabird to many of the population, yet to a golfer it represents the term for getting a ball into the appropriate hole, using only a restricted and prescribed number of hits or strokes. It is a form of shorthand used to express particular characteristics of the game. The footballer talks of 'offside' and 'pass-back' decisions, the tennis player of 'lobs' and 'aces' and the cricketer of 'silly mid-off' and 'maidens'. Each is an important differentiation to be made within the game for those who are connoisseurs and those who hope to be. Part of the game is the language used to describe it and an individual will not be accepted as a fan, a player or an expert without its acquisition.

Sports and leisure activities provide only one example of subcultures evident within society, and those relating, say, to the youth of the population provide another valuable instance. Along with wearing the *right* clothes with the *right* labels, and going to the *right* venues with the *right* people or group, there is the need to use the *right* phrases or sayings which form the 'language' of the moment for that group and which differentiate members from those of other gangs. Of course, it is not only the young who have such specific criteria for group membership, for most people would understand the characteristics associated with the 'yuppy' and the 'wrinkley'! The nature of employment, too, proffers the opportunity for the development and use of a specific linguistic shorthand, and whether it is an architect extolling the virtues of 'perpendicular' over 'Norman' constructional styles, the geologist discussing 'platetechtonics' or 'sedimentary rock formation' or the computer analyst's 'bit', 'byte' and 'ram', every occupational group does it.

It has a value to the group, of course, in that it provides a rapid indicator of who is 'in' or 'outside' of the group, that is, who is 'one of us' and therefore may be admitted to the benefits brought by membership. The fake, or pretender, can usually be identified as an interloper and dealt with appropriately because of his or her inability to interpret and respond to questions posed. It similarly represents one aspect of the 'ceremony' of induction to the group, a hurdle to be overcome prior to acceptance into the group entity, and provides evidence that not just any old 'novice' can perform at a level deemed satisfactory to the standards imposed by the group members. It may serve to elevate the status of the group in the eyes of society by exhibiting the 'ultra-technical' nature of the content of activities and/or discussions, thereby excluding the faint-hearted or otherwise unsuitable candidate from even considering an attempt to apply for membership! Yet, in other situations, it may serve to engender mystique and intrigue, or enhance the power potential of the group, because of this exclusivity of understanding of intrinsic activities, their processes and characteristics as evinced by the terminology used.

Of course, there is a down-side to the use of linguistic shorthand and one aspect of this may be *because* it is only understood by those within the circle. The technical nature evinced may deter what may have been very willing and capable 'converts', as demonstrated by those who refuse to involve themselves in, for example, computers, because of a lack of understanding of terminology used. Some individuals may be unwilling to offer more than a passing attempt towards competency or literacy, because they feel overwhelmed by the language used by the expert or teacher. It may be considered to be beyond their level of understanding and therefore novices may avoid further exposure. For others, inattention and disinterest—even boredom—may be the response of the uninitiated, who feel excluded from the group but do not deem the gains to be of a sufficient level to impress them with the values to be awarded on achievement, or find the area of focus of little relevance or worth within their current experiences of life and living. Anxiety may be engendered on the part of the novice, or temporary participant within group activities, thereby inhibiting understanding further and reducing optimum levels of performance. Fear of exposure as 'incompetent' and therefore increasing feelings of vulnerability, may prevent continual requests for clarification or explanation. Self esteem and confidence levels plummet as the novice gets further and further behind in the expected outcomes associated with the activity, merely because the foundations supplied by this initial learning have not been successfully laid and hence application to practice cannot be understood and

therefore internalized. Similarly misunderstandings may occur, as both parties infer a different meaning to terminology utilized. At the most innocent level:

First person:	I had a great round today! Best ever.
Second person:	Good, I'm pleased.
First person:	Did myself a bit of good with the boss, too. I could see he was impressed when I hit an albatross at the fourth.
Second person:	I do wish you wouldn't go shooting. You know I don't like it—it's cruel! Anyway, I thought you were playing golf today?

Medical terminology and categorization represents just one more example of a linguistic shorthand, which has been developed and is utilized by just one more professional group, and, as such, should be of no more importance or significant than 'computer-speak'. As a form of *intra-professional communication* it is therefore of value, but only in situations where the categories utilized and the parameters of each can be agreed. In mental health care, the Dean *et al* (1983) study, amongst others, has signified that this is not so, and therefore its value as a shorthand means of communication is suspect. Semanticity is not evident.

Similarly, categorization and diagnosis may be suggested as the facilitator of advances in knowledge and treatment. If every client was viewed as 'truly' unique, groups of individuals eliciting 'similar problems' would not be available to researchers, and hence no common biopsychosocial evidence would be collated upon which to formulate, test and evaluate hypotheses relating to aetiology, course, treatment response or prognosis. Within somatic health care, such patterning of problems does tend to be demonstrated by individuals, and advances have been forthcoming within the area. It cannot be demonstrated to have been as successful within the field of learning disability, where even today, aetiology of problems experienced is only discernible in one-third of those affected, or within mental health care, where progress within this area is equally slow. Whilst not experienced or authoritative within the sphere of learning disability, we believe that a substantial reason for the singular lack of success within the investigation of mental health problems may have been directly due to the penchant evinced, by those involved, for looking for differences rather than similarities both within the client group and in relation to those considered mentally well within society. There is still no definition of the line at which 'wellness' ends and 'madness' begins and no indication of the degree to which problems associated with 'severe mental illness'—hallucinations and delusional ideation—truly exist within the 'well' population, but never come to the notice of specialist services. Certainly one Dutch study (Romme *et al.*, 1992) would suggest that a large number of individuals experience auditory hallucinations but have learned to manage the experience and hence have never come to the attention of the 'experts'. One has to question their abilities to participate effectively in daily life and living, for, if they 'cope' well, perhaps management strategies should become a higher priority than the currently utilized first line of treatment, via drugs. We feel it may be a point worth pursuing, not only to elicit the true meaning of the terms 'normal' and 'mentally well', for the value of self-control of such symptomatology cannot be overestimated, both for the client and resource utilization in general.

The similarities between 'normal', 'normal under adverse conditions', 'somatically sick' and 'mentally unwell' have been demonstrated in other chapters, and probably the prime examples are those of hallucinations and delusional ideation. Perhaps if there were to be a concentration on a specific problem and its incidence, the various situations in which this one problem is exteriorized and the common biopsychosocial features that link such problem development—in other words the similarities, not the differences—rather than an emphasis on delineation of 'mental illnesses', which have often very fine dividing lines artificially drawn, more may have been discovered about the field of psychiatry. Perhaps the focus of providing a diagnostic label has inhibited mental health care rather than enhanced its development.

The client may feel great relief and comfort in the award of a 'diagnosis', of course, but that must be heavily dependent upon what that diagnosis is and his or her understanding of the term. On occasions, it may legitimize the individual's own feelings, observations and thoughts surrounding current levels of functioning, emphasizing the 'real-ness' of perceptions and providing evidence to validate or excuse reduced/aberrant performance. It may, because it is a doctor offering the label, serve to reinforce the belief that such problems are associated with 'illness', 'disease', and 'conditions', and not lifestyle or living, and hence may be beyond one's own sphere of influence or control. Amelioration or cure of these problems is then assumed to be the doctor's role and responsibility, and is expected to be achieved via a pill, potion or prescribed procedure. At a time when the biggest killers in Western society may be considered to be self inflicted or society induced, the above is a dangerous belief. Cardiovascular and respiratory disease (including cancers), and trauma and violence are in some degrees preventable and are certainly not amenable to a 'quick fix' cure. Similarly, those problems engendering the greatest psychosocial distress—depression, anxiety and substance misuse—are difficult to cure medically and require life adjustment and management. Therefore, cure by the doctor may be an unreasonable expectation evinced by the client and an impossible and irrational position assumed by the doctor.

Returning to the original focus of attention, that is, to the quality and value of professional–lay interactions, we asserted that health problems 'belong' to individuals seeking assistance and that they should have a right to know the facts—as well as the doctor's opinions—about their health status and needs. Unfortunately, the terminology utilized to describe the individual's problems 'belongs' to the health care professionals and is either incomprehensible or poorly understood by those outside of the occupational subculture. Whilst it is useful to use an appropriate and agreed linguistic shorthand, in the form of diagnosis and categorization, within intra-professional communication, it is the responsibility of the professionals to ensure that the facts are imparted to the client, with skill, with honesty and using a shared, common language. In recognizing the potential enthusiasm of the client for a name for his problems, and the fact that a 'rose by any other name' would still be a rose, there is no reason why that should not be provided. However, emphasis should be laid upon the real meaning of the diagnostic label to the client, in respect of aetiology, continuing effects on health and wellbeing both of the individuals and significant others, treatment options, their relative values and limitations, and, of course, prognosis. In essence, it should assume, and be presented, in its true light—magicless and only of academic interest, and not the centre of importance or attention.

In the absence of the above, the 'remainder' of the client may become lost from view and individuals become—as is still too frequently seen—of secondary importance to their health problems. They assume the identity of an 'appendix', a 'schizophrenic' or 'obsessive'. The person becomes superfluous, and yet health problems, and resolution or amelioration of those problems, are only logically able to be viewed from the position of their effect upon life, hopes, ambitions, expectations and norms. When the 'treatment' proves more distressing, painful or debilitating than can be anticipated as a benefit or advantage to the client, the label has to assume second place to the ethical–moral issues of comfort, dignity and peace of mind. Treatment should not be undertaken at any cost, for the balance must always be weighed in regard to the client's wishes and advantage against prescribed and automatically evoked action.

Sometimes, too, professionals may not look beyond the label in regard to added or further health problems, elicited by the client and hence miss highly significant changes in the individual's health status:

A 45-year-old woman had a long history of migraine, which had been diagnosed and successfully treated by her general practitioner, using prophylactic and symptomatic medi-

---

cation. When the frequency and nature of the attacks altered substantially, she returned to the GP for advice and further assistance. He duly changed the medication previously prescribed, asserting that she had developed a tolerance to it. She became progressively more distressed as the headaches worsened and created profound impairment in her ability to perform everyday activities.

A further consultation elicited another change in medication, but before the prescription could be filled, the lady suffered a *grand mal* epileptic seizure in the street. Taken to Accident and Emergency, a full neurological examination was performed and a provisional diagnosis—later confirmed—of a cerebral tumour, temporal lobe was made.

We have to admit that the above example is only one of many within our repertoire of such errors and hence must remain high on our list of concerns related to the use of diagnostic labels. Similarly, some labels remain with the client forever, long after their relevance or significance is passed:

Twenty years ago, Tom was diagnosed as schizophrenic. For over 15 years he has 'been well controlled' on oral phenothiazines and supported by his wife at home. He is a hard worker, who rarely misses a day from his painting and decorating job.

Not so long ago, Tom twisted his back and attended his GP. He was prescribed anti-inflammatory medication and advised to rest for at least a week. He was given a 'sick-note' and instructed to return one week later. Unfortunately his employer mislaid his sick-note and, in response to Tom's wife's request for a replacement, was duly sent the certificate, which on this occasion identified the cause of his absence from work, not as 'back injury', but as 'schizophrenia'.

In response to the example of Tom's experience and recalling the previous concern expressed regarding the lack of definition and parameters associated with mental health, Becker's (1964) questions are appropriately reproduced:

Who applies the label of deviant to whom?

What consequences does the application of the label have for the person labelled?

Under what circumstances is the label of deviant successfully applied?

In Tom's situation, the psychiatrist has labelled him as deviant and he is never to be allowed to forget it. His employer has long since stopped singling him out as 'fragile' or 'different' to his colleagues, mainly one would suspect because he has never provided any evidence to support the perception—his health record is better than that of most of his co-workers from all accounts.

The neighbours are totally unaware of his previous medical history and whilst most would consider him 'no great mixer' because of his apparent disinterest in local get togethers, all consider him a nice fellow, and a good and helpful neighbour. It was, indeed, only because of his wife's anger at the error outlined above and the fact that she sought advice as to the action available to her in the situation, that longstanding professional curiosity was satiated by the conversation. Of course Tom is 'deviant' and not 'sick' because of the continuing public perception of this thing 'schizophrenia'. Violence and frightening behaviour may be the automatic associations made with regard to this individual who is considered different to the rest of society and therefore is suspect and to be avoided. Tom, because the label was not broadcasted to the neighbourhood, has not been adversely treated by his peers or other residents of the area. He is not 'too different' to them—he adheres to the broad parameters applied to health and 'normality' and therefore responses remain within similarly constructed parameters and limits. Has he been successfully labelled as 'deviant'?

Of course, Goffman's (1983) exposition clearly identifies the manner in which the perception of 'differentness' serves to preclude full acceptance of the individual by the society in which he resides

and there are many examples of this, including the difficulties encountered by Jewish and non-white immigrants. The otherwise healthy adult, who needs a wheelchair to facilitate mobility, often describes the approach taken by some members of the public, as they talk over his head, to a walking adult accompanying the lesser mobile person, or down to him, in a manner suggestive of his having a brain deficit, rather than difficulty in walking. Facial scarring may evoke similar responses, and the elderly, isolated and slightly eccentric cat-loving spinster may acquire the label of 'local witch'. 'Differentness' which is visible or which becomes known to others, provides discredit and loss of status and value. The words of Szasz (1961), Laing (1967) and Scheff (1984) facilitate an appreciation of the theories of the influence of labels upon behaviours associated with 'mental illness'. There is no doubt, of course, of the effect of an authoritatively delivered, negative descriptor upon the individual's perception of himself and others present, especially when such a comment is forthcoming from one so respected in society as is the teacher, the doctor or the judge. There is always, though, someone in a 'high position' within any society or subculture who is considered powerful enough, and influential enough, to have such an effect:

Matron told me—on several occasions and frequently with an audience—that I would never make a 'daffodil', the term of approval applied to nurses who not only qualified via the School of Nursing but did so by exhibiting a slavish adherence to the unwritten rules of presentation—of self, the ward, paperwork, professional relationships, etc.

I remember that the first time she applied such a 'death sentence' was the day I forgot to *underline* the patient's names on the evening report. To me, it was unimportant, the quality and accuracy of the comments alongside each name being the area that I had focused energy and attention upon. To Matron, it was the first indicator of the slippery slope via which I was destined to descend. A ladder in a stocking, a blood-stained apron, hair falling down from a starched cap and the like were the elements of performance on which I seemed to be judged. Of course the fact that all were gained via emergency activity with a patient who was bleeding to death and I'd not had time to change yet, was no excuse!

Unfortunately, Matron had a lot of friends amongst the older Ward Sisters and I remember her comments upon entering the ward where I was working, as she informed the Sister that my performance was 'lacking'. From that point on, I would be 'singled out' and it seemed, at 18 years old, that whatever I did would be wrong or inadequately carried out. I seriously began to question my choice of profession.

It wasn't until I worked with Sisters who, being of the younger element and less influenced by Matron's comments, that my confidence returned and I began to enjoy the wards again. I actually got good ward reports, which really mattered to me.

Many years later, as a Senior Tutor I met up with one of the older Ward Sisters I'd worked for, many years before and now also a Senior Tutor. She remembered me, when I introduced myself, and, upon hearing of my present position, promptly commented—and loudly—that, 'they'd promote *anybody* these days'.

Whilst I could laugh at her opinions now, I wondered how many more inexperienced students she had decimated in this way. In saying that, they really made me what I am, for whilst sticking to my principles of what was/wasn't important, I did work ten times harder just to prove them wrong!

This could not happen now—or could it? The label ascribed via the authoritative or 'expert' figure still adheres, but we agree with Pickerill's (1992) assertions regarding the relatively detrimental nature of labelling by the health professionals. In a detailed analysis, in relation to those experiencing the effects of learning disability, Pickerill asserts that the informal, lay response to 'differentness' is the point at which labelling occurs and any reaction to such a label is already deeply ingrained and well established, before any formal label is able to be applied. If an individual is visibly 'odd', overtly different or inexplicable in terms of 'norms', society itself will ascribe the label and the potential for a secondary deviation, dependent or provoked solely by that societal response. Whatever the terminology utilized by formal diagnostic labels, the rose by any other name is still a rose. Whilst the edict issued from the elevated position of the doctor may confirm the 'oddness', perhaps society's reaction to 'differentness' has already done the damage.

THE MENTAL HEALTH PERSPECTIVE

The position within mental health care, relating to the sphere of terminology and diagnostic categorization is, at best, tenuous. In essence, labels ascribed by the professionals are an everyday part of lay language, and yet semanticity is lacking. There is dispute between professionals both with regard to the automatic assumptions that may be implicit in such a label and when that label may legitimately be awarded. Diagnostic categories, therefore, do not assist greatly in advancing the boundaries of knowledge regarding 'mental illness' because agreement in criteria cannot be exacted. Even the professionals and the law do not agree, with much dispute in relation to the degree to which deviations within mental health status may be regarded as 'illness' and which are the result of ineffective learning about life and its traumas. None of this bodes well with regard to the value of a linguistic shorthand method of intra-professional communication. And yet mental health professionals persist in using such labels, despite the paucity of their value to the professional and the client, who continues to be perceived via stereotypical pictures associated with varying degrees of 'madness', as portrayed by the media and internalized by society. So what are the broad categories in use and what treatment can be offered via the medical profession?

THE MENTAL HEALTH JIGSAW

You may recall our previous assertions relating to the fact that a problem of one sphere of function will have deleterious effects upon all aspects of function, and that serious repercussions are therefore evident in all elements of life and living. Categorization may be seen—though less than definitive in description—to encompass problems of all spheres and activity, in other words:

Problems of affect + Problems of behaviour + Problems of cognition = Diagnosis (Fig. 10.1)

This is the format utilized, therefore, in the following brief outline of commonly encountered diagnostic categories, with their variations. Criteria employed relate to the DSM IIIR (American Psychiatric Association, 1987) classification system.

Mood disorders

Problems associated with lowered mood are required to be present for two weeks before a diagnosis of *major depressive episode* is awarded (Fig. 10.2). Similarly, such feelings are necessarily evident for most of the day and nearly every day during this period, and represent an obvious departure from previous status. Concomitant

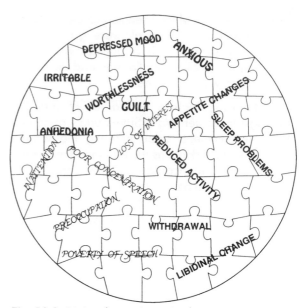

Fig. 10.2 *Major depressive episode.*

with lowered mood is a loss of joy in life, a reduction in pleasure related to all activities and loss of interest. Self perception is often related to inadequacy of function and worthlessness and may achieve delusional proportions, whilst guilt may be evident as a result of these feelings or past activities or events.

Anxiety and fear—for one's own health, for the wellbeing of others and for the future in general—may be experienced, as may irritability and loss of control.

Facial expression reflects sadness, eye contact may be lost and there is often tearfulness, or evidence of recent and prolonged crying. Movement levels may demonstrate retardation or, conversely, agitation, as the individual paces, wrings the hands, pulls or rubs skin, clothing, hair and other objects. Appetite is often poor, resulting in lowered energy levels, constant fatigue and weight loss, though on occasions 'comfort' eating may be elicited. The fatigue is compounded via sleep problems, with falling to sleep (initial insomnia), waking during sleep (middle insomnia) and early morning wakening (terminal insomnia), all common complaints. Again, on occasions, sleep may be seen to be excessive (hypersomnia), with frequent day time 'naps' or longer periods of night time sleep.

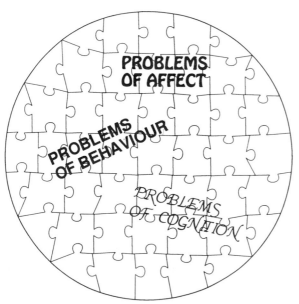

Fig. 10.1 *Aggregation of problems to provide a diagnosis.*

Cognitively, the individual frequently experiences a difficulty in thinking, inattention and problems related to concentration. Thinking is slow and preoccupied, often with somatic health or death and dying, with the belief expressed that all would be 'better off' if the individual was dead. Speech is slow and monotone, and often considerably reduced in amount, at times to the point of mutism. Commonly, where delusional ideation and hallucinatory experiences occur, there is a reflection of the sad, negative mood within content (mood congruence), more rarely is there incongruence.

Variations on the themes of depressed mood are commonly diagnosed. Episodes, for example, may be single or recurrent, or may be elicited in conjunction with episodes of intense psychomotor activity and elevated mood, as a *bipolar disorder*. It may be evinced at all stages of life. In children, problems associated with agitation, rather than retardation, and somatic health are more commonly seen. Hallucinations are usually auditory in nature and mood congruent. Adolescents often demonstrate overtly antisocial behaviour, examples being negativism, aggression, withdrawal and psychoactive substance use. The 'leanings' of adolescence are greatly exaggerated and often completely out of character. Exteriorization of problems associated with depression in the elderly population may be confused with those of organic impairment and hence precise diagnostic techniques are required to elicit the true picture.

Major life changes, which evoke feelings of stress and inadequacy, may precede depressed mood. Loss of a loved one—death, divorce, separation—or some other important element of life—a job or property—may precipitate difficulties, as may chronic, somatic ill-health. Leaving school, changing work place, childbirth and retirement may all evoke stress and hence problems of this nature.

A *manic episode* (Fig. 10.3), conversely, demonstrates problems for the individual which are almost at the opposite end of the continuum, for mood is persistently, and inappropriately, elevated, thus presenting an infectiously euphoric face to the world. The over optimistic and expansive approach to life engendered, prompts

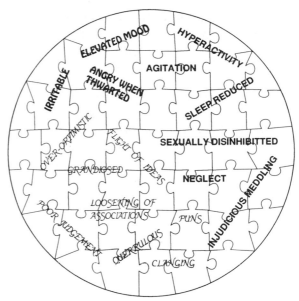

Fig. 10.3 *A manic episode.*

pleasure-seeking activities and disinhibited behaviour, which if thwarted, may provoke irritation and anger.

There is a pronounced increase in motor activity which is goal directed and yet which demonstrates no appreciation of the implications or repercussions of actions. The individual exhibits well-intentioned—though none the less irritating—and continual meddling and interference in whatever interaction or event takes his or her fleeting attention or interest. Sleep pattern is disturbed, with an apparent reduced need for prolonged periods of rest. Two or three hours will furnish the individual with limitless energy and unrestrained activity. Social convention and inhibitions are thrown to the wind as the individual follows the immediate desire and therefore tactless, offensive and, often, sexually frank behaviour ensues.

The individual finds no time for the basic activities of eating or self care, being far too preoccupied with the environmental- and thought-provoked stimulation of his surroundings. Work activities and social relationships inevitably suffer.

The individual exhibits grandiosity, in the form of grossly inflated beliefs concerning his own characteristics, abilities and experiences, and presents, therefore, as self opinionated and arrogant. Flight of ideas reflects in pressurized, loud and rapid speech, which often becomes incoherent and unintelligible. As thoughts race, the individual displays distractibility and frequent shifts in attention towards external stimuli. In turn speech shows evidence of word selection via sound rather than meaning, in rhymes and clang association, and silly jokes and puns.

Manic episodes may similarly be precipitated by psychological stressors, but may also be a problem following treatment to alleviate depressed mood, that is, antidepressant medication and electroplexy. Mood aberrations are a frequently observable feature where psychoactive substances are in use.

Anxiety

The diagnostic category of *generalized anxiety disorder* (Fig. 10.4) is reserved for those individuals

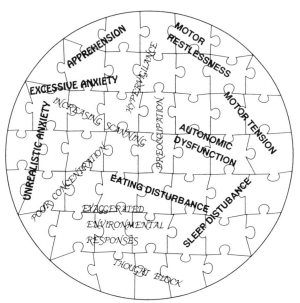

Fig. 10.4 *Generalized anxiety disorder.*

who experience excessive or unrealistic anxiety and apprehension, relating to two or more life activities or circumstances, on more days than not during a six-month period. Depressed or irritable mood may feature due to the individual's per-

ceived sense of inadequacy to meet current needs to perform.

Somatic experiences reflect the hyperarousal of the sympathetic innervation of the autonomic nervous system and hence are observed in all spheres of function. Muscle tension gives rise to shaky, aching muscles and general feelings of fatigue. Shortness of breath, difficulty in breathing and rapid, shallow function may feature via the respiratory system, and light-headedness, dizziness, and palpitations are mediated via the cardiovascular system, as are cold, clammy—or alternatively flushed—skin characteristics. The gastro-intestinal problems associated with dysphagia, nausea, diarrhoea and 'butterflies' often serve to reduce the desire for food. An increased desire to micturate is also a common complaint. Sleep is disturbed, with problems often experienced in going off to sleep, or in remaining so, and therefore feelings of fatigue are compounded.

There is a preoccupation with the areas of concern, and therefore inattention and poor concentration may be complaints. Thought blocks may be elicited and words 'lost' within explanatory dialogue. The individual's perceptual functions are on a high state of alert, and hypervigilance and hyperattentiveness to environmental nuances are observable, via exaggerated responses to minor changes and cues in the surroundings.

Anxiety is a common element of many diagnoses. In children and young adults, for example, *separation anxiety disorder* may be seen following detachment from a loved one. Such youngsters demonstrate a need for familiar surroundings, clinging behaviour and often somatic symptomatology, such as nausea, vomiting, diarrhoea and headaches. In older children, dizziness, palpitations and fainting may occur. Fears of harm befalling the loved one and of never being reunited are commonly expressed, and the youngster is often afraid to go to sleep alone, with bad dreams and nightmares creating further disturbance.

Avoidant disorder of childhood and adolescence may similarly be diagnosed where social anxiety is a problem. This child is withdrawn, shy and embarrassed in unfamiliar company and yet sociable and happy with those known to him. The problem is rarely seen in isolation, and often accompanies a generalized anxiety disorder, or an *overanxious disorder*, where problems associated with a preoccupation and concern with future or past events is seen. The child worries about his/her competence in a variety of situations and the perceptions of others regarding his/her performance are a major concern. The somatic problems associated with autonomic arousal are frequently observed.

Panic attacks, or relatively short-lasting and discrete periods of intense fear and terror, may occur without any obvious precipitating event or as an integral feature of other anxiety-provoking situations. *Phobias* represent a persistent and focused fear of a specific situation, event or object which evoke the autonomic anxiety response. There is a recognition of the unreasonable nature of the fear but continued avoidance of the stimulus wherever feasible. Intense anxiety is elicited if exposure occurs, and an integral aspect of the phobia is often related to the possibility of humiliating oneself during such an exposure. Where the stimulus is a commonly encountered one within everyday life and living experiences, work and social routines and relationships may be significantly impaired.

Post-traumatic stress disorder may occur following the experience of a situation encompassing characteristics of terror, intense fear, helplessness and fear of life. Traumas beyond the comprehension and believed physical endurance of many, for example, rape, combat, earthquakes and torture, may engender a recurrent re-living of the trauma, an avoidance of stimuli associated with it or an emotional detachment from the world. Recurrent nightmares may further disturb already difficult sleeping patterns. Irritability, loss of control and aggression may be problems, as may generalized and exaggerated responses to environmental cues. Withdrawal, diminished interest, poor attention and concentration spans may all be experienced.

Obsessive compulsive disorder is the term reserved to describe the problem compilation associated with obtrusive, repetitive thoughts and the physical manoeuvres instigated to eradicate, neutralize or prevent that thought content from occurring. The obsessive thoughts are recognized

as belonging to, and generated by, self and initially behaviours may be resisted as senseless or unreasonable activities. Anxiety and tension created by resistance may be seen to be released only by the performance of the stereotyped, ritualistic movements which commonly include handwashing, touching, checking and counting procedures. The problems may be seen to begin in childhood, adolescence or the early adult years.

Problems associated with somatic health status

Hypochondriasis (Fig. 10.5) is the category utilized to refer to an amalgam of problems engendered by an unwarranted fear or belief that one has a somatic disease, although no actual evidence is found upon medical evaluation to support such a belief. The fear may be accompanied by frustration and anger in response to the inability of medical practitioners to support the individual's fears with a concrete somatic diagnosis and their apparent disbelief with regard to problems expressed. Depressed mood may similarly be evidenced, again in response to the above, but also in relation to the persistent sensations and perceptions experienced.

Clients may, because of their beliefs, present

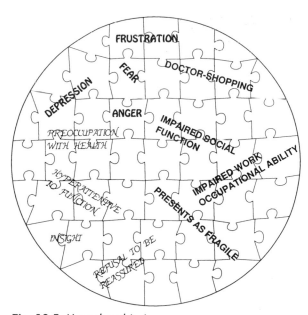

Fig. 10.5 *Hypochondriasis.*

themselves as 'delicate' or 'fragile' in health and indulge in 'doctor-shopping', trailing from expert to expert in the hope of recognition and diagnosis of symptomatology, and may eventually end up as bedridden. Several body systems may be included within the focus of attention at any one time, or, conversely, the perceived signs and symptoms may be transposed from one system to another. Social and occupational functioning may be affected to a greater or lesser degree, dependent upon the intensity of the beliefs or fears and the nature of the symptoms expressed.

Whilst the belief regarding the somatic disorder may be intense, it is not of delusional proportions, in that the client may consider medical suggestions of exaggeration of symptoms as a possibility, and indeed that such symptoms do not exist at all. Uncertainty, whilst possibly elicited, does not, however, reassure the client of no abnormality existing. The individual demonstrates a preoccupation, therefore, with the functions, or perceived sensations related to the area of the body under focus.

There are many variations on the theme of somatically orientated problems ranging from *malingering*, where there is an intentional production or excessive exaggeration of health problems, which is motivated by external incentives, such as avoiding work, legal prosecution or obtaining drugs, to *non-compliance with medical treatment*, due to denial of the illness, religious beliefs and value judgements made in regard to the relative values of treatment. Whilst neither in themselves can be attributed to 'mental illness', they may usefully be seen to form the parameters of somatic health related problems.

Body dysmorphic disorder is exhibited as an excessive preoccupation with an imagined, or real but slight, body defect, in an individual who appears 'normal'. Focus of preoccupation may be related to imagined wrinkles, spots or lumps, or the size, shape and symmetry of features. Repeated medical advice and assistance is sought to correct the supposed flaws. Such ideation may assume delusional levels as a separate *delusional disorder—somatic subtype*.

Conversion disorder is the term describing the problems associated with a loss or alteration in some aspect of bodily function which, whilst suggestive of underlying somatic pathology, is put forward as a physiological expression of a psychological desire or conflict. It has been suggested that exteriorization of the problem in a physical form fulfils two different motives or needs for the client. The first relates to achievement of a 'primary gain', by preventing the need for a conscious awareness of the psychological conflict. An individual may witness a traumatic event and, rather than admitting or acknowledging the trauma, unconsciously 'develops' a blindness, or the person who fears hurting a loved one, following an intense argument, may develop a paralysis of an arm. The symptom may therefore also supply an 'insurance policy' against the occurrence of feared activity and offer a potential solution to the continuance of such a psychological conflict. Similarly a 'secondary gain' may be achieved via the provision of a legitimate reason for avoidance or prevention of a traumatic situation or event. Examples may be seen in the situation whereby a wife who had been about to leave her husband is unable to do so when he develops a paralysis of both legs, or that of the soldier unable to fire his weapon because of a hand paralysis. There are, of course, oft-quoted examples of 'glove' and 'stocking' paralysis—that is a loss of function over a discrete, symmetrical area which is physiologically impossible—convenient aphonia, blindness and anosmia development, though it must always be borne in mind that symptoms are not consciously produced. *La belle indifference*, an apparent lack of concern regarding the problem, may be a feature.

Individuals who exhibit recurrent, multiple somatic health complaints over a period of several years which, upon medical investigation, are not apparently caused by physiological abnormality, may be considered to be experiencing *somatization disorder*. Descriptions of symptomatology may be vague or delivered in dramatic or exaggerated form, and medical assistance has often been sought on numerous occasions over many years. Problems may be considered to reflect neurological dysfunction, as paralyses, paraesthesias and blindness, cardiovascular manifestations, as chest pain and dizziness, gastro-intestinal pathology, via abnormal pain or bowel dysfunction, and female reproductive function, as dysmenorrhoea, or sexual dysfunction, as pain or sexual indifference. Anxiety or depressed mood is frequently elicited and life or relationship difficulties often a feature.

Complaints solely related to the experience of pain, which, again, are unable to be accounted for by medical findings, may acquire the diagnosis of *somatoform pain disorder*. The presence, within the environment, of some conflict-evoking stimulus may be readily demonstrated, or, conversely, such pain may be seen to facilitate avoidance of an unpleasant activity or situation. Often the symptoms develop immediately after a traumatic experience, and the individual refuses to consider a psychological aetiology as a potential feature.

Schizophrenia

The problems that are experienced by an individual in the combination diagnosed as *schizophrenia* (Fig. 10.6), need to have been in evidence

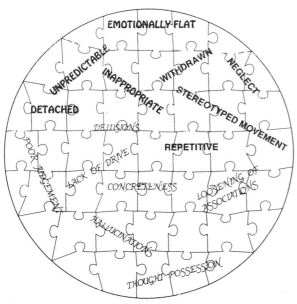

Fig. 10.6 *Schizophrenia.*

for a minimum period of six months, within *DSM IIIR* (American Psychiatric Association, 1987) categorization in order to fulfil criteria indentified. This may include symptomatology which is put forward as indicative of three phases associated with the development of the overall picture of presentation, namely *prodromal*, *acute* and *re-*

sidual symptoms. The former and latter of the three phases are essentially the same and, in reality, demarcation of separate developmental stages may only be observable in retrospect. In essence the phases reflect the increasing–plateauing–decreasing nature of problem severity.

Within prodromal/residual phases, significant others describe features which indicate a clear deterioration from previous levels of the individual's performance and suggest an apparent change in personality characteristics. Affect may be blunted, shallow and inappropriate to events. Behaviour is often described as 'odd' or 'peculiar', with evidence of hoarding or collecting activities (often rubbish unassociated, unconnected items) which may assume great importance to the individual, or talking to himself in public. The individual isolates himself from previous interactions, relationships and activities and therefore deterioration of previous roles and functions are observed. Self neglect is evident in all spheres of personal and social care, and the individual exhibits a lack of energy, interest and drive. Speech may be poor in quantity and content, often eliciting vagueness, circumstantiality and over elaboration. Odd beliefs may be indicated within speech content, which are not reflective of the culture prevailing, and misperceptions and illusions may be frequent. A minimum of two of the above problems must be present to warrant diagnosis as prodromal/residual symptoms of schizophrenia.

The acute, active phase of the diagnosis is very precisely defined, and must adhere to *one* of the three sets of criteria defined, for a minimum period of one week, that is, either:

1 Must demonstrate at least *two* of the following:
    (a) Flat, or inappropriate affect
    (b) Catatonic behaviour
    (c) Delusions
    (d) Loosening of associations
    (e) Hallucinations—must be of more than a fleeting nature, experienced several times a day for a week, or several times a week for several weeks

or,

2 Bizarre delusions, for example related to thought possession, or control of behaviour by outside agencies

3 Prominent hallucinations, commonly of an auditory nature and often related to one or more voices, conversing or commenting upon the individual's behaviour or actions

Self care, relationships and occupational spheres of activity demonstrate considerable deterioration over previous or anticipated levels of performance. *DSM IIIR* identifies four 'types' of schizophrenia, which, whilst conceded to be less than stable over time and variable with regard to treatment implications and prognosis, are based upon the predominant features evident upon clinical evaluation.

Catatonic type is indicated by gross disturbances in both behaviour and cognition. Stupor may be evident, whereby the person elicits a decreased level of reactivity to the environment and its stimuli, and is often associated with muteness and a drastic reduction in motor activity, sometimes to the point of total immobility. Conversely, *catatonic excitement* may be evident, or there may be a rapid transition from one extreme to the other, from stupor to purposeless, excited motor activity. Neither seem to be provoked by environmental stimuli. An apparently motiveless resistance to the desires or instructions of others may be exhibited, termed *negativism*, and a *rigidity* of stance or position may similarly be observed. *Catatonic posturing*, where the individual voluntarily assumes obviously uncomfortable and bizarre positions and which he may maintain for prolonged periods, may also be a feature.

The *disorganized type* is characterized by grossly inappropriate affect, bizarre behaviours, which may include grimaces, mannerisms and stereotyped movement patterns, and severe loosening of associations and incoherence. Delusions and hallucinatory experiences may be less persistent and more fleeting and fragmentary than are experienced by other individuals.

The problems usually linked with schizophrenia—flat or inappropriate affect, disorganized behaviour and loosening of associations—are not evident within the *paranoid type*. Delusions, which are systematized and may be related to one or more themes, and related auditory hallucinations are the essential features here, with anger, argumentativeness and aggression all possible. Anxiety may be unfocused where demonstrated. Behaviour may appear to be precise and consciously thought out, particularly where interactions with others are concerned, where there is a total absence of warmth and a stilted, formal manner is assumed.

Where the individual fails to meet the criteria determined by any of the above three categories, the term *undifferentiated type* may be utilized.

When no evidence of a prodromal stage is demonstrated and similar symptomatology appears following events of an intensely stressful nature, the diagnosis of *brief reactive psychosis* may be made. Affect may be intense and rapid shifts may be observed. Behaviour may be catatonic or disorganized in nature, and cognition demonstrates features of incoherence, loosening of associations, delusions and hallucinatory experiences. The symptomatology resolves within a relatively short period, and always within one month.

Schizophreniform disorder is said to demonstrate identical symptomatology to that of schizophrenia, but the duration of problems experienced does not exceed six months, with a full return to the levels of premorbid functioning evident after that time. Similarly where a mixture of symptomatology associated with both a mood disorder and schizophrenia are evident, the term *schizoaffective disorder* may be applied.

On occasions, significant others involved in relationship with an individual experiencing a 'psychotic disorder', may similarly exteriorize and share the delusional ideation exhibited by the 'client'. In a sort of contagion, the 'well individual' will demonstrate an extinction of the belief system when separated from the primary person, and there has often been a very close relationship in the past, which has been 'undiluted' because of reduced social contact with others, outside of the situation. Diagnostic category utilized to indicate such an aetiology is one of *induced psychotic disorder*.

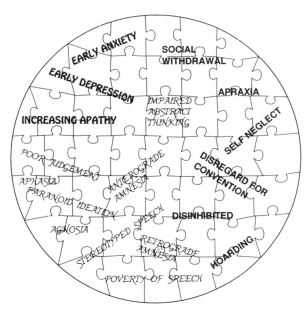

Fig. 10.7 *Dementia.*

Dementia

Whilst acknowledging the fact that the term 'dementia' (Fig. 10.7) may be used by many to infer a progressive and unremitting course and eventual severe cognitive impairment as the prognosis, *DSM IIIR* clearly describes the term in relation to the presenting clinical picture rather than its outcome. Clear statements indicate the potential degree of reversibility as dependent upon aetiology and early recognition and treatment.

The individual may present as anxious or depressed within the early stages of deterioration, as a response to the awareness and appreciation of the deficits arising in previously efficient functioning. This may result in withdrawal from social interaction, excessive organization of activities and overelaboration of details relating to events experienced in an attempt to conceal memory problems and intellectual difficulties. Psychosocial stressors impact severely upon the already struggling individual, with further deterioration as its result. Paranoid ideation may engender anger and its verbal and motor consequences. Diagnosis is made only when intellectual impairment is of sufficient *degree* to provoke deterioration in occupational and social functioning.

Primary problems relate to the impairment of short- and long-term memory and the implicit difficulties of vast gaps in personal and common knowledge. Difficulties are evinced within abstract thinking, with the individual unable to identify similarities or differences in objects or situations, and impairment in the ability to define words and concepts. Judgement is therefore unreliable. There may be a failure to recognize everyday objects, despite intact sensory pathways, as agnosia, and similarly an inability to perform motor activities, despite intact understanding and motor function, as apraxia. Constructional activities, for example reproducing three-dimensional figures, may also create difficulties for the individual. Significant others frequently observe an accentuation or alteration in previous personality characteristics.

Where neurological disease, for example, cerebral tumours, infections and metabolic dysfunctions, and trauma, via head injury, have been excluded, problems which develop insidiously and which show a progressively deteriorating course may be diagnosed as a *primary degenerative dementia of the Alzheimer type.* Evidence to support such a diagnosis may be commonly observable after the age of 50 years, when it is termed 'presenile', or after 65 years of age, when it is labelled 'senile' in nature. On occasions, delirium, delusions or depression may be significant individual and predominating features, and hence the word is appended to the overall diagnosis.

Dementia-related problems may also be seen within an overall pattern of abrupt onset, patchy degrees of deterioration in intellectual function and a step-wise, rather than gradual, progression and course. *Mutli-infarct dementia* is due to cerebral and systemic vascular disease which results in small, but multiple, areas of cerebral tissue softening and death, hence the pattern of deterioration seen. Neurological signs are evident, often with a concomitant deterioration in physical function. Dysarthria, dysphagia and a characteristic small-stepped gait may be observed. Physical examination reveals problems associated with circulation, for example, hypertension or heart disease. As with Alzheimer-type problems, significant delirium, delusions or depression may be demonstrated and therefore the main category is amended to indicate this. Lability of mood, with sham tears alternating with laughter, is a generally encountered problem.

Psychoactive substance dependence

Eleven classes of substances are identified as commonly used, on a non-medical basis, to achieve a change of mood or behaviour within *DSM IIIR* namely:

1 Alcohol

2 Amphetamines, or other similarly acting sympathmomimetics

3 Caffeine

4 Cannabis

5 Cocaine

6 Hallucinogens

7 Inhalants

8 Nicotine

9 Opioids

10 Phencyclidine (PCP) and other similarly acting arylcyclohexylamines

11 Sedatives, hypnotics and anxiolytics

Dependence (Fig. 10.8), despite the specific substances utilized, elicits common features, as well as some individual differences, and must be evident for a minimum period of one month to meet criteria awarded.

Whilst mood problems may be demonstrated, particularly in relation to depression, anxiety, irritability, anger and lability, it is often unclear as to the degree to which this is induced by substances used or was pre-existing, and in some instances, a precipitant factor in, initial use. A large, increasing amount of time is spent in activities relating to substance procurement, use and recovery from use, which may provoke withdrawal both from social situations and role performance. Indeed there may be occasions where,

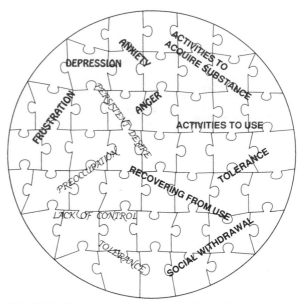

Fig. 10.8 *Psychoactive substance dependence.*

during daily activities and occupational pursuit, the individual is observed to be intoxicated. Though cognizant of the problem and its detrimental effects on biopsychosocial functioning, the individual is unable to control his or her intake of the substance and is in fact aware of developing a tolerance for it, requiring increasing amounts to achieve the desired effects.

Some substances induce characteristic symptoms of *withdrawal* from use. These may relate to mood, in the form of depression, anxiety and irritability, psychomotor agitation, sleep disturbance and fatigue, as with, for example, amphetamines and cocaine. In withdrawal from alcohol, sedative, hypnotic and anxiolytic substances, problems experienced may include autonomic nervous system hyperactivity. Each substance, barring cannabis, hallucinogens and phencyclidine, which are not identified as evoking withdrawal symptomatology, produces a characteristic pattern of features associated with abrupt cessation of use.

Delirium may be a sequelae associated with the use of cocaine, amphetamines, phencyclidine and similar acting preparations. Rapidly developing, and often of brief duration, delirium may be heralded by emotional disturbances of anxiety, fear, irritability, depression, anger, euphoria or apathy, which may be consistent in exteriorization or fluctuate rapidly and unpredictably as lability. There may be a reduced level of consciousness, psychomotor retardation or acceleration and/or sleep disturbance which is frequently demonstrated in the form of insomnia or excessive day-time somnolence. The individual experiences a reduced ability to maintain or shift attention, with a concomitant reduction in reactivity to the environment. Thinking may evidence disorganization, irrelevancy and wandering, as indicated by the nature of speech and there is often disorientation to time, place and person. Memory difficulties and perceptual disturbances may similarly present, and, as delirium may occur in relation to a wide, and varied, number of health-related problems, diagnosis is dependent upon use of an evoking substance within the preceding 24-hour period.

Organic delusional disorder may be a feature of amphetamine, phencyclidine (and related substances), cannabis, cocaine and hallucinogen preparations. The former, for example, may evoke a highly organized paranoid state, with ingrained persecutory delusions, as may cannabis and cocaine. Whilst hallucinations may be exteriorized, they are a less prominent symptom. Where hallucinations are equally or more prominent, a diagnosis of *hallucinosis* may be added to, or substituted for, that of delusional disorder, as may be seen related to alcohol ingestion. On occasions, a *post-hallucinogen perception disorder* may be seen, where there is a re-living of one or more of the perceptual symptoms experienced during use, following cessation of use. Macropsia and micropsia, halos surrounding objects or people, and intensified, or flashes of colour may all be reported and cause distress. Hallucinogens and phencyclidine, and related substances, may similarly engender a *mood disorder* within one or two weeks of the substance use, persisting for more than 24 hours following cessation of its use. An enveloping depressed, elevated or expansive mood provides the predominant problem and, as with delirium, delusional and hallucinatory disorders, requires a history of substance use to enable the award of this diagnosis category, due to the same features being displayed in relation to a number and variety of different aetiological factors.

CONCLUSION

The above provides a mere outline of the major diagnostic categories utilized within *DSM IIIR* and, with those identified within specialist sections, for example relating to sex and gender and sleep, offer an insight into labels applied within mental health care. Continuing concern remains with regard to the numerous aetiological factors which may result in the exteriorization of the same problem—or symptom—and the very fine dividing lines drawn between diagnostic entities may be validated within the sketch provided and the plea for a review in regard to similarities within, rather than to differences between, categories is renewed. The care worker will hear such terminology used and be an integral part of professional dialogue relating to diagnostic categories and, whilst we are sceptical, rather than unconvinced, of its value in real terms as any form of linguistic shorthand, we offer it here only to facilitate understanding of colleagues.

FURTHER READING

Barker, P.J. & Baldwin (Eds) (1991) *Ethical Issues in Mental Health*. London: Chapman & Hall.

Rumbold, G. (1993) *Ethics in Nursing Practice*. London: Baillière Tindall.

Soothill, K., Henry, C. & Kendrick, K. (Eds) (1992) *Themes and Perspectives in Nursing*. London: Chapman & Hall.

REFERENCES

American Psychiatric Association (1987) *Diagnostic and Statistical Manual of Mental Disorders*, 3rd edn, revised. Washington: APS.

Becker, H.S. (1964) *The Other Side: Perspectives on Deviance*. New York: The Free Press.

Brown, R. (1973) *A First Language: the Early Stages*. Cambridge, MA: Harvard University Press.

Campaign for Freedom of Information (1992), The Right to Know Bill (Proposals), Campaign for Freedom of Information.

Dean, C., Surtees, P. & Sashidharan, S. (1983) Comparison of research diagnostic systems in an Edinburgh community sample. *British Journal of Psychiatry*, **142**, 247–256.

Department of Health (DH) (1991) *The Patient's Charter: Raising the Standard*. London: HMSO.

Goffman, A. (1983) *Stigma: Notes on the Management of a Spoiled Identity*. Harmondsworth: Penguin.

Gostin, L. (1983) *A Practical Guide to Mental Health Law: The Mental Health Act 1983 and Related Legislation*. London: MIND.

Laing, R.D. (1967) *The Politics of Experience and the Bird of Paradise*. Harmondsworth: Penguin.

Pickerill, C.J. (1992) An examination of the effects of labels upon persons with an intellectual disability. Unpublished Ms.

Romme, M.A.J., Honig, A., Noorthoorn, E.O. & Escher, A.D.M.A.C., (1992) Coping with hearing voices: an emancipatory approach. *British Journal of Psychiatry*, **161**, 99–103.

Scheff, T.J. (1984) *Being Mentally Ill: A Sociological Theory*. New York: Aldine.

Stockwell, F. (1984) *The Unpopular Patient*. London: Croom Helm.

Szasz, T.S. (1961) *The Myth of Mental Illness*. New York: Hoeber-Harper.

United Kingdom Central Council for Nursing, Midwifery & Health Visiting (UKCC) (1992) *Code of Professional Conduct*. London: UKCC.

United Kingdom Parliament Acts (1984) *Data Protection Act, Elizabeth II 198 Ch. 35*. London: HMSO.

United Kingdom Parliament Acts (1990) *Access to Health Records Act*. London: HMSO.

World Health Organization (1988) *International Classification of Disease*. Geneva: WHO.

PERSONALITY DISORDERS

Tony Thompson and Peter Mathias

AIMS

i) To introduce and analyse the concept of personality disorder
ii) To define and categorize personality disorders

KEY ISSUES

Characteristics and traits
Involvements of judicial system
Impulsive personality disorder
Histrionic disorder
Avoidant personality disorder
Dependent personality disorder
Anankastic personality disorder
Habit and impulsive disorder
Pathological disorder
Pathological fire raising
Pathological stealing
Enduring personality change

Identify, analyse and assess factors causing distress and illness	Promote health, provide direct care and make interventions	Manage care programmes and services
Be critical, analytical and accountable, continue professional development	Counter discrimination, inequality and individual and institutional racism	Work within and develop policies, laws and safeguards in all settings
Understand influences on mental health and the nature/causes of disorder and illness	Know the effects of distress, disorder, illness on individuals, groups, families	Understand the basis of treatments and interventions

'All this is madness, cries a sober sage:
But who, my friend, has reason in his rage?'
'The ruling Passion, be it what it will,
The ruling Passion conquers reason still!'
Alexander Pope, Moral Essays, Epistle III

INTRODUCTION

The concept of personality disorders is amongst the most challenging to all those with interest in the mental health field. Many of the arguments which seek to further studies in this area revolve around deviance theory and labelling processes which tend to invite substantial critics from opposers of these concepts. Nurses and others studying this field can be tempted to dismiss some of the ideas as a means by which repressive and intolerant societies seek to control those who do not conform to social norms. This would be an extreme view; it would also be unfortunate as the fact remains that nurses and other workers are likely to encounter patients who have experienced personal suffering as a result of personality defects. Likewise they will encounter those from whose resulting 'disorder' society suffers. Within the caring services, professionals associated with mental health of adults are most likely to see personality disorder expressed in the terms of the diagnosis antisocial personality. Indicative of some of the traits of such a personality includes the failure to adapt to working in a consistent and responsible manner, irresponsible practices of parenthood, the inability to maintain and enjoy sexual attachment, possible criminal activity, generalized irritability, physical aggression, impulsivity, lying and disregard for the safety of either themselves or others. In some instances these personality or behavioural traits are seen alongside a bright, charming and interesting personality.

The demands on mental health services brought about by someone displaying one or more of these characteristics is great. They are also prone to subjecting people working within these services to question their relevance. Quite often personality disorders are not marked by any consistent disorder of thought, perception or mood. People who display such disorders are often in full command of their behaviour and yet there is no defect of reasoning or any overt or measurable attribute that might make destructive behaviours more probable or predictable. Such people do not often regard themselves as ill and indeed it was only in the middle of this present century that the possibility of illness was considered.

In the most sensational cases of disorder it is likely that the judicial system will be involved and very often justice is seen by the general public to be compromised as they may not be convinced that the nature and quality of an act associated with a disordered personality was committed by someone who knew what he or she was doing was wrong or was suffering from a defect of reason so as not to know. It is in the area of serious offenders that conflicting views as to the care and treatment of offenders really comes to the fore. It is within the prison hospital service and the special hospital service that successful treatment can present the professional charged with the custodial responsibility with powerful dilemmas. Many public safeguards are built into the care programmes associated with treatment in these two institutional facilities. However, it is often the case that therapy and treatment required is of a long-term nature. This usually includes ongoing medical supervision and multifaceted therapies including that of medication. The enforcement of these requirements involves treatment designs and methods that general medicine and health and social care is not necessarily either equipped for nor inclined to attempt to adopt. Despite many efforts to ensure that the most sensational of cases do not remain a public risk, the same public remains generally dissatisfied with the way in which mentally ill offenders are handled by the courts. It is sometimes not realized by society at large that mental health professionals are not likely to be able to predict violent or criminal behaviour any more accurately than lay persons.

The evidence that professionals rely on is usually a past history of violent or uncontrolled behaviour and if they conclude that someone is likely to repeat such behaviour they are then dependent upon the development of services which will allow them to identify reasonable options for care. However, it remains a hard fact that the criminal justice system is still largely responsible for providing some degree of care for people who have offended and many of these may not necessarily fall into the category of criminal and are more likely to be offenders who are mentally ill. This undesirable state of affairs creates many problems within the prison and special hospital systems, particularly as the aims of both are to some extent inextricably linked. It may be worth reflecting here on some of the aims of the prison service which it is expected to accomplish when incarcerating criminals:

Prevention of further crime together with safeguarding the public

Reform or rehabilitation

Deterrents

Revenge

It is likely that imprisonment actually only achieves the first of these aims. There is conflicting evidence whether the other aims actually occur or whether they just fit a variety of personal, political and social viewpoints. It is against this backcloth that it is likely that in the United Kingdom, Health Authorities and Local Authorities will develop specialized services for the provision of 'forensic' or secure units where offenders with mental health problems will be able to receive appropriate care and treatment.

DEFINING PERSONALITY DISORDER

These tend to be persistent disorders of the mind which may or may not include significant impairment of intelligence and which are likely to result in abnormally aggressive or seriously irresponsible conduct.

Whether a person is diagnosed as having a personality disorder is often dependent upon a process known as psychopathology in which previous behaviour and conduct is considered in a retrospective manner. It has become conventional within organized services to include certain traits which are associated with people known to have a psychopathic personality. These include the person lacking the ability to feel a sense of guilt for the consequences of their actions, a lack of empathy with others is often combined with impulsive behaviour and a continuing need for excitement. Whilst often possessing charm alongside the ability to manipulate, psychopaths are liable to exploit others purely for their own gain. There can be a history of a lack of long-term loving relationships due to inability to receive or to demonstrate meaningful affection. The inadequate personality is usually depicted as someone who is unable to cope with the demands of daily life within emotional, intellectual and physical boundaries. It can be seen that the concept of personality disorder has to be viewed within a broad range of personal and social situations. They can represent extreme deviations from the way in which the average individual from a particular culture actually perceives, thinks and feels when they are relating to others. It is most important that when assessing what is meant by personality disorder the professional should consider as many aspects of personal function as possible. Nurses and others are a most useful resource in this situation as they can form a valuable source of information themselves together with the ability to collect relevant data from informants.

Rubrics of disorder

The disharmony of attitudes and behaviour associated with personality disorder, for example arousal, impulse control, style of relating to others and affectivity, means that it is unlikely that a person is diagnosed as having a personality disorder before the age of 16 years as the onset of problems tend to occur in late childhood or adolescence, being fully manifest in adulthood. The results of a personality disorder usually come to the attention of mental health services because of the division between the overt behaviour and the prevailing social values and norms; this is usually manifested in:

Disregard for the feelings of others

Irresponsible action regarding normal social roles, values and rules

Low tolerance to frustration and a low threshold for discharging aggression which may include violence

The inability to learn from experience including the effects of punishment

A tendency to blame others and to offer plausible and other rationalizations or excuses for the behaviour which brings the person into conflict with the community

---

People who have one or a combination of these features in their personality who come into contact with formal mental health services may at some time or another find themselves with the following labels or classifications attached to them:

Amoral

Antisocial

Asocial

Psychopathic

Sociopathic personality

Differing cultures will develop different criteria regarding the social norms associated with this particular phenomena. It is likely that within services in the United Kingdom particularly the presence of more than one of these traits or behaviours previously mentioned would have to be manifest before the evidence was considered to be diagnostic.

Impulsive personality disorder

This type of disorder can present particular problems for mental health services because of the tendency to act without consideration for the consequences coupled with instability of mood. The person tends to have a reduced ability to forward plan life's events and periods of intense anger can lead to violence particularly when an impulsive act is criticized by someone in authority.

Histrionic disorder

The features associated with this disorder can include a searching for appreciation by others, self indulgence and persistent manipulative behaviour. The following characteristics may be present either singly or in combination:

Dramatization of emotions

Shallow and labile moods

Influenced by suggestibility from others or by events

Preoccupying concern with physical attraction

Performing actions which result in the person being the centre of attention

---

Avoidant personality disorder

This disorder tends to be associated with anxiety which tends to be related to a hypersensitivity to criticism and the potential for rejection. The characteristics of such a disorder includes the following:

A feeling of being personally unappealing and inferior to peers

Constant feelings of tension and apprehension

A fear of being rejected or isolated in social situations

A reluctance to be involved with a peer group without a perceived guarantee of being welcomed and liked

---

Dependent personality disorder

This is usually associated with features which include perceiving oneself as incompetent, helpless and feeble. People who present to Mental Health Services with this disorder are likely to be characterized as weak, compliant and inadequate, lacking vigour and showing little capacity for life enjoyment. There is an excessive dependence on others with an unwillingness to make even reasonable demands on people that might be depended upon. In a therapeutic situation, particular problems can arise because of the associated expression of feeling uncomfortable or helpless when alone and the fear of inability to care for oneself. There may also be a preoccupation with fears of being abandoned by a person in a close relationship and subsequently being left to care for oneself.

Anankastic personality disorder

This is typified by perfectionism that overcomes the completion of tasks. The person may express feelings of excessive doubt, caution, stubbornness and rigidity in thinking. There is likely to be an inability to relax and the tension which often is associated with this disorder can be coupled with conflict in relation to sexual drive. What can often be seen as a virtue in relation to a person's occupation, that is, conscientiousness and a preoccupation with productivity, can become excessive to the extent that pleasure within interpersonal relationships is excluded. The person with this type of disorder who is in a formal relationship with Mental Health Services may well have a history that points towards an obsessive or compulsive disorder which may include unwelcome thoughts or impulses intruding into their mind.

Habit and impulsive disorder

These disorders are manifested in repeated acts that have no clear, rational motive or reason, and are likely to harm the person's interests and those of other people. The person with this type of disorder often shows behaviour associated with impulsive action which they conceive as difficult or impossible to control. There is no accurate evidence of causation of these conditions and whilst there might be broad similarities they do not necessarily have particularly important features attached to each condition. It is conventional to exclude the habitual or excessive use of alcohol or drugs as it is to exclude the impulse and habit disorders involving sexual or eating behaviour which may be seen to be problematic to either the person involved or to other people. Amongst the more frequent disorders likely to be encountered in professional services are those associated with the following:

Pathological gambling

This usually manifests as frequent and repeated gambling activities which can dominate the person's life to the detriment of his or her social, professional and family attachments. This stressful disorder may result in a person's home and job being placed at risk, the acquisition of excessive debt leading to a vicious circle of social breakdown or law-breaking activities in order to obtain financial resources for further gambling together with evasion of debt repayment. It is not unusual for this disorder to result in a repeat of gambling activity which was responsible for creating adverse consequences such as disruption of family life and general impairment of well-being.

Pathological fire raising 'pyromania'

This is a disorder which is often a characteristic of people who find themselves in institutional services such as the prison service and special hospital service. The history is usually one of multiple axe or attempts at setting fire to property without apparent motive, together with a preoccupation with objects related to fire and burning. The person may report an intense satisfaction in watching fires burn, together with feelings of increasing tension just before the act and excitement immediately after the act has been perpetrated.

Pathological stealing 'kleptomania'

People who cannot resist impulses to steal certain objects, which are not required for personal use or gain, may present with a history of increasing tension before stealing, together with a sense of gratification either during or immediately after they have committed the act. The person usually acts by themselves and following the act, the person may express anxiety, distress and guilt; however, this may not prevent a repetition of theft.

Enduring personality change following catastrophic experience

It is a sad fact that some people are exposed to excessive and prolonged stress. This stress is profound and sometimes horrific. It can result in a person's behaviour changing to the extent that they become a different person in their outlook than they were prior to the event occurring. This condition has become easier to understand now that the media are able to transmit images of the types of stressful situations which some people have to endure. Examples of this would include people who have been tortured, those who have experienced disasters, people who have been exposed to prolonged life-threatening circumstances, those that have been taken hostage and subsequently suffered long periods in captivity with the threat of death being an ever present stress. Mental health professionals and those working within the learning disability field are increasingly working in situations, particularly in Eastern Europe and former communist block countries, where people may have experienced stress so extreme, that it becomes understandable that this has a profound effect on their personality, for example, those associated with concentration camps and orphanages which are deprived of stimulation and contact. It is a diagnosis which can usually only be safely made in adults when there has been a personality change present for at least two years and cannot be attributable to pre-existing personality disorder or to a mental disorder other than post-traumatic stress syndrome. It is usual for the extent of the personality change to be conveyed by someone who knows the person before the event and some of the more obvious features include:

Social withdrawal

Feelings of hopelessness

A constant state of anxiety and feeling under threat

The hostile or mistrustful attitude towards society

CONCLUSIONS

The classification and the aetiology of personality disorders remain controversial and to some extent, obscure. Traditionally, research has been focused on the relative effects of genetics and environmental factors, commonly portrayed as the nature versus nurture theory. It is likely that there is overlap in both areas. The term personality disorder is used in two quite different ways. Firstly, to describe the individual who has a neurotic personality trait but does not suffer from a full-blown neurosis (neurotic personality disorder). Such a person may complain continually of anxiety or depression, and their emotional instability may create havoc in the area of interpersonal relationships, thereby causing unhappiness and disruption to the lives of those around them. More commonly, the term is synonymous with psychopathic disorder. The *ICD 10* (WHO, 1992) classification of mental and behavioural disorders describes a specific personality disorder as a severe disturbance in the character and constitution together with behavioural tendencies of the individual, usually involving several areas of the personality and nearly always associated with considerable personal and social disruption. Personality disorder tends to appear in late childhood or adolescence and continues to be manifest into adulthood. They tend to be conditions that are not attributable directly to brain damage or disease and other psychiatric disorders have been excluded. The following criteria may be apparent:

Overt disharmonious attitudes and behaviour likely to involve several areas of function including affectivity, arousal, impulse control, ways of perceiving and thinking, and style of relating to others

Any abnormal behaviour pattern is likely to be

enduring and not limited to episodic events regarded as a mental illness

The abnormal behaviour patterns tend to be pervasive and maladaptive to a broad range of personal and social situations

These manifestations tend to appear during childhood or adolescence and continue into adulthood

The disorder leads to considerable personal distress but this may only become apparent later in its course

The disorder is usually, but not invariably, associated with its significant problems in occupational and social performance

---

It can be seen, therefore, that both therapeutic intervention and specific diagnosis has to be set against criteria with regard to social norms and rules and therefore can be different depending upon the culture.

The definition of personality disorder is often carried out retrospectively by reflecting on past behaviours and conduct. Within therapeutic communities, a gross personality disorder can be extremely disruptive. This may be seen by the person possessing much charm but combining this with manipulative ability. Those persons considered to be psychopathic may exploit others for their own gain. There appears to be an inability to receive or offer affection in a meaningful way.

Direct nursing intervention as part of the treatment of people with a personality disorder is extremely taxing. It is necessary in many cases for confrontation to take place but because of the poor interpersonal skill development, both the timing and structure of any confrontation has to be extremely well considered. Whilst treatment utilizing group techniques can be effective, it is not unusual for the person with this type of disorder to relinquish their place in the group before real progress can be achieved.

Highly structured and consistent nursing supervision is necessary, particularly if undertaking cognitive or behavioural management techniques as a way of meeting the challenge relating to control and direction. This is particularly so if

such challenge is viewed as threatening to people presenting with a personality disorder. Therapeutic contracting with people experiencing personality disorder is not easy. A high level of both personal and professional maturity is demanded of the nurse both in their understanding of personality disorder and its outward manifestations. Goal-directed therapies rely upon the client having the intellectual ability to pursue the process alongside the professionals. It is probably in this area of care that professional staff really get to understand the nature of teamwork and team solidarity is absolutely essential for each member to be able to relate his or her own experience and feelings and attitudes towards someone with a manipulative personality.

Personality disorders are enduring patterns which may be considered schizoid, compulsive, histrionic and antisocial or paranoid. Therapeutic intervention is difficult because the person may not experience any real need for change as, providing the particular lifestyle is not threatened, there may be little or no associated anxiety.

FURTHER READING

Brooking, J. (1986) *Psychiatric Nursing Research*. Chichester: Wiley.

Brooking, J., Ritter, S. & Thomas, B. (Eds) (1992) *A Text Book of Psychiatric and Mental Health Nursing*. Edinburgh: Churchill Livingstone.

Charry, D. (1983) The borderline personality. *Association of Family Practitioners*, **3**, 195–202.

Hyman, S.E. (1988) *Manual of Psychiatric Emergencies*. Boston: Little, Brown.

Gross, R.D. (1990) *Psychology. The Science of Mind and Behaviour*. Sevenoaks, Kent: Hodder & Stoughton.

Porritt, L. (1990) *Interaction Strategies. An Introduction for Health Professionals*. Edinburgh: Churchill Livingstone.

REFERENCE

WHO (1992) *The ICD-10 Classification of Mental and Behavioural Disorders: Clinical Descriptions and Diagnostic Guidelines*. Geneva: World Health Organization.

PSYCHOSOCIOECONOMIC FACTORS IN SUICIDE

Colin Pritchard

AIMS

i) To explore the psychosocioeconomic factors associated with suicide
ii) To compare two types of self-destructive behaviour 'psychiatric related' and 'stress related'
iii) To consider how to reduce the rate of suicide

KEY ISSUES

Definition of suicide
Historical/cultural variations
Aetiology
Psychiatric related
Psychosocioeconomic factors
Deliberate self-harm (parasuicide)
Intervention

Identify, analyse and assess factors causing distress and illness	Promote health, provide direct care and make interventions	Manage care programmes and services
Be critical, analytical and accountable, continue professional development	Counter discrimination, inequality and individual and institutional racism	Work within and develop policies, laws and safeguards in all settings
Understand influences on mental health and the nature/causes of disorder and illness	Know the effects of distress, disorder, illness on individuals, groups, families	Understand the basis of treatments and interventions

INTRODUCTION

What is suicide? The answer may appear obvious; suicide is when a person dies by his or her own hand. However, as in law, to determine suicide there has to be both the 'Act' and the 'Intent', and to complete the suicide, a fatal 'Outcome'. Thus the Act may be unequivocal, a person takes a gun and shoots him or herself, but was this decisive 'outcome', death, intended? How do we know?

In English law, suicide has to be proved, with evidence that both act and intent were directly linked to the outcome, and some believe that it is this burden of proof that partially accounts for comparatively low suicide rates in Britain compared with most of Europe (Chambers and Harvey, 1989). The evidence required mainly centres around the issue of intent, hence the importance placed upon some form of communication from the deceased, that is 'the note'. Statements to other people from the deceased, if verified, are often acceptable, and are usually drawn from relatives or professionals, who can claim to have knowledge about the person's state of mind. Where it becomes problematic is when either intent or the act is unclear, for example a road accident, a drowning, a fall—all of which may have been accidental, in spite of the fact that the person was said to be depressed or even contemplating suicide. Such complexities may have contributed to the ambiguities which surrounded a number of deaths in the electronics industry, aptly chronicled by Collins (1990) as an 'open verdict', and it is easy to see how speculation can arise in such situations.

These difficulties in proving suicide may be further complicated by coroners who, when it is a question of a balance of judgement, may prefer to record a different verdict in order to save the family distress in what is still a socially stigmatized event (Chamber and Harvey, 1989). This prompts some to wonder whether there are serious doubts about the accuracy of recording suicide, which may lead to underreporting (Kolmos and Bach, 1987; O'Carrol, 1989). However, on balance, research on annual figures has demonstrated that at national level, the data are reasonably reliable (Holding and Barraclough, 1978; Sainsbury,

1983; Kolmos and Bach, 1987; Kleck, 1988; Speechley and Stavarky, 1991), not least because any 'errors' tend to be consistent over time in the same culture. This applies to the particularly difficult area of determining adolescent suicide, with the understandable tendency of coroners to minimize family anguish, though careful analysis shows that even here, the figures are reasonably stable (Males, 1991). Hence the use of the annual suicide rate of a country can be taken as an accurate indicator of improvements or worsening in those environmental factors associated with suicidal behaviour (Durkheim, 1952; Brenner, 1983; Pritchard, 1992). Thus our definition will remain simple; suicide is when a person kills themselves, though the reasons why they should take this extreme course is often complex and multi-causal, and is the core question which we will explore.

The importance of suicide can be gauged by simple comparison with statistics which attract far more public concern and media interest, that is murder. In 1990 for every homicide in the UK, there were 11.2 suicides, 4,463 to 413 murders, including all the Northern Irish terrorist-related deaths. Indeed, in six of the last eight years, suicide in Northern Ireland exceeded the total murder rate. Suicide is also the second highest cause of death amongst young men under 25, and in view of its association with mental disorder, we can continue to consider suicide as the 'psychiatric emergency'.

HISTORICAL/CULTURAL VARIATIONS IN SUICIDE

Suicide has been known throughout the whole of recorded history but what has changed over the centuries, has been the different social and cultural attitudes towards suicide, which still influence current perspectives. In Greco-Roman times suicide was often related to an 'honourable' course of action, often to escape the humiliation of capture by the enemy, for example, Cleopatra wished to avoid 'riding in young Octavian's triumph', a response that is still associated with the Samurai tradition in Japan. In Rome, where if Tacitus, Seutonius and Plutarch are to be believed, under the Caesars, political opponents were given the option of suicide, rather than execution, and thereby reducing the economic penalty to their families. None the less, there was a degree of ambivalence about suicide as, according to Gibbons, suicides were buried with their right hand chopped off, though there were no further sanctions, as happened in later Christian times, when such people were buried outside hallowed ground.

Interestingly, there is no direct injunction, or indeed comment, about suicide in either the Old or New Testaments. The closest we come to any disapproval is when Saul, after his defeat by the Philistines, seeks to kill himself, and asks help of his guard who apparently horrified by the suggestion, turns his sword against himself; a very 'Roman' attitude, yet 400 years pre-Rome. The Jews, however, appeared to accept suicide as being related to madness, but the self-massacre by the defenders of Massada, who first killed their families and then themselves rather than fall into the hands of the conquering Vespasian in AD 70, still evokes ambivalent admiration. Judas Iscariot is probably the only unequivocal suicide in the New Testament, yet his death is recorded without comment.

The Christian Church, however, began to express concern about suicide as a false martyrdom, and the heresy of the fifth century Donatists was seen as an affront to God, as the act of despair was a denial of the potential grace of God. This theological point still appears to underpin the Church's disapproval of suicide. From the fourth or fifth century, suicide was considered a kind of heresy and then a crime, and in Britain it was not until 1961 that the act, completed or attempted, was decriminalized.

Throughout the Roman Catholic Church, however, suicide is still a cardinal sin, though there is significantly greater understanding and compassion than yester years, but the old German word for suicide, 'Selbstmord' or self-murder, reflects how many feel about the phenomena. Except for apparent 'rational' suicide, a point to which we will return, such as the elderly Koestler who killed himself when his chronic irreversible illness seemed to be insupportable, suicide still carries a considerable social and professional stigma (Fremouw *et al.*, 1990; Usher, 1991). It

should be remembered, however, that to assist in a person's suicide is still an indictable offence.

Shakespeare, whilst obviously English, but can be claimed for Renaissance Western Europe, gives us classical insight into attitudes about suicide that still prevail into modern times. His *Hamlet* speech of 'to be or not to be, that is the question', as the Prince ponders whether it is better to 'bear the slings and arrows of outrageous fortune' or to die, is essentially restrained by religious scruples as God had 'fixed his cannon against self-slaughter'. We would argue that one factor in the great genius of Shakespeare was his psychological authenticity, and it is noteworthy that, of his 38 plays, suicide was an issue in 11 of them. They died for honour, oft tinged with revenge, for example in *Julias Caesar*; for love in *Romeo and Juliet*; for jealousy in *Othello*; for remorse in *Macbeth*, all similar reasons reported by Durkheim in the late-nineteenth century and in any old Asylum record book (Durkheim, 1952. Only in *Hamlet* and *King Lear* do we come close to mental illness when the now blind, destitute and betrayed Gloucester, who clearly intended to die, was saved by his son, on recovering ponders whether he was mad at the time or whether he had been led astray by a 'thousand nose-some fiend', reflecting the association of mental disorder with demonic possession.

Attitudes towards suicide in the Western world continue to be influenced by the Judaeo-Christian traditional position, and there continues to be a sense of stigma and shame, with an ambivalent oscillation between sympathy and shock. However, in the Islamic tradition there continues to be greater consistency in attitudes towards suicide. This appears to be because in the Koran, and therefore in Islam, there is a direct prohibition and sanctions levelled against suicides, something that does not occur in the Bible. Consequently, the taboo against suicide remains, which can have practical ramifications in terms of assessment and intervention for clients and families from Islam who may have a mental illness.

In the broad Hindu faith there is also a taboo against suicide, especially against suicide in men. However, 'altruistic' suicide is acceptable in the Hindu tradition, but there are other differences from the Western profile, especially in relation to gender (AIIMS, 1986). It may be, therefore, that this may account for the differential level and patterns of suicide in the case of people from Islamic and Asian countries, living both in Asia and in Europe (Soni Raleigh *et al.*, 1990). It is worth mentioning here, that unlike Eurocentric societies, there is an honourable Hindu tradition associated with the bereaved committing suicide, and whilst there is not a great deal of research, women from the Hindu tradition appear to die at almost twice the rate as men, which is virtually the opposite for most 'westernised' societies, including Japan.

With respect to people from a Chinese background, recent data from mainland China (WHO, 1991), Hong Kong (Pritchard, 1993) and Singapore (Kok, 1988), where they have a major Chinese community, show a more mixed gender picture. In mainland China, women clearly die more frequently than men, but apart from youth female suicide in Hong Kong (Pritchard, 1993) it appears that Hong Kong Chinese have a profile closer to the westerner. What is unequivocal, however, is that mental disorder in the Chinese culture appears to be even more stigmatized than amongst Europeans. Interestingly, variations occur when people from different ethnic backgrounds migrate. Usually, first generation immigrant suicide levels are closer to their country of origin than the average for the host society, thus American Hispanics have a significantly lower rate than the average American, but second and third generations rates appear to grow closer to that of the dominant culture country (Sorenson and Golding, 1988; Kok, 1988; Vernon and Phillpe, 1988). Yet at the same time there is evidence for real differences in suicide in the various cultures, seen in studies based upon migrant ethnic minorities over generations.

With respect of Afro-Caribbeans, we do not know of any specific study in Britain that looked at differential rates, though Holinger (1987) found significantly lower suicide rates for both male and female Afro-Americans than Whites. Why this might be is open to debate and is explored elsewhere (Pritchard, 1994). The practical implication is that in a multicultural world, people of different ages, religions and ethnic traditions will probably have a varied response to ideas surrounding suicide and mental illness than the dominant Eurocentric model. And in practice we need to remember that what we know of the suicide complex has probably been learned from western studies and we should be alert to possible age and gender variations in people from traditions other than European.

AETIOLOGY OF SUICIDE

The factor most often associated with suicide is mental illness, mainly depression. Suicide is the morbidity associated with mental illness, and it has been found that between 80 and 90% of all suicides, had, or were in the process of, a severe mental illness, predominately depression (Barraclough and Hughes, 1987; Arato *et al.*, 1988; Marttunen *et al.*, 1991). In study after study, be it in relation to mode of death (Heim and Lester, 1991), age or gender (Kreitman, 1988), or psychosocial factors (Platt, 1984; Allebeck, 1988; Rich *et al.*, 1989), it is depression that is the prevailing theme. Of course, within depression there are the triggers of hopelessness, despair, sense of worthlessness and rage (Beck and Steer, 1991; Beck *et al.*, 1990; Brittlebank *et al.*, 1990), with a seeming plethora of emotions and reactions, brilliantly captured by Keats—'at war with all the *frailty* of grief, of rage, of fear, anxiety, revenge, remorse, spleen, hope, but most of all, despair'.

It is for this reason we reject the traditional division between suicide and attempted suicide/ parasuicide, or what is increasingly called deliberate self harm, and postulate two working categories, 'psychiatric-related' and 'stress-related' suicide (Pritchard, 1993). As will be seen, whilst there remains a degree of overlap, by considering suicidal behaviour in this way, we hope to determine the priority areas for intervention, and to reinforce the importance of the interactive pressures upon the client, family and the professionals.

PSYCHIATRIC-RELATED SUICIDE

Affective depressive disorder

The classic symptoms of the affective depressive disorder are a disturbance of mood with a prevailing sense of profound misery and sadness, and a disturbance of cognition so that the world is perceived as consistently dismal, with no apparent positives, and/ or a translation of everything into self-defeating hopeless negatives. There are patterns of 'physical' symptoms, for example disturbance of sleep and early waking, loss of appetite, weight, and a diurnal variation of mood and energy, where the person usually feels worse in the early morning, can be a particularly 'dangerous' time and so demoralising for the person. The symptoms are outlined in the internationally agreed *Diagnostic and Statistical Manual III*, commonly described as *DSM III*:

---

1 A change of mood, involving feelings of sadness, apathy and/or loneliness

2 A neglect self-concept, with feelings of guilt, self-blame, self-reproach

3 A loss of interest in usual activities and in sex—a general loss of energy

4 Problems with sleeping and eating (appetite can be either poor or increased)

5 Trouble concentrating

6 Psychomotor retardation or agitation

These physio-psychological feelings can lead to a crucial mixture of hopelessness, despair and worthlessness, which appears to be the psychological dynamic associated with suicide. It is experienced as psychically intensively painful, and qualitatively, very different from the 'normal' depression or feeling low, and we are reminded that Dante's description of Hell was the abandonment of hope. Not surprisingly, therefore, people with a depressive affective disorder are 80 times more likely to die by suicide than people without depression (Barraclough and Hughes, 1987). So whenever we see depression, we should always consider it being linked with aggression, albeit against one's self.

The experience might be described as a vortex of depression, as the person's profound mood disturbance of misery and sadness includes worthlessness and guilt with a sense of anger, as the person is overwhelmed and self-blaming:

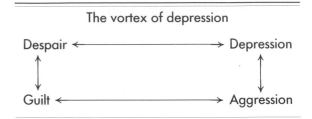

The vortex of depression

Despair ⟷ Depression

Guilt ⟷ Aggression

Schneideman (1988) offers a useful psychological interactional model which describes the subjective experience of the person. There is 'perturbation' (psychical distress), with a sense of psychological 'constriction', a sense that there is 'no option' that is, no sense of any alternative to the misery, and, if there is a 'penchant for action', then self-destructive behaviour is a real possibility. These four features emerged from a content analysis of thousands of suicide notes, and in this sense have a particular significance. Regretfully, Schneideman has not empirically tested these elements and his work has therefore less 'validity' than say the work of Beck (1967), though intuitively, it seems to be a useful practical guide. Beck, however, has a long-established empirical approach to depression and subsequent suicide (e.g. Beck *et al* 1985), with the key theme to note after the depressed mood being the sense of hopelessness that might well subsume Schneideman's category minus the penchant for action. The value of Beck's work is that, whilst based in the USA, it closely paralleled the work of the British research psychiatrist, the late Max Hamilton, and both research teams developed clinical rating scales which were found to match each other and demonstrably provide the *DSM III* with empirical underpinnings (Beck and Steer, 1991).

The schizophrenias

People suffering from schizophrenia are also at risk from self-destructive behaviour, though not as frequently as people suffering from the affective disorders—the dynamic appears to be different. The greatest danger is linked to the person either having an hallucinatory command to kill him or herself, or having a self-denigratory delusion. However, it also appears to be a secondary danger with people with long-standing or recurrent schizophrenia, as if their morale and self-esteem is eroded over time (Cheng *et al.*, 1990; Cohen *et al.*, 1990). Indeed they may well appear as depressed and of course, where ever there is a mixture of schizophrenic and affective symptoms, the risk of self-damaging behaviour is heightened, and suicide lies at the end of the continuum (Prasad and Kumar, 1988; Peterson and Bonger, 1990). Impressionisticly, people who have survived three or four serious psychotic episodes appear to been ground down by their experience, undermining any hope or optimism. One man, known to the author, explained the drabness he had experienced after finding himself 'virtually unemployable' once they 'knew I'd been in hospital'. To 'live on social security benefits alone, means being condemned to permanent house arrest'! This reflects many people's experience chronicled by Patmore (1987), who recognizes the importance of 'occupation' for any person chronically disabled, especially by mental illness, a point to which we shall return.

Substance misuse: alcohol and drugs

Some would argue that substance misuse involving alcohol and drugs is not strictly 'psychiatric'. However, they are included in the *International Diagnostic Manual* and alcohol and drugs are very frequently linked to suicidal behaviour (Platt and Robinson, 1991), thus it is appropriate to include them in this section.

It would be easy to digress and explore the attributable causes of either alcohol or drug misuse, for certainly they appear to be both a response to psychosocioeconomic pressures (Plant, 1989; Janlert and Hammarstrom, 1992), and often found in conjunction with depressive illness (Sournia, 1990). However, as so often is the case, human beings are not like the text book 'neat and tidy' categories, as was found amongst young adult clients in the Probation and Social Service Departments caseloads. Despite belonging to a non-specialist workload, there was a significant overlap with a drug–alcohol/mental illness axis compounded by poverty (Pritchard *et al.*, 1993),

which was similar to the very mixed picture of men in British prisons (Gunn *et al.*, 1991). El-Guebaly (1990) has argued for the concept of a 'dual diagnosis', as he found that between 30 and 65% of people with alcohol problems who enter rehabilitation programmes also had a formal psychiatric disorder.

What seems to happen is people sometimes use drugs or alcohol to relieve their actual or borderline depression. People along the continuum of psychosocial despair associated with drug or alcohol misuse probably feel reactively depressed, or respond to a sense of extreme low self-esteem, and impulsively become involved in deliberate self-harm with fatal consequences. The danger with misuse of either substance is that they are mind-influencing and impair judgement. Experienced workers in the field will relate cases where people have died from apparent 'accidental' overdose or a particularly large injection which has led, via choking following vomiting, to their death. This can give rise to speculation as to whether there was a degree of 'intent' in the outcome, as there appeared to be a 'risk-taking' element in the person's behaviour—the almost classical 'Russian Roulette' especially amongst younger people (Miller *et al.*, 1991; Graham and Burvill, 1992). Taking an over-view of the research there are suggestions that frequent or heavy use of either drugs or alcohol, significantly increases the likelihood of suicide in a person with depression, especially adolescents (Crumley, 1990; Miller *et al.*, 1991; Merrill *et al.*, 1992) whilst Murphy and Wetzel (1990) found that one in four completed suicides also involved either drugs or alcohol problems. In other words the presence of alcohol or drug use, quite independent of dependency, adds to the uncertainty of a situation and probably compounds the risk of impulsivity and therefore of death.

Physiological factors

For us, the etiological debate about 'nature (genetics) versus nurture (social)' is sterile as the evidence appears, overwhelmingly, that they are interactional. For example, a person with a high constitutional loading for schizophrenia, may well have two parents with the condition yet two people in three will remain free of the syndrome. Thus it appears that 'vulnerability', be it endowed or psychosocial, is stretched to breaking point by life events (Quinton and Rutter, 1988; Oliver, 1988). This biopsychosocioeconomic approach has been developed into a model which merits the further exploration of Mann and Arango (1992), who neatly juxtapose all factors into what they call a stress–diathesis model. Crucially, it acknowledges the two-way interaction between the physiological and the psychosocial environment. They include some interesting research that suggests that serotonin metabolism may predispose to either suicidal ideation and behaviour, or aggressive and impulsive behaviour (e.g. Bourgeois, 1991; Golden et al., 1991). However, the work is in its early stages, but theoretically it may lead to either biochemical tests to indicate level of suicide risk within a potentially identified psychosocial stress complex, or, for some types of depressive/suicidal situations, treatment. However, when reviewing psychiatry over the last 50 years, in spite of the undoubted advances, wise practitioners realize that there is still much to learn, and that individual cases will always confound the research, which though identifying patterns of behaviour, is based upon analysis of group samples, which leaves considerable variation in individuals.

PSYCHOSOCIOECONOMIC FACTORS

The following psychosocioeconomic factors are relevant to 'psychiatric-related suicide', though as Fig. 12.1 shows, the greater the non-psychiatric factors present in an individual situation, the greater the likelihood of the suicide risk being 'stress-related'.

Gender

Throughout the Western world, men kill themselves more often than women. The ratio ranges from about 1.5:1.0 to 4:1, but broadly averaging at about two and a half males to every female suicide (WHO, 1992). Thus, in terms of practical risk, men are more likely to die by their own

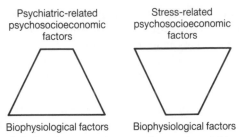

Fig. 12.1 *Psychosocioeconomic factors in suicide.*

hand. However, Kushner (1989) presents data which resolve the apparent anomaly that females have twice the rate of formal depression, yet have half the suicide rate. He contrasts levels of deliberate self harm (attempted suicide) in the USA, with suicide rates, along the gender divide. He makes the point that there is almost an inverse matching, as the women's greater frequency of deliberate self harm, of about two to one male, is the reverse of completed suicides. Thus he suggests, the combined figures of suicide added to deliberate self harm, are so similar that they cancel out the gender divide. If this is so, it is probably an indication of the distress associated with the depression, but affected by differences in gender approaches to violence, seen in the differences in the mode of deaths.

It has been found that males use more violent methods to kill themselves (MaClure, 1987), especially in the use of firearms in the USA and Australia (Heim and Lester, 1991; Males, 1991). The media in Britain have noted an increase in suicides amongst farmers, who probably have greater access to weapons than any other group, save the police/military, in the UK. Women, on the other hand, will predominantly use drugs, whilst men are more likely to hang or drown themselves or use car exhausts. In countries with dense populations and high rise building, men are more likely to throw themselves from skyscrapers than women (Peng and Choo, 1990). Thus it might be argued that here is an other example of men suffering from the inherent sexism of Western society, as males are socialized into more assertive and violent behaviour, which when directed against themselves, is more fatal (Kushner, 1989). The UK male to female suicide ratio averages 3.32:1, though as will be seen this partly

Suicide in the UK by age and gender in 1990 (rates per million population)								
Age	General	15–24	25–34	35–44	45–54	55–64	65–74	75+
Males	126	122	172	175	171	142	141	194
Females	38	21	41	46	55	55	63	59
Ratio	3.32	5.81	4.20	3.80	3.11	2.58	2.24	3.29

reflects the worsening suicide position for men as women's fatalities have been reduced over the past two decades:

However, do not underestimate the degree of seriousness in women, simply because they have lower completed suicides, for despite the very welcome recent improvements in the reduction of female suicides in Britain, younger women did not enjoy the same degree of improvement (Pritchard, 1990). It was suggested that the under 30-year-old woman's attitude to her place in the socioeconomic arena has changed, which may well work through into new statistics by the end of the decade.

As mentioned earlier, we must also remember to differentiate between clients from a 'European/ Western' background and those from Asia, the Orient and Islam. This again shows just how complex is suicide, as the professional has to make client-specific judgements, guided, but not directed, by the best research information available.

Age

The next most important social variable is that of age. With each successive decade, the suicide rate increases proportionately, and, with the exception of Ireland and Norway, this is the case throughout the Western world (WHO, 1992). Indeed, the over 64-year-olds, virtually in *every* country of the world, have a higher rate than any other age group, and in the majority of the world, the over 75s lead the 'league table' of proportion of suicide deaths by age. The figures above show the age and gender suicide rates extrapolated for the UK in 1990.

At first sight it might be easy to assume that as people get older, as they are borne down by life's difficulties in terms of physical as well as mental illness, suicide may appear 'rational'. This is a dangerous potentially 'ageist' position, as recent studies show variations in elderly suicides (Pritchard, 1992a) which appear to be linked to the relatively higher degree of *psychosocial* factors, as victims experience neglect, isolation and rejection (Vogel and Wolfersdorf, 1989). Indeed, we can be unequivocal, the isolated, depressed, 'psychiatric' or 'stressed' elderly (75 years plus) person carries a particularly high level of suicide risk.

The increase over the years, in most of the developed nations is quite dramatic and raises serious policy and practice questions. For example, countries with lower average rates than Britain, such as Italy, Spain and Greece, have higher levels of over 75-year suicide than the UK (Pritchard, 1992b). Beware therefore of the 'ageism' assumption, that if you were a 75-year-old plus you might consider suicide. It has to be remembered that the current elderly belong to a generation with greater traditional values when the norm was that 'the almighty had fixed his canon against self-slaughter'. What are the pressures that make this generation take such a drastic step?

Adolescents

First the 'reassurance', adolescents compared with other age groups usually have the lowest suicide rate. Indeed it is noteworthy that the 122 rate for the 15–24-year-old is *double* the 'normal' rate when Britain does not suffer a recession (Pritchard, 1992b). Children's suicide (5–14 years) is extremely rare, usually seldom above one per million in the age band per annum.

On reflection it is easy to see why the death rate

is relatively so very low. Prior to young adult-hood, children and adolescents are simply not competent in knowing what is fatal and so often, distressed adolescents are flying from, rather than to an outcome. This is typified in Shakespeare's King John where the young Prince Arthur throws himself from the battlements, but to escape. He acknowledges the risk, but as his situation has become intolerable, he believes that God's justice will bear him up, but if not then he will dare the risk. However, this is not to deny the potential seriousness of the adolescent's distress (Kerfoot, 1984) but suicide under 18 is relatively very rare. However, De Chateau (1990), in a 30-year follow-up study of children previously attending child guidance, found that more than 4% had died from suicide, which was higher than would have been expected. This is yet another area of ambiguity, for whilst completed suicide in the age group is rare, this is not the case for deliberate self harm. Within a cohort of 2,181 adolescents nearly 4% were involved in self-destructive be-haviour without prior indication and a third of youngsters with known suicidal ideation went as far as damaging themselves (Kosky et al., 1990). The risk of death is perhaps slight but the ramifi-cations upon the young person and their families can be profound. We shall return to the problem of adolescents when we come to discuss deliber-ate self harm.

Physical illness

An obvious linking problem is that of physical illness. Studies over the years have found a small but on occasions significant finding of the presence of a physical illness, usually of a chronic nature amongst suicide victims (Barraclough and Hughes, 1987). However, it is again too easy to make the simplistic jump to such conditions as cancer. For example, Stensman and Sundqvist-Stensman (1988) found a non-significant presence of physical illness amongst 416 consecutive suicides in Sweden. Allebeck and Bolund (1991) examined the archetypal assumption about suicide and people with cancer. Whilst there was a higher proportion of suicide attempts in people suffering from malignant disease, proportionately

it was far lower than those with a mental illness, drug/alcohol problem or 'personality disorder' (Allebeck, 1988; Stiefel et al., 1989). What appears to be the key is the degree of pain control in such situations and probably the extent to which there are supports for the patient in their social networks.

A new association of physical illness and suicide has emerged with the advent of the acquired immune deficiency syndrome (AIDS). It has been found that the risk of suicide increases not only in people with AIDS (Marzuk et al., 1988), but on first learning that they are HIV positive (Schneider et al., 1991). Consequently, most reputable HIV testing centres now insist upon a counselling support service to anyone undertaking the test. The HIV dimension can be further complicated when combined with nega-tive social circumstances such as found amongst homeless young people (Cohen et al., 1991; Kruks, 1991), with increased risks of 'survival' prostitution, drug and alcohol misuse which can be literally, a fatal mixture (Yates et al., 1991).

Bereavement

Another factor that may contribute is the impact of bereavement upon surviving members of the family, not only amongst elderly survivors. People are more likely to be involved in suicidal behaviour within 12 months of a key bereavement and often around the anniversary of the pivotal death (Clayton, 1982; Barraclough and Hughes, 1987; Fasey, 1990). Evidently, if the person was already child free and elderly, it is more likely that there will be a greater degree of objective isolation and loneliness, with possible less psycho-social support. These are features which *may* account for the proportionably higher Italian and Spanish figures who have a stronger pro-elderly tradition compared with British figures. Whilst the above range of factors has been found to be statistically associated with suicide, there is a degree of over-lap with deliberate self harm which is especially strong in the following areas, which again emphasizes that one always has to make specific client-focused judgements both in terms of assessment and intervention.

Social factors

A person living alone can be at risk in the presence of the above factors, particularly depression. Equally, being isolated is another factor, for if others are not around then there is no one to intervene or stop people from killing themselves. It is, however, the subjective sense of loneliness and isolation which is so important, as noted earlier (Vogel and Wolfersdorf, 1989). Marriage appears to 'protect' against suicide, and single people are more likely to die than those with a partner, but being divorced accentuates the risk of suicide (Kreitman, 1988).

Homelessness has been found to be a factor, which may partly be due to the fact that one major feature leading to becoming homeless is having a mental illness (Appleby and Desai, 1985; Hammond and Wallace, 1990; Lister, 1991). Indeed it may be argued that suicide can be a sequelae of poor, or an absence of adequate, care in the community following discharge of previously long-term mentally ill people (MIND, 1974; NFS, 1988). Former patients tend usually to be older, whereas the young homeless can be at double risk (Cohen *et al.*, 1991) though there is a different dynamic, often being associated with previous family disruption (Powers *et al.*, 1990).

Not surprisingly, for a person in *any* age group to be homeless exposes one to a whole range of '—pitiless storms, and, how shall your houseless heads—defend you from such seasons as these—' (*King Lear*). To complete the quote 'take physic pomp; expose they-self to what wretches feel', would take us into the issue of an under-funded social policy, which in this context would be a digression, yet clearly what we 'can afford' for our NHS and Social Services is highly relevant to the kind of service we offer to citizens who are mentally ill (Pritchard, 1992c). Nevertheless, in the presence of homelessness, stress-related depression and possible suicide complicates an already fraught situation in which drug/alcohol misuse, previous physical and sexual maltreatment, family disruption, crime and delinquency is a cocktail indicating severe psychosocial disruption.

Unemployment

Brenner (1983) built upon earlier work and demonstrated a connection between suicide and unemployment. The interaction appears that, with people who would deal with their lives perfectly competently, redundancy makes them vulnerable, reflecting Freud's classic aphorism that 'work binds people to reality'. The majority of people find their identity, self-esteem and sense of worth confirmed or enhanced by the job they do; conversely in the vast majority of cases, unemployment undermines these positives (Warr, 1987). The association has not been without controversy, as some feel such a link is 'political' and in times of recession, few Governments in any country are likely to welcome such news. Platt (1984) explored the issue in a seminal review and subsequent national and international work has confirmed his conclusion, that there is an unquestioned association between increases in suicide and recession. This link has been found throughout Europe (Pritchard, 1990, 1992b) North America and Australasia (Pritchard, 1992b). One confirming feature was that such a statistical association was not found internationally during the 1960s and early 1970s, but emerged at times of recession (Pritchard, 1990). What happens is that there is a gap between jobs available and the number of people seeking work, which can be described as a 'gap of despair'. Some people apply for 50, 70 or a even 100 jobs and may not even receive an acknowledgement. Based upon the psychosocial impact of the 1980s recession, we have to conclude that for the UK, structural unemployment, centring upon three million people being jobless, is likely to continue to the end of the millennium. Its relevance for practice will become self-evident, for there is overwhelming evidence that unemployment damages people's health, both physical and mental (Whitehead, 1990). Our work contributed to confirming the association between suicide and recession but we also found that whilst suicide had risen nationally by almost a third, it rose even faster in the three most affluent employment regions. This was apparently due to the sense of isolation and stigma experienced by jobless people in Greater London, the south-east and

Male suicide in England and Wales by age, 1974–1990 (rates per million population)								
Year	General	15–24	25–34	35–44	45–54	55–64	65–74	75+
1974	95	58	106	114	154	159	189	196
1990	121	117	160	171	164	133	136	194
Ratio	1.27	2.02	1.51	1.50	1.06	0.84	0.72	0.99

East Anglia. To be unemployed in Liverpool or Middlesbrough may be a bad experience, but there is nevertheless a degree of understanding and sympathy, whereas unemployed people in Winchester, Reading or Norwich are described as work-shy, as few appreciate that at the height of the recession even these areas had a ratio of vacancies to jobless of more than 1:15. The grave situation facing the most affluent areas of Britain, is that there is a ratio of 1:20 between notified vacancies and the number of jobless, and in September 1992 it reached an alarming 1:50+ in Greater London (Dept Employment, 1992), a level that even exceeded the Northern Irish average, which has been the highest in the UK and amongst the worst in Europe.

Male suicide has increased since 1973, the year of the oil crisis, which first triggered unemployment in the west. The general rate is the national rate per million male population and the ratio between 1974 to 1990 is equivalent to a 27% rise, which was down on the 1988 level (Pritchard, 1990). It can be seen however, that youth suicide, between the ages of 15–24, doubled, reaching unprecedented heights. Indeed in Scotland and Northern Ireland youth suicide was higher than the average Anglo-Welsh deaths, which has never happened before. The work of Jackson and Warr (1988) illustrates the ramifications of unemployment, especially long-term and the classic review by Platt (1984) still merits close consultation. Both will remind practitioners what Whitehead (1990) demonstrated from a range of socio-medical studies, that unemployment damages *both* physical and mental health. It would seem therefore that unemployment will continue to be a factor requiring consideration in both assessment and intervention terms for some considerable time to come.

Psychological factors

From the nineteenth century onwards, efforts to understand the psychological predisposition and triggers of suicide have attracted considerable research interest. The neo-Freudian notion of 'turning aggression against the self' (Freud), and the behavioural school's concept of 'learned helplessness' (Seligman) have contributed useful insights. Increasingly there has been a merging of previously disparate schools, now come together, exemplified since 1981 in the *British Journal of Behavioural Psychotherapy*, a title which would have been anathema to the antagonists of the pre-1970s. Perhaps the most promising line of enquiry and intervention comes from the broadly 'cognitive behavioural' school with contributions from Kelly's 'construct theory', Lazarus's 'multi-modal approach' and Beck's 'cognitive psychology' which led to a British classic by Hawton *et al.* (1989). The strength of the approach is that it focuses upon the perception and experience of the individual and how he or she perceives and interprets the situation, and suggests client-specific problem-solving techniques. It has been found, particularly from studies of people involved in deliberate self harm (DHS) compared to non-DHS people, who may also be depressed, that those involved in suicidal behaviour are poor at problem solving. They interpret the world as constrained, both currently and in the foreseeable future, which becomes frankly aversive and hopeless. At the same time they appear to have a restricted armoury of personal problem-solving devices (McLeod *et al.*, 1992).

McLeod and his colleagues explore some very promising work described as 'dialectical behavioral therapy' (Linehan *et al.*, 1987, 1992) which attempts to focus specifically upon those emotional features that contribute to Beck's category of 'hopelessness'. Once again we quote the master observer of the human experience 'how weary, stale, flat and unprofitable seam to me all the uses of this world' (*Hamlet*), and the dynamic of action and anger 'I am one whom the blows and buffets of this vile world hath so incensed I am reckless what I do to spite the world' (*Macbeth*). It is a truism, that wherever there is depression there is often aggression (Paykel *et al.*, 1975), as the recklessness is turned against themselves. One might speculate that the anger and frustration that occurs following life events such as unemployment perhaps follows the classic flight or fight divide, the 'fighters' damage others, seen in crime and delinquency statistics (Home Office, 1992), whilst the 'fliers' damage themselves?

Previous deliberate self harm

One factor that is a high statistical indicator of the risk of suicide, is deliberate self harm. Whilst we disagree with McLeod *et al.* (1992) preference for the term 'parasuicide' (Kreitman and Phillip, 1969), there is no disagreement concerning the overlap between suicide and DSH nor the likelihood that the two phenomena are essentially different but meet in an interaction.

Almost half the people who die from suicide have a history of previous self harm (Barraclough and Hughes, 1987; King and Barraclough, 1990), though it should be noted that slightly more than half had *no* DSH history (Allgulander and Fisher, 1990), emphasizing, if such emphasis is needed, the need for specific judgements in respect to the individual's situation. However, as mentioned previously, drugs/alcohol misuse/dependency increases the likelihood of both repeated DSH and a completed suicide (Miller *et al.*, 1991; Bayatapour *et al.*, 1992). Let us briefly turn to this problematic area of DSH and the possible overlap with completed suicide.

DELIBERATE SELF HARM

Aetiology of deliberate self harm (parasuicide)

Incidence, gender and age

The incidence of deliberate self harm (DSH) is difficult to establish though the greatest single reason for acute medical female admissions in England and Wales was drug over-dosage, which exceeded 100,000 per annum (DHSS, 1984), whilst it was the second highest reason for male *medical* admissions, the highest being for heart conditions (Hawton and Catalin, 1987). Determining the numbers of people involved in DSH shares some of the same recording problems as with suicide, as there may be an understandable 'protective' reluctance to acknowledge the self-damaging behaviour (Kreitman, 1977).

Estimates of DSH in the USA have ranged from 120 to 730 per hundred thousand population (Fremouw *et al.*, 1990) which, based upon the latest USA suicide rates (1990) would be equivalent to 58 DSH's per completed suicide. However, these gross ratios are markedly affected by age and gender. Unlike suicide, there is a preponderance of female over male DSH of about 2:1, and it occurs far more frequently in younger people, especially the under 30s. Recent figures in Europe concerning DSH have shown a very wide range, the highest female DSH rate was 5,950 per million population (Platt *et al.*, 1992), contrasting with a rate of 117 suicides in France, a ratio of 51:1. The lowest rate was in Spain, 950 DSH compared with 40 per million suicides, equivalent to 24:1. These extrapolations, however, do not take into account the marked variation between the age bands, as the under 24-year-olds have about three times the DSH rate of the 55-year-olds and older, hence for any estimate of these ratios in Britain we must consider the age and gender factors.

Based on the number of *all* drug overdose admissions in England and Wales (approximately 133,000) we would add a further 10% for other methods of DSH. This would yield a figure of approximately 146,000 per annum. This would be a ratio of about 37 DSH to one suicide. However if we 'corrected' for age and assumed 60% of

DSH was under 30, the ratio of DSH to suicide rises to 97:1.

However, a further complication in regard to the age factor is that recent research in relation to elderly DSH has shown that, whilst DSH is less frequent amongst the elderly, where it occurs, for every four people involved in DSH one died from suicide (Merril *et al.*, 1990), adding further emphasis to the risk of suicide amongst elderly people.

Psychiatric factors

Unlike suicide, where formal psychiatric illness is clearly established, the main problems appear to be related to people with personality disorders, alcohol difficulties and not infrequently drug misuse (Kreitman and Foster, 1991).

Intent

Perhaps the most difficult feature to determine is whether or not the person intended to die. Beck *et al.* (1974) developed a very useful 'intent scale' which is still useful, and aids us understand the person's particular circumstances. It would appear that if the individual was not isolated at the time of the DSH; or did not take precautions to avoid discovery; or did not premeditate the act; or believe that the method was fatal, then 'intent' seems to be low and is different from the suicide constellation.

Repetition

As mentioned above, previous DSH is both associated with completed suicide, but also further repeated DSH. Thus if a person has been involved with more than one DSH episode, the likelihood is that they will repeat again. Buglas and Horton (1974) prediction of repeat scales, along with the Beck intent instrument, have been used over the years. They noted six key factors associated with repetition; these were problems in the use of alcohol, diagnosis of 'sociopathy' (often interchangeable for personality disorder), previous in-patient and out-patient psychiatric treatment, not living with family, and previous DSH.

Kreitman and Foster (1991) developed this work and identified 11 elements:

1	Previous DSH
2	Personality disorder
3	Frequent alcohol consumption
4	Previous psychiatric treatment
5	Unemployment
6	Belonging to social class 5
7	Drug abuse
8	Criminal record
9	Violence, either given or received
10	Aged between 25 and 54
11	Single/widowed or divorced

When set alongside suicide factors, it can be seen that there is a different profile but with an increasing overlap in regard to the psychosocial factors. However, Kreitman and Foster still found that even if a person had an accumulative score of eight or more, 60% did *not* repeat the DSH within two years. Thus, as in most cases when dealing with people, the various scales can only be used as a guide to assist the professional in making an *informed* judgement about a specific individual in a particular circumstance. It may be easy, however, for some practitioners to became somewhat 'case-hardened' in respect to DSH and dismissively put it down to a 'cry for help'. Yet we should never forget that DSH is an extreme action, and apart from the real risk to the person, is indicative of a very self-defeating method of dealing with life problems. In an excellent review, McLeod *et al.* (1992) bring together both epidemiological studies, with recent psychological treatment developments, and juxtapose a cognitive behavioural therapy approach to deal with the person's psychological state. The following list might help to differentiate suicide from DSH and as will be seen, the lower down the order, the greater the overlap (see table on opposite page).

Differentiating suicide from DSH (+ degree of strength of association)

Suicide	*DSH*
1 Psychiatric illness—affective disorder, some schizophrenia	Mainly personality disorder
2 Wishes to die	No decision, probably not
3 Males 2:1 females	Females 2:1 males
4 Alcohol / drug misuse ++	Alcohol / drug problems
5 Age, increases with each decade highest in 75+ year olds. Statistically rare under 16 years	Mainly younger people, especially under 30s. Not uncommon in adolescents
6 Previous DSH (47%)	Previous DSH
7 2% of DSH die in next year	Don't, *but* 10% of DSHs finally die from suicide
8 Physical illness, chronic pain	Not prevalent
9 Violence and gender, male assailants women recipients	More emotional violence and possible 'gains'
10 All social classes	More social class 4 and 5
11 Unemployed +	Unemployment
12 Divorce +	Divorce
13 Living alone, isolated	Living without relatives, overcrowding
14 In spring and autumn	No seasonal variation

INTERVENTION

It is argued that modern integrated treatment of psychiatric disorders is at a stage similar to kidney dialysis, as people can be maintained in the community providing the availability of a kidney machine and appropriate backup services. So, too, in the mental health field, as there is empirical evidence that we can offer effective treatment, providing it is based upon an interdisciplinary integrated approach.

Suicides, as well as DSH, are human tragedies, involving individuals and their families, and making major demands upon health and community services. Effective intervention therefore is imperative. There are grounds to share the Government's recent optimism, heralded in the White Paper *Health of the Nation* (1992) which seeks to reduce by a third suicide related to psy-

chiatric illness. We shall briefly review the forms of intervention.

Suicide is the 'complication' of psychiatric disorder, especially the affective mood disorders, therefore we need to treat the basic affective disorder. There is evidence that an integrated approach that aims at lifting the depression, improving clients' self-esteem and maintaining their personal and social networks, is effective in terms of treating the underlying depression and influencing those interactive psychosocial factors (Weismann, 1981; Corney and Clare, 1983; Gottleib, 1983; Beck, 1988; Jack, 1988; De Man and Labreche-Gauthier, 1991; McLeod *et al.*, 1992). This demands the availability of the whole treatment armamentum of health and community services, which includes psychiatrist, social workers, community psychiatric nurses, general practitioners (very important as they provide more psychiatric care in the community than anyone else), residential and half-way house staff and last, but by no means least, engages both individuals and their families as active allies in their own treatment.

In terms of the schizophrenias, again an integrated approach that uses chemotherapy to control the core symptoms, aided by a appropriately trained counselling support service to assist communication within the family and assist maintaining socioeconomic networks, and where appropriate, social skills training (Hogerty et al., 1986; Doane, 1986; Faccinani et al., 1990; Holmes-Elber and Riger, 1990). In particular the development of 'family management of schizophrenia', sometimes described as the Fallon approach (Fallon, 1985), sees people in their total environment, and recognizes that the majority of people with schizophrenia invariably depend upon their families. There have been some very promising results in terms of improving family relationships and reducing hospital re-admissions (Leff and Vaughan, 1985; Kuipers, 1987). What this group of therapists has appreciated, and what the Schizophrenia Fellowship has been urging for years, is to take the families into partnership, or as Lefley and Johnson (1990) say, 'Families as allies in the treatment of the mentally ill'.

In respect of the stress-related suicide, an improved social policy is needed to reach out to people under socioeconomic pressures, especially vulnerable men, who are often reluctant to admit the need for help. There is good evidence that carefully targeted care in the community can enhance the quality of people's lives and be an effective bulwark against the dangers of suicide, maintaining contact over time, and crucially, being accessible to clients and their families (Parry and Schapiro, 1986; Gibbons and Butler, 1987; Jack, 1988; Emerick, 1990). In addition there is a need for occupation, as well as employment initiatives (Patmore, 1987), for it is vital that we do not leave the mentally ill alone, isolated and neglected, for whose self-esteem would not evaporate or brood about a sense of worthlessness, if we were made to feel 'like shadows left wandering in the day'?

One group, who are often more neglected than the mentally ill, is the families of those people who have died from suicide. It is as if we as professionals compound their loss by our sense of failure/guilt, and so often cease contact far too soon. We need to acknowledge that bereavement, especially following a suicide, damages people's health (Pennebaker and O'Heeron, 1984; Barraclough and Hughes, 1987; McIntosh and Wrobleski, 1988). In the USA there are a range of 'survivors' self-help groups, who are relatively rare in Britain, yet we have long known about the potential abnormal grief reaction in families of suicides (Bunch and Barraclough, 1971), so we should be active in encouraging the development of such support groups.

Suicide, it has been argued, is the ultimate rejection (Pritchard, 1993). If we fail to respond to the needs of some of our most disadvantaged citizens, the mentally ill, then we fail the Churchillian test of being a civilized society. We now have a better scientific understanding of this bitter human condition, which should improve our therapeutic art. We need to match empathy with analysis, in our continued search for an improved service, and perhaps for the first time in human history we 'can cleanse the stuffed bosom of that perilous stuff that weighs so heavy upon the heart'.

CONCLUSIONS

Suicide remains the 'psychiatric emergency' as people with a mental disorder are 80 times more likely to kill themselves than non-mentally ill people. Modern research shows that there are important psychosocioeconomic factors associated with suicide which can have a serious bearing upon identification, prevention and intervention with the suicidal individual. Suicidal behaviour is seldom 'neutral' in its impact, which can affect the individual's family, factors that should be considered in relation to assessment, prevention and subsequent intervention plan.

The research cited in this chapter is drawn from all Western countries, and the brief comparisons between British and Continental data is relevant as community mental health work will increasingly include people from mainland Europe. The research, however, is predominantly 'eurocentric' and special attention is required when working with people from Asian and Islamic communities, as the evidence indicates significant differences in patterns of suicide amongst them.

Two types of self-destructive behaviour are postulated, 'psychiatric-related' and 'stress-related' suicide, though there are overlaps that create complex practice dilemmas. Suicide is schematically discriminated from 'deliberate self-harm' (parasuicide/attempted suicide) but both similar and dissimilar elements are identified.

It will be argued that the annual toll of suicides in Britain, which exceeds the murder rate by ten to one, can, with an appropriate multidisciplinary and integrated approach, be significantly reduced. The practice approach of the author reflects this integrated strategy, which reminds us that people are not like text books, and even the most experienced professional can feel overwhelmed by the pressures of operating in problematic areas.

FURTHER READING

Books are always helpful, as is the present text in that they synthesize material. The weakness is that they reflect the relatively narrow perspective of the author/editors. It is therefore recommended that students should get into the professional habit which will inform their practice, and by getting access to the following journals: *The American Journal of Psychiatry*, *The British Journal of Psychiatry*, *The British Journal of Social Work*, and, though slightly more difficult but ideal for the suicide theme, *Suicide and Life Threatening Behaviour*.

REFERENCES

Allebeck, P. (1988) Predictors of completed suicides in a cohort of young men: Role of personality and deviant behaviour. *British Medical Journal*, **297**, 176–178.

Allebeck, P. & Bolund, C. (1991) Suicides and suicide attempts in cancer patients. *Psychological Medicine*, **21** (4), 979–984.

AIIMS (1986) Suicide attempts and suicides in India: Cross-cultural aspects. *Acta Psychiatrica Scandinavia*, **32** (2), 64–73.

Allgulander, C. & Fisher, L.D. (1990) Clinical predictors of completed and repeated self-poisoning in 8895 self-poisoning patients. *European Archives Psychiatry Neurological Science*, **239** (4), 270–276.

Appleby, J. & Desai, P.N. (1985) Documenting the relationship between homelessness and psychiatric hospitalisation. *Hospital Community Psychiatry*, **36** (7) 732–737.

Arato, M., Demeter, E. & Somogyi, E. (1988) Retrospective psychiatric assessment of 200 suicides in Budapest. *Acta Psychiatrica Scandinavia*, **77**, 454–456.

Barraclough, B. & Hughes, J. (1987) *Suicide: Clinical and Epidemiological Studies*. Croom Helm.

Bayatpour, M., Wells, R.D. & Holford, S. (1992) Physical and sexual abuse as predictors of substance use and suicide among pregnant teenagers. *Journal Adolescent Health*, **13**, (2), 128–132.

Beck, A.T. (1967) *Depression: Clinical, Experimental and Theoretical Aspects*, New York, Harper Row.

Beck, A.T. (1988) *Cognitive Therapy and Depression*, 2nd edn. Chichester: Wiley.

Beck, A.T. & Steer, R.A. (1991) Relationship between the Beck Anxiety Inventory and the Hamilton Rating Scale with anxious outpatients. *Journal Anxiety Disorders*, **5** (3), 213–223.

Beck, A.T., Schulyer, D. & Herman, I. (1974) Development of suicidal intent scales. In Beck, A.T., Resnik, C.P. & Lettiere, D.J. (Eds) *The Prediction of Suicide*. Bowie, Maryland: Charles Press.

Beck, A.T., Steer, R.A. & Garrison, B. (1985) Hopelessness and eventual suicide: A 10 year prospective study of patients hospitalised for suicidal ideation. *American Journal Psychiatry*, **142**, 559–563.

Beck, A.T., Steer, R.A. & Skeie, T.M. (1990) Panic disorder and suicide ideation and behaviour: Discrepant findings in psychiatric out-patients. *American Journal Psychiatry*, **148** (9) 1195–1199.

Bourgeois, M. (1991) Serotinin impulsivity and suicide: a review. *Human Psychopharmacology*, **6** (Suppl.) S31–S36.

Brenner, M.H. (1983) Mortality and economic instability: detailed analysis for Britain and comparative analysis for selected countries. *International Journal Health Service*, **13**, 563–620.

Brittlebank, A.D., Cole, A. & Hassanjay, F. (1990) Hostility, hopelessness and deliberate self-harm. A prospective follow-up. *Acta Psychiatrica Scandinavia*, **81** (3) 280–283.

Buglas, D. & Horton, J. (1974) A scale for predicting

subsequent suicidal behaviour. *British Journal Psychiatry*, **125**, 168–174.

Bunch, J. & Barraclough B. (1971) The influence of parental death anniversaries upon suicide dates. *Social Psychiatry*, **6**, 193–199.

Chambers, D.R. & Harvey, J.G. (1988) Self inflicted death 1971–1985. In Moller, H.J. & Schmidtke, R. (Eds) *Current Issues in Suicidology*. Berlin. Springer.

Chambers, D.R. & Harvey, J.G. (1989) Inner urban and national suicide rates, a simple comparative study. *Medicine Science Law*, **29** (3) 182–185.

Cheng, K.K., Leung, C.M. & Lam, T.H. (1990) Risk factors of suicide amongst schizophrenics *Acta Psychiatrica Scandinavia*, **81** (3) 220–224.

Clayton, P.J. (1982) Bereavement. In Paykel, E.D. (Ed.) *Handbook of Affective Disorders*. Edinburgh: Chuchill Livingstone.

Cohen, L.J., Test, M.A. & Brown, R.L. (1990) Suicide and schizophrenia: Data from a prospective community treatment study. *American Journal Psychiatry*, **147** (5) 602–607.

Cohen, E., MacKenzie, R.G. & Yates, G.L. (1991) HEADASS, a psycho-social risk assessment instrument: Implications for designing effective intervention programmes for runaway youth. *Journal Adolescent Health*, **12** (7), 539–544.

Collins, T. (1990) *Open Verdict: An Account of 25 Mysterious Deaths in the Defence Industry*. Sphere.

Corney, H. & Clare, A.W. (1983) The effectiveness of attached social workers in the management of depressed women. *British Journal Social Work*, **13** (1), 57–74.

Crumley, F.E. (1990) Substance abuse and adolescent suicidal behaviour *Journal American Medical Association*, **273** (22), 3051–3056.

De Chateau, J. (1990) Mortality and aggressiveness in a 30 year follow-up study in child guidance clinics in Stockholm. *Acta Psychiatrica Scandinavia*, **147** (6) 761–765.

De Man, A. & Labreche-Gauthier, L. (1991) Suicide ideation and community support: an evaluation of two programmes. *Journal Clinical Psychology*, **47** (1), 57–60.

Department Employment (1992) *Employment Gazette*. December. London: DoE.

Department Health (1992) *The Health of the Nation: A strategy for England*, DoH. London: HMSO.

DHSS (1984) *The Management of Deliberate Self-Harm* LA–SSL 84: London, HMSO.

Doane, J.A. (1986) The impact of individual and family treatment on the affective climate of families of schizophrenics. *British Journal Psychiatry*, **148**, 279–287.

Durkheim, E. (1897) Translated by Spaulding, J.A. & Simpson, G. (1952) *Suicide: A Study in Sociology*. London: Routledge Kegan Paul.

El-Guebaly, A.M. (1990) Substance abuse and mental disorders; The Dual Diagnosis concept. *Canadian Journal Psychiatry*, **35** (3), 261–267.

Emerick, R.M. (1990) Self-help groups and former patients: relationships with mental health professionals. *Community Psychiatry*, **41** (4), 401–407.

Faccinani, C., Mignolli, G. & Platt, S. (1990) Service utilisation, social support and psychiatric status in a cohort of patients with schizophrenia. A 7-year follow-up. *Schizophrenia Research*, **3** (2), 139–146.

Fallon, I.R.H. (1985) *Family Care of Schizophrenia*. London: Guildford Press.

Fasey, C.N. (1990) Grief in Old Age: A Review of the literature. *International Journal Geriatric Psychiatry*, **5**, 67–75.

Fremouw, W.J., Perczel, M. & Ellis, T.E. (1990) *Suicide Risk: Assessment and Response Guidelines*. Oxford: Pergamon Press.

Gibbons, J.S. & Butler, J.P. (1987) Quality of life of 'new long stay' psychiatric in-patients, the effect of moving into a hostel. *British Journal Psychiatry*, **151**, 347–354.

Golden, R.N., Gilmore, J.H. & Corrigan, M.H.N. (1991) Serotonin, suicide and aggression: Clinical studies. *Journal Clinical Psychiatry*, **52** (12), (Suppl.) 61–69.

Gottleib, B. (1983) *Social Support Strategies*. New York: Sage.

Graham, C. & Burvill, P.W. (1992) A study of coroners' records on suicide in young people 1986–1988 in Western Australia. *Australian New Zealand Journal Psychiatry*, **26** (1) 30–39.

Gunn, J., Maden, A. & Swinton, M. (1991) Treatment needs of prisoners with psychiatric disorders. *British Medical Journal*, **303**, (6798), 338–341.

Hammond, T. & Wallace, P. (1990) *Housing for People Who are Severely Mentally Ill*. London: NFS.

Hawton, K. & Catalin, J. (1987) *Attempted Suicide*, 2nd edn. Oxford: Oxford University Press.

Hawton, K., Kirk, J. & Clark, D.M. (1989) *Cognitive Behaviour Therapy for Psychiatric Problems*. Oxford: Oxford University Press.

Heim, N. & Lester, D. (1991) Factors affecting choice of method for suicide. *European Journal Psychiatry*, **5** (3), 161–165.

Hogerty, G.E. *et al.* (1986) Family psycho-education, social skills training and maintenance chemotherapy in the after care of schizophrenics. *Archives General Psychiatry*, **43**, 633–642.

Holding, T.A. & Barraclough, B. (1978) Undetermined deaths—suicide or accident? *British Journal Psychiatry*, **13**, 542–549.

Holinger, P. (1987) *Violent Death in the United States*. New York: Guildford Press.

Holmes-Elber, P. & Riger, S. (1990) Hospitalisation and the composition of mental patients social networks. *Schizophrenia Bulletin*, **16** (1), 157–164.

Home Office (1992) *Digest of Criminal Statistics*. London: HMSO.

Jack, P.R. (1988) Personal networks, support mobilisation and unemployment. *Psychological Medicine*, **18**, 397–404.

Jackson, P. & Warr, P. (1988) Adapting to the unemployed role: a longitudinal investigation. *Social Science Medicine*, **25** (11), 1219–1224.

Janlert, U. & Hammarstrom, A. (1992) Alcohol consumption among unemployed youths: Results from a prospective study. *British Journal Addiction*, **87**, 703–714.

Kerfoot, M. (1984) Suicidal behaviour: adolescents and their families. In Wedge, P. (Ed.) *Social Work–Research Into Practice*. London: BASW.

King, K. & Barraclough, B. (1990) Violent death and mental illness. A study of a single catchment area over eight years. *British Journal Psychiatry*, **156**, 714–720.

Kleck, G. (1988) Miscounting suicides. *Suicide Life Threatening Behaviour*, **18** (3), 219–236.

Kok, L.P. (1988) Race, religion and female suicide attempters in Singapore. *Social Psychiatry Psychiatric Epidemiology*, **23** (4) 236–239.

Kolmos, L. & Bach, E. (1987) Sources of error in registering suicide. *Acta Psychiatrica Scandinavia*, **336** (76), 23–43.

Kosky, P., Silburn, S. & Zubrick, S.R. (1990) Are children and adolescents who have suicidal thoughts different from those who attempt suicide? *Journal Mental Disorders*, **178**, 38–43.

Kreitman, N. (ed.) (1977) *Parasuicide*. London: Wiley.

Kreitman, N. & Phillip, A.E. (1969) Parasuicide'. *British Journal Psychiatry*, **115**, 746–747.

Kreitman, N. (1988) Suicide, age and marital status. *Psychological Medicine*, **18**, 121–128.

Kreitman, N. & Foster, J. (1991) The construction and selection of predictive scales with particular reference to parasuicide. *British Journal Psychiatry*, **159**, 185–192.

Kruks, G. (1991) Gay and lesbian homeless/street youth: Special issues and concerns. *Journal Adolescent Health*, **12** (7) 515–518.

Kuipers, L. (1987) Research in expressed emotion. *Social Psychiatry*, **22**, 216–220.

Kushner, P. (1989) *Self-Destruction in the Promised Land: A psycho-cultural Biology of American Suicide*. New York: Rutgers University Press.

Leff, J. & Vaughan, C. (1985) *Expressed Emotion in Families*. London: Guildford Press.

Lefley, H.P. & Johnson, D.L. (1990) *Families as Allies in the Treatment of the Mentally Ill*. American Psychiatric Press.

Linehan, M.M. (1987) Inter-personal problem solving and parasuicide. *Cognitive Therapy Research*, **11**, 1–12.

Linehan, M.M., Armstrong, H.E. & Heard, H.I. (1991) Behavioural treatment of chronically parasuicidal borderline patients. *Archives General Psychiatry*, **48** (12), 1060–1064.

Lister, J. (1991) At the sharp end of care. In Page, M. & Powell, R. (Eds) *Homelessness and Mental Illness: The Dark Side of Community Care*. London: Concern.

McLeod, A.K., Williams, J.M.G. & Linehan, M.M. (1992) New developments in the understanding and treatment of suicidal behaviour. *Behavioural Psychotherapy*, **20**, 193–218.

MaClure, G.M.S. (1987) Suicide in England and Wales 1975–84: Mode of death. *British Journal Psychiatry*, **150**, 309–314.

McIntosh, J.L. & Wrobleski, A. (1988) Grief reactions among suicide survivors: An exploratory comparison of relationships. *Death Studies*, **12** 21–29.

Males, M. (1991) Teen suicide and changing cause-of-death certification. *Suicide Life Threatening Behaviour*, **21** (3), 245–259.

Mann, J.J. & Arango, V. (1992) Integration of neurobiology and psychopathology in a unified model of suicidal behaviour. *Journal Clinical Psychopharmacology*, **12** (2) (Suppl.) 2S–7S.

Marttunen, M.J., Aro, H.M. & Lonnqvist, J.K. (1991) Mental disorders in adolescent suicide: DSM III–R Axes I & II diagnoses in suicides among 13–19 year olds in Finland. *Archives General Psychiatry*, **48** 834–839.

Marzuk, P.M., Tierny, H. & Tardiff, K. (1988) Increased risk of suicide in persons with AIDS. *Journal American Medical Association*, **259** (9), 1333–1337.

Merrill, J., Milner, G., Vale, A. & Owens, D.J. (1992) Alcohol and attempted suicide. *British Journal Addiction*, **87** (1), 83–89.

Miller, N.S., Mahler, J.C. & Gold, M.S. (1991) Suicide risk associated with drug and alcohol dependency. *Journal Addiction Disorders*, **10** (3), 49–61.

MIND (1974) *Coordination or Chaos? The Run-down of Psychiatric Hospitals*. London: MIND.

Murphy, G.E. & Wetzel, R.D. (1990) The life-time

risk of suicide in alcoholism. *Archives General Psychiatry*, **47** (4), 383–393.

NFS (1988) *Mental Hospital Closures*. London: National Schizophrenia Society.

O'Carrol, P.W. (1989) Validity and reliability of suicide mortality data. *Suicide Life Threatening Behaviour*, **19**, 1–16.

Oliver, J.E. (1988) Successive generations of child maltreatment *British Journal Psychiatry*, **153**, 543–553.

Parry, G. & Shapiro, D.A. (1986) Social supports and life events in working class woman. *Archives General Psychiatry*, **43**, 315–323.

Patmore, C. (1987) *Living After Mental Illness: Innovations in Services*. London: Croom Helm.

Paykel, E.S., Prusoff, B.A. & Meyers, J.K. (1975) Suicide attempts and recent life events. *Archives General Psychiatry*, **32**, 327–333.

Peng, K.L. & Choo, A.S. (1990) Suicide and parasuicide in Singapore. *Medicine Science Law*, **30** (3), 225–233.

Pennebaker, J.W. & O'Heeron, R.C. (1984) Confiding in others and illness rates amongst spouses of suicide and accidental death victims. *Journal Abnormal Psychology*, **93**, 473–476.

Peterson, L.G. & Bonger, B. (1990) Repetitive suicidal crises: Characteristics of repeating and non-repeating suicidal visitors to a psychiatric emergency service. *Psychopathology*, **23** (3), 136–145.

Plant, M. (1989) The epidemiology of illicit drug misuse in Britain. In MacGregor, S. (Ed.) *Drugs and British Society*. Basingstoke: Macmillan.

Platt, S. (1984) Unemployment and suicidal behaviour: A review. *Social Science Medicine*, **19**, 93–115.

Platt, S. & Robinson, A. (1991) parasuicide and alcohol: A 20 year survey of admissions to a regional poisoning treatment centre. *International Journal Psychiatry*, **37** (3), 159–172.

Platt, S., Bille-Brahe, U. & Kerkhof, A. (1992) Parasuicide in Europe: The WHO? EURO multicentre study on parasuicide I Introduction and preliminary analysis for 1989. *Acta Psychiatrica Scandinavia*, **85** (2), 97–104.

Powers, A.L., Eckenrode, J. & Jaklitsch, B. (1990) Maltreatment among runaway and homeless youth. *Child Abuse Neglect*, **14**, 87–98.

Prasad, A.J. & Kumar, N. (1988) Suicidal behaviour in hospitalised schizophrenics. *Suicide Life Threatening Behaviour*, **18** (3) 265–269.

Pritchard, C. (1990) Suicide, unemployment and gender. Variations in the Western World 1964–1986. Are Anglophone women 'protected' from suicide? *Social Psychiatry Psychiatric Epidemiology*, **25**, 73–80.

Pritchard, C. (1992a) What can we afford for the NHS? An analysis of Government expenditure 1974–1992. *Social Policy Administration*, **26** (1), 40–54.

Pritchard, C. (1992b) Changes in elderly suicides in the USA and the developed world 1974–87: comparison with current homicide. *International Journal Geriatric Psychiatry*, **7**, 125–134.

Pritchard, C. (1992c) Is there a link between suicide in young men and unemployment? A comparison of the UK with other European Community Countries. *British Journal Psychiatry*, **160**, 750–756.

Pritchard, C. (1994) *The Ultimate Rejection: A Psycho-Social Study of Suicide*. London: Open University (in press).

Pritchard, C., Cotton, A., Cox, M., Godsen, D. & Weeks, S. (1993) Mental illness, drug and alcohol misuse and HIV risk behaviour in 214 young adult (18–35 yrs). Probation clients: implications for policy, practice and training. *Social Work Social Science Review*, **3** (2), 150–162.

Pritchard, R.A.H. (1989) Women and the valuing of work. A comparison between gender in a Northern and Southern City. Unpublished dissertation, University of London R.H.B.N.C.

Quinton, D. & Rutter, M. (1988) *Parenting Breakdown: The making and breaking of inter-generational links*. London: Avebury.

Rich, C.L., Fowler, R.C. & Young, D. (1989) Substance abuse and suicide. The San Diego study. *Annals of Clinical Psychiatry*, **1** (2), 79–85.

Quinton, D. & Rutter, M. (1988) *Parenting Breakdown: The Making and Breaking of Inter-generational Links*. London: Avebury.

Sainsbury, P. (1983) Validity and reliability of trends in suicide statistics. *World Health Statistics Quarterly*, **36**, 339–348.

Schneider, S.G., Taylor, S.E. & Hammen, C. (1991) AIDS-related factors predictive of suicidal ideation of low & high intent among gay and bisexual men. *Suicide Life Threatening Behaviour*, **21** (4), 313–328.

Schneideman, E.S. (1985) *Definition of Suicide*. New York: Wiley Inter-Science.

Soni Raleigh, V., Bulusu, A. & Balarajan, R. (1990) Suicides among immigrants from the Indian subcontinent. *British Journal Psychiatry*, **156**, 46–50.

Sorenson, S.B. & Golding, J.M. (1988) Suicidal ideation and attempts in Hispanic and non-Hispanic whites: Demographic and psychiatric disorder issues. *Suicide Life Threatening Behaviour*, **18** (3), 205–218.

Sournia, J.C. (1990) *The History of Alcoholism*. Oxford: Blackwell.

Speechley, M. & Stavarky, K.M. (1991) The adequacy of suicide statistics for use in epidemiology and public health. *Canadian Journal Public Health*, **82** (1) 38–42.

Stensman, R. and Sundqvist-Stensman, U. (1988) Physical disease and disability amongst 416 suicide cases in Sweden. *Scandinavian Journal Social Medicine*, **16** (3), 149–153.

Stiefel, F., Volkenandt, M. & Breitbart, W. (1989) Suizid und krebserkrankung. *Scweizter Medinzine Wochenschriber*, **119** (25), 891–895.

Usher, J. (1991) *Women and Madness*. Brighton: Harvester Wheatsheaf.

Vernon, M. & Phillpe, A. (1988) Suicidal pathology in migrants. *Psychiatric Psychobiology*, **3**, 115–123.

Vogel, R. & Wolfersdorf, M. (1989) Suicide and mental illness in the elderly. *Psychopathology*, **22**, 202–207.

Warr, P. (1987) *Work, Unemployment and Mental Health*. Oxford: Oxford University Press.

Whitehead, M. (1990) *The Health Divide: Inequalities in Health in the 1980s*, & Townsend P. *Poverty*. Harmondsworth: Penguin.

Weisemann, M.M. *et al.* (1981) Depressed patients. Results after one year treatment with drugs, and/or inter-personal psycho-therapy. *Archives General Psychiatry*, **37**, 401–405.

World Health Organization (1991) *Annual Statistics*. Geneva: WHO.

Yates, G.L., Mackenzie, R.G. & Swofford, A. (1991) A risk profile of homeless youth involved in prostitution and homeless youth not involved. *Journal Adolescent Health*, **12** (7), 545–548.

13

ELDERS AND MENTAL HEALTH

Ruth Prime

AIMS

i) To show how images of elders can affect mental health
ii) To explore issues of race and culture
iii) To distinguish between various mental disorders affecting elders
iv) To identify aspects of good practice

KEY ISSUES

Images, attitudes, beliefs
Race and culture
Acute confusional states
Chronic confusional states
Depression
Dementia
Risk

Identify, analyse and assess factors causing distress and illness	Promote health, provide direct care and make interventions	Manage care programmes and services
Be critical, analytical and accountable, continue professional development	Counter discrimination, inequality and individual and institutional racism	Work within and develop policies, laws and safeguards in all settings
Understand influences on mental health and the nature/causes of disorder and illness	Know the effects of distress, disorder, illness on individuals, groups, families	Understand the basis of treatments and interventions

INTRODUCTION

Although generally unacknowledged, perhaps one of the best indicators of society's attitude to ageing is the difficulty encountered in attempting to find terminology which does not carry pejorative undertones to describe women over 60 and men over 65. A range of terms is in current use—pensioners, old age pensioners, retired people, senior citizens, elderly people, older people and elders. There seems to be an uncomfortable feeling when addressing the issue of ageing. In contrast there is no problem with youth. The terms adolescents and young people are used with ease, and as we move up the age range the term middle aged gains currency.

In this chapter the term 'elders' will be used and an attempt will be made to show how the images of elders presented throughout life affect beliefs, attitudes and behaviour towards them and in turn how these attitudes, beliefs and behaviour can affect their mental health. It must be remembered, however, that elders come from different backgrounds, have different lifestyles and age at different rates. In addition in a multicultural, multiracial society there are elders of different ethnic origins, who will be referred to as black and minority ethnic elders. This group of elders suffer from society's attitude to elders in general as well as 'racism', which has further implications for the state of their mental health.

MENTAL HEALTH

The term mental health is almost always associated with mental ill health or mental disorder, particularly in reference to elders. Mental health is about having a sense of wellbeing and living life as fully as possible. A combination of physical, social, economic, psychological and emotional factors influences wellbeing throughout life but may become more of an issue as people grow older.

Images, attitudes and beliefs

In this society youth is glorified and age denigrated. The images presented by the media, in particular newspapers, television and advertising, and even children's books, subscribe to this negative image and we should not forget Shakespeare's much glorified seven ages of man, which in reality is tantamount to an onslaught on elders—'sans teeth, sans eyes, sans taste, sans everything'.

Society as a whole sees elders as economically unproductive, financially dependent, a drain on the health service, physically unattractive, figures

of fun, difficult, and unable to make decisions for themselves. In short, elders are seen as problems and are treated as such. However, there is evidence that attitudes are changing.

There are numerous sayings used to describe elders which reflect negative attitudes:

You can't teach an old dog new tricks

No fool like an old fool

Gone past it

Past the sell-by date

Over the hill

Going to seed

Long in the tooth

What do you expect at your age?

Why do you want to do that at your age?

No spring chicken

A look at some of the beliefs about black and minority ethnic people will help to highlight the additional disadvantages for black and minority ethnic elders. Black and minority ethnic people are often seen as of:

Low intelligence

Aggressive

Suspicious

Uncultured

They are also seen as having a chip on their shoulder, a ghetto mentality and as people who 'look after their own'. The latter is apparently a positive statement but has negative consequences for black and minority ethnic elders and their carers.

IMPLICATIONS

The effects of this general negativism are far reaching and have implications for policy makers, the medical profession, elders themselves and those involved in caring for elders (care workers).

Policy makers focus on problems, low income, poverty, mental deterioration. The assumptions appear to be that these issues are inevitable not preventable. The medical profession largely focuses on dysfunctioning and disability and some GPs are reluctant to have elders on their case-loads.

Social services focus mainly on the provision of practical help. Emotional needs are not usually addressed and social workers, by and large, see work with children and families as having a higher status than work with elders. There is much rhetoric about elders' rights, choice and empowerment but not enough action. In addition insufficient attention is given to the needs of the carers of elders.

Elders are part of society so it is not surprising that they consciously or unconsciously accept this negativism and although not everyone is affected in the same way, there are many who fear the process of ageing, the loss of youth and the loss of status in society. They are also inclined to believe that ill health is inevitable and untreatable so do not seek help. The picture is one of negative self image leading to self neglect, poor physical health and poor mental health.

Care workers

All workers involved in the care of elders must acknowledge that workers are part of a society which subscribes to ageism and racism. It is incumbent therefore on each individual worker to examine his or her beliefs and attitudes towards ageing and race. Workers must understand how personal and institutional racism works. Moreover they must be committed to a positive approach.

Issues of race

Race must not be confused with culture as so often happens. Issues of race are concerned with:

> The combined use of prejudice and power against people from black and minority ethnic communities.
>
> The creation of differential access to housing, employment, education, social services and health services.
>
> The resulting racial harassment and hostility.
>
> The consequential devastating impact on the mental health of the recipients.

Culture

Issues of culture are concerned with the specific mores that characterize a group of people and which are passed from one generation to another. Account must be taken of:

> Attitudes and beliefs
>
> Kinship system
>
> Music
>
> Food
>
> Religion
>
> Political systems
>
> Class systems
>
> Lifestyles

In attempting to illustrate the need for and the value of a positive approach it would be helpful to look at some of the commonest causes of confusion in elders—confusional states, depression and dementia. Before doing so, however, a word of warning. Being positive is not to deny that elders do go through biological changes from 50 years onwards. Physical changes do occur as part of the ageing process and can involve all the organs and functions of the body. Each individual, however, ages at a different rate because of genetic inheritance and life experience.

Confusional states

One of the most frequently misused terms in reference to elders is 'confused', and is often used as synonymous with dementia. Everyone has lapses of memory but when elders forget there is a tendency to jump to conclusions regarding the elder's state of mind. There seems not only to be an expectation of confusion in elders, but also an acceptance. Consequently treatable conditions go undiagnosed and untreated.

Confusion is not a disease, it is a symptom. One of the commonest causes of confusional states is physical illness but social and environmental factors do play a part. Confusional states can be acute or chronic. In the following pages checklists are given which highlight the key features and characteristics of different conditions in order to help in their differentiation at assessment. Table 13.1 compares acute confusional states, Alzheimer's disease and multi-infarct dementia.

Acute confusional states (ACS)

The most outstanding feature of ACS is the suddenness and rapidity of onset. The level of confusion can be quite alarming and is illustrated later in a chart demonstrating the differences and similarities between ACS and dementia. A summary of the causes of ACS follows:

Acute confusional states
Onset: sudden and rapid
Causes

1   *General disorders*
Anaemia (poor diet iron deficiency resulting in lack of oxygen to the brain)

Cerebral vascular disease (stroke, an interruption of blood supply to the brain)

Infection (particularly chest and urinary)

Cardiac condition

Diabetes (uncontrolled)

Constipation

Dehydration

2   *Medication (drugs)*
Prolonged use of or incorrect dosage of antidepressants, cardiac drugs and anti-parkinsonian drugs (e.g. digoxin, artaine, mogadon)

Reaction of one drug on another

Mixture of drugs and alcohol

Exclusion of food not being observed when taking certain drugs

3   *Other causes*
Change of environment

Recent bereavement or loss

Isolation

Loneliness

Chronic confusional states

While the onset of acute confusional states is sudden and rapid in chronic states the onset is slow and insidious. The likelihood of going unnoticed is therefore greater. Among conditions causing chronic confusional states are thyroid gland deficiency and vitamin B_{12} deficiency. The condition may occur over a period of years but with treatment can be reversed.

An incorrect diagnosis of confusional states can be sometimes made through miscommunication or misinterpretation of what is seen or heard by elders who have:

Communication problems due to language problems or speech impairment

Visual impairment

Hearing impairment

Depression

The commonest functional mental disorder encountered in surveys of elderly populations is depression. The majority of elders, however, do not suffer from depression but, of those who do, a significant number suffer severe depression, but depression is often undiagnosed in elders.

Causes There appears to be general agreement that a number of factors can contribute to depression in elders. There is some evidence to support the view that biological changes in the brain could be a factor; other factors are physical ill health, loss, racism, bad housing, fear, hostile environments and past experiences.

Although physical illness and depression are closely related at all ages, the relationship appears to be more pronounced in elders. Illness such as arthritis which produce high levels of pain and disability and give rise to dependency are particularly liable to give rise to depression. The diagnosis and treatment of physical illness, the alleviation of pain and measures to aid and maintain independence are vital in the prevention of depression.

Loss can also affect all age groups but appears to play a more significant part in the lives of elders. Some losses are preventable, others are not, but elders can be helped to adjust and adapt to some situations.

Summaries of the causes, symptoms and treatment of depression follow:

Causes of depression

1   Physical illnesses which give rise to severe pain or are handicapping leading to dependency:
    Arthritis

    Strokes

    Heart conditions

2   Loss of:
    Income

    Mobility

    Functional ability

    Independence

    Dignity

    Role identity

Status (in society and in the family, a major loss for some minority ethnic elders)

Confidence

Self image

Youth

Loved ones/social contacts

Dreams (the unfulfilled dream of returning home is also a great loss for black and minority ethnic elders)

Home (having to accept residential care)

3   Other factors
    Racism

    Bad housing

    Hostile environment

    Fear

    Past experiences

Symptoms of depression

1   Lowering of mood
    Markedly lower than normal

    Variable—often lowest in the early mornings

2   Abnormal lowering of physical activity
    Frittering away energy in purposeless non-productive activity—agitation

    Loss of weight

    Loss of appetite

    Loss of sexual desire

    Pre-occupation with bodily functions, e.g. palpitation, constipation, pain

    Altered sleep patterns

Self reproach, guilt, unworthiness, poor concentration, hallucinations

Suicidal thoughts

Treatment of depression

Alleviation, e.g. improve housing, finance

Manipulation of environment

Improve physical health

Foster independence (aids adaptation, education)

Minimize isolation and loneliness

Establish trusting relationship to disclose emotional problems, e.g. loss, racism

Encourage to talk

Listen

Deal with racism

Work with other disciplines

Determine needs and wishes of carers

Determine carers understanding of situation

Counselling

Drug therapy—antidepressants

ECT

Prevention is possible

Dementia

Dementia, an organic mental disorder causing a lowering of the usual level of mental ability, is the main organic mental disorder in elders. While it is normal to suffer a daily loss of brain cells from an early age, in dementia the loss is accelerated well beyond the normal rate. Dementia occurs in 5% of people over the age of 65 and 20% over the age of 80. There are several types of dementia but the most common are Alzheimer's disease (AD) and Multi-infarct dementia (MD).

Dementia

1   Alzheimer's disease (AD)
    Accounts for approximately 55% of all cases

    A dramatic increase in the rate of death of cells in the cortex (top layer) of the brain

    More common in women

    Cause unknown

    In small number of cases heredity

    Deficiency of brain chemical-acetylcholine

    Abnormal concentration of aluminium in the brain

2   Multi-infarct dementia (MD)
    Hardening of the arteries which supply the brain with blood

    Arteries thicken and narrow in a patchy fashion

    Different parts of brain get an impoverished supply of blood

    Insufficient oxygen and glucose to brain

    Manifested in mini-strokes

    Accumulation of mini-strokes lead to dementia (larger strokes do not)

    Causes: high blood pressure, obesity, lack of exercise, cigarette smoking, excessive animal fat in the diet

    More common in men

PRACTICE

A range of issues has been discussed. In the final analysis, however, concern must be centred on practice. Throughout the chapter reference has been made to implications for practice which will now be summarized and one implication will be further developed as it is of extreme important in

Table 13.1 *Similarities and differences between acute confusional state and dementia*

	Acute confusional state	Alzheimer's disease	Multi-infarct dementia
Onset	Sudden and rapid	Slow and insidious	Slow and insidious
Sex	Both	Commoner in women	Commoner in men
Age of onset		Commonly 65+	45+
Cause	Acute medical cause	Loss of brain cells general	Loss of brain cells patchy
Course	Short duration—reversible	Progressive and global	Progressive but intermittent
Orientation	Loss of sense of time and place. Worse at night variability unusual Disorientation very irregular and unpredictable can vary from minute to minute		
Thought processes	Disorganized, drifting in and out of drowsy state. The mind tends to wander and concentration becomes impaired	Impoverished Difficulty in understanding what is going on. Inability to take a global view. Difficulty in interpreting sensory input, e.g. the word 'undress' may not be interpreted or if interpreted the action may not be completed. Inability to concentrate. Loss of memory for recent events. Inappropriate recall of long-term memory	
Sleep patterns	Disturbed	Normal sleep but clock may be wrong	
Visual perception	Misinterpretation of what is seen (visual illusions) sees things that are not there (Hallucinations)	Less common and are not as vivid or disturbing	
Changeability of emotions	Feeling of fearfulness, anger, loss of temper, sudden tears sudden laughter	Poverty of emotions or apathy. Does not feel or express emotions as before. Loss of personality (often late)	
Physical signs and symptoms	Related to underlying cause	Absent or few and late on	Related to minute strokes e.g. weakness of one side, blackouts, falls
	Restlessness and unease	Settled, apart from aimless wandering or searching	

working with elders who are affected by dementia—management.

Implications for practice

1 Awareness of the effects of negativism (ageism and racism)

2 Understanding the impact on elders

3 Understanding the effect on self

4 Change of attitudes, beliefs and behaviour—positivism

5 Prevention

6 Promotion of good health

7 Early medical diagnosis

8 Appropriate treatment

9 Holistic assessments
   (a) Gather information

Physical environment of home and neighbourhood

Financial factors

Health factors—how functioning is affected

Elder's abilities to carry out personal care, household tasks, etc.

Formal networks

Informal networks (friends, neighbours)

Emotional and psychological needs

Past history

Communication—language, speech impairment, hearing impairment

Issues of race

Issues of culture

Hobbies and interests

Risk factors

Carer's needs, abilities, perception and wishes

Elder's perceptions and wishes

(b) Evaluate information gathered

Making sense of the whole is the key to this vital stage of the process and needs skills and objectivity

(c) Draw conclusions

(d) Decide on action

Action can range from simple to complex

Involve other disciplines where appropriate

Call care planning meeting where appropriate, involve pertinent people including carers, elders and relatives

Draw up package of care stating what is to be done by whom and within what time limit. Design package to give maximum help with minimum intrusion and confusion

(e) Implement decision

(f) Monitor and review

10 Counselling—a vital aspect of the package often neglected

11 Provision of appropriate resources

12 Management

MANAGEMENT

Elders who suffer from Alzheimer's disease (AD) are first and foremost people who have the same basic needs as the rest of the population and are entitled to be treated with equal dignity and respect. They are therefore entitled to live as full a life as possible; but because AD is an irreversible and progressive condition, in addition to the usual management techniques applied in caring for frail elders, special measures are needed. Three of these measures will be discussed—reality orientation (RO), reminiscence and management of risk.

Reality orientation

Reality orientation (RO) technique is useful in helping Alzheimer sufferers who are not making use of their remaining faculties but it is unlikely to help those who are suffering from severe dementia. RO consists of the repeated presentation of facts with positive reinforcement and encouragement—facts such as time of day, date, meal times, news events, etc. The objective is to help individuals to be in touch with reality, albeit for a short while. Other measures include the use of signs, labels and colours; where language is a problem, symbols can be used.

Reminiscence

Reminiscence is a pastime in which most people, particularly elders, indulge. However, in the treatment of dementia reminiscence has therapeutic value. By stimulating the memory to recall past and often pleasant events, elders are helped to improve their confidence. Care workers should be aware that unpleasant memories can also be evoked and skill will be needed to deal with the consequences. Workers must also be aware that all elders do not reminisce about the same sorts of things. Elders born and brought up in the West Indies or Asia will certainly not recall memories of sleeping in air raid shelters, the camaraderie of life during the war or dancing at the Hammersmith Palais. Workers must therefore be sensitized to the cultural and regional differences when working with groups of elders.

Management of risk

In attempting to keep dementia sufferers in the community and to enable them to live as full and independent a life as possible, a high degree of risk is inevitable. For carers and workers understandably, one of the most difficult aspects of care is coping with 'risk'.

Defining risk

Longman's dictionary defines 'at risk' as a situation or circumstance where loss, injury, etc. are possible. 'Taking risks' is defined as placing one's self in a dangerous situation liable to mischance. Both definitions are pertinent in working with vulnerable groups, where the mischance can lead to physical, emotional and psychological abuse, neglect, injury and even loss of life. However, risk can be estimated, that is to say taken in the light of a wide range of knowledge. In calculating risk some assessment must be made of the possibility of failure, the degree of which must be estimated and taken into account before a venture is embarked upon.

The combination of disorientation, memory loss and personality changes in dementia sufferers give rise to the following elements of risk:

Risk from self and to others

Risk from carers

Risk to carers

Risk from the community/neighbourhood

Risk from self and to others. Risk from self can take the form of self neglect, danger from fire, and wandering.

Self neglect entails failure to eat properly, keep warm, dress adequately or take medication. These risks can be minimized with proper support and supervision.

Danger from fire is a major risk not only to self but also to others and creates dilemmas for care workers. Measures such as switching off cookers from the mains when the elder is left on his or her own, removing matches, etc. appear to some to be in conflict with the rights of the individual. Common sense must in the end prevail in balancing risk and need.

Wandering is the most problematic risk of all but the nature of the wanderings must be considered. Where the person goes, at what time of day, and for what length of time are among factors which help to determine the level of risk and the nature of the preventative response if any.

Risk from carers. Although high priority is given to the independence of the individual it is obvious that total independence is impossible. The extent to which elders depend on carers can vary from minimal to extreme. Carers can therefore be subjected to varying degrees of physical and emotional stress. The tolerance level to stress of each individual is different and can fluctuate in relation to variables such as ill health and emotional needs. Conflict between the needs of carers and the needs of elders can heighten the risks to which the elders may be exposed.

Assessing the needs and abilities of carers is crucial in the assessment and management of risks.

Risk to carers. All the determinants to elders from carers indirectly put carers at risk. Firstly, if carers subject those for whom they are caring to physical abuse they put themselves at risk legally. Secondly, when on account of stress they subject elders to emotional or physical abuse, they may suffer from guilt, remorse and depression. Moreover, there is the risk of physical and emotional abuse to carers from those for whom they care—risks which should not be underestimated.

Risks from the community/neighbourhood. Attitudes to elders vary from neighbourhood to neighbourhood and in individuals within the neighbourhood. Elders, particularly the most vulnerable, can be exposed to physical attacks, robbery and black and minority ethnic elders can be subjected to racial harassment.

The management of risk must take account of all the above elements but the key is the assessment process through which the risk factors and potential dangers to elders and carers can be identified.

Finally, care workers need clear guidelines and supportive mechanisms to enable them to manage risk sensibly and effectively. This chapter would not be complete without a few points to be considered when working with black and minority ethnic elders. Many of these points have been discussed throughout the text but it is helpful to summarize them:

Points to consider when working with black and minority ethnic elders

1 Communication
Different language

Lack of differentiation and nuances in respect of emotion

Literal translation can lead to misinterpretation

Sign language can be misleading

2 Difference in presentation
Depression best documented

Presentation in terms of physical illness rather than feelings/emotions
Instead of agitation, worthlessness, guilt, etc. complaints of headache or sore stomach for which no physical reason can be found

3 Racism—contributory factors
Low income, poor housing, etc. more characteristic of ethnic minorities

Hostile environment—isolation (e.g. in day and residential care)

Loss of self-esteem

Lack of positive self image

Loss of opportunities

4 Changes in family patterns lead to:
Loss of role

Loss of kinship support

Loss of long cherished dreams (e.g. dream of returning home)

5 Religious beliefs
Often misinterpreted

6 Cultural differences
Often used negatively

CONCLUSIONS

Negative stereotyping has made a major contribution to the creation of a dependent ageing population. With the population over 65 years continuing to rise, particularly in the over 80 age group, it is imperative that urgent steps are taken to change negative attitudes, beliefs and behaviour towards elders. A climate of *positivism* must be created in order to foster good health, both physical and mental, and independence as far as possible.

In such a climate the mental health of elders will be enhanced and society will benefit from the wealth of knowledge, skills, ideas and energy which lie unharnessed in the community.

SOURCES AND FURTHER READING

Atkin, K. (1991) Community care in a multiracial society—incorporating the user view. *Policy and Politics*, **19**, (3) 159–166.

Caines, R. (1986) The culture factors in mental health. *Social Work Today*, 10 February.

DHSW (1988) *Working with Older People*. Milton Keynes: Open University.

Gearing, B., Johnson, M. & Heller, T. (Eds) (1988) *Mental Health Problems in Old Age*. John Wiley. Milton Keynes: Open University.

Jacques, A. (1992) *Understanding Dementia*, 2nd edn. Edinburgh: Churchill Livingstone.

Marshall, M. (1990) *Working with Dementia: Guidelines for Professionals*. Venture Press.

Norman, A. (1982) *Mental Illness in Old Age: Meeting the Challenge*. London: Centre for Policy on Ageing.

Norman, A. (1985) *Triple Jeopardy: growing old in a second homeland*. London: Centre for Policy on Ageing.

Norman, A. (1987). *Aspects of Ageism: A Discussion Paper*. London: Centre for Policy on Ageing.

Rack, P. (1982) Race, Culture and Mental Disorder. London: Tavistock.

Squires, A. (Ed.) (1991) *Multicultural Health Care and Rehabilitation*. Sevenoaks, Kent: Age Concern.

III

INTERVENTION AND TREATMENT

Nurses and other practitioners intervene, or manage interventions which draw insight and inspiration from a wide range of disciplines, as well as their own practice. Developing the framework developed in Part II, this section reflects a bio-psycho-social approach to health and ill health. It examines the historical, spiritual and biological context of treatment and explores interventions from mental health promotion to a comprehensive analysis of enduring mental health problems.

Canst thou not minister to a mind diseas'd;
Pluck out from the memory a rooted sorrow;
Raze out the written troubles of the brain

Shakespeare, *Macbeth*

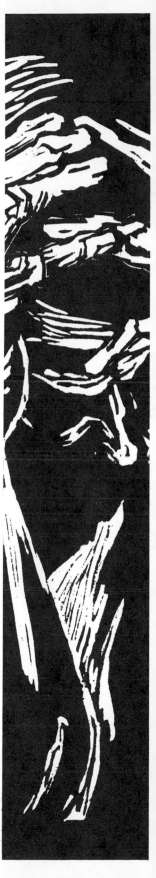

14

MANAGING INTERVENTIONS

Tony Thompson and Peter Mathias

AIMS

i) To provide an overview of nursing interventions

| Identify, analyse and assess factors causing distress and illness |
| Be critical, analytical and accountable, continue professional development |
| Understand influences on mental health and the nature/causes of disorder and illness |

KEY ISSUES

Successful intervention
Models of nursing

Promote health, provide direct care and make interventions	Manage care programmes and services
Counter discrimination, inequality and individual and institutional racism	Work within and develop policies, laws and safeguards in all settings
Know the effects of distress, disorder, illness on individuals, groups, families	Understand the basis of treatments and interventions

The effective implementation of national community care programmes and how these are reflected in the local community care proposals will, in the end, depend entirely upon the personal effectiveness of those people who manage to intervene successfully at an appropriate time in the client's life. The person who manages the intervention will design proposals around what they consider feasible and so increase the chances of the professional intervention being successful. Other contributors to this textbook reinforce the notion that a person comes into contact with professional mental health services often because they are encountering a specific crisis in their lives. Whatever the triggers for this crisis the chances of a successful outcome depends not only on the person's own coping strategies but also on the effectiveness of the intervention which aims to support them in their vulnerability and to identify and use the variety of resources identified throughout this book. Quite often the most effective professional intervention is that which can respond rapidly to an escalating crisis and which manages to restore a balance as quickly as possible. As part of this rapid response the professional who manages to intervene has to manipulate a number of variables in order to provide effective action wherever and whenever the crisis manifests.

Mental health nurses are in a particularly strong position to provide a response that is flexible and immediate. The registered mental health nurse is a specialist who functions within a professional and academic framework designed to provide care and treatment to the people with mental illness and to contribute to prevention and to health promotion. The way in which they intervene in the interests of client care, and how they equip and deploy valuable human resources, are important for health gain.

It is likely that the professional input will revolve around a key worker system. The compatibility of worker and client is of paramount importance and therefore the client should be involved with either the selection or allocation of this worker. Amongst the skills required are:

Effectively utilizing professional preparation skills when assisting clients to cope with crisis

Providing accountable support and care in a positive and confident manner

Being a focus of professional contact for service users and other carers

Endeavouring to ensure that the service user is registered with available services such as the general practitioner

Effectively and efficiently helping with planning and subsequent monitoring of care delivery as identified as part of an overall care package

---

Wherever services are placed, effective intervention should be provided in the least restrictive setting possible and it should operate within a quality standard framework that is capable of being continuously monitored and reviewed. In recent years nurses have increasingly pursued and searched for models upon which to base their practice. These models are approximations to reality and therefore are constructed by nurses as part of their search for coherent intervention strategies and as a means of evaluating any innovation with respect to other interventions such as primary care and transition programmes. Whatever the construct used, it usually has to match the need to implement practice in a wide range of settings that suits the client's particular environment. The use of models of nursing as a way of implementing concept-based or theory-driven practice has been well documented (Roper *et al.*, 1983; Orem, 1985; Aggleton and Chalmers, 1986).

Contemporary practice can be led by ideas but the pragmatic implementation tends to revolve around the following areas of service user needs:

Valued employment

Satisfying leisure

Access to appropriate services

Comfortable accommodation

Sufficient finance

Pursuing self help and self advocacy

Overcoming stigma

Support within the domiciliary setting

Recognizing the need to be sensitive to gender, cultural and ethnic differences

Ensuring personal safety

Whatever the construct utilized by the professional, the possibility of a successful outcome for intervention will rely on meeting the needs and co-ordinating the service in an effective way. Amongst the attributes required to make this intervention would be the capability of taking a broad perspective of services but at the same time having the confidence to take action based upon the skilled delivery of individualized care. In describing the profound effect of the work of Peplau, Barker (1993) draws attention to the way in which her emphasis on nursing as a 'human response to illness' assisted him in perceiving nursing as a 'human' philosophy, built on interpersonal processes.

In Barker's excellent description of Peplau's impact he refers to the way in which her views have led psychiatric nursing out of the confinement of custodial care into a theory-driven professional practice (Carey *et al.*, 1989). The theory explored by Peplau has been developed over the years in the contemporary psychiatric nurse's framework around the therapeutic use of interpersonal relationships. There can be little doubt that Peplau's work which, although sometimes described as a model by others, is more concerned with the identification of common elements in explanatory theory and the use and influence of an individual's presence, perception and experience. Fundamental to successful nurse/client interaction is the use of accurate observations and explanatory concepts when making practical or clinical judgements, it is these which Peplau sees as determining the nursing intervention. It is these types of views that reinforce the need for the professional intervention to use any construct in a creative and questioning way. In contemporary mental health practice, such organized ways of thinking and acting tend to reflect:

The concept of health gain

Deliberate and effective nursing intervention

Recognition of the holistic view of the person and their interaction with the environment

---

Nursing intervention aims to utilize relevant research as a way of underpinning the nursing activity. The intervention is co-ordinated in order to increase the chances of creative practice being perpetuated. The simple aim of the intervention should be to produce high quality care delivery.

The intelligent use of any constructed framework for intervention has to promote the ability and authority in the practitioner together with being able to modify and adapt his or her model as new knowledge associated with experience and practice emerges. Theories and models of contemporary mental health nursing do little more than offer a challenge to the development of a knowledge base but they are important as they reinforce the need for critical evaluation of nursing activity within practical settings, wherever those settings may be. They offer a framework of understanding which enable nurses to plan rationally and implement nursing care which informs further interventions.

The advantages of reflecting on this type of theory as a means of informing practice are apparent and include making the aims of service provision relevant to the range of individual needs. It then should follow that intervention and its effective management will start through an objective assessment of human need. These approaches will be particularly important in the future when professionals may have to assess the elements of provision and make judgements around the notion of health or social care needs. At the level of everyday practice these judgements can be complex and it is not simple to separate these needs into polarized elements. The confident use of theories to underpin intervention can assist interdisciplinary teams working within mental health because it can help clarify aims, determine priorities and define boundaries for skilled practice.

A good intervention is one that enables the practitioner to identify client strengths and effective coping skills rather than focusing narrowly on problems and deficits. Of course this does not mean that the handicapping conditions which can accompany someone with a mental health problem have to be ignored, but it does encourage clients to be active partners in the intervention and allows them to shape their own programme of care by developing strengths within partnership and their living situation. These principles mean that the professional obligation towards someone with a mental health problem is never confused or neglected. It also means that the professional relationship is reinforced by means of effective intervention and it will mean that at times the professional has to assert authority in order to provide for the long-term interest of the service user and their carers. The use of effective intervention techniques is closely associated with professional attitude as well as constructing rational plans for achieving satisfactory outcomes and conditions in the process of care. Professional, informed and educated techniques of intervention will reinforce the conventional wisdom found within psychiatric nursing in that people who are prone to problems are inextricably interwoven as part of a fabric of a system and are subject to change as their circumstances and environment change around them. The ultimate aim of intervention is to manipulate the situation to the advantage of the service user and to alter the balance in order to achieve positive long-term health and social care gains.

The roles, skills and competence of mental health nurses are discussed in detail by Johnson and Smith (Chapter 2), Moxham (Chapter 31) and Sines (Chapter 32). These roles and skills are set within the historical context of treatment by Lyttle (Chapter 15) and in the context of service provision by the chapters in Part 4. Farine (Chapter 20) explains the basis of physical interventions and treatment. In the other chapters in Part 3, Repper and Cooney (Chapter 19) consider how the needs of people with enduring problems can be met, Evans (Chapter 16) examines interventions designed to promote health, Marshall (Chapter 17) describes and evaluates cognitive

behavioural therapy, and Narayasamy (Chapter 18) considers the provision of spiritual care.

FURTHER READING

Barker, P.J. & Baldwin, S. (1991) *Ethical Issues in Mental Health*. Chapman & Hall.

Collister, B. (1988) *Psychiatric Nursing: Person to Person*. E. Arnold.

McFarland, G. (1992) *Nursing Diagnoses and Process in Psychiatric Mental Health Nursing*. Lippincott.

Milne, D. (1993) *Psychology of Mental Health Nursing: A Problem Solving Approach*. Macmillan.

REFERENCES

Aggleton, P. & Chalmers, H. (1986) *Nursing Models and the Nursing Process*. London: Macmillan.

Barker, P. (1993) The Peplau legacy. *Nursing Times*, **89** (11).

Carey, E.T., Noll, J., Rasmussen, I. & Hildegard, A. (1989), Peplau: psychodynamic nursing. In Marriner-Tomy, A. (Ed). *Nurse Theorists and Their Work*, 2nd edn. St Louis: C.V. Mosby.

Orem, D. (1985) *Nursing: Concepts of Practice*. New York: McGraw-Hill.

Roper, N., Logan, W. & Tierney, A. (1983) *Using a Model for Nursing*. Edinburgh: Churchill Livingstone.

15

A BRIEF HISTORICAL ACCOUNT OF APPROACHES TO TREATMENT

Jack Lyttle*

AIMS

i) To provide a historical account of approaches to treatment as an introduction to subsequent chapters

ii) To examine the implications of recent trends in care (for mental health nursing)

KEY ISSUES

Humanitarian approaches

The development of physical treatments

Non-physical approaches based on understanding of mind

Identify, analyse and assess factors causing distress and illness	Promote health, provide direct care and make interventions	Manage care programmes and services
Be critical, analytical and accountable, continue professional development	Counter discrimination, inequality and individual and institutional racism	Work within and develop policies, laws and safeguards in all settings
Understand influences on mental health and the nature/causes of disorder and illness	Know the effects of distress, disorder, illness on individuals, groups, families	Understand the basis of treatments and interventions

'Canst thou not minister to a mind diseas'd;
Pluck from the memory a rooted sorrow;
Raze out the written troubles of the brain';
Shakespeare: Macbeth Act V Scene III

HISTORICAL BACKGROUND

An examination of the history of psychiatric treatment reveals a complex fabric in which inhumanity, compassion, superstition and scientific innovation are closely interwoven. Ancient records reveal that mental disorder has been recognized and treated for thousands of years. Egyptian medical papyri of around 1500 BC say of senility that 'The heart grows heavy and remembers not yesterday' (Henderson and Batchelor, 1962), and dream interpretation was practised in Ancient Egypt as long ago as 2900 BC (Jones, 1983).

The Old Testament records Saul's depression and attempt to commit suicide (Samuel 1:5–10) and the Ancient Greeks formally recognized mental disorder in their writings. Plato (Republic Bk XI c. 13) instructed 'If anyone is insane let him not be seen openly in the city, but let the relatives of such a person watch over him at home in the best manner they know of, and if they are negligent let them pay a fine'.

During the time of Hippocrates the mentally disordered visited the Temple of Aesculapius—the god of healing—where prayers were offered and sleeping overnight in the Temple brought relief.

The second century AD saw the emergence of chains, flogging, incarceration and starvation—often in the belief that the mentally disordered were possessed. Medieval Europe left the treatment of mental disorder to priests, and superstitious beliefs in witchcraft were used to justify the segregation and brutal ill-treatment of those persons who aroused concern or alarm as a result of disordered behaviour or beliefs. (Szasz (1973) has suggested that 'the concept of mental illness serves the same social function in the modern world as did the concept of witchcraft in the late Middle Ages'.) Holy wells and springs were the subject of pilgrimages in medieval times in the hope of effecting relief of mental disorder. One such was St Fillan's Well in Scotland, mentioned by Sir Walter Scott:

'Thence to St Fillan's blessed well
Whose spring can frenzied dreams dispel
And the crazed brain restore'.
Marmion, Canto i, 29

Similar healing wells and springs were used in France, Finland, Belgium, Germany and England and, in modern times, the bathing of the sick at Lourdes remains an important adjunct to the spiritual exercises.

Many people who experienced learning disability or psychosis were abandoned to live as outcasts: 'When civilization grew in the Western world it grew behind walls—in castles and monasteries and small crowded cities; and the outcasts lived in the forests—madmen and idiots, lepers and escaped slaves, outlaws and felons' (Jones and Fowles, 1984).

In 1377 the Bethlehem Hospital in London was used to house mental patients, giving rise to the terms 'Bedlam' and 'Tom O'Bedlam', the latter term being used to describe the mentally handicapped or psychotic.

'The country gives me proof and precedent
Of Bedlam beggars who with roaring voices...
Enforce their charity'.
Shakespeare: King Lear, Acts III & IV

The sixteenth century saw mass burnings of witches and heretics, the Attorney General of Lorraine (who burned 900 'witches') explaining that 'Whatever is not normal is due to the Devil', though one courageous doctor protested about current theological doctrines asking 'Do figments like these move us to the torturing of harmless women?' (Szasz, 1973).

By the seventeenth century many European cities had institutions for 'the debauched, spendthrift fathers, prodigal sons, blasphemers, men who seek to undo themselves, libertines' (Szasz, 1973). Bedlam, the Narrenturm in Vienna, the hôpital general in Paris, all incarcerated the mentally disordered under conditions of great barbarity. A visitor to Bedlam in 1753 said 'I saw a hundred spectators making sport of the miserable inhabitants, provoking them into furies of rage' (Seymer, 1956), such a visit being vividly portrayed in the Hogarth engraving 'The Rake in Bedlam' (1735).

This lack of respect for the mentally disordered was even extended to royal personages. When George III suffered attacks of maniacal excitement no hesitation was evinced in knocking him down, and one attendant boasted that he knocked him 'flat as a flounder' (Henderson and Batchelor, 1962). 'Treatment' largely consisted of restraint, bleeding, purging and beating, though attempts to use 'medication' were sporadically employed. Sydenham treated mania by prescribing a concoction which would have aroused the envy of any witch doctor—it contained the flesh and blood of vipers, wine, honey and 61 other ingredients (Henderson and Batchelor, 1962). Many herbs were believed to be efficacious in the treatment of melancholia and other disturbances, and the substances used included chrysanthemum, saffron, rosewater, marigolds, carnations, moonwort, hellebore, lavender, gentian, opium and cannabis.

The latter part of the eighteenth century saw the emergence of an era of humane reform. Pinel in France and Tuke in England pioneered extensive reforms—removing chains and initiating coherent attempts at treatments—though historians have often over-idealized both the men and their approaches. Even Pinel believed in the efficacy of 'short sharp shocks' and the regime at the Salpetriere included the 'douche ascendante' which was a stream of cold water directed on to the anus of the naked, seated, unsuspecting patient (Jones, 1983). Pinel also observed that 'If (the madman) is met by a force convincingly superior he submits without opposition or violence. This is a great and invaluable secret in the management of well regulated hospitals' (Szasz, 1973). It has also been suggested that Pinel struck off the chains of his patients, not in response to

humanitarian instincts, but because the revolutionary National Assembly wished patients to be freed as a political gesture. 'Man is born free but everywhere he is in chains' wrote Rousseau, and Pinel may have hastily endorsed the revolutionary spirit by freeing his patients. His hospital was certainly visited twice in 1793 by Couthon, the hostile and powerful president of the Paris commune. Michel Foucault (1967) sees Pinel not as a philanthropist but as a prudent survivor.

In 1796 William Tuke opened the Retreat at York, a Quaker community, which used 'soft and mild persuasion' to treat the mentally disordered and explicitly rejected coercion and intimidation. The Retreat foreshadowed many therapeutic community principles as self-restraint and control were encouraged by an atmosphere in which the esteem of others was something to be concerned about. Despite this innovative approach the Retreat primarily offered 'moral management'; that is, the emphasis was on promoting an awareness of good and evil, of right and wrong, though it was thought that the emotions were best controlled rather than expressed or discussed.

Despite these humanitarian developments, fear and restraint played a major part in 'treatment' well into the nineteenth century. Patients were restrained in immobilizing chairs, spun to the point of collapse in revolving chairs, purged, starved and beaten. Boats and bridges were constructed which would break up and force patients to swim to the shore, and ducking chairs and cages were used to plunge pinioned patients into icy water.

The nineteenth century saw the introduction of drugs into the network of fast developing mental hospitals. Potassium bromide was widely used as a sedative, hypnotic and anticonvulsant, though excess led to bromism—a state of toxic confusion. Around the same time (the 1830s) chloral hydrate was introduced as a sedative and hypnotic, and paraldehyde was introduced in the 1880s. It will be noted that the drugs mentioned all have a sedative effect and excessive reliance on preparations like these may simply 'place the bars of Bedlam and the locked doors *inside* the patient' (Laing, 1964). The first barbiturate (Veronal— another sedative) was introduced in 1903 and reliance on sedatives continued until the 1950s when the first *neuroleptic* drugs (i.e. the pheno-thiazines) were introduced.

In 1933 Sakel introduced *insulin therapy* in the belief that the hypoglycaemia associated with carefully induced insulin coma would somehow interrupt abnormal neural connections in the brain. Insulin therapy brought about improvements but it was increasingly suspected that these improvements were the results of the increased staff/patient interactions in the insulin unit rather than of any biochemical adjustments. As research cast greater suspicion on the rationale of insulin therapy it went into decline and disappeared in the late 1950s.

In 1935 Moniz introduced *psychosurgery* (prefrontal leucotomy) for the management of crippling fears, obsessions and anxiety, and was awarded the Nobel Prize for Medicine in 1955 (he was shot in the spine by a leucotomized patient rendering him paraplegic). In 1938 Cerletti and Bini introduced electroplexy (electroconvulsive therapy or ECT)—still a major treatment for some types of mood disorder.

The 1950s saw an expansion of the range of psychotropic drugs available, and chemotherapy became more sophisticated, many of the drugs introduced then still being in frequent use (e.g. the phenothiazines).

Treatments mentioned so far aim at bringing about some change in the physical functioning of the patient and are therefore referred to collectively as *physical methods of treatment* (e.g. chemotherapy, electroplexy and psychosurgery). Many other treatments aim to restore functioning without physical intervention; that is, they treat mental disorder by mental means, and treatments of this nature (psychotherapy and behaviour therapy) are collectively described as *non-physical methods of treatment*.

Non-physical approaches date back to the dream interpretations of the Ancient Egyptians and the 'temple sleep' of Ancient Greece but psychotherapy, as we know it, was first associated with Antoine Mesmer (1734–1815) who coined rather bizarre theories of 'animal magnetism' and saw all illnesses (physical and mental) as a result of disturbances in the flow of 'magnetic fluid'. 'Mesmerism' was soon discredited but the fact remains that many of his patients improved dra-matically, not as a result of animal magnetism, but because Mesmer was giving (albeit inadvertently) effective psychotherapy. He was a tall, charismatic individual with piercing eyes, and he made a practice of speaking commandingly to his overawed patients and suggesting that symptoms would disappear—as they often obligingly did. Long after 'animal magnetism' had been forgotten, the memory of the power of suggestion lingered on.

In 1843 an Edinburgh dentist, James Braid, coined the term '*hypnotism*', leaning heavily on some of Mesmer's techniques, and Charcot and Janet later used the technique of hypnosis in the study and treatment of hysteria.

In 1882 Freud began to use hypnosis to gain access to troublesome thoughts and wishes which had been repressed by his patients but was soon to abandon hypnosis as the techniques of psycho-analysis were fully worked out by him. The aim of psychoanalysis is the uncovering of unconscious conflicts and repressed experiences and Freud soon began to use three major techniques. The first technique is *free association* by the patient (the patient is encourged to verbalize his stream of consciousness, to speak aloud any thoughts entering his mind, no matter how trivial, irrelevant, stupid or obscene they seem to him). The second technique is the formation and analysis of *transference relationships*; that is, critical early experiences are re-enacted as the patient 'transfers' emotions associated with them on to the psychoanalyst. Transference relationships may be positive or negative as the patient transfers love or hate felt for parents or significant others on to the therapist. The therapist may respond with *counter-transference* when he responds to feelings of resentment with hostility or responds to progress with feelings of pleasure. Psychoanalysts work with the transference relationship as an aid to understanding the patient's feelings and as a method of gaining awareness of repressed conflicts. The third technique used in psychoanalysis is *interpretation* by the therapist who may interpret dreams and 'slips of the tongue', and in particular will emphasize the relationship between present feelings and past experiences. Sometimes patients will recall past experiences with a considerable discharge of previously buried emotions. This discharge of emotions is often of an intensity which is surprising and disturbing to the patient; the discharge is called a *catharsis*. Cathartic experiences are often experienced as therapeutic by the patient as they may 'purge' the unconscious of troublesome repressed material and provide an increase in insight. Some of Freud's early followers broke away to establish variants of orthodox psychoanalysis and this group of dissenters is often collectively referred to as the *Neo-Freudians*.

Alfred Adler (1870–1937) rejected Freud's view of sexuality as the prime mover of human behaviour and established the school of *individual psychology* which emphasizes consideration of the individual's 'lifestyle' and uses re-education to establish healthier patterns and goals. Adler introduced the term 'inferiority complex' and suggested that feelings of inferiority were a creative force since they led to striving for superiority.

C.G Jung (1875–1961) also disagreed with Freud's view of sexuality and developed his own system of *analytical psychology* which emphasizes *individualism*—an innate striving for self-realization. Jung described libido as natural energy which first and foremost serves the purposes of life and which flows between the opposing poles, 'the opposites'. Many opposites can be described, for example introversion and extroversion, thinking and feeling, consciousness and unconsciousness. The natural movement of the libido (or life energy) is backwards and forwards—a movement of psychic tides. Jung called forward movement (which satisfies the demands of the conscious) *progression*, and backward movements (which satisfy the demands of the unconscious) *regression*. Progression is concerned with the active adaptation to one's environment and regression with the satisfaction of one's inner needs. Regression may be a restorative phase, as in a return to a dreamy state after a concentrated period of directed mental activity. Regression is therefore not always 'a bad thing' but is in many ways as natural a counterpart to progression as sleeping is to waking.

Jung's view of the unconscious was that it is more than a mere repository of primitive and infantile urges. The unconscious is the matrix of consciousness and in it are to be found the germs of new possibilities—the seeds of new ways of being. Jung also introduced the concept of the *collective unconscious*, a deeper stratum of the unconscious than the individual or personal unconscious, the unknown material from which our consciousness emerges. Jung suggested that the collective unconscious is shaped and influenced by the remote and distant experiences of mankind. Intellectually we are in some ways like a group of savages huddled round the comforting light and heat of the fire of conscious reason, but beyond the flickering shadows of the unconscious lies the dark (but rich) forest of the collective unconscious. This tendency to experience and apprehend life in a manner conditioned by the past history of mankind Jung called *archetypal*, and recurring symbols or motifs in art and literature (archetypes) are expressions of the primordial collective unconscious. The threatening devouring mother figure is an example. This archetype occurs throughout the history of mankind, from cave paintings to the ancient goddesses Ishtar and Isis, Kali, the Oedipus myth, the witch figure of the Middle Ages and children's fairy tales. Archetypes indicate the presence of primordial hopes, fears, wishes and instincts, and myths, in particular, are a direct expression of the collective unconscious.

Jungian therapy never loses sight of the constructive elements which can always be found in mental disorder and sees every neurosis as having an aim—an attempt to compensate for a one-sided approach to life and a voice proclaiming the existence of a side of the personality which has been neglected or repressed. Every neurosis thus has its secret strengths and the belief in the regulatory functions of the 'opposites' emphasizes that the mentally disordered are not irretrievably stranded on some alien psychic shore but are still involved in a process of psychic travel or movement. Regressive movement always has the potential to become progressive movement, and negative movement will inevitably be followed by positive movement, as light follows dark. Effective care facilitates this movement and the therapist may act as a guide on the journey.

Jung's writings are sometimes dismissed as being obscure, mystical and irrelevant to modern psychotherapy; this is, to say the least, unfortunate, as Jung's writings contain core ideas which have heavily influenced many other schools of thought. Above all Jung offers a view of psychic functioning which is positive and optimistic, and provides a much needed counterbalance to some rigid 'medical model' views of mental disorder which tend to reduce the individual to a sterile list of 'medical' symptoms, and offer little more than sedation, hospitalization and crippling loss of self-esteem. Description is a necessary first step in all sciences but in some approaches to psychiatry it has become an end in itself. Jung encourages us not only to say 'how' in describing behaviour and feelings but to ask 'why'. The warmly humanistic Jungian approach with its recognition of each individual's capacity for positive personal growth incorporates attitudes which will be an asset to any health care professional.

Otto Rank (1884–1939), also seceded from the ranks of the 'orthodox' Freudians (in 1929), examined separation anxiety and experimented with short-term therapy (orthodox Freudian or Jungian analysis usually takes some years). He introduced the concept of 'birth trauma' as the precursor of all later anxiety and this theory has a modern counterpart in Janov's theory of neurosis as a symbolization of primal pain due to the denial of primal needs.

Wilhelm Reich (1897–1957) developed 'character analysis' exploring the relationship between bodily tensions and posture, 'character armour' and psychological defences. Reich had a somewhat chequered career (he was expelled from the International Psychoanalytical Association because he was a Communist and was then expelled from the Communist Party because he was a psychoanalyst), though Reichian therapy continues in a modified form as 'bio-energetics'.

Erich Fromm (1900–1983) emphasized the interaction between the individual and society and the outcomes of stress and loneliness in industrial society, and *Karen Horney* (1885–1952) stressed the individual's need for security and also emphasized cultural and situational determinants of neurosis.

Harry Stack Sullivan (1892–1948) developed a system of psychotherapy which explored the interpersonal relationships of his patients, and *Fritz Perls* (1894–1970) devised *Gestalt therapy* in which the patient is asked to personify the warring parts of his body and mind and invent a dialogue in which they could come to agreement, completing the gestalt (or wholeness).

Perls used an approach that diverged from the techniques of psychoanalysis and his approach is an example of what became a rapidly expanding alternative school of thought—the *humanistic* approach to psychotherapy—which emphasizes the uniqueness of the individual and adopts a person-centred approach to life's difficulties.

The humanistic approach acquired new impetus when *Carl Rogers* introduced *client-centred therapy* which became a major influence in the 1950s. This approach does not emphasize insight and does not use transference relationships. Diagnosis, interpretation and direction are avoided and the 'client's' capacity for personal growth and self-regulation is recognized and encouraged. Rogers prefers the term 'client' to 'patient' as he does not believe that persons in therapy are 'sick' or 'ill' and the term 'client-centred' is used as therapy centres around the client's perceptions, and not those of the therapist, who does not interpret or direct as would a psychoanalytically orientated therapist. Many humanistic therapists are critical of 'insight-directed' therapies, emphasizing that there is a risk that the 'patient' may be said to develop 'insight' when he agrees with the therapist's interpretation of his problems.

The humanistic approach to psychotherapy was broadened in the 1960s when *Eric Berne* introduced 'transactional analysis', which focuses on the interpersonal 'transactions' of the client. The humanistic approach 'demedicalized' psychotherapy as many humanistic approaches do not consider a qualification in medicine to be necessary (or indeed relevant) to the practice of psychotherapy. Rogers has even stated that a training in psychology may be a disadvantage as it may produce a tendency to see persons as objects to be dissected or experimentally manipulated (Rogers, 1951, 1961). The important prerequisite for effective therapy is seen to consist of the personal philosophy of the therapist which outweighs 'theory' and 'technique'. Attitudes of *warmth*, *empathy*, *acceptance* and a belief in the client's capacity for *personal growth* are seen as the critical dimensions of the therapist.

Client-centred therapy (sometimes described as Rogerian therapy) also brought psychotherapy from the consulting room into the community at large. Lay counsellors trained in the Rogerian approach are using it effectively in schools, colleges and in industry. In Britain, the National Marriage Guidance Council (founded in 1948) has relied largely on the Rogerian approach while accepting recently the Masters and Johnson programme for brief sexual therapy (Parry-Jones, 1983).

A third non-physical approach to treatment consists of *behavioural psychotherapy*, which uses techniques derived from classical (Pavlovian) and operant (Skinnerian) conditioning. This approach rejects consideration of unconscious conflicts and instead focuses on behaviour—those activities which can be *observed*. The emphasis is thus not on the private inner world of thoughts, feelings and emotions (though these are not denied) but on the public, observable and measurable realm of behaviour. This approach considers mental disorder as maladaptive patterns of learned behaviour which can be 'unlearned' by a process of 'counter-conditioning'. Learned behaviour is any behaviour present in the mature organism which was not present at birth. We are not born neurotic but learn to be neurotic (largely by processes of conditioning) and can learn to respond with adaptive behaviour to previously troublesome conditioned stimuli.

Techniques used include *systematic desensitization* which constitutes an effective treatment for phobic anxiety. The rationale is that the patient has become 'sensitized' to certain stimuli (insects, heights, public places) just as the asthmatic may have become sensitized to foreign proteins. As the asthmatic may be desensitized by giving graduated doses of the troublesome substances, so may the phobic be desensitized by gradual exposure to the troublesome environmental stimulus, thus overcoming 'social allergies'. Thus the person with a phobic fear of spiders would first be taught relaxation techniques and would then be desensitized by approaching anxiety-evoking situations arranged in a hierarchical order (from least anxiety-evoking to most anxiety-evoking). For example, the patient may commence by looking at photographs of spiders and may then progress to models of spiders (looking and then handling)—dead spider sealed in jar—dead spider in open jar—live spider in sealed jar—live spider in open jar—entering a dusty basement where spider webs are in evidence. The patient would not move on to the next step in the hierarchy until anxiety associated with the previous step had been reduced.

The technique of *flooding* (implosion) confronts the patient with the most anxiety-evoking stimulus without a graduated approach. These techniques create a situation whereby the patient who has become conditioned to associate troublesome stimuli with responses of anxiety now associates these stimuli with responses of relaxation (counter-conditioning).

Other techniques include operant conditioning, whereby the frequency of adaptive behaviour is increased and the behaviour strengthened (reinforced) by arranging desirable consequences for these behaviours while maladaptive behaviours are decreased in frequency and strength by ensuring that no rewarding consequences follow them (for example, simple behaviour modification programmes and token economy programmes).

The range of behaviour therapy techniques is very diverse and most are successful in rapidly reducing or extinguishing certain types of troublesome responses (notably anxiety responses), though in practice techniques may be only loosely related to learning theory (Parry-Jones, 1983). In chapter 17 Marshall describes the cognitive behavioural approach to therapy which draws on both behavioural and cognitive understanding.

Group therapies offer psychotherapeutic intervention to a small group of individuals and aim to create a group climate of mutual support and understanding in which the individual feels free to offer his/her difficulties to the group for discussion. Listening to others reduces feelings of isolation and alienation and promotes willingness to actively consider faulty approaches to living. Problems are shared, troublesome feelings are worked through in a climate of support and encouragement and new solutions are formulated. The success of the group approach is underlined by its use in groups like Alcoholics Anonymous, Phobics Anonymous, self-help groups for depressed housewives, persons with drug problems and the use of group techniques in management and educational settings.

The *encounter group* invites the participant to 'encounter self' and began as a sensitivity-training technique for 'normals'. The emphasis is on the 'here and now' aspects of human feelings and the aim is to increase awareness. The peer group dominates the proceedings rather than the authority of the group conductor, and participants are not allowed to conceal feelings behind the convenient social façades of etiquette, privacy or 'good manners'. Stark emotional confrontations may occur and openness and emotional honesty are regarded as essential. The desired outcome is increased personal growth. The often ruthless exploration of previously 'taboo' intimate areas may be experienced as very disturbing by some participants, and the result may be a distinctly 'bad experience' (an 'encounter group neurosis' has been described). Prospective participants are advised to consider this course of action carefully; participation involves some personal risk and the experience may be very rewarding but simultaneously very punishing.

Encounter groups aiming at an increase in 'human potential' by confrontational emotional techniques have drawn upon the techniques of sensitivity training, gestalt therapy, transactional analysis and, above all, the philosophy and approach of Rogers.

Encounter groups are often regarded with attraction by mental health care professionals and can indeed heighten self-awareness and enable the participant to approach life difficulties (personal or those of others) with increased awareness and confidence. Prospective members should, however, ask the following questions carefully:

1 Have I carefully considered why I want to join?

2 Are my expectations of this group realistic?

3 Am I prepared to fully embrace the intimate climate of such a group?

4 Is the group I am considering joining being conducted for bona fide reasons and by a suitably experienced/qualified person?

If the answers to all four questions are 'yes' then the result may be a rewarding and enriching experience; if not, careful consideration is suggested.

Consideration of the plethora of psychotherapeutic interventions available may tend to induce little else other than confusion in the student's mind. This is unnecessary. The similarities between approaches are more marked than the differences. Total embrace of any one school of thought may be injudicious for the student but all have something to offer. For example, Freud suggests that we are not always conscious of the reasons for our behaviour and consideration of underlying forces may be fruitful. The nurse should also be able to recognize transference relationships when these (inevitably) develop between her and her patients. Cathartic experiences should not be nervously suppressed—they are usually very therapeutic.

Adler suggests that inferiority complexes may serve a positive function as they may generate positive attempts to compensate. Jung supplies the view that psychic functioning is never static— we must not complacently categorize our patients as 'withdrawn' or 'aggressive' or 'self-defeating'— psychic movement is continual and no one is 'frozen' in a negative state. Rank emphasizes that short-term therapy may be effective and Reich underlines the importance of the relationship between physical tensions and posture and emotional state. Fromm highlights the importance of the social background and sees man as a figure in an increasingly critical urban landscape. Gestalt therapy (Perls) emphasizes the importance of attempting to unify thinking, feeling and being, while Rogers (client-centred therapy) indicates that the would-be therapist need not recoil from offering psychotherapy on the grounds of lack of therapy/qualifications but should consider his/her view of other persons as the most appropriate starting point.

The behavioural approach reveals that the reasons for many troublesome problems are not particularly complex and that relatively brief interventions may produce satisfactory results. The group approach reveals the fact that the means of resolving common difficulties is available in any ward or out-patient department and that intervention need not be either prolonged or interpretative.

The beginner is often tempted to opt for one 'school' or the other (to the exclusion of alternative viewpoints). This would be unfortunate as the approach adopted by many effective therapists is *eclectic* (drawing upon more than one school of thought). The 'purist' may achieve intellectual vigour at the expense of practical efficacy and is at risk of developing a rigid frame of reference which will help some of the clients some of the time, but will be of little help to most of the clients for most of the time. The risks of the 'purist' stance are perhaps best described by Ogden Nash:

'I give you now Professor Quist,
A conscientious scientist,
Trustees exclaimed—he never bungles
And sent him off to distant jungles,
Camped by a tropic riverside,
One day he missed his blushing bride,
She had, a guide informed him later
Been eaten by an alligator.
Professor Quist could not but smile,
You mean, he said, a crocodile'.

Many mental health care professionals profess to have open minds whereas the aforesaid area is only slightly ajar; this is unfortunate as awareness of the range of psychotherapeutic interventions available will greatly enrich perspectives on mental disorder. Analytical or interpretative approaches should only be used once the appropriate post-basic training has been undertaken and the novice should resist the temptation to offer sweeping interpretations. Despite this proviso, an awareness of the interpretative models contributes greater understanding of human behaviour and emotions, and the student should not regard interpretative writings as a 'taboo' area but should try to enhance his/her understanding by considering each of the major perspectives.

The nurse should, for example, be able to recognize transference relationships and cathartic experiences and should be able to approach nurse/patient relationships with a broad awareness of psychodynamics, and increased sensitivity to the emotional responses of self and others. Non-directive approaches are eminently suitable for use by nursing staff, as are some variants of the humanistic approach.

EDITORS' NOTE

In helping to produce responses to life difficulties and illness and distress nurses may draw on a range of methods and approaches to mental health. They will take part in or support patients through physical treatments originating in bio-medical approaches and experience. They may also participate in programmes that draw on understanding from learning theory and its application in behavioural approaches. They may be active in helping people offset the effects of illness through social skills training programmes or they may themselves become expert in one or more of the other psychological approaches such as cognitive therapy, client-centred therapy, personal construct theory, and transactional analysis. These activities will take place from a base in a variety of services and settings from primary care to perhaps the special hospital and will involve variously health promotion, care and case management and direct intervention through the use of personal helping skills.

Other chapters provide ideas and information relevant to nursing intervention but do not deal in depth (except for cognitive behavioural therapy) with specific psychological approaches and therapies such as cognitive therapy, client-centred therapy, social skills training, personal construct theory, transactional analysis and others of a similar nature. The further reading list contains references to general readers through which a more detailed understanding of the various approaches can be obtained. Expertise in these areas can only be obtained through specialized study and practice.

* FOOTNOTE

This chapter is taken from the first edition, *Mental Disorder* (1986), and includes an Editors' Note (p. 321) for the purposes of this volume.

FURTHER READING

Jones, W. (1983) *Ministering to Minds Diseased—A History of Psychiatric Treatment*. London: Heinemann.

Laing, R. (1964) *The Divided Self*. Harmondsworth: Pelican.

Nolan, P. (1992) *A History of Mental Health Nursing*. London: Chapman & Hall.

Parry-Jones (1992) The development of the psychotherapies. A brief historical overview. In Weller, M. & Eysenck, M. *The Scientific Basis of Psychiatry*, 2nd edn. London: Saunders.

Patterson, C.H. (1986) *Theories of Counselling and Psychotherapy*, 4th edn. Cambridge, Philadelphia: Harper & Row.

Szasz, T. (1973) *The Manufacture of Madness*. London: Paladin.

REFERENCES

Foucault, M. (1967) *Madness and Civilisation*. London: Tavistock Publications.

Henderson, D. & Batchelor, I. (1962) *Henderson and Gillespie's Textbook of Psychiatry*, 9th edn. Oxford: Oxford University Press.

Jones, W. (1983) *Ministering to Minds Diseased—A History of Psychiatric Treatment*. London: Heinemann.

Jones, K. & Fowles, A. (1984) *Ideas on Institutions—Analysing the Literature on Long-Term Care and Custody*. London: Routledge & Kegan Paul.

Laing, R. (1964) *The Divided Self*. Harmondsworth: Pelican.

Parry-Jones, W. (1983) The development of the psychotherapies. In Weller, M. (Ed.) *The Scientific Basis of Psychiatry*. London: Baillière Tindall.

Rogers, C. (1942) *Counselling and Psychotherapy*. Boston: Houghton Mifflin.

Rogers, C. (1951) *Client-Centred Therapy—Its Current Practice, Implications and Theory*. London: Constable.

Rogers, C. (1961) *On Becoming a Person—A Therapist's View of Psychotherapy*. London: Constable.

Seymer, L. (1956) *A General History of Nursing*. New Zealand: Faber.

Szasz, T. (1973) *The Manufacture of Madness*. London: Paladin.

16

PROMOTING OPTIMUM HEALTH AND DEVELOPMENT

A LIFE SPAN PERSPECTIVE

Margaret Evans

AIMS

i)   To outline the nurse's role in promoting health and development—historical and modern perspective

ii) To define the concepts of health promotion, health education, prevention and health protection

iii) To discuss the prevention of mental ill-health in children and adults

iv) To discuss the promotion of optimum health and development in childhood—meeting basic needs

v)   To evaluate child health surveillance and immunization programmes

vi) To identify ways in which the optimum health and development of adults is compromised

vii) To discuss the promotion of optimum health of the elderly

viii) To identify obstacles to prevention and health promotion

KEY ISSUES

The nurse's role in the promotion of health
The prevention of mental ill-health
   Identifying the problem
   Promoting optimum health and development in childhood
   Child health surveillance
   Adolescents
   Fitness and mental health
   Illicit drug use
   Sexual practices
   Road accidents
Occupational health
Promoting optimum health of the elderly
Obstacles to prevention and health promotion

Identify, analyse and assess factors causing distress and illness	Promote health, provide direct care and make interventions	Manage care programmes and services
Be critical, analytical and accountable, continue professional development	Counter discrimination, inequality and individual and institutional racism	Work within and develop policies, laws and safeguards in all settings
Understand influences on mental health and the nature/causes of disorder and illness	Know the effects of distress, disorder, illness on individuals, groups, families	Understand the basis of treatments and interventions

'By health I mean the power to live a full adult, living, breathing life in close contact with what I love ... I want to be all that I am capable of becoming'.
Katherine Mansfield

'The main social targets of Governments and the WHO in the coming decades should be the attainment by all citizens of the World by the Year 2000 of a level of health that will permit them to lead a socially and economically productive life. Primary health care is the Key to attaining this target!'
WHO, 1977

Many people die prematurely or suffer debilitating ill-health from conditions that are to a large extent preventable. Initially, the responsibility for health lies with each individual but the increasing dominance of preventable diseases means that health professionals have responsibilities to assist individuals to achieve full potential.

The education and training of health professionals must, therefore, take into consideration the need to appeciate that disease, prevention and health promotion are as important as disease management and the provision of high quality care.

THE NURSE'S ROLE

Nurses have unparalleled opportunities to advise individuals, families and communities and to help them to overcome obstacles to achieving optimum health and development. These obstacles to human potential may be 'biological, environmental, societal, familial or personal' (Seedhouse, 1986).

In the days of Florence Nightingale, the obstacles to health potential were bad hygiene, poor nutrition and poverty and she saw health in terms of prevention and eradication of disease because of the conditions she observed around her. It was her aim that nurses both in hospital and community should help people overcome the obstacles of the day. In 1891, she wrote in one of her letters, 'I look forward to the day when there are no nurses of the sick, only nurses of the well' (Nightingale, 1891).

The World Health Organization views health promotion as an important activity for all health professionals. The Declaration of Alma-Ata reads:

Primary health care includes all health care professionals involved in the delivery of care to individuals and communities. Nurses, therefore, play an increasingly important role in the challenge of achieving WHO targets by the year 2000.

The Government White Paper, *The Health of the Nation*, acknowledges that the role of the health professional is crucial to the successful achievement of the Government's overall goal of 'adding years to life' and 'adding life to years' (DH, 1992).

The United Kingdom Central Council also acknowledges the importance of health promotion and illness prevention. To be admitted to the UKCC Professional Register, nurses must demonstrate competence in 'the identification of health related learning needs of patients and clients, families and friends and in the ability to participate in health promotion (UKCC, 1986).

Despite the fact that nurses routinely interact with patients and clients and are in a privileged position to promote health, they often fail to capitalize on the opportunities. In the past, nurse education lacked a framework for health promotion and nurses were not taught the necessary concepts and skills to enable them to function as health promoters. They were taught within a medical framework which embodied the principles of diagnosis, treatment and cure (Syred, 1981). Studies by Faulkner and Ward (1983) and Macleod Clark *et al.* (1987), highlighted the lack of interpersonal skills training in the traditional curriculum. The ability to listen, to deal sensitively with questions and to respond appropriately to client needs is fundamental to effective health promotion.

Project 2000 pre-registration nurse education is based on a health model which places emphasis on health promotion and disease prevention and the fundamental health promotion skills are included in the curriculum.

Health promotion

Downie *et al*. (1990), identified the overall goal of health promotion as 'the balanced enhancement of physical, mental and social facets of positive health, coupled with the prevention of physical, mental and social ill-health'. A great many individuals and agencies have a part to play in achieving the overall health promotion goal.

According to Tannahill (1985b), health promotion comprises three overlapping spheres of activity, health education, prevention and health protection.

Health education

All health professionals who work with the public will as part of their everyday work, teach, inform, advise and counsel their patients/clients individually or in groups. In this way all health professionals are 'health educators' (Ewles and Simnett, 1985).

Smith (1979) defines health education as a 'communication activity aimed at enhancing positive health and preventing or diminishing ill-health in individuals and groups through influencing the beliefs, attitudes and behaviour of those with power and the community at large'.

The cardinal principle of health promotion is empowerment. Health education seeks to empower by providing necessary information and helping people to develop skills and self-esteem so that they feel they have significant personal control. Good preventive services and a healthy environment shaped by health protection policies will also contribute to the process of empowerment.

Health education has many orientations and Downie *et al*. (1990) refers to disease-orientated health education which is aimed at preventing specific diseases with success being measured by achieving morbidity and mortality target rates. This orientation assumes that major preventable diseases such as cardiovascular disorders and malignancies are best dealt with by specific prevention programmes aimed at reducing relevant

risk factors. This is a negative focus and people will be less likely to change their lifestyle on the strength of some 'intangible future benefit' (Downie *et al*., 1990). The disease-orientated module is also 'expert' dominated, people are expected to comply even though they may not agree with the diagnosis or see the appropriateness of the prescription.

The health-orientated health education model cited by Downie *et al*. (1990) has a dual focus. Its aim is to enhance positive health as well as to prevent ill-health. Physical, mental and social dimensions of health are recognized in the model. Due to the positive focus people are more likely to adopt a more healthy lifestyle. They like to do things that are appealing and enjoyable and give tangible and speedy results. This model acknowledges underlying circumstances including social factors and therefore contributes to a holistic view of health and its determinants and can be applied to individuals or a whole community. The public are involved in identifying health factors and priorities and in shaping and securing action.

Prevention

Central to prevention is the notion of reducing the risk of occurrence of illness, injury, disability or handicap and is usually classified into primary, secondary and tertiary prevention.

This classification focuses on disease and treatment of ill-health and Alderson (1976) identifies the shortcomings of this focus for secondary prevention. If this is defined as 'the treatment and cure of established disease' then just about everything a doctor does could be construed as prevention when in fact treatment is aimed at the prevention of certain consequences of ill-health (Downie *et al*., 1990).

The benefits of the traditional classification can be preserved and the drawbacks minimized by describing instead Downie's (1990), four foci for prevention as follows:

---

1 Prevention of the onset or first manifestation of a disease process, or some other first occurrence, through risk reduction, e.g.
   (a) The avoidance of a first unwanted pregnancy through contraception.

(b) Accident prevention through reducing hazards or risk-taking behaviour.

(c) Rubella vaccination to reduce the risk of foetal abnormality.

2 Prevention of the progression of a disease process or other unwanted state, through early detection when this favourably affects outcome, e.g.

(a) Screening for premalignant changes in the cervix.

(b) Detection of an unwelcome foetus at a stage which permits termination of pregnancy.

(c) Early detection of foetal abnormality through ultrasound, foetoscopy, amniocentesis, AFP, or chorion villus sampling followed by termination of pregnancy if necessary.

3 Prevention of avoidable complications of an irreversible, manifest disease or some other unwanted state, e.g.

(a) Early detection of PKU or hypothyroidism.

(b) Prevention of pressure sores or urinary tract infection in victims of multiple sclerosis.

(c) Arrangements for the adoption of an unwanted child.

4 Prevention of the reoccurrence of an illness or other unwanted state, e.g.

(a) Efforts to prevent a second heart attack.

(b) Efforts to prevent a second unwanted pregnancy.

(c) Efforts to prevent a further suicide attempt.

This system of classification may not be ideal, but it does embody the philosophy and practice of prevention (Downie et al., 1990).

Health Protection

The third overlapping sphere of activity identified by Tannahill (1985) comprises 'legal or fiscal controls, other regulations and policies and voluntary codes of practice aimed at the enhancement of positive health and the prevention of ill-health' (Downie et al., 1990). Examples include

legislation concerning the wearing of seat belts in cars; the sale of alcohol and tobacco to minors; drinking and driving; the control of communicable diseases, and health and safety at work.

It is widely accepted that health problems associated with alcohol and tobacco in a society correlate with the levels of use of these drugs in that society and that over time, usage is inversely related to real price (ASH et al., 1988; FCM, 1988). Despite occasional health-motivated increases in duty, smoking and drinking are cheaper in real terms than 40 years ago when there was much less information about the ill-effects of the practices. Deterrent increases in tobacco taxation are not overall in the national interest since the tobacco revenue is the country's third largest source of income. The calls for increases, therefore, fall on deaf ears which often stems from the enormous power of vested interests over public policy making. Big business can oppose pro-health policies and perpetuate unhealthy ones in the interest of profit.

Other health protection policies address the full range of the prerequisites for health identified by WHO in the Strategy for Health for all by the year 2000. These are:

Freedom from the fear of war

Equal opportunities for all

Satisfaction of basic needs
Food
Basic education
Water and sanitation
Decent housing
Secure work and a useful role in society

Political will and public support

The UK Government has expressed strong support for the strategy which legitimized health promotion, notably through the Ottowa Charter (WHO, 1986), and is centred on certain key principles:

The promotion of equity in health

The impact on health of policies and services outside the health sector

The need for fruitful intersectoral collaboration

The importance of multidisciplinary collaboration

Community participation

Primary care and health promotion may be seen as twin pillars of the Health for All (HFA) strategy and according to Tannahill (1988) it makes good sense to try to strengthen the bridging between these two pillars by further developing health promotion in the primary care setting.

THE PREVENTION OF MENTAL ILL-HEALTH

Identifying the problem

'More than five million people consult their GP each year because of mental ill-health. It is a leading cause of illness and disability and accounts for about 14% of certificated sickness absence, 14% of NHS in-patient costs and 23% of NHS pharmaceutical costs. The cost in human misery and suffering to individuals and their families is incalculable!'
Department of Health, 1992

Depression is the commonest form of mental ill-health in the community today and is sometimes associated with, but is twice as common as, anxiety alone. Depression and dementia are also prevalent in the elderly and are progressively disabling. More serious conditions such as schizophrenia and affective psychosis are less common.

Even though the exact cause or causes of abnormal depression is not known, those at greatest risk are young to middle age working-class women. Recent negative life events involving loss are the most clearly identified risk factors but are not the only ones. Vulnerability factors in the presence of a life event markedly increases the risk of depression. One of these is the lack of a confiding relationship (Wing, 1982).

Suicide is the third leading cause of death among 15–34-year-olds and parasuicide is the second commonest reason for emergency medical admission. Some important general features emerge from overall patterns of suicide that point to the scope for their prevention. Most suicides occur in middle age with the highest rate among men over 60 years who are either widowed, divorced or single. It is more common among manual than non-manual groups and the rate is high among people with alcohol problems. Suicide rates also increase in times of recession in particular among self-employed businessmen. Alcohol is implicated in up to 65% of suicide attempts. Excessive drinking is also associated with depression, anxiety, eating disorders and personality problems.

Both suicide and parasuicide are much more common among the unemployed living in areas of multiple deprivation and 40% of those who commit suicide have a history of parasuicide. If it is possible to identify those parasuicide at risk of committing suicide, it has implications for prevention. Controlling the availability of methods for committing suicide may also help to reduce death rates. The majority of people who commit suicide have suffered a depressive illness and have contacted their GP in the month beforehand.

Bereavement counselling has been shown to be effective in preventing a deterioration in the mental health of older widows and widowers who are at risk of suicide. Counselling services such as the Samaritans provide a valuable service although the effect on suicide rates is difficult to ascertain.

About 150,000 people suffer from schizophrenia in the UK and this results in a heavy burden of care on families, the community and health and social services. On the basis of current knowledge, little can be done to prevent the onset of schizophrenia but a great deal can be done to minimize the resulting disability.

One of today's biggest public health challenges is the prevention of mental ill-health in an expanding population of older people. Fifteen per cent of over 70-year-olds and 20% of over 85-year-olds suffer from dementia.

The scope for prevention is limited for Alzheimer-type dementia but high blood pressure is implicated in the multi-infarct kind of dementia. Reducing blood pressure in middle age may, therefore, not only reduce the risk of coronary heart disease but may possibly reduce the incidence of dementia.

Physical and mental health are often interlinked. Serious and continuing physical illness may lead to depression, anxiety state or social handicap and it is known that severely mentally ill people have extremely high rates of deaths from cancers, respiratory and cardiovascular disease.

Children and adolescents are also vulnerable to physical, intellectual, emotional, social or developmental disorders. The scope for the prevention of mental ill-health in children was outlined in two major reports (WHO, 1977; RCGP, 1981). Some of the most exciting possibilities are in the field of mental handicap/learning disabilities and Jacobson et al. (1991) identified the following measures aimed at reducing or preventing mental ill-health in childhood:

The reduction of unwanted and unplanned pregnancies through the provision of family planning and abortion services

Antenatal screening and the offer of termination of pregnancy for the prevention of Down's syndrome and spina bifida. Newer techniques such as gene mapping and sampling will offer more opportunities in future

Avoidance of smoking and heavy drinking during pregnancy to prevent retardation of foetal growth and development

Prevention of premature births

Prevention of birth injuries

Screening for phenylketonuria and congenital hypothyroidism to prevent impaired intellectual development

Immunization against rubella and measles

Other preventative measures are concerned with reducing environmental lead which may cause intellectual impairment in children and monitoring other food additives which may contribute to hyperactivity in children.

Child abuse

In 1988, the first national survey of Child Protection Registers was carried out in England and Wales. Approximately 40,900 children and young people were on the Registers in March 1988, representing a rate of 3.5 children per thousand in the population under 18 (Jacobson et al., 1991). Of these, 37% were on the register in the 'grave concern' category, 28% under 'physical abuse', 15% under 'sexual abuse' and 13% in the neglect category.

It is known that children most at risk of physical abuse tend to come from multiple deprived families, where young parents live in overcrowded conditions. Sexual abuse can occur in any social group. Public and political concern about individual abuse cases has led to more clearly defined ways of managing the care of children following hospital admission to minimize the damage to 'at risk' children.

The Cleveland inquiry into child abuse generated a report in 1988 which recommended training and co-ordination of a wide range of professional activities (Cleveland, 1988). Following the publication of this report the Department of Health issued further guidance for interagency collaboration and the regulations regarding Child Protection were further tightened and are now embodied in the Children Act (DH, 1989).

Preventative measures are directed at social issues which may make a positive contribution to the prevention of physical abuse. Early identification of parents at risk and the provision of emotional support and occasional substitute child care may be life-saving in an emergency. If, for any reason, biological parents are unable to look after their children, long-term fostering and, preferably, adoption is the best means of preventing later emotional disorders in childhood (RCGP, 1981).

Emotional disorders affect about 5% of children and associated risk factors include overprotective parents, families with severe marital problems or ambivalence about a pregnancy (RCGP, 1981). Over protectiveness may result from past experience of miscarriage or cot death

(SIDS) or it may be the response of anxious parents to a disabled child. Early recognition of the problem followed by child-centred counselling may be helpful.

Conduct disorders in older children and adolescents has trebled in the last 20 years, particularly among 14–17-year-old boys and are twice as common in inner city as in rural areas. Different research approaches have identified some aspects of inner cities that may predispose children and their families to mental ill-health:

Higher inner city rates are not simply due to high population density or urbanization. City living on its own is not a sufficient explanation (Newman, 1973, 1975).

Rates of delinquency vary widely within the inner city. Children living above the fifth floor in housing estates have higher levels than those living on lower floors (Richman, 1977).

Schools have a protective effect on scholastic achievement attendance and delinquency rates (Rutter, 1979).

Psychological adversity in the family places it at risk of having children with psychiatric disorder. The direct adverse effects on parents are likely to be indirectly exerted on the children.

Recognition of these predisposing factors has led to the identification of potential public health action in:

Improved building design with more security and privacy.

Better supervision and planning, together with control of alcohol at sporting venues.

Improved leisure facilities.

Improved school organization. Preschool education has a favourable effect on children's emotional and intellectual development.

Major obstacles to effective primary prevention are the continuing social inequality, poor housing, unemployment and unequal access to health and resources that prevail in this country. The number of children growing up in poverty is increasing, as the gap between the rich and poor in both income and health widens (Smith, 1986).

Recognition of the emotional needs of children has fostered the trend to allow parents to stay with their children in hospital and to participate actively in their care. Despite the awareness that hospital admission is a frightening experience for many children, hospitals still admit too many who could be treated on an out-patient or day-care basis.

Nurses who are involved in child health surveillance, who provide follow-up care after discharge from hospital, who help in the management of children with special needs or work in schools should be experienced in children's nursing and properly trained to meet the physical, psychological, developmental and social needs of all children in their care.

The health of children and their parents is inextricably linked. Parents' health and behaviour have an impact on their children. Parents who smoke or drink heavily are more likely to produce children who do likewise. It is also known that postnatal depression and family disharmony or parental neglect and abuse can have a profound effect on children's wellbeing and development.

Children may also have an impact on their parents' wellbeing. There is evidence that bringing up a mentally handicapped child takes a toll of the mental health of parents, especially the mother (Romans-Clarkson et al., 1986).

Rearing healthy children can also have adverse effects on the mental health of their mothers. A small study which investigated the impact of caring for preschool children on the health of 102 mothers found that in the main, the brunt of all child care was borne by the mothers, who spent 70% of their 15-hour working day with their children. This left little time for relaxation and was associated with symptoms of emotional upset in most mothers (Graham, 1986).

Promoting optimum health and development in childhood

'Children's physical, emotional, social and intel-

lectual needs must all be met if they are to enjoy life, develop their full potential and grow into participating, contributing adults'.
Pringle, 1980

Health in childhood is shaped by influences acting long before birth and childhood itself. Children born to manual workers are less likely to survive infancy and early childhood and those brought up in deprived inner city areas are more at risk of conduct and other emotional disorders. Children's physical and mental health can be significantly affected by their parents family planning practices as well as by events which may take place during pregnancy and around birth.

Any commitment to health prevention in childhood must consider the factors that promote or compromise the health of the parents who are responsible for the healthy development of their children.

The basic needs of children

Pringle (1980), identifies four basic emotional needs which have to be met from the beginning of life to enable a child to grow from helpless infancy to mature childhood. These are the need for love and security, for new experiences, for praise and recognition, and for responsibility. During the different stages of growth, the ways in which these needs are met will change.

Meeting the child's need for love and security is the most important because it provides the basis for all later relationships, within the family as well as friends, colleagues and eventually the child's own family. Love and security will facilitate the healthy development of the child's personality and his or her ability to care and respond to affection and later to becoming a loving, caring parent.

This need is met within a continuous reliable, loving relationship initially with a mother and father and later extending to other contemporaries and adults. A stable family life will provide the child with the security of a familiar place and known routines ensuring continuity and predictability in an ever-changing world. It also provides a sense of personal continuity, a past as well as a future, and a coherent and enduring identity.

If a child's intelligence is to develop satisfactorily the need for new experiences must be met. These facilitate the learning of how to learn and learning that mastery brings a sense of achievement. The ability to learn depends not only on inborn capacity but also on environmental opportunity and encouragement. The emotional climate of the home as well as parents' support and aspirations can foster, limit or impair mental growth (Pringle, 1980).

Play enables the child to learn about the world and provides a means of coping with and resolving conflicting emotions. The quality of the child's language environment is crucial to intellectual development and the ability to reason and think and to develop relationships. In formal education, the child's progress will be affected by the teachers attitudes, values and beliefs. Teachers have the opportunity to preserve and awaken the child's curiosity and joy in learning about new things.

To grow from a helpless infant into a self-reliant, self-accepting adult requires a great deal of emotional, social and intellectual learning which is accomplished by the child modelling himself on the adults caring for him. The most effective incentives are the praise and recognition from adults who love the child and whom he in turn loves and wants to please. The level of expectation must be geared to the individual child's capabilities and stage of development.

Most children will spend half their working life for at least 11 years in school. Teachers will, therefore, play a vital role in meeting the child's need for praise and recognition. The time spent in school is the ideal opportunity to establish a favourable attitude to learning and to improve a child's self-esteem and attitude to effort and achievement.

The need for responsibility is met by allowing children to gain personal independence at first, through learning self-care activities and the exercising of ownership of personal possessions. With increasing maturity, responsibilities will be extended to more important areas, ultimately allowing them freedom for their own actions and the ability to accept responsibility for others. Increasing independence must develop within negotiated parameters. They are helped by knowing what is expected and permitted and the reason for any rules imposed in their interests or the interests of others.

If children's basic needs are unmet, the consequences can be wider ranging. Prisons, mental hospitals and schools for the maladjusted contain a high proportion of individuals who in childhood were unloved and rejected. Anger, hate, lack of concern for others and an inability to make mutually satisfactory relationships are common reactions to having been unloved and rejected.

A child growing up in an unhappy home is also liable to become emotionally disturbed or anti-social. A quarrelling, inadequate or disturbed parent makes a poor adult role model. Parental hostility has a particularly harmful effect on a child's later development especially on his ability to give, as an adult, unselfish loving care to his own children. Parental hostility also perpetuates itself from one generation to another (Rutter and Madge, 1976).

If children are not exposed to new experiences, it will adversely affect their intellectual development and will result in the apathy, restlessness and frustration frequently seen in adolescents with nothing to do and nowhere to go. There is little freedom or safety for children to explore or experiment without adult supervision, and older children looking for the excitement of new experiences may turn to mindless vandalism and destruction.

Praise and recognition are almost always given for achievement rather than effort and this disadvantages children who are intellectually less able, are culturally disdvantaged, emotionally neglected or maladjusted. Whatever successes they achieved demand far more effort and perseverance, yet they receive less reward because they achieve less. The encouragement and expectations of parents and teachers have a most powerful influence on a child's progress.

Children who do not have the opportunity to exercise responsibility will fail to develop a sense of responsibility for themselves, for others or for material possessions. When such children leave school, they often drift into jobs which give them little, if any, responsibility and will heighten their feeling of alienation and rejection.

Parents make a very positive contribution to their children's emotional and physical develop-

ment. A small study found that 80% of the mother's activities recorded in a diary were concerned with her child's nutrition and health. This reinforces other research into more specific aspects of child health which shows that parents deal with 90% of childhood illnesses themselves and that general participation in the use of preventative services such as child health clinics can improve both their effectiveness and efficiency.

The increasing number of women in paid employment is likely to have major implications for child health and development. Nurseries can offer an acceptable solution for the families where both parents are in paid employment or for single parents. The lack of state-provided nurseries in the UK reflects the long standing British concern about the potential adverse effects that separation from the mother may have on the child as well as the possible adverse effects of the nursery itself.

Available evidence to date shows that separation of a child from its mother is not harmful in itself and that emotional disturbances in children are more likely to originate from family discord (Tizard, 1986). There is no evidence that day care nurseries are damaging to children and high-quality care confers some social advantages on the attenders.

It is widely agreed that preschool education has a favourable effect on children's emotional and intellectual development and attendance at nursery schools in England has increased over the last decade from 28% of under fives in 1977 to 48% in 1988.

The most detailed research on the direct impact of schooling has been conducted on children of junior and secondary school age and there is compelling evidence that some schools have a protective effect on scholastic achievement, attendance rates and even delinquency rates (Rutter, 1979).

In a major controlled study of 12 schools in Inner London, the following factors were significantly associated with successful achievement at school and low delinquency rates:

A good mix of intellectually able and less able pupils

The use of reward and praise

An attractive school environment

Encouragement for children to participate in the running of the school together with firm leadership and participation by the teaching staff

Teachers' attitudes and behaviour

Growing recognition of the school's role in promoting the health and development of children has resulted in the integration of health education throughout the curriculum. The importance of encouraging pupils of all ages to participate actively in their own learning about health is now recognized.

The School's Council programmes are founded on three main principles:

The success of the educational approach depends on fulfilling social and emotionally defined outcomes as well as medical objectives.

The programmes need to be integrated right across the curriculum.

Learning, in general, and health-related behaviour, in particular, are enhanced by methods geared towards promoting a child's self-confidence and decision-making skills.

The aim is to allow students ultimately to make informed choices about health-related behaviours. Evaluation of this approach has shown increases in confidence and self-awareness among students and wide acceptance by teachers throughout the country (Bolam, 1985; Thacker, 1985).

Child health surveillance

The Health Visitors' Association (HVA) has identified four essential components of surveillance:

Screening tests to detect specific disorders

Health promotion support

Developmental screening

Developmental assessment

Screening tests for hypothyroidism and phenylketonuria in the newborn have been shown to be effective. Other potentially effective tests for problems such as undescended testes, congenital dislocation of the hip and hearing and visual impairment require clear guidelines for implementation. The WHO has concluded that screening tests for hearing and visual impairment are of proven efficacy. Visual and hearing impairments are common problems in childhood. About 4% of children age 5–7 years have moderate visual impairment and 6% of 7-year-olds have significant hearing loss (Anon, 1986).

Untreated visual impairment such as squints can result in permanent damage and subsequent reading difficulty. Children with untreated hearing impairment are more likely to be educationally and psychosocially handicapped than normal children at the age of seven years. Screening at repeated intervals is essential, because one normal result may be followed by the detection of subsequent abnormalities, for example, short-sightedness is not usually apparent before the age of seven years.

Health promotion support

Health Visitors and GPs are important sources of advice and support for parents of preschool children but it is not known whether this advice beneficially affects health outcomes. Information on some health-related trends in childhood is now sufficiently detailed to initiate intervention studies on the effects of advice from health professionals in these areas. It is known for example, that although the average height of children continued to increase between 1972 and 1980, there is still scope for improvement as children from less well-off families remain shorter than children from well-to-do families (Tanner, 1986).

Developmental screening and assessment

Even though developmental screening was introduced more than 25 years ago, there is still no reliable information on which tests are valid, effective and reliable, when it is best to do them and how much emphasis should be placed on their results (Alberman, 1986). Delay in achieving developmental milestones is a poor predictor of subsequent abnormality and most children who start walking or talking late turn out to be normal. Development is a dynamic process and children can learn new skills throughout childhood. Carrying out developmental screening can also create anxiety among parents and children.

The publication of *Health for All Children: A Programme for Child Surveillance* in 1989 brought together representatives from all relevant professional bodies in a joint working party on child health surveillance (Hall, 1989). The working party reviewed the scientific basis for each component of the surveillance programme and produced a consensus report on what the content of such programmes should be. They recommended examinations in the neonatal period, at discharge or within 10 days; then at 6 weeks; 8 months; 21 months; 39 months; five years and periodically throughout the school years.

Procedures considered to be essential and scientifically well founded include checks for Congenital Dislocation of the Hip (CDH) and testicular descent; screening for hearing and visual impairment; height; weight; listening to the heart at five years as well as immunizations at the appropriate times. They also stressed the importance of health promotion and taking notice of parental concerns at every stage including parents' worries about behaviour.

Promoting the optimum health of adolescents

Adolescence is a time of uncertainties, experimentation and change. The improved nutritional status of children has been accompanied by an increase in growth and weight and a reduction in the age of onset of puberty. This earlier sexual maturity, an increase in permissiveness, easy access to alcohol, tobacco, drugs, fast cars and sexually transmitted diseases, have together contributed considerably to the current problems of our adolescent children and young adults (Forfar, 1988).

The National Curriculum requires the 11–14-year-olds to understand the processes of human conception, the physical and emotional changes that take place during adolescence and the need to develop a responsible attitude to sexual behaviour. They must also study the ways in which HIV affects the healthy functioning of the human body.

Adolescence is an anxious time for handicapped children due to the increased dependence during childhood and concern over the degree of independence possible in adulthood.

Parents often find it difficult to accept the maturation of a dependent child, denying emerging sexuality and failing to face up to the fact that the adolescent might consider a life away from them. These difficulties are compounded by the poor services available to both physically and mentally handicapped children when they leave school.

Medical services continuing the care of the adolescent must understand their needs. The handicapped child has the same needs as a normal child, but his or her difficulties are often exacerbated. The family should have access to the normal forms of support as well as the special support that may be required because of the handicap.

Promoting the optimum health of adults

Mortality rates in adolescence and early adult life are comparatively low in the UK, but beyond the age of 45 mortality rates from coronary heart disease, strokes and cancers are much higher than those for many other European countries (House of Commons Committee of Public Accounts, 1989). Over 50% of all deaths before the age of 85 years are attributed to cancers and heart disease.

There is good reason to believe that many of the deaths from these causes are potentially avoidable. Although success in prevention tends to increase the need for caring services for our older population, there is little doubt that it postpones the onset of disabling conditions and enriches the quality of life overall.

Coronary heart disease and stroke
Coronary heart disease (CHD) is the leading cause of death in the UK and in 1988 accounted for about 180,000 deaths among British men and

women. Each year, 100,000 people suffer a stroke and in 1988 nearly 69,000 people in England and Wales died of a stroke (KF, 1991). In 1989, the NHS spent £10 million on trying to prevent CHD and over £500 million on treatment.

Evidence suggests that the disease process begins early in life and those with the highest death rates are men and women in the manual classes and men and women of Asian origin. Intensive research carried out over the past 15–20 years has shed more light on the risk factors in heart disease. These include the classical risk factors—cigarette smoking, blood cholesterol, diet and high blood pressure—as well as other factors such as physical inactivity, obesity and diabetes.

Cigarette smoking

Smoking is estimated to be responsible for one in four of all deaths from CHD (RCP, 1983). The risk of developing heart disease in middle age is more than three times as great for someone who smokes more than 20 cigarettes a day than for a non-smoker. Giving up smoking is of major importance in reducing the risk of heart disease and those who have already had a heart attack can halve their future risk of another by stopping smoking.

Cholesterol and diet

The higher the cholesterol level in the blood the greater the risk of heart disease (Rose and Shipley, 1986). There is good evidence that the amount of saturated fat in the diet is an important determinant of cholesterol levels. A reduction in cholesterol levels can be achieved through a reduction in total fats and saturated fats, an increase in polyunsaturated fats and an increase in dietary fibres.

High blood pressure

High blood pressure is a major contributory factor in both heart disease and stroke (WHO, 1982). The higher the blood pressure, the greater the risk of heart disease. Blood pressure is influenced by a combination of factors such as genetic factors, obesity, heavy drinking and a high dietary salt intake.

Various reports have concluded that salt intake in the UK is too high and that salt is an important, potentially reliable determinant of high blood pressure. A moderate reduction of 3 g a day would lower systolic blood pressure by an average of 5 mmHg, in people with 'normal' blood pressure and 7 mmHg in people with high blood pressure. Such a reduction across the whole UK population would be expected to reduce the incidence of stroke by more than a quarter and coronary heart disease by 15%.

Obesity and diabetes

Obesity is associated with heart disease and probably contributes by increasing the risk of high blood pressure and diabetes and by raising blood cholesterol levels. For each 6 kg excess in weight there is an associated 4 mmHg increase in blood pressure. In 1985, 36% of men and 31% of women were classed as overweight and a further 8% of men and 15% of women were obese.

Between 1 and 2% of the population has diabetes, about 90% of which is related to overweight and obesity and is thus potentially preventable (*Lancet*, 1985). Dietary policies that will not only reduce blood cholesterol levels but also obesity and thus diabetes offer most scope for prevention.

Physical activity

Regular exercise is not only enjoyable, but makes a major contribution to health and fitness at all ages. The effects of moderate, rhythmic and regular exercise such as brisk walking, running or swimming have been studied in people up to the age of 70 years and has a number of demonstrable effects:

Improved cardiovascular function

Better tolerated and sustained work effort

Improvement in muscle size and strength and ligament strength which improves muscle function which helps to maintain posture thus protecting against joint instability and injury and back pain

---

Maintenance of fitness is beneficial to all ages but is critical in elderly people and can mean the difference between independence and institutionalization. Although some decline is inevitable in old age, there is evidence that about 20% or more is due to disease and is thus recoverable at any age (Muir-Gray *et al.*, 1985). If the central goal for health in old age is the promotion of independence and autonomy, then the maintenance of stamina, suppleness and strength through physical activity is an integral part of this process (King's Fund, 1991).

Fitness and mental health

Available evidence suggest that:

Physical fitness results in significant improvement in measures of self-confidence and self-esteem

Exercise has an antidepressant effect which has been most reliably demonstrated in the short term among mildly or moderately depressed people in both hospital- and community-based population

A number of poorly controlled trials show an association between exercise and a reduction in anxiety

Randomized controlled trials have shown that exercise can reduce the immediate physiological response to stress

Research in brain chemistry shows that one of the immediate effects of exercise may be an increase in the brain levels of endorphins—a heroin-like substance which may have an anti-depressant and possible anti-anxiety effect

---

Alcohol

Over 90% of Britons drink and most enjoy alcohol without endangering themselves or others. In 1988 almost as much was spent on alcohol in the UK as on clothes, and alcohol accounted for the equivalent of half of consumer spending on food.

The range of medical, social and emotional damage caused by alcohol is vast but hard to quantify accurately. In 1988 nearly 60% of deaths from cirrhosis and chronic liver disease occurred before the age of 65 years and over 1,500 deaths on the roads were estimated to be alcohol linked. The risk of developing cirrhosis of the liver, cancer of the oesophagus and alcohol dependence increases directly with the amount of alcohol drunk and the number of years of excessive drinking.

Available evidence suggests that young people are drinking more often, and starting to drink at an earlier age. Per capita alcohol consumption is clearly the best predictor of a wide range of alcohol-related harm. This increase in per capita alcohol consumption is almost always followed by corresponding increases in death rates from cirrhosis of the liver, convictions for public drunkenness and drinking and driving, as well as first admissions to psychiatric hospitals for alcohol dependence.

Unlike cigarette smoking, alcohol presents a challenge—how to minimize the harm without jeopardizing the benefits. The WHO has recommended three main methods of achieving these aims:

Fiscal measures to maintain the price of alcohol above that of inflation

Controls on the availability of alcohol through licensing restrictions

Public and professional education

It is suggested that these aims can be achieved by interdepartmental government co-ordination, increases in alcohol tax, closer monitoring of licensing and advertising, improved education, training and treatment services and random breath testing. The most detailed implementation strategy so far comes from the Scottish Health Education Co-ordinating Committee (SHECC) (1985) and the Health Education Advisory Committee for Wales (HEACW) (1986) reports which have laid out clear plans for action by a wide range of agencies from Government and the NHS to local authorities, industry and trade unions, the media, voluntary organizations and the courts.

Illicit drug use

There has been a rapid growth in drug use since

the late 1970s. Between 1973 and 1988 the number of new narcotics addicts notified to the Home Office increased nearly seven-fold. The number found guilty or cautioned for drug offences increased two-fold overall, with more than a six-fold increase in the number of offences associated with heroin. The number of police seizures for heroin increased by more than 13-fold and for cocaine it increased five-fold (Jacobson *et al.*, 1991).

The use of illicit drugs is not confined to any particular lifestyle or socioeconomic group. Some information from national studies indicates that most heroin users start in their late teens and early twenties, the majority are male, unemployed and from socially deprived areas (Pickin and St Leger, 1993).

It will be impossible to eliminate illicit drug use due to the availability of drugs on the black market. Jacobson *et al.* (1991) identify three realistic goals:

To reduce experimentation with potentially hazardous illicit drugs

To help those who are dependent on drugs to stop or reduce the harm associated with use

To minimize the harm associated with continued drug use

These goals may be achieved by:

Reducing the supply and demand for illicit drugs

Discouraging the more hazardous forms of drug use

Introducing supportive socioeconomic measures aimed at reducing the deprivation associated with a high risk of misuse.

Internationally, attempts have been made to control the supply of drugs by crop substitution and control of trafficking. At national level, there is better policing and drugs law enforcement as well as tighter controls on the prescribing of narcotic drugs. These measures will only be partly successful and it is estimated that only about 10% of the total amount of heroin available on the black market is confiscated (Advisory Council on the Misuse of Drugs, 1984).

Two approaches aimed at reducing demand involve educational initiatives to reduce experimentation and support for users who wish to stop drug misuse. The mass media approach must be aimed at young people, parents and professionals. The best education initiatives are those which put legal and illegal drugs into a realistic social and cultural context and encourage young people to develop sufficient knowledge and self-confidence to make an informed decision.

If the illicit use of drugs cannot be eradicated, measures must be taken to reduce drug-related harm. It is very crucial to minimize the spread of HIV/AIDS through intravenous drugs misuse and the common practice of sharing syringes and needles. The long-term outcome of needle exchange schemes in reducing the risk of spreading HIV/AIDS, hepatitis B and other infections is not yet known. What is known already is that needle exchange schemes are inadequate to meet identified needs.

There is an urgent need for local treatment and rehabilitation services which are totally inadequate at present. Outside London, long-term rehabilitation is largely left to voluntary agencies. It is hoped that further Government funding will be made available to transfer hospital-based treatment schemes to community and primary care.

Sexual practices

Acquired immune deficiency syndrome (AIDS) is the most serious worldwide threat to public health to emerge in the last 10 years (Jacobson *et al.*, 1991). In the UK, there were more than 9,100 reported cases by March 1990. Fifty-six per cent of these have already died. In 1988, it was estimated that the cost of hospital treatment for HIV/AIDS patients ranges between £20 and £30 million (Wells, 1986). This does not include costs incurred in the community or the potentially prohibitive costs of using drugs such as Zidovudine AZT prophylactically.

Prevention of HIV/AIDS requires changes in

lifestyle. Evidence so far confirms that HIV cannot be transmitted by normal social or occupational contact (Greddes, 1987). Follow up studies over two years shows that household and non-sexual close contacts of AIDS patients have not become HIV positive. Health care workers who have accidentally exposed themselves to HIV-infected blood run a much lower risk of becoming HIV positive than becoming hepatitis B infected which occurs in 6–30% of staff accidentally exposed to the virus.

HIV can be transmitted through semen, blood and blood products and cervical and vaginal fluids. The commonest route of transmission is sexual. In the UK, up to 1990, 80% of AIDS cases occurred in the homosexual/bisexual population. The pattern was similar for Netherlands, Denmark, Sweden, Norway and Germany. In Spain and Italy, over 60% of AIDS sufferers were intravenous drug users. In Scotland in 1990, the majority of HIV positive individuals were intravenous drug users and it is expected that newly diagnosed cases of AIDS in the intravenous drug users population will soon exceed the numbers of homosexual suffering from AIDS.

In many African countries heterosexual transmission is the most important route and an equal number of men and women have developed AIDS. This mode of transmission is also becoming more common in the UK and other countries. Heterosexual transmission occurs both from men to women and women to men. Having multiple partners and sex with prostitutes is associated with a high risk of becoming HIV positive. The presence of genital ulcers and sexually transmitted diseases such as gonorrhoea and syphilis increase the risk of transmission.

In 1986, 44% of people with haemophilia A and up to 60% of severe haemophiliacs who needed multiple transfusions were HIV positive (UK Haemophilia Centre, 1986). Prior to 1986, transfusions of blood and blood products were the second most important source of HIV infection in the UK. In 1985 screening of all donors and heat treatment of blood products were introduced.

A national strategy for limiting the spread of HIV/AIDS already involves a combination of educational and public health measures aimed at the screening and heat treatment of blood and blood products and limiting intravenous drugs use and needle sharing. Advice and information is aimed at reducing the number of sexual partners and the use of barrier methods of contraception, together with the avoidance of sexual practices which involve the exchange of infected body fluids.

Changes in sexual behaviour would need to be substantial if it is expected to influence disease trends, but a reduction in the number of sexual partners and widespread use of barrier methods of contraception are realistic goals.

Road accidents

The cars we drive, the way we use our roads and motorways and the influence that transport policy has on us can adversely affect our health as do cigarettes, alcohol, drugs or diet.

In 1988, over 5,000 people died and nearly 63,500 were seriously injured on the roads in Great Britain. Thirty-six per cent of the deaths were under 25 years and road accidents were the single most important cause of death in 5–24-year-olds, representing over two-thirds of all accidental deaths of this age group.

It is impossible to know the true cost of road accidents to society but in 1987, 115,000 years of lives were lost due to road traffic accidents in England and Wales, compared with 393,000 from cancers and 205,000 from coronary heart disease in the same period.

The Department of Transport estimated in 1987 that 20% of all road fatalities were alcohol associated. Young men between the ages of 20 and 24 years were the most likely to be convicted of drink/drive offences and the highest conviction rates are in summer.

The commonest injury in all road users is head injury. Motor-cyclists are now less likely to be admitted to hospital with head injuries than other road users and this is most likely due to almost full compliance with the law which requires riders of two-wheeled motor vehicles to wear crash helmets. Increasingly, pedal cyclists are also wearing crash helmets.

Excessive speed is responsible for a high proportion of accidents. The Transport Road Research Laboratory (TRRL) estimates that high speed directly accounts for 10–20% of accidents. A 1983 TRRL survey showed that:

40% of cars and up to 90% of coaches and HGVs exceeded the speed limit on motorways.

50% of vehicles exceeded the speed limit in residential areas. As many as two-thirds of young male car drivers claimed to drive regularly at speeds of over 70 mph.

The most striking fall in deaths or serious injuries in the last decade occurred in car users following legislation which made the use of seat belts mandatory in the front seats of cars and light vans in 1981. Similar legislation for back seat passengers is now in force.

Occupational health

Work-related diseases and injuries are preventable because they are caused by identifiable agents in, or aspects of the working environment (Jacobson et al., 1991). Over the last 20 years the incidence of work-induced injuries has fallen steadily. This may be due in part to shorter working hours and increasing unemployment.

The implementation of the Health and Safety at Work Act (1974) has played a role in this decrease in work-related injuries. The Act placed new, enforceable responsibilities on employers to provide a safe and healthy workplace as well as maintaining high standards of monitoring and evaluation of control measurement.

In the manufacturing and construction industries there has been a significant and sustained increase in reported major injuries and even more in accident rates—a 43% increase for construction and 33% for manufacturing from 1981 to 1985. According to the Health and Safety Executive these figures must reflect a real deterioration in safety standards (Health and Safety Executive, 1985).

Much progress has been made in reducing the occupational risks that caused life-threatening illness such as asbestos-related lung cancer, mesothelioma and bladder cancer caused by aromatic aminos used in the rubber and dyestuffs industries. There are now stringent controls on the permitted concentration of asbestos fibres in the workplace and blue asbestos is banned completely.

Two years after the Employment Medical Advisory Service (EMAS) confirmed the findings of early research, the British Rubber Manufacturers Association in collaboration with relevant trade unions and the Health and Safety Executive published a guide which recommended immediate control of all dust and fumes (RPRA, 1982).

In 1950 the WHO and the International Labour Organization (ILO) identified the aims of occupational health as 'the promotion and maintenance of the highest degree of physical, mental and social wellbeing of workers in all occupations by prevention of departures from health, and controlling risks' (WHO, 1950). The WHO European strategy for health for all by the year 2000 embodies this principle (WHO, 1985).

During the past 10 years more emphasis has been placed on broader preventive measures which promote awareness of occupational hazards and general health promotion issues. Concern has been expressed that today's working population may be experiencing adverse physical and psychosocial effects of new electronic technology. Repetitive strain injuries and visual problems are common among VDU operators. New legislation is being introduced in 1993 to ensure operators are given breaks from operating keyboards and reading the monitors. Employers must face the challenge of minimizing occupation stress by planning the working day in such a way that the workforce are stimulated to participate to the extent which ensures job satisfaction.

A WHO collaborative study in the prevention of heart disease was able to demonstrate that a simple, factory-based programme of advice on diet, smoking and exercise could significantly reduce heart disease. Heartbeat Wales is actively pursuing this kind of intervention. Advice and education about a healthy lifestyle is being backed up with workplace policies which ensure that a wide range of healthy foods are available in work canteens and smoking control policies and the provision of exercise and showering facilities enable employees to act on the advice they are given. Increasing evidence of the adverse effects of passive smoking has led to litigation by nonsmokers. The provision of smoke-free workplaces is now top priority for most employers.

Promoting optimum health of the elderly

Improved standards of living and child health earlier this century, together with better nutrition, prevention and health care, have all helped to ensure that by the 1990s the life expectation for a woman is 82.4 years and for a man 78.5 years.

The retired population now forms about 16% of the community. Two-thirds of retired people are women and 80% of carers of the elderly are also women. By the age of 85 years, women outnumber men by four to one.

A realistic objective for the elderly is to be able to live long, disability-free lives and any assessment of health needs must consider five important dimensions:

The ability to perform activities of daily living

Mental health

Physical health

Social function

Economic function

This multidimensional assessment of the elderly provides the information necessary to develop policy that meets the needs of the clients.

The prevalence of ill health increases with age and in the UK 7 out of 10 people over 75 years suffer from chronic ill health such as arthritis and joint problems, respiratory disease, cataracts and dementia. Major studies of the over 65s show that up to threequarters of elderly people see themselves as healthy for their age. Over 80% were able to perform activities of daily living (ADL) and only a minority suffered severe functional incapacity. When mental function was included in the assessment the majority among the over 65s who were able to perform activities of daily living without assistance was reduced to 54% (OPCS, 1989). A qualitative study showed that elderly people held a positive view of themselves and

their abilities (Finch, 1986). It is possible that some of the loss of functional capacity associated with ageing is avoidable and should act as a stimulus to develop appropriate policies for both elderly people and their carers.

It is Government policy to support elderly people so that they may live independent lives in their own homes (DHSS, 1981). This is also the goal of statutory and voluntary agencies as well as the elderly people themselves. The WHO has subdivided the overall goal into six key objectives (WHO, 1983):

To prevent unnecessary loss of functional capacity

To maintain the quality of life in old age by preventing distressing symptoms

To assist elderly people to live in their own homes and to prevent unnecessary admissions to residential care

To prevent the breakdown of informal networks of care particularly families

To prevent unnecessary decline in functional capacity and quality of life if admission to long-stay care is essential

To prevent iatrogenic disease, including the distress that can be caused by inappropriate interventions in old age

---

To achieve these objectives support must be available through relevant health care, social and welfare policies and a commitment to health promotion. There must be a successful integration of prevention, treatment and rehabilitation.

Hospital and specialist services have a considerable role to play in preserving and improving the functional capacity of elderly people. Among those over 65 in England, there are over 1,000 operations a week for cataracts, 500 prostatectomies and 500 hip replacements while large numbers of patients receive surgical or gynaecological repair and are treated for angina, diabetes or rehabilitation from stroke.

Promoting autonomy in old age, involves

income, housing, transport and communication policies and their impact will have a major effect on the ability of elderly people to function independently in the community. State pensions form the major source of income for retired people and one-third of pensioners are so poor that their resources are near or below the Income Support level. Elderly people are more likely to live in old, dilapidated housing. About half are owner-occupiers and there was an increase in the number of owner-occupied homes deemed unfit between 1971 and 1981. In the same period improvement grants to owner occupiers decreased by 28%.

Good health in old age depends largely on the avoidance of disease when younger and the promotion of physical activity in old age. Research shows that some of the loss of fitness in old age is not inevitable and results from disease rather than from the ageing process itself. Maintenance of fitness is beneficial to health at all ages but is critical in elderly people and can mean the difference between independence and institutionalization. As people get older, there is a steady decline in the capacity to do physical work and maximum oxygen capacity, muscle bulk and strength decrease by about 1% per year. Although some of this decline is inevitable, there is evidence that about 20% is due to disease and is, therefore, recoverable at any age. Such an improvement in physical fitness might extend the period of independent living in old age by eight or nine years (Shepherd, 1985).

Independence and autonomy must be the desired aim of every elderly person. The maintenance of stamina, suppleness and strength through physical activity will be an integral part of this process. The elderly themselves together with their families and friends have a key role in maintaining a good quality of life. There is increasing recognition of the need for emotional and social support that primary health care professionals can give elderly people.

Voluntary and statutory provision in the community promotes the independence and autonomy of the elderly but limited resources may mean that leisure facilities, adult education activities, day centres and luncheon clubs may be sacrificed to enable meals on wheels and other essential services to be provided. The implementation of the NHS Community Care Act in April 1993 will hopefully acknowledge the needs of this ever growing population.

It is important that health professionals do not become overprotective even though the elderly may be very vulnerable in particular to iatrogenic health problems which may be one of the commonest preventable problems in old age. The elderly receive a disproportionate amount of all drug prescriptions and they are especially vulnerable to doctors who over-prescribe medicines. They are more likely than other groups to receive repeat prescriptions and in one study, up to 28% of repeat prescriptions to the elderly were deemed unnecessary (Williamson & Chopin, 1980). Studies of admissions of elderly people to hospital suggest that at least 10% are associated with the over-prescription of drugs particularly benzodiazepines, diuretics and digoxin (Age Concern, 1977).

Research that has demonstrated the existence of undetected disease in elderly people questions the value and practicability of establishing screening programmes for them. Interest in screening has now broadened from the detection of disease to assessment of functional capacity and social need. Results from trials so far, suggest that Health Visitor assessment and intervention on a regular basis does not have much impact on levels of disability but can increase use of appropriate services and reduce the need for hospitalization. There is no firm evidence yet that screening adds to an elderly person's quality of life. Recent convincing evidence supporting a social rather than a medical approach to screening among elderly people showed that assessment and provision of simple aids significantly improved functional status (Hart *et al.*, 1990).

The rising prevalence of mobility problems makes the provision of appropriate housing very important. Inappropriate housing can lead to social isolation and consequent poor mental and physical health. Good public transport systems are very important to the elderly as they cannot walk far and only a few may have access to a car. Lack of good transport networks will limit access to recreational activities, social support networks and health care facilities.

Obstacles to prevention and health problems

Major obstacles to effective prevention and health promotion are the continuing social inequality, poor housing, unemployment and unequal access to health care resources that prevail in this country. Almost all health indicators confirm the association between the prevalence of ill health and poor social economic circumstances.

In 1981, the death rate was twice as high in the lowest social classes as in the highest. The number of children growing up in poverty is increasing as the gap between the rich and poor widens (Smith, 1986). The expectation of life for a child with parents in Social Class V is over seven years shorter than for a child whose parents are in Social Class I.

The reduction of inequalities in health is the first of the WHO European targets for health for all (WHO, 1985). All 32 European states are signatories to this document and have endorsed the aim that by the year 2000 health inequalities should be reduced by 25%. Historically, major advances in health reflect the fact that intrinsically desirable changes in social circumstances tend to be those that favour good health. Past improvements in health have been a by-product of a rising standard of living indicating that the kinds of housing, environments, types of employment, leisure activities and diet to which people with greater choice have access are generally beneficial to health.

The link between deprivation and ill-health is irrefutable. The relationship offers four broad approaches to prevention:

The economic approach aims to increase wealth and to redistribute resources as to reduce the deprivation

Risk factor reduction aims to sever the link between deprivation and ill-health by promoting behaviour change

The educational approach aims to promote a better educated community especially among the most disadvantaged

The community development approach aims to

---

support and promote self-esteem and autonomous action among the most deprived groups in the community

---

Once the burden of socioeconomic disadvantage is reduced, efforts to reduce specific risk factors, to promote a better educated community or to promote community action among disadvantaged groups will become more effective. It is reasonable to suppose that given the greater freedom of the middle classes and a greater command of resources, the lower classes would be more responsive to health information and education.

The Government's overall goal is to secure continuing improvement in the general health of the population by:

Adding years to life by increasing life expectancy and reducing premature deaths

Adding life to years by increasing years lived free from ill health, reducing or minimizing the adverse effects of illness and disability, promoting healthy lifestyles, physical and social environments and overall, improving quality of life *DH, 1992*

These goals will be achieved by:

Considering the health dimensions when developing policies

The active promotion of physical environments conducive to health in the home, in schools, at work, on the roads, at leisure, in public places

Increasing knowledge and understanding of the way people's lifestyle affects their health

Meeting the health needs of local population and receiving the most appropriate balance between health promotion, disease prevention, treatment, care and rehabilitation

---

If these goals are achieved, health for all by the year 2000 may yet become a reality.

SUMMARY

Many people die prematurely or suffer debilitating ill health from conditions that are to a large extent preventable. Although initially the responsibility for health lies with each individual, health professionals clearly have responsibilities to assist individuals to achieve full potential. The education and training of health professionals must take into consideration the need to appreciate that disease prevention and health promotion are as important as disease management and the provision of high-quality care.

Nurses have unparalleled opportunities to advise individuals, families and communities to help them to overcome obstacles to achieving optimum health and development. This is reflected in the Government White Paper, *The Health of the Nation* (DH, 1992), which acknowledges that the role of the health professional is crucial to the successful achievement of its target.

The goal of health promotion is the balanced enhancement of physical, mental and social facets of positive health coupled with the prevention of physical, mental and social ill health, and physical and mental health are often interlinked. The major obstacles to effective prevention and health promotion are the continuing social inequality, poor housing, unemployment and unequal access to health care resources.

FURTHER READING

Department of Health (1992) *Immunisation Against Infectious Diseases*. London: HMSO.

Ewles, L. & Simnett, I. (1992) *Promoting Health: A Practical Guide to Health Education*. Chichester: Wiley.

Hull, D.M.B. (Ed.) (1992) *A Programme for Child Health Surveillance*. Oxford: Oxford University Press.

Nutbeam, D. (1986) Health promotion glossary. *Health Promotion*, **1**(i), 119–127.

Nutbeam, D. & Catford, J.C. (1984) Towards a definition of health education and health promotion. *Health Education Journal*, **43** (2×3), 38.

Nutbeam, D. & Catford, J.C. (1986) Health promotion in action: practical ideas for programme implementation. *Health Promotion*, **1**(2), 187–190.

Pickin, C. & St Leger, S. (1993) *Assessing Health Needs Using the Life Cycle Framework*. Buckingham: Open University Press.

Seedhouse, D. (1986) *Health: The Foundation for Achievement*. Chichester: Wiley.

Seedhouse, D. & Cribb, A. (1989) *Changing Ideas in Health Care*. Chichester: Wiley.

Towes, K., Tilford, S. & Robinson, Y. (1990) *Health Education: Effectiveness and Efficiency*. London: Chapman & Hall.

Townsend, P., Davidson, N. & Whitehead, M. (1990) *Inequalities in Health*.

World Health Organization (1985) *Targets for Health for All. Targets in Support of the European Regional Strategy for Health for All*. Copenhagen: WHO.

REFERENCES

Advisory Council on the Misuse of Drugs (1984) *Prevention: A report*. London: HMSO.

Age Concern (1977) Profiles of the elderly—their health and health services. Age concern research publication No 2. Survey, Age Concern.

Alberman, E. (1986) Prevention and health promotion. *British Medical Bulletin*, **42**(2), 212–216.

Alderson, M. (1976) *An Introduction to Epidemiology*. London: Macmillan.

Anon (Editorial) (1985) Insulin dependent? *The Lancet*, 12 October, 809–810.

Anon (Editorial) (1986) Developmental surveillance. *The Lancet*, 26 April, 950–952.

Action on Smoking and Health (ASH) (1988) *An Introduction to Epidemiology*. London: Macmillan.

Bolam, R. (1985) *Active Tutorial Work Training and Dissemination: an Evaluation*. Oxford: Health Education Council/Blackwell.

Cleveland (1988) Report of the inquiry into child abuse in Cleveland (1987) CM 412. London: HMSO.

Department of Health and Social Security (DHSS) (1981) *Growing Older*. London: HMSO.

Department of Health (DH) (1989) *Children Act*. London: HMSO.

Department of Health (DH) (1990) *National Health Service, Community Care Act*. London: HMSO.

Department of Health (DH) (1992) *The Health of the Nation: Strategy for Health in England*. London: HMSO.

Downie, R.S., Fyfe, C. & Tannahill, A. (1990) *Health Promotion Models and Values*. Oxford: Oxford University Press.

Ewles, L. & Simnett, J. (1985) *Promoting Health: A Practical Guide to Health Education*. Chichester: Wiley.

Faulkner, A. & Ward, L. (1983) Nurses as health educators in relation to smoking. *Nursing Times*, **79**(15). Occasional papers No 8.

Faculty of Community Medicine (FCM) (1988) *Alcohol: The Prevention of Problems Related to Its Use*. London: FCM.

Finch, H. (1986) Health and older people. Research report No 6. London: Health Education Council.

Forfar, J.O. (Ed.) (1988) *Child Health in a Changing Society*. British Paediatric Association/Oxford University Press.

Graham, H. (1986) Caring for the family. Research report No 1. London: Health Education Council.

Greddes, A.M. (1987) Risk of AIDS to health care workers. *British Medical Journal*, **292**, 711–712.

Hall, D.M.B. (Ed.) (1989) *Health for all Children: A Programme for Child Health Surveillance*. Oxford: Oxford University Press.

Hart, D. & Bowling, A. (1990) Locomotor disability in very elderly people: value of a programme for screening and provision of aids for daily living. *British Medical Journal*, **301**(6745), 216–220.

Health Education Advisory Committee for Wales (1986) *Dealing with alcohol problems in Wales*. Cardiff: HEAW.

Health and Safety at Work Act (1974).

Health and Safety Executive. *Health and Safety Statistics 1985–6*. London: HMSO.

House of Commons Committee of Public Accounts, Session 1988–1989. Twenty-sixth report: coronary heart disease. London: HMSO.

Jacobson, B. (1991) *The Nations Health: A Strategy for the 1990s*. London: King's Fund.

Jacobson, B., Smith, A. & Whitehead, M. (1991) (Revised Edition). London: King's Fund.

King's Fund (1991) *The Nation's Health: A Strategy for the 1990s. A Report from an Independent Multidisciplinary Committee*. London: King's Fund.

Macleod-Clark, J. (1987) Helping patients and clients to stop smoking. Assessing the effectiveness of the nurse's role. Research Report No 19. London: HEA.

Muir-Gray, J.A. *et al.* (1985) The risks of inactivity. In Muir-Gray, J.A. (Ed.) *Prevention of Disease in the Elderly*. Edinburgh: Churchill Livingstone.

Newman, O. (1973) *Defensible Space*. London: Architectural Press.

Newman, O. (1975) Reactions to the 'defensible space' study and some further findings. *International Journal of Mental Health*, **4**, 48–70.

Nightingale, F. (1891) Letter to Mr Frederick Verney on the teaching of health at home in Buckinghamshire County Council (1911). Reproduction of a printed report originally submittd to the Buckingham County Council in the year 1992, containing letters from Miss Nightingale on health visiting in districts, pages 17–19. Re-quoted from Hinchcliff *et al.* (1989), *Nursing Practice and Health Care*. London: Arnold.

Office of Population Censuses and Surveys (OPCS) (1989) *General Household Survey—1986*. London: HMSO.

Pickin, C. & St Leger, S. (1993) *Assessing Health Need Using the Life Cycle Framework*. Buckingham: Open University Press.

Pringle, M.K. (1980) *The Needs of Children*, 2nd edn. London: Hutchison.

Royal College of General Practitioners (RCGP) (1981) Prevention of psychiatric disorders in general practice. Report from General Practice No 20. London: RCGP.

Richman, N. (1977) In *Child Psychiatry: Modern Approaches*. Oxford: Blackwell Scientific.

Romans-Clarkson, S.E. (1986) Impact of a handicapped child on mental health of parents. *British Medical Journal*, **293**, 1395–1397.

Rose, G. & Shipley, M. (1986) Plasma cholesterol concentration and death from coronary heart disease: 10 year results of the Whitehall study. *British Medical Journal*, **293**, 306–307.

Royal College of Physicians (1983) *Health or Smoking? A Following Report*. London: Pitman Medical.

Rubber and Plastics Research Association for Great Britain (1982) *Clearing the air*. London: Rubber and Plastics Research Association.

Rutter, M. & Madge, N. (1976) *Cycles of Disadvantage*. London: Heinemann.

Rutter, M. (1978) *Changing Youth in a Changing Society*. Cambridge, Mass.: Harvard University Press.

Rutter, M. (1979) *Fifteen Thousand Hours. Secondary Schools and Their Effects on Children*. Cambridge, Mass.: Harvard University Press.

Scottish Health Education Coordinating Committee (1985) *Health education in the prevention of alcohol-related problems*. Edinburgh: SHECC.

Seedhouse, D. (1986) *Health: The Foundations for Achievement*. Chichester: Wiley.

Shepherd, R. (1985) The value of physical fitness in preventive medicine. In Evered, D. & Whelan, J. (Eds) *The Value of Preventive Medicine*. CIBA

Foundation Symposium 110. London: Pitman Medical.

Smith, E.A. (1979) In Sutherland, J. (Ed.) *Health Education. Perspectives and Choices*. London: Allen & Unwin.

Smith, R. (1986) Whatever happened to the Black Report? *British Medical Journal*, **293**, 91–92.

Syred, H. (1981) The abdication of health education by hospital nurses. *Journal of Advanced Nursing*, **6**(1), 27–33.

Tannahill, A. (1985) What is health promotion? *Health Education Journal*, **44**, 167–168.

Tannahill, A. (1988) Health for all by the year 2000. Promoting health in East Anglia. In *Promoting Health in East Anglia, Conference Report*. Cambridge: East Anglian Regional Health Authority.

Tanner, J.M. (1986) Physical development. *British Medical Bulletin*, **42**(2), 212–216.

Thacker, J. (1985) Extending developmental group work to Junior/Middle schools: an Exeter project. *Pastoral Care*, **Feb**, 5–13.

Tizard, B. (1986) *The Care of Young Children—Implications of Recent Research*. London: Thomas Coram Research Unit.

UK Haemophilia Centre (1986) Prevalence of antibody to HTLV-III in haemophiliacs in the UK. *British Medical Journal*, **293**, 175–176.

United Kingdom Central Council (UKCC) (1986) *Project 2000—A New Preparation for Practice*. London: UKCC.

Wells, N. (1986) *The AIDS Virus. Forecasting its Impact*. London: Office of Health Economics.

Williamson, J. & Chopin, J.M. (1980) Adverse reaction to prescribed drugs in the elderly: a multi-centre investigation. *Age and Ageing*, **9**, 73–80.

Wing, J.K. (1982) Epidemiology of depressive disorders in the community. *Journal of Affective Disorders*, **4**, 331–345.

World Health Organization (WHO) (1950) *Occupational Health*. Third Report. WHO Technical Report Services No. 135. Geneva: WHO.

World Health Organization (WHO) (1977) *Child Mental Health and Social Development*. WHO Technical Report Services No. 613. Geneva: WHO.

World Health Organization (WHO) (1978) *Report of the International Conference on Primary Care*. Alma Atar USSR. Geneva: WHO.

World Health Organization (WHO) (1982) *Prevention of Coronary Heart Disease*. Report of a WHO expert committee. Technical Report Services No. 678. Geneva: WHO.

World Health Organization (WHO) (1983) *Objectives of Health Promotion in the Elderly*. Copenhagen: European Regional Planning Group, WHO.

World Health Organization (WHO) (1985) *Targets for Health for All—Targets in Support of the European Regional Strategy for Health for All*. Copenhagen, WHO.

World Health Organization (WHO) (1986) *Ottawa Charter for Health Promotion*. Geneva: WHO.

17

COGNITIVE BEHAVIOUR THERAPY

Sue Marshall

AIMS

i) To offer an introduction and overview of cognitive behaviour therapy
ii) To provide examples which illustrate aspects of the cognitive behavioural approach

KEY ISSUES

Collaborative, active, problem centred and educational process.

Techniques developed from the behavioural and cognitive schools of therapy.

Theoretical underpinnings of cognitive behaviour therapy.

Assessment as a critical first step.

Enabling the client to overcome a range of mental health difficulties.

Providing individuals with an 'inoculation'.

Identify, analyse and assess factors causing distress and illness	Promote health, provide direct care and make interventions	Manage care programmes and services
Be critical, analytical and accountable, continue professional development	Counter discrimination, inequality and individual and institutional racism	Work within and develop policies, laws and safeguards in all settings
Understand influences on mental health and the nature/causes of disorder and illness	Know the effects of distress, disorder, illness on individuals, groups, families	Understand the basis of treatments and interventions

INTRODUCTION

The purpose of this chapter is to offer an introduction to cognitive behaviour therapy. It is aimed at providing an insight into the theory and methods associated with cognitive behavioural approaches to therapy. It is not intended as an inclusive review of all the techniques used by cognitive behaviour therapists or of the related literature. It is intended to sensitize readers to the depths and diversity of cognitive behaviour therapy; but it is not a procedural manual. There are other texts which are readily available that cover this (Hawton *et al.*, 1989; Blackburn and Davidson, 1990; Stern and Drummond, 1991).

The chapter will, however, provide material that may inform practitioners who are skilled in the use of cognitive behavioural approaches; and for those yet to develop those skills it will give some insight into the background and efficacy of this approach when working with people who have, or are vulnerable to the development of, mental health diffficulties. Like other therapies, cognitive behaviour therapy requires supervision by someone experienced in its practice and should not be attempted just on the basis of reading this introduction.

The chapter is structured so that after an overview of cognitive behavioural therapy has been provided, particular attention will be paid to the technique of self instructional training. This has been chosen for description because of its importance to the practice of cognitive behavioural therapy.

Throughout this chapter examples will be given that will illustrate aspects of the cognitive behavioural approach to therapy. These examples will not include extensive biographical, clinical or background information—they will simply act as explanatory vignettes that highlight a particular point.

A glossary of terms is provided at the back of the book to help both in deciphering the jargon associated with cognitive behavioural therapy and as a reference resource.

A DEFINITION OF COGNITIVE BEHAVIOUR THERAPY

Cognitive behaviour therapy has been variously described (Meichenbaum, 1977; Dryden and Golden, 1986; Blackburn and Davidson, 1990), but is best viewed as representing an approach encompassing a range of specific techniques. A definitive description is therefore not possible and it is better to conceptualize it as an amalgam of a number of techniques taken from the cognitive and behavioural approaches to therapy. The efficacy of cognitive behavioural therapy has been demonstrated in connection with a range of psychological difficulties; for example in helping adults and children who experience self control problems (Meichenbaum and Goodman, 1971; Novaco, 1975), helping those who have suffered a traumatic event that has left them with difficulties in coping (Foa *et al.*, 1991), those people who suffer with depression (Biram and Wilson, 1981), or those who suffer with anxiety-related difficulties (Salkovskis and Warwick, 1986). It has been shown to be more effective than alternative therapies in the treatment of these and other psychological difficulties (Rush *et al.*, 1977; Foa *et al.*, 1991; McCullough, 1991; Morse *et al.*, 1991).

Before embarking on a description of the elements of the practice of cognitive behavioural therapy, an understanding of the theoretical concepts that underpin the therapy is vital. Blackburn and Davidson (1990), describe cognitive approaches and behavioural approaches to therapy as sharing much in common but they highlight how a cognitive approach utilizes a mediational model whereas behaviour therapy is based on a stimulus response model.

THEORETICAL UNDERPINNINGS OF COGNITIVE BEHAVIOUR THERAPY

Central to behavioural approaches to therapy are stimulus response models. These are non-mediational theories of learning (Skinner, 1953). They propose that the exhibition of behaviour is based on learning that is founded on the development of a bond between a particular stimulus event and a particular response. This bond is developed and maintained by a process of reinforcement simply. If an activity is reinforced the likelihood of it occurring again will be increased. Conversely, if it is not reinforced then it will ultimately disappear from that person's repertoire of behaviours. Appendix 1 (p. 361) contains an overview of some of the fundamental aspects of behavioural approaches to therapy and is designed to be read at this point by those new to the approach.

Such theories do not allow for the interjection of any kind of cognitive processes. In these models it is the response strengthening effect of the behaviour that is primary in promoting learning not the information conveyed in the event. Thorndike (1898) first describes this as the law of effect. It describes how a behavioural response is more or less likely to occur depending on whether it produces a pleasing or irritating state of affairs for the individual. The difficulty here is that what is pleasing or irritating for one individual need not be so for another individual. Reinforcement cannot be equated with reward. Thorndike argued that behaviours that elicit a pleasing response are more likely to be repeated. This is too simplistic and suggestive of a straightforward relationship in which a response that is pleasurable results in the development of a bond and hence learning. There may may be evidence for this in purely theoretical terms, but in practice it is problematic because the notion of pleasure is subjective or value laden. When we begin to look critically at this issue the waters become quite murky; what is reinforcing for one individual need not be so for another.

According to the stimulus response model the individual who is described as socially anxious will behave in a particular way because reinforcing consequences act directly and automatically to strengthen overt responses. They will therefore avoid situations that, through a process of association, have become linked with unpleasant sensations and feelings. The link between stimulus and response is direct, there is no mediating thought interpreting these events. Yet if we accept that pleasure and irritation are both subjective then the stimulus response model begins to lose its power as an explanatory model when considering complex human behaviour. What is

the explanation for why some individuals, on entering a crowded room, feel perfectly at ease, while others hover outside with their hand tentatively on the door handle summoning up the courage to sneak into the room as unobtrusively as possible? What accounts for the two quite different responses to what is apparently the same stimulus? It is possible to construct an argument that highlights a difference in individual learning history which accounts for these differences and indeed that is what some have done (Wolpe, 1982), but consideration needs to be given to a different theoretical perspective which can more readily accommodate such differences in behaviour. An approach that recognizes individual differences in behavioural response to the effects of a range of reinforcers is required. Such a model would go hand in hand with an integrated approach to therapy.

A mediational model maintains there is an interaction between the way the individual thinks, feels and behaves. The individual's observable behaviour is the result of the way the person constructs events in his or her environment. Construction occurs through a process of cognitive mediation. Cognitive mediation in learning arose from the early work of Tolman (Tolman, 1932). His experimental work with rats led him to postulate that cognitive factors are important in the development and maintenance of new behaviours. Tolman argued that internal representations of events are crucial when considering the person's behaviour. An example of this is Novaco's cognitive or mediational model of anger (Novaco, 1975). He proposes that an individual perceives events as being aversive and responds in an angry way in response to a set of assumptions. It is these assumptions that mediate between the event and their behaviour. If an individual has an expectation that an event is likely to be frustrating, threatening or insulting, this expectation will mediate between their thoughts and feeling in such a way that their behaviour will reflect their expectation. It is the information conveyed to the individual by the event that is primary in promoting learning.

If the mediation model is adopted to explain behaviour then it is possible to include a whole range of explanatory variables, including the role of expectation and anticipation. Take again an example of individuals who are fearful in social situations. These individuals are likely to report that they dread some terrible disaster befalling them when they are in a public place. For example, they will often report how they think they are likely to faint or lose control in some way and as a result make a fool of themselves in front of a crowd of people. It is their anticipation of what may happen that is critical in the maintenance of their difficulties. Their thoughts mediate between events and their behaviour or response to those events.

This relationship is illustrated in the diagram below which contrasts the traditional behavioural model in which there is no mediation between stimulus and response; with a representation of Tolman's model, in which cognitive variables intervene between the stimulus and the response:

A representative of mediational and non-mediational models for describing behaviour

S -------------------------------------- R
STIMULUS   RESPONSE
A crowded room   Walking away

S ------------------ M ------------------ R
STIMULUS   MEDIATION   RESPONSE
A crowded room   'I will   Walking away
                       lose control'

The diagram illustrates how, through a process of mediation, the behavioural response to a stimulus is formed. That response will be different across individuals but will also be different within individuals if the circumstances change.

Rotter and Hochreich (1975) refer to this intra-individual difference as the person's psychological situation. They argue that it is not enough to know details of the situation or settings in which the stimulus occurs; in addition we need to know how the person interprets the stimulus before we can make sense of the observable response. Knowing about the person's psychological situation will not effect the observable behaviour but it may help to make some sense of it and to

explain why an individual behaves in such a way. An individual's behaviour pattern will become established because over the course of events, he or she observes the differential consequences of different types of responses and through this process of observation is encouraged to engage in particular activities. Rotter and Hochreich (1975) refer to this as reinforcement value; there is here some recognition of the subjective nature of reinforcement. Taking Novaco's model and using as an example individuals who anticipate that another person is intent on threatening their security, if in the past these individuals have observed a model behaving in a particular way they are likely to respond in that same way if they consider that the model has been successful in their display of behaviour.

Although mediational models of learning appear to have more common sense appeal, it is important to consider if there is sufficient theoretical evidence for them. A major theme in psychology, particularly in response of any critique of the use of scientific and experimental methodology in the gathering of data, has centred around the nature, collection and interpretation of data. Depending on the school of psychology or the perspective adopted, what is acceptable as data varies, with alternative methods of collection and interpretation tending to be rejected and their validity denied. For some, the data of self report and introspection are not substantive and should therefore not be allowed. A radical behaviourist may consider all this talk of mediating processes as unscientific and non-sensical. Indeed Wolpe (1982) describes a cognitivist view as a demonstration of 'loose thinking'. Such a dismissive approach to alternative perspectives should be treated with caution; a critical approach is called for in respect of evidence both for and against a particular perspective. Ericsson and Simons (1981) present a detailed historical account in which they argue cogently for cognitions to be accepted as valid.

It is essential that the practitioner has a grasp of what underlies the theory of any particular therapy. It may be argued that this is particularly the case when considering cognitive behaviour therapy. For if cognitive behaviour therapy is essentially an educative process, then its aim is to enable the client to use the skills that form the basis of the therapeutic intervention by the practitioner. Without a good grasp of the underlying theory the practitioner will not be able to engage fully in this element of the therapy.

AN INTEGRATED APPROACH TO UNDERSTANDING BEHAVIOUR

Social cognitive theory combines behavioural and cognitive principles. It recognizes the importance of observational learning and self reinforcement and can be broadly considered to represent mediational models of learning. Social cognitive models that account for behaviour acknowledge both behavioural and cognitive elements of psychological theory. The behavioural elements are based on the stimulus response model for which it is possible to gather data which may be called more or less objective. Leaving aside the issue of the interpretation of that data for now, we will accept that observable behaviour offers relatively objective data. Additionally Ericsson and Simons (1981) have made a case for the data for the cognitive element to be taken seriously. This is made easier by a consideration of the human information processing model. This has become very influential in contemporary psychology. It attempts to account for all aspects of human cognition and argues that from an investigation of these elements we will gather some evidence that will advance our understanding of behaviour. There are many excellent introductory descriptions of the human information processing model (Baddeley, 1976; Reed, 1981) but for our purposes it is sufficient to have an overview of the main tenets of the model.

Cognitive processes are argued to occur as a series of events. Information from the environment passes through a series of stages before being stored into long-term memory. Given the plethora of information in the environment, some selection is necessary. This selection is proposed to take place in response to a range of processes; the selection results in the individual focusing attention and heeding particular bits of information from the surroundings. This process of selection occurs automatically and it is this that accounts for differences in the way the same event is 'seen' by two different people in two different ways. It is this difference that is the focus of cognitive behavioural therapy.

HISTORICAL BACKGROUND

It has been demonstrated that cognitive behaviour therapy has its theoretical roots in two camps—the behavioural and the cognitive approaches to therapy. The apparent differences in these two approaches have been highlighted in the preceding description of mediational and non-mediational models. Their amalgamation may seem an unlikely marriage. Several dates in the history of behaviourism are worthy of note in a consideration of why this integrated approach developed.

The seminal work of Pavlov with his description of classical conditioning was published in 1927 (Pavlov, 1927). Thorndike (1896) had described the law of effect and Watson and Rayner (1920) demonstrated the practical application of these new theories. In 1938 Skinner had published *The Behaviour of Organisms*, in which he identified the role of operant conditioning in learning. By the 1950s and 1960s these theories began to be incorporated into clinical work and to form elements of behaviour therapy. This work proliferated in the 1960s and by the 1970s operant and classical techniques of behaviour therapy had become firmly established. Behaviour therapy was the treatment of choice for a whole range of difficulties, including simple phobias and sexual dysfunction. It gained credence beyond the field of mental health and showed itself to be effective in working with people with mental handicaps (Ayllon and Azrin, 1968).

Despite seeming to be a panacea, failures in behaviour therapy started to be recognized. It became increasingly apparent that behaviour therapy, even if delivered competently, did not always achieve the success that was anticipated. Finally Foa and Emmelkamp (1983) edited a book concerned with treatment failures. This work highlighted failures across a range of difficulties including obsessions, phobias, problems of addiction, sexual dysfunction and relationship problems.

Foa and Emmelkamp (1983) identified several types of failure. These were relatively small in number and could be put under several headings: amongst these failures were inaccurate diagnosis of the problem which resulted in the inappropriate application of a treatment, inaccurate application of the selected technique, and poor generalization of the newly acquired behaviour to settings beyond the 'treatment room'. They argued that part of the difficulty is the attempted imposition of a homogeneous technology, namely behaviour therapy, upon a heterogeneous group of psychological difficulties, that is, practitioners were trying to use a standard technique to help people who have a range of difficulties, the difficulty having to fit in with available treatment, rather than the treatment being designed to fit the presenting problem.

An issue that is not explicitly dealt with relates to the permeation of cognitive elements into behaviour therapy and vice versa. Wolpe (1982) described how many cognitive therapists utilize behavioural techniques but fail to recognize their importance. Meichenbaum (1977), in describing work done by Wolpe in the area of systematic desensitization, highlights how Wolpe appears to fail to take full account of the cognitive elements in a behavioural approach to therapy. These are just two examples amongst many, of how the apparently distinct approaches of cognitive and behaviour therapy are in reality, often integrated. Blackburn and Davidson's claim that a major difference between cognitive therapy and behavioural therapy is that behavioural approaches uses behavioural techniques exclusively, whereas cognitive therapy uses both behavioural and cognitive techniques. Blackburn and Davidson (1990) demonstrate how these artificial distinctions are still influential today. It is important to identify both elements in therapy and not be wooed into thinking that behavioural techniques are somehow secondary to cognitive techniques and need not be referred to.

THE NATURE OF COGNITIVE BEHAVIOUR THERAPY

Some essential components

Cognitive behavioural therapy is problem centred, it deals with the here and now, with the current difficulties that the client is experiencing. It is undertaken in a spirit of collaboration in which the client has a central role to play, not only in the revelation of the nature of the problem, but also in the completion of the tasks which the therapeutic encounter identifies as being important. Without a commitment by the client to therapy there is unlikely to be any change in the nature of the client's difficulties. The therapy is aimed at influencing the underlying pathology which is causing the distress to the individual, the nature of this pathology relates to the way the individual interprets their world and how they behave in it. If the individual persistently thinks that events in their life happen because they are unable to influence them positively and as a result of this way of thinking about the world they withdraw from social contact, then a whole range of psychological problems may become apparent. The person may start to feel depressed, they may be anxious about social contact, they may behave aggressively when they are in anxiety-provoking situations or feel quite unable to cope with the every-day demands of living. By engaging in cognitive behavioural therapy they may be enabled to cope with these demands.

Cognitive behaviour therapy is an educational process that is concerned with identification of difficulties with the client and the development of skills to help the client deal with their difficulties in an adaptive way, that is a way in which they do not resort to behaviour that isolates them from their peers or effects their self esteem in such a way as to prevent them from engaging in ordinary school activities.

It is structured and time limited, with the client being aware of both the intended structure and format and of the expectations in respect of the time commitment. Unlike other psychotherapeutic techniques there is no 'hidden agenda' or use of paradoxical techniques (Cade, 1979). Such techniques would be contrary to the ethos in which cognitive behaviour therapy should be conducted.

As has already been highlighted, amongst the necessary basic skills which are important for carrying out cognitive behaviour therapy is an understanding of the theoretical background of the approach to therapy. Without such an understanding it would not be possible to engage in a therapeutic alliance with a client which is vital to the participation in cognitive behavioural therapy. In addition to knowing the theory behind the practice of cognitive behaviour therapy it is essential that the therapist has the necessary skills to enable the client to make the changes they identify as important to them.

Some essential skills

These skills will include those identified many times before in other texts (Rogers, 1951; Truax, 1963); they are genuineness, warmth and empathy. Rogers (1961) considers these qualities as affording the 'mainspring of change'. In addition Rogers describes 'unconditional positive regard' as central to client-centred therapy in ensuring change for the client. This could not readily be ascribed to the therapist who adopts cognitive behavioural therapy as their model for treatment. Although cognitive behaviour therapy is client centred in that it aims to address and explore issues that are identified by the client, it is more directive and challenging than Rogerian therapy. This directive element of cognitive behaviour therapy is made apparent in the goal-directed nature of cognitive behaviour therapy. In some situations it may even be described as prescriptive. During the course of cognitive behaviour therapy goals and outcome are identified, these will include aspects of behaviour or cognition which the client seeks to change. The way this change is achieved is via a process of engagement in a series of tasks that are identified in collaboration with the therapist. In order for the client to achieve these goals it will be necessary for the therapist to challenge the client and to ask them explicitly to provide evidence for constructing their world in a particular way. In challenging the client, the therapist aims to encourage change; the notion of unconditional positive

regard as described by Rogers (1961) does not rest easily with this more challenging approach. That is not to say that the role of the therapist is to disregard what the client reports or to make him feel foolish because of what he reports, clearly such behaviour would be unacceptable.

Cognitive behaviour therapy can be used for a wide range of difficulties and the literature has consistently demonstrated its comparative efficacy. It also has utility in offering inoculation against the recurrence of future difficulties. Meichenbaum has shown that by learning the techniques of cognitive behaviour therapy some individuals can be enabled to recognize and avoid situations that may cause them difficulties (Meichenbaum, 1986). It may be used when working with groups and with individuals. There is evidence for its efficacy in the treatment of children, adults, older adults and people with learning disabilities (Kendall and Branswell 1985; Lindsay, 1986; Zerhusen *et al.*, 1991; McCullough, 1991; Stern and Fernandez, 1991; Reeder, 1991).

What follows is an overview of the practice of cognitive behaviour therapy. It may read as though it were a cook book offering a quick and easy way to deal with a range of difficulties, but this is a misperception and it cannot be over emphasized that as with any therapy there must be a complete assessment. Only after the assessment processes have been embarked upon can any therapeutic intervention be considered.

Aspects of Assessment

Assessment should be the first stage of any therapeutic intervention, it should not be seen as a 'one off' but as a continuous and integral part of the therapeutic process. The material gathered during assessment will inform therapy and changes may be made in response to the findings of the evaluative aspects of assessment. The main object of the initial stages of assessment is to get a broad overview of the problem as the client perceives it, the focus of which becomes increasingly narrowed as primary difficulties are identified.

In the spirit of collaboration it is important that the therapist seeks the client's view and description of the problem. This process may highlight several difficulties which the client is currently experiencing and it may be that they have to identify which of these difficulties is a priority for them. On occasions this primary difficulty will not be what has been identified by the referring agent. This presents an early challenge to the therapist's commitment to working in collaboration and partnership with the client. Often this can be overcome and therapy can proceed using the priorities identified by the client. Occasionally, however, there may be a dilemma for the therapist. Individual clients may be referred because they are engaging in a behaviour that is potentially damaging, yet they may seek to highlight another problem as being the primary problem in their view. For example a young woman may be referred because of an eating problem that has reached such a stage as to cause concern about her physical and psychological wellbeing. However, she may consider that her tension headaches are the primary difficulty. On further questioning it may become apparent that these headaches are unrelated to the eating difficulties. She may admit to them being infrequent and unrelated to exacerbation in her eating problem. Despite this she may insist that before she can address the issue of eating she needs to overcome these tension headaches. This will present an early challenge to the therapist who must deliberate between working on the problem for which the person has been referred and working on the problem the client identifies as of primary concern. Such debates are particularly problematic when the therapist is attempting to establish a therapeutic alliance which has collaboration as a central theme.

In such cases it will be necessary to negotiate and in some cases compromise. Where there is a refusal to address a major problem, particularly one in which the client is damaging himself or herself, the therapist must question if an approach that is firmly grounded in collaboration and that requires full participation is the therapy of choice. It is these issues that should be addressed during the course of supervision. Once an agreement has been reached about which problems to tackle and in which order to tackle them, the therapist needs to elicit some infor-

mation about the nature of the problem. This will include information related to aspects of frequency, intensity, nature, duration and sense of the problem (Herbert, 1987). Using these headings as guidelines for gathering material the therapist will gain information that relates not just to the observable aspects of the problem—the behaviour—but also information related to the cognitive aspects of the problem. The client will be asked what sense they make of the problem, what they think about the problem, and also what they think about when the problem is manifest. It may be that eliciting this material is challenging for the therapist and they may have to work hard to engage the client in this process. Some clients may misunderstand the purpose of this line of questioning and may begin to take a pseudo-psychoanalytical line offering explanations related to their unconscious. Such misunderstandings offer the therapist the opportunity to educate the client both about the nature of cognitive behaviour therapy and about the proposed link between thoughts, feelings and actions.

In addition to information about the difficulties, the therapist should spend time gathering material related to the individual's living and working circumstances. This should include an exploration of who else is involved with the maintenance of the problem—would anyone benefit from the continuance of this difficulty; what are the secondary gains for the individual? If the client is being reinforced for engaging in this behaviour for which he or she now seeks help then there will be a conflict of interests which may interfere with the motivation to change. If other people do appear to be directly involved then they may need to be involved in therapy at some stage.

By the end of the first session the therapist should have gathered material related to the primary problem that the client identifies as the area where they would like to attempt change. Additionally, the therapist will have material in relation to the problem in respect of its frequency, intensity, nature, duration and the sense the individual makes of it. Material related to demographic details, to work and home life will also have been gathered. Therapists should have also taken time to describe cognitive behaviour therapy and to identify for the client what expectations they have for the therapy. Finally, therapists should close with a review of the session, including their understanding of what work is to be undertaken. They should ensure some agreement from the client that he or she is willing to participate in the therapy and have an understanding of the commitment in terms of time and effort. Cognitive behaviour therapy requires the client to make changes, many of which may provoke discomfort and anxiety, but unless the client is prepared to engage in these changes the therapy will not be successful.

Assessment tasks may be summarized as follows:

Gather material related to:

Demographic factors

Work situation

Family and social life

Nature of the identified problem
F requency
I ntensity
N ature
D uration
S ense

Give material related to:

Nature of cognitive behaviour therapy
C ollaborative
A ctive
P roblem centred
E ducational

The need for self monitoring—and how to do it

Agree an agenda

Identify the primary and secondary problems

Outline the structure and time scale for therapy

After assessment—what next?

The initial stage of assessment will highlight the problems the client wants to work on. If there are several problems it may be necessary to prioritize them and to agree, with the client, which problem should first be addressed. After this the prac-

titioner will need to select from a whole range of techniques which fall under the rubric of cognitive behaviour therapy. The techniques should be chosen to match problems that have been identified during assessment. The basis of selection will be that the essence of cognitive behaviour therapy is to challenge the assumptions and expectations that currently inform the individual's behaviour and to teach the individual a range of techniques, both behavioural and cognitive, which will enable him or her to do this. The techniques chosen will match the problem which has been identified. In making this choice the practitioner must be mindful of the complex nature of mental health difficulties and should be flexible in selection.

The techniques may be categorized under four broad headings, these are: problem-solving skills, cognitive-restructuring skills, personal-effectiveness skills and inoculation skills. Within each of these broad headings several specific skills can be identified. Some of these specific skills appear under more than one heading, the reason for this being that skills such as self instruction, self monitoring and self reinforcement have general utility and can be used to address a range of difficulties at different times.

Problem-solving deficits may be apparent in the individual's description of occasions when he or she has not known how to respond to a particular situation. Typically the situations will include interpersonal behaviour, work-related behaviour, aspects of social behaviour, financial difficulties and problems associated with actual or threatened loss. Individuals may recognize that the solutions they come up with are maladaptive; for example they may lose their temper, or they may avoid situations in which they anticipate problems may arise. Clients may describe themselves as being indecisive and unable to make a decision or to find a solution for an every-day problem; their solutions will often include resorting to maladaptive behaviour, for example binge eating or behaving aggressively.

Problem-solving deficits can be addressed using the following techniques:

Self-instructional training to identify the nature of, and possible solutions to, the problem

Self monitoring to ensure evaluation of chosen solution to the identified problem

Self-reinforcement skills

In many cases individuals experience difficulties because of the way they are interpreting events. Beck *et al.* (1979) identified errors in logic in people suffering from depression. These errors include arbitrary inferences, catastrophizing, personalization, selective abstraction and overgeneralization. They inform the person's view of the world and as a result they have a mediating effect on behaviour. Although Beck highlighted these errors in people suffering from depression similar errors have been found in other groups of people, for example those suffering from anxiety-related problems and relationship difficulties can often display similar errors in the way they interpret events (Beck and Emery, 1989). He also identified them as occurring in the healthy population; automatic thoughts need not have a negative content but they become problematic at the point at which they have a negative effect on behaviour and affect.

The crucial issue in the practice of cognitive behaviour therapy is that the practitioner assists the client in the identification of the errors of logic that they persistently engage in. These may not fit neatly into Beck's categories but it will be possible to detect a cognitive style that is effecting the way the client interprets events. For example, through a process of self monitoring, it may become apparent that clients who are fearful in social situations are consistently searching their environment for evidence to reinforce their view of themselves as being personally ineffective. They will concentrate on small and often trivial details from all the incoming material and in doing so they may misinterpret the meaning of events. This process would be analogous to Beck's description of selective abstraction. What it is called for, however, is far less important than identifying the persistent errors that inform the clients' world view and enabling them to challenge their maladaptive cognitive style in order that they can set about cognitive restructuring.

Cognitive restructuring can be achieved through the implementation of the following techniques:

Self monitoring to enable the client to identify errors of logic

Self instructional training in challenging these identified errors in logic

Education regarding the nature of the link between thoughts, feelings and behaviour

---

For many people, difficulties are manifest in their inability to assert themselves and to have their needs met, which results in a feeling of personal ineffectiveness. Personal effectiveness can be addressed using the following techniques:

Assertiveness training

Social skills training

Relaxation skills training

Self reinforcement to encourage the use of the newly acquired skills

Self monitoring to enable reassessment of personal effectiveness

Self instructional training in the use of self talk to guide the client in the use of adaptive behaviours

---

Inoculation against the reoccurrence of difficulties is an important part of cognitive behaviour therapy. This can be achieved through the proactive and continued use of a range of skills including self monitoring, self instruction and self reinforcement. The potential for inoculation highlights how cognitive behaviour therapy can be used to promote mental health as well as offering methods for coping with current difficulties.

Cognitive behaviour therapy is essentially an educative process. The role of the practitioner is to enable clients to identify and acknowledge their difficulties and to develop ways of ameliorating them. It is a process of passing on of skills and as part of this there will, of necessity, be a process of self monitoring and record keeping by the client. The purpose of the self monitoring is to provide the material for the practitioner and client to work with in order to embark upon other aspects of cognitive behaviour therapy. It is also essential in providing material with which to demonstrate the link between thoughts, feelings and behaviour. The recognition of this link is a critical first step in the whole process of cognitive behaviour therapy. In order for cognitive restructuring, personal effectiveness, problem solving and inoculation to be successful, this link must be recognized by the client. If that recognition comes through a process of self monitoring it will be more meaningful because it will be born of personal experience.

Self monitoring

Self monitoring can be achieved through various means. The principal method is through the use of some kind of diary. In order for this to have any use it is important for it to be structured. Ensuring the client uses a structured approach serves a learning function beyond the client's immediate needs and can assist in the inoculation process. If clients need to use their newly acquired skills at some point in the future they will readily recall the structure that was previously used if it has been used consistently—they will have gone through a process of over learning and the skill will become relatively automatic.

The diary need not be written—for some clients this will not even be an option if they have limited literacy skills. An alternative is for the client to use some kind of audio tape, for example, a hand-held dictaphone can be used. The content and structure of the diary will vary depending on the nature of the client's difficulties. It is also likely to vary at different stages in the therapy. The structure of the diary should allow for the recording of some specific material but this will invariably be centred on a structured analysis of the individual's difficulties.

As has already been highlighted, information related to frequency, intensity, nature, duration and sense of the problem should be obtained both during the assessment session and as an ongoing process through the diary. The diary should be structured in such a way as to access material

related to these parameters. The frequency of episodes will be readily available if a record is kept each time an episode is experienced. Obtaining this information will, therefore, be relatively straightforward.

The individual must then be enabled to record material related to the other parameters. The intensity of the difficulty needs to be defined in some way so as to make recording as objective as possible. This objectivity should only be viewed as important in terms of the individual—it is not meant to be a reliable measure that can be used across a group of people. The therapy is about individual change and as such all measures, unless they are those of standard questionnaires, relate to the individual.

In measuring intensity it may be possible to employ one of several measures—these include visual analogues or as a variation on that theme, 'bar charts' can be used (Fig. 17.1). The labelling of the points on the scale should be altered to suit the needs of each client; they should be written using the words the client uses to describe the intensity of their problem. More than three points to the scale can be used if it is thought necessary. The bar chart can be used to enable the client to give some degree of differentiation within each category. It may be that the client feels a good deal of discomfort but not enough to place him or her in the 'so bad I can't stand it' category. In this

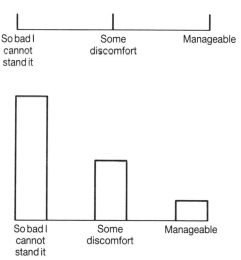

Fig. 17.1 *Two examples of methods of recording the intensity of the problem.*

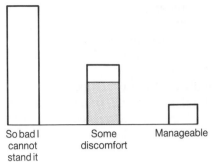

Fig. 17.2 *An example of how to introduce finer detail into the recording of intensity of the problem.*

A	Antecedents	What happened before the problem?
		What were you thinking before the problem occurred?
B	Behaviour	What did you do and what did you think?
C	Consequences	What happened as a result of your actions and what did you think?

case the person can shade the middle box to represent the level of intensity. Additionally, the height of the shading can vary according to the relative degree of intensity; in this way each category could be viewed as having an internal axis (Fig. 17.2).

It may be helpful to use a standard questionnaire to elicit detailed information about the relative intensity and nature of the individual's difficulties, for example, The Beck Anxiety Inventory (Beck, 1990) measures the severity of anxiety in adolescents and adults. It evaluates both cognitive and physiological symptoms of anxiety. It is useful in that it gives both reliable and valid information in relation to an individual's condition and in doing so augments the material gathered through self report. Such information is particularly important when writing reports in that it is objective and can be used as comparative data. Such questionnaires are commercially available.

The nature of the problem refers to what the problem is like. It is about the observable behaviour and the related cognitions. If, for example, the person is having self-control problems then the nature of the problem will be concerned with actions such as banging doors, changes in body posture and tone of voice. It will also relate to what the person is thinking about before, during and after the incident.

In order for this material to be recorded, clients should be introduced to the notion of a functional analysis. They should be given the acronym A B C as a way of recalling what it is they are to record:

These three factors give vital material about the nature of the client's difficulties. Duration will be relatively easy to record and may be included as part of the intensity recording.

The sense of the problem is concerned with the cognitive aspects of it. The cognitions associated with the problem behaviour, both those preceding and recognized as a consequence of the problem, will be recorded together with a description of what happened.

The diary should, therefore, include a visual representation of the intensity of the episode. There should be material related to the A B C of the problem giving a description of the nature and sense of the problem. Taken together this will provide the client and the practitioner with a great deal of material on which to work.

If the diary is taped then the verbal reports should be structured in the same way so that the material can be used in the therapy sessions. The diary should be used from the assessment session throughout the contact. It represents a baseline record and can be used at various stages as a way of evaluating progress and change and on the basis of this evaluation any alteration in therapy may be embarked upon.

For the diary to be effective the practitioner must give clients sufficient information to enable them to keep a record of behaviour, thoughts and feelings. Without adequate information clients may be made to feel deskilled and foolish. Some clients may even default on their appointments or withdraw because they feel unable to complete

An example of a diary entry.

Antecedent	Behaviour	Consequences
I was finishing work for the morning and was getting ready to go to lunch. I was thinking I had a great deal of work to get through that day.	I shouted persistently and aggressively at a friend on the telephone who had phoned to change an appointment.	I thought I had behaved badly but that I rushed to finish work so I could make our appointment.

the task. Behavioural techniques such as shaping and offering positive reinforcement should be used to guide clients in their early efforts at diary keeping. It is important to be sensitive to clients when asking them to complete a diary and to recognize what a difficult task it may be. It should be borne in mind that there is always a potential danger in asking clients to keep diaries; they may think that they have to record what you as the practitioner want to read, and they may think that there are 'right' answers. This good subject effect has been shown to influence the outcome of experiments performed in the psychology laboratory and it should be considered when asking individuals to keep accounts of their thoughts, feelings and behaviour (Rosenweig, 1986).

During the initial assessment session, clients should receive instruction on how to keep a diary so that by the time they return for the second interview they will have some material from which to work. This material gathered before this second session will act as a baseline because it will have been gathered before any therapeutic intervention has begun. Over the course of time, as the therapy progresses, the client will need to keep a diary which is focused on the cognitive aspects of their problem. This diary can be kept in the same way as the A B C diary but increasingly more material related to cognition will be required. There are many examples of the various ways that thought diaries can be kept (Blackburn, 1987; Kirk, 1989; Stern and Drummond, 1991).

Self regulation through self instruction

Amongst the techniques employed by the practitioner while working on the client's problems as demonstrated through diary entries is self instruc-tion. Self-instructional training occupies a central role in cognitive behaviour therapy. It is a broad term which describes a technique in which the individual is trained to talk to themselves in a way that decreases their maladaptive behaviour and increases their adaptive behaviour. Meichenbaum (1977) refers to this as learning to engage in 'healthy talk'. It is the basic technique which is elaborated in other aspects of cognitive behaviour therapy; for example the process of cognitive restructuring, challenging negative assumptions and engaging in self reinforcement all take place via self talk.

Bandura (1969) argued that self regulation is especially important in cases where change is attempted on a behaviour that is maladaptive but reinforcing for the client. If the newly acquired adaptive behaviour is practised in an environment in which there is only weak reinforcement then change is unlikely to occur. An example of such behaviours could be the individual who engages in obsessive behaviours 'behind closed doors', in such a way as to make reinforcement from the environment limited. For example, a client may report how, before they can leave their home, they feel compelled to engage in rituals. These rituals may include obsessively washing, checking doors and windows, dressing and redressing. The person who engages in such behaviour gets very little obvious positive reinforcement for engaging in such behaviour. They will describe a feeling of relief of anxiety if they do engage in the ritual but will often be able to keep their problem hidden away from significant others who potentially can provide feedback to them. The practice of self regulation and self reinforcement is particularly important in such cases. Other examples may be the person who suffers with bulimia but hides it from the people around them, or the person who is dependent on alcohol.

It should not be assumed, however, that self regulation via self instruction only has utility with difficulties that are somehow hidden from those around the client. Self instruction has been demonstrated to be effective in enabling generalization of change (Meichenbaum, 1977). Generalization refers to the process whereby skills that are acquired in one specific area can be used to guide and inform behaviour in another situation. This is particularly important when considering complex and pervasive mental health difficulties. Examples include individuals who suffer with social anxiety which pervades a whole range of situations and the client who has a pervasive depression that is not reactive to any particular situation. These clients will need to be enabled to use skills across a range of situations. They will benefit from being taught skills which have demonstrable advantages in that they generalize more readily.

The issue of generalization has been closely studied during investigations into methods of behaviour change with people with learning disabilities. This group of people presents the practitioner with major difficulties in ensuring the maintenance and generalization of newly acquired skills. There is a great deal of evidence to demonstrate that training people with learning disabilities to use self-instructional techniques overcomes problems of maintenance and generalization (Whitman *et al.*, 1987). The importance of these findings is not only in highlighting the utility of self-instructional training, but also to demonstrate that as a therapeutic technique self-instructional training need not be limited to individuals who have well-developed verbal skills. Indeed Meichenbaum has proven the utility of self-instructional training with a group of people with schizophrenia (Meichenbaum, 1969). However, as with any technique, practitioners should not be seduced into the assumption that the approach they favour will work for every individual and although the weight of evidence is such that it suggests self-instructional training has broad utility there are examples of treatment failures (Oei *et al.*, 1991).

Self-instructional techniques are based on the experimental work of the Soviet psychologists Luria and Vygotsky (Luria, 1961; Vygotsky, 1962). They demonstrated verbal control over motoric behaviour, arguing that internal dialogue influences behaviour. Self-instruction techniques exploit this proposed relationship, providing the individual with a dialogue which will effect behaviour in such a way as to ensure positive outcomes. By altering the content of the internal dialogue the client can influence not only behaviour but also affect. This is the central element of cognitive behaviour therapy. Beck (1976), in identifying errors in logic that are apparent as automatic thoughts, simply uses different terminology in describing what is essentially internal dialogue. He outlined the therapeutic process concerned with challenging these automatic thoughts and in doing so utilized many aspects of the model of self-instructional training. The terminology may be different but the principles are the same—the object of the cognitive element of cognitive behaviour therapy is, through a process of self regulation, to monitor and influence an individual's internal dialogue in such a way as to ensure adaptive behaviour takes place rather than maladaptive behaviour.

The details of self regulation may vary but the principles remain constant. They can be usefully thought of as a series of stages in which clients learn to recognize the link between their internal dialogue and their behaviour. This is followed by a challenge to the dialogue and replacing it with adaptive self talk. This finally enables the clients to influence their own behaviour.

In order to create this change in behaviour and affect, the client must first be enabled to recognize the link between thoughts and feelings and behaviour. It is not enough for the practitioner to simply tell the client that this link exists, nor is it sufficient to cite the research evidence. Although both of these are important, the client needs to experience the link. This can be achieved through encouraging clients to monitor their thoughts, feelings and behaviour and to record their findings in a diary. The structure and function of a diary has been described above. The purpose initially is to highlight this link so that the client can make sense of the therapy.

The early stages of self monitoring help to sensitize the clients to their internal dialogue. For many this will come as an important revelation, for some it will be something akin to a religious conversion experience in which they suddenly recognize the power they have to influence their own behaviour. For others it will merely confirm what they had suspected. Importantly for many clients it will legitimate a process that they have already engaged in, that is, trying to talk themselves into a positive frame of mind in order to influence their behaviour.

Once clients have begun to make the link between internal dialogue and behaviour then they need to go through a process of challenging and restructuring their cognitive style. They should be encouraged to do this through a process of self talk, during which they recognize the negative self talk, challenge its underlying assumptions and substitute positive self talk.

A course of cognitive behaviour therapy will last a variable length of time depending on a number of factors, for example the nature of the problem, the frequency of contacts, and the opportunities available to clients to practise their newly acquired skills. During the course of therapy the client and the practitioner should continue to work in a collaborative way in an effort to overcome the difficulties identified by the client. If the initial assessment and formulation of the problem is accurate then the practitioner should be confident that cognitive behaviour therapy will assist clients in overcoming their difficulties and in addition it will help them to avoid similar difficulties in the future.

FURTHER READING

Beck, A.T. (1976) *Cognitive Therapy and the Emotional Disorders*. New York: Meridian.

Blackburn, I.M. & Davidson, K. (1990) *Cognitive Therapy for Depression*. Oxford: Blackwell Scientific.

Dryden, W. & Golden, W.L. (1986) *Cognitive-behavioural Approaches to Psychotherapy*. London: Harper & Row.

Hawton, K., Salkowskis, P., Kirk, J. & Clark, D. (1989) *Cognitive Behaviour Therapy for Psychiatric Problems. A Practical Guide*. New York: Oxford University Press.

Meichenbaum, D. (1979) *Cognitive-behaviour Modification. An Integrative Approach*. New York: Plenum.

REFERENCES

Ayllon, T. & Azrin, N. (1968) *The Token Economy: A Motivational System for Therapy and Rehabilitation*. New York: Appleton-Century-Croft.

Baddeley, A. (1976) *The Psychology of Memory*. New York: Harper Row.

Bandura, A. (1969) *Principles of Behaviour Modification*. New York: Holt Reinhart Winston.

Beck, A.T. (1976) *Cognitive Therapy and the Emotional Disorders*. New York: Meridian.

Beck, A.T. (1989) *Cognitive Therapy and the Emotional Disorders*, 2nd end. New York: International University Press.

Beck, A.T. & Emery, G. (1989) *Anxiety Disorders and Phobias: a Cognitive Perspective*. New York: Basic Books.

Beck, A.T. (1990) *The Beck Anxiety Inventory*. Sidcup: The Psychological Corporation.

Beck, A.T., Rush, J.A., Shaw, B.F. & Emery, G. (1979) *Cognitive Therapy for Depression*. New York: Guildford Press.

Biram, M. & Wilson, G.T. (1981) Treatment of phobic disorders using cognitive and exposure methods: A self-efficacy analysis. *Journal of Consulting and Clinical Psychology*, **49**, 886.

Blackburn, I.M. (1987) *Coping with Depression*. Edinburgh: Chambers.

Blackburn, I.M. & Davidson, K. (1990) *Cognitive Therapy for Depression*. Oxford: Blackwell Scientific.

Cade, B. (1979) The use of paradox in therapy. In Walrond, I. & Skinner, R. (ed.) *Family and Marital Psychotherapy: A Critical Approach*. London: Routledge & Kegan Paul.

Dryden, W. & Golden, W.L. (1986) *Cognitive–Behavioural Approaches to Psychotherapy*. London: Harper & Row.

Ericsson, K.A. & Simons, H.A. (1981) Sources of evidence on cognition: An historical overview. In Merluzzi, T.V., Glass C.R. & Genest, M. (Eds) *Cognitive Assessment*. New York: Guildford Press.

Foa, E. & Emmelkamp, P. (1983) *Failures in Behaviour Therapy*. New York: Wiley.

Foa, E., Rothbaum, B.O. & Murdoch, T.B. (1991) Treatment of post traumatic stress disorder in rape victims: a comparison between cognitive–behavioural procedures and counselling. *Journal of Consulting and Clinical Psychology*, **59** (5), 715.

Hawton, K., Salkovskis, P., Kirk, J. & Clark, D. (1989) *Cognitive Behaviour Therapy for Psychiatric Problems. A Practical Guide.* New York: Oxford University Press.

Herbert, M. (1987) *Behaviour Treatment of Children with Problems: A Practice Manual.* London: Academic Press.

Kendall, P.C. & Braswell, L. (1985) *Cognitive–Behaviour Therapy for Impulsive Children.* New York: Guildford Press.

Kirk, J. (1989) Cognitive–behavioural assessment. In Hawton, K., Salkovskis, P., Kirk, J. & Clarke, D. (Eds) *Cognitive Behaviour Therapy for Psychiatric Problems: A Practical Guide.* New York: Oxford University Press.

Lindsay, W.R. (1986) Cognitive changes after social skills training with young mildly handicapped adults. *Journal of Mental Deficiency Research.* **30**, 81.

Luria, A. (1961) *The Role of Speech in the Regulation of Normal and Abnormal Behaviours.* New York: Liveright.

McCullough, J.P. (1991) Psychotherapy for dysthymia. A naturalistic study of ten patients. *Journal of Nervous and Mental Disease,* **179** (12), 734.

Meichenbaum, D. (1969) The effects of instructions and reinforcement on thinking and language behaviours of schizophrenics. *Behaviour Research and Therapy,* **7**, 101.

Meichenbaum, D. (1977) *Cognitive–behaviour modification. An Integrative Approach.* New York: Plenum.

Meichenbaum, D. (1986) *Stress Inoculation Training.* New York: Pergamon.

Meichenbaum, D. & Goodman, J. (1971) Training impulsive children to talk to themselves: A means of developing self control. *Journal of Abnormal Psychology,* **77**, 115.

Morse, C.A., Dennerstein, L., Farrell E. & Varnavides, K. (1991) A comparison of hormone therapy, coping skills training, and relaxation for the relief of premenstrual syndrome. *Journal of Behavioural Medicine,* **14** (5), 469.

Novaco, R. (1975) *Anger Control: the Development and Evaluation of an Experimental Treatment.* Lexington: Heath & Company.

Oei, T.P., Lim, B. & Young, R. (1991) Cognitive processes and cognitive behaviour therapy in the treatment of problem drinking. *Journal of Addictive Disorders,* **10** (3), 63.

Pavlov, I. (1927) *Conditioned Reflexes.* New York: Oxford University Press.

Reed, S.K. (1981) *Cognition: Theory and Application.* Monterey: Brooks Cole.

Reeder, D.M. (1991) Cognitive therapy of anger management: theoretical and practical considerations. *Archives of Psychiatric Nursing,* **5** (3), 147.

Rogers, C.R. (1951) Client-centred Therapy: Its Current Practice, Implications and Theory. Boston: Houghton Mifflin.

Rogers, C.R. (1961) *On Becoming a Person: A Therapist View of Psychotherapy.* London: Constable.

Rosenzwig, R. (1986) *Freud and Experimental Psychology: The Emergence of Idiodynamics.* New York: Academic Press.

Rotter, J.B. & Hochreich, D.J. (1975) *Personality.* Glenorew: Scott Foreshaw.

Rush, A.J., Beck, A.T., Kovacs, M. & Hollon, S.D. (1977) Comparative efficacy of cognitive therapy and pharmacotherapy in the treatment of depressed outpatients. *Cognitive Therapy and Research,* **1**, 17.

Skinner, B.F. (1938) *The Behaviour of Organisms.* Englewood Cliffs. Prentice Hall.

Skinner, B.F. (1953) *Science and Human Behaviour.* New York: Macmillan.

Stern, R. & Drummond, L. (1991) *The Practice of Behavioural and Cognitive Psychotherapy.* Cambridge: Cambridge University Press.

Stern, R. & Fernandez, M. (1991) Group cognitive and behavioural treatment for hypochondriasis. *British Medical Journal,* **303**, 1229.

Thorndike, E.L. (1898) Animal intelligence: an experimental study of associative processes in animals. *Psychological Monographs,* **2**, 223.

Tolman, E.C. (1932) *Purposive Behaviour in Animals and Men.* New York: Appleton.

Truax, C.B. (1963) Effective ingredients in psychotherapy: An approach to unravelling the patient–therapist interaction. *Journal of Counselling Psychology,* **10**, 256.

Vygotsky, L. (1962) *Thought and Language.* New York: Wiley.

Watson, J.B. & Rayner, R. (1920) Conditioned emotional responses. *Journal of Experimental Psychology,* **3**, 1.

Whitman, T., Spence, B.H. & Maxwell, S. (1987) A comparison of external and self instructional teaching formats with mentally retarded adults in vocational settings. *Applied Research in Developmental Disabilities,* **8**, 371.

Wolpe, J. (1982) *The Practice of Behaviour Therapy,* 3rd edn. New York: Pergamon.

Zerhusen, D., Boyle, J. & Wilson, W. (1991) Out of darkness: group cognitive therapy for depressed elderly. *Journal of Psychosocial Nursing and Mental Health Services,* **29** (9), 16.

BEHAVIOURAL ASPECTS OF THERAPY

Sue Marshall

AIMS

i) To provide a brief overview of fundamental aspects of behavioural approaches to therapy
ii) To serve as an introduction to Chapter 17 on cognitive behaviour therapy

KEY ISSUES

Origins of the behavioural approach
Classical conditioning
Operant conditioning
Reinforcement
Behavioural programmes

Identify, analyse and assess factors causing distress and illness	Promote health, provide direct care and make interventions	Manage care programmes and services
Be critical, analytical and accountable, continue professional development	Counter discrimination, inequality and individual and institutional racism	Work within and develop policies, laws and safeguards in all settings
Understand influences on mental health and the nature/causes of disorder and illness	Know the effects of distress, disorder, illness on individuals, groups, families	Understand the basis of treatments and interventions

Before an individual can consider using cognitive behavioural therapy he or she must have a working knowledge of both behavioural and cognitive elements in therapy. The major thrust of this appendix is to give a relatively detailed account of how used together, these two approaches to therapy can offer a powerful tool in enabling some people with mental health difficulties to overcome their problems successfully. What follows is a brief overview of some of the fundamental aspects of behavioural approaches to therapy, it is given in order that the worker may be made aware of the complexity of using a behavioural approach in therapy and not consider it an easy option when working with people with mental health problems.

Behavioural approaches to therapy are based on the laboratory work of Pavlov (1927) and Skinner (1953). They are concerned with observable events and assessment of behaviour is made by considering only what can be observed. Radical behavioural approaches take no account of unconscious desires, or of individuals' thoughts and feelings about what is going on around them. The focus of this appendix is to suggest that such radical approaches should be replaced by integrated therapy which takes account of the individuals' thoughts about their difficulties. Integrated approaches do, however, use techniques that originated in the seminal work of the early behaviourist and it is important to recognize these origins.

Pavlov identified a process of learning based on reinforcement. What he described as classical conditioning demonstrated that through a process of association it is possible to establish a link between events that would under other circumstances be quite unconnected. Pavlov established such a link between the sound of a bell and salivation as a physiological response in preparation for food. This link was established by presenting food to a dog immediately after ringing a bell. Over a period of time and a number of such events the dog learned to associate the sound of the bell with the presentation of food. Once the association had been learned by the dog the sound of the bell alone would be sufficient to elicit salivation. This response would continue for a certain period of time but in the continued ab-

sence of the presentation of the food then the salivation response would eventually disappear.

A whole set of terminology has developed around conditioning. This terminology is used to describe the various elements that are necessary for classical conditioning to occur. In the example given above the conditioned stimulus is the bell, the unconditioned stimulus is the food and the conditioned response is salivation on presentation of the bell.

For classical conditioning to be possible there are several conditions that must be met, one of which is that there must be temporal contiguity between the stimulus to be conditioned and the unconditioned stimulus. This means that the sound of the bell must be followed almost immediately by the presentation of food. If this does not happen then the link will not be formed.

The role of classical conditioning in mental health difficulties is not clearly identified. It has been argued that classical conditioning is an element in the development of phobias (Eysenk and Rachman, 1961), although this is not entirely clear and other workers would argue that the process involved in the development of phobias is a more complex matter involving processes other than classical conditioning.

Operant conditioning offers more in terms of both an explanatory framework and a therapeutic tool when working with people with mental health difficulties. Operant conditioning was first described by Skinner (Skinner, 1953).

Within the field of mental health, behavioural techniques that rely on aspects of both operant and classical conditioning can be used to enable people to cope with a whole range of difficulties. Assessment forms a crucial aspect of such work and focuses on identifying the function of an individual's behaviour and what is responsible for maintaining the maladaptive behaviour. To complete an assessment can be a lengthy and complex process, the nature of which is the subject of other texts. Only some aspects of the process can be covered here.

Much of Skinner's early work was done with animals (Skinner, 1953). Through his experimental laboratory work he identified that actions in animals could be learned because of the effect those actions have on the environment. He found that if an animal is reinforced for an action it performs, then there is an increased probability of the action being performed again. Skinner went on to identify various 'schedules of reinforcement'. These have particular importance for workers using behavioural techniques therapeutically. He discovered that if reinforcement is offered intermittently then the strength of the learned association between an action and the response elicited by that action is greater than if reinforcement is offered each time the behaviour is performed. Therefore the link is more difficult to break than if reinforcement has been offered on each occasion that the behaviour has been performed. In practical terms this means that when behavioural programmes are designed the role of intermittent reinforcement has to be carefully considered during the assessment phase of work. The aim of many programmes will be to decrease the frequency of an identified target behaviour and to increase the frequency of the adaptive behaviour using a system of offering positive reinforcement for exhibition of the adaptive behaviour and offering nothing for the maladaptive behaviour. Under such conditions if the individual is able to elicit some positive reinforcement for engaging in the maladaptive behaviour intermittently, then the outcome of the programme may be unpredictable. This source of reinforcement may be difficult to control and has a potential for undermining what may otherwise be an adequate behavioural programme.

An example of the role of intermittent reinforcement may be the case of an individual who is depressed and as a result of this is not doing very much. This person may be passive and withdrawn and as part of treatment could be started on a behavioural programme aimed at increasing level of engagement in those activities that have been previously identified as adaptive. The success of this programme depends on many things, one of which is the absence of intermittent reinforcement for relative inactivity. If, therefore, a neighbour intermittently offers to take on the responsibility for doing the shopping, because the person is not feeling well, then this may be sufficient to prolong that individual's difficulty and in doing so may undermine the programme.

Within an institutional setting the potential sources for intermittent reinforcement are legion and need to be carefully considered and identified before any programme is embarked upon. Intermittent reinforcement can, however, establish strong links when used therapeutically—it need not always be something that creates difficulties for the practitioner.

This issue of potential for intermittent reinforcement highlights a whole range of important aspects of using behavioural approaches when working with individuals, with consistency in approach being amongst them. In order for behavioural techniques to be used effectively to describe maladaptive behaviours and to increase adaptive behaviours a programme must be written in such a way that it can be applied consistently. Without consistency in the delivery of reinforcement there will be limited potential for developing the link between a stimulus and a response. If it has been identified that a target behaviour should be responded to in a particular way then that should be the case invariably or intermittently if that is the requirement of the programme. A programme should specify under what circumstances a reinforcer should be delivered. These circumstances may change as the programme is evaluated and reviewed.

When designing a behavioural programme it is important to give consideration to the nature of the reinforcement that is being offered and to embark upon a process of surveying potential reinforcers. This can be done in a variety of ways, the most obvious being by simply asking the individual what they enjoy doing, who they like doing things with, and under what circumstances they find various activities pleasurable. It is essential that consideration be given to who will be delivering the reinforcer because this may effect its potential power. If, for example, we enjoy walking with a particular member of our family or a friend then the attention that we are receiving from that individual during the walk will be a variable in making the activity reinforcing. On the other hand, if we are given the opportunity of engaging in the same activity with another person then that element of the activity is changed and the reinforcement value of the activity may be significantly altered. Where it is not possible to get the information from the individual then the practitioner will need to conduct a reinforcement survey. This may be the case when working with someone who is depressed or who has long-standing mental illness that has resulted in the person being withdrawn and passive. A reinforcement survey is a process whereby a sample of potential reinforcers is presented to the individual and an assessment of their relative value is made based on the person's reaction to them. The reinforcers are not all presented at the same time, but over a period of time and over a number of trials. The hypothesis would be that individuals respond favourably to those reinforcers they rate most highly. They would be offered access to the reinforcer for engaging in a target behaviour. Their engagement or otherwise would serve as an indication of the value they attach to a particular reinforcer. It may, of course, also be possible and less time consuming to gather this information from someone who knows the person well.

The recognition of the role of the deliverer of the reinforcer has been illustrated by work examining the role of the various elements of token economy system (Ayllon and Azrin, 1968). A token economy is a method of structuring an environment in order to reinforce individuals for engaging in identified target behaviour. It has been used with people suffering with long-term mental health difficulties who, as a result of these difficulties, have lost some skills in performing activities of daily living, for example they may have stopped taking care of their personal hygiene. In such a case the target behaviour may be washing or cleaning teeth. The individual would be reinforced for engaging in the target behaviour. The reinforcer would be a token which could be exchanged at a later time for a range of other things. Each target behaviour would have a value given to it and each token would represent a particular value. At face value it would appear that the success of a token economy is based on the individual acquiring tokens to be exchanged for other objects, usually consumable. However, recent work has demonstrated that the efficacy of token economy is based on the social interaction that takes place during the handing over of the tokens. The most powerful aspects of token economy are suggested to be the feedback, guidance and social contact that indi-

viduals get as a result of the system (Falloon *et al.*, 1984; Hall and Baker, 1986). These are important findings because they demonstrate that behavioural techniques can be effective by simply using existing human resources and further more that the nature of relationships within an environment can have a demonstrable effect on the behaviour of individuals.

This has implications not only for the use of behaviour therapy as an intervention but also as a proactive or health-promoting technique. If individuals are offered reinforcement in their daily lives then it influences their ability to respond to their environment. In the absence of reinforcement, it has been argued that the individuals are at risk from developing learned helplessness—a state which some workers identify with depression (Brown and Harris, 1978; Seligman, 1973). Negative reinforcement refers to a situation where, if a desired behaviour is demonstrated, an unpleasant stimulus is removed.

Negative reinforcement has been particularly associated with learned helplessness. Seligman (Seligman, 1973) has argued that learned helplessness is a common feature of depression. It arises from individuals' persistent inability to avoid unpleasant events. Negative reinforcement is not accessible to them from their environment. Over time they give up trying to elicit reinforcement from their surrounding. This leads to a person who is apathetic, passive and withdrawn. In a situation where the person had been given reinforcing feedback from their environment then, Seligman argues, they would be less likely to develop learned helplessness. They would be better able to elicit reinforcement from their environment.

The manipulation of the environment is a crucial element of behavioural work. This is a relatively new development in the therapeutic use of behavioural theories although the early laboratory work of Skinner clearly showed how by manipulating the environment the experimenter could observe different responses from the individuals. Traditionally, workers have considered the consequences of events as being of primary importance (Lyttle, 1986), and have paid little attention to the antecedents of the behaviour. This preoccupation can result in a narrow focus for behaviour therapy and the potential to blame the individuals for their own difficulties. If a practitioner is working with someone who persistently behaves in a particular way and that assessment of the behaviour focuses on the results or consequences of the behaviour, then material related to what may have prompted the behaviour will not be available during the assessment and analysis stage of the intervention. The setting events may not be considered and aspects of the environment may go unconsidered. It could be that individuals are engaging in behaviour that is entirely adaptive given the circumstances in which they live. An example might be individuals who are misusing drugs. They could be responding to a set of circumstances which are causing them distress. The only strategy available to them may be to misuse drugs. Similarly, self control and anger management problems will be assessed as the result of some individual difficulties. The outcome of an assessment which concerns itself entirely with the individual will inevitably identify the source of the difficulties as being located within the individual. An assessment that takes account of the setting events has the potential for recognizing the role of the environment in effecting and promoting maladaptive behaviours which may become part of a mental health problem.

Setting events and cues to behaviour can be manipulated and offers a rich source of interventions for the worker. Take as an example an individual who describes suffering from panic attacks which affect his or her capacity to do every-day things like go to the shops. When assessing the individual's needs it will be important to identify exactly what happens before, during, and after the panic attack. This will be done by using the procedures of functional assessment, that is, making an assessment of antecedents and consequences of the behaviour as well as gathering detailed information about what happens during the panic attack. Information related to the antecedents will yield information about the setting events of the behaviour, for example the individual may describe the preparation for going out on the shopping trip. The preparation may be elaborate and include a whole range of behaviours which make the person feel secure and safe and able to go out. It may be that these preparations

merely serve to heighten anxiety and in fact increase the probability of a panic attack. By manipulating these preparatory routines it may be possible to enable the person to go out without having to rely on these props, thereby increasing feelings of personal control and also to reduce the anticipatory anxiety which the person experiences and which may translate into a panic attack.

There may be occasions when the setting events for a particular behaviour may not be clear. There is increasingly a recognition that antecedents may be both proximal and distal. This means that a behaviour may be prompted by events that are closely linked in terms of time, that is, proximal. Other behaviours may be prompted by events that are more distant in time, that is, distal. In the case of distal antecedents it may be difficult to use a strictly behavioural approach in assessment of the person's behaviour and it would be appropriate to consider additional elements in the assessment process, for example cognitive aspects of the behaviour.

REFERENCES

Ayllon, T. & Azrin, N. (1968) *The Token Economy: A Motivational System for Therapy and Rehabilitation.* New York: Appleton-Century-Croft.

Brown, G.W. & Harris, T. (1978) *Social Origins of Depression. A Study of Psychiatric Disorder in Women.* London: Tavistock.

Eysenck, H.J. & Rachman, S. (1961) *The Causes and Cures of Neurosis.* London: Routledge & Kegan Paul.

Falloon, L.R., Boyd, J.L. & McGill, C.W. (1984) *Family Care of Schizophrenia.* New York: Guildford.

Fao, E.B., Rothbaum, B.O. & Murdock, T.B. (1991) Treatment of part traumatic stress disorder in rape victims. A comparison between cognitive-behavioural procedures and counselling. *Journal of Consulting and Clinical Psychology*, **59** (5), 715.

Hall, J.N. & Baker, R.D. (1986) Token economies and schizophrenia: a review. In Kerr, A. & Snaith, R.P. (Eds). *Contemporary Issues in Schizophrenia.* London: Gaskell.

Lyttle, J. (1986) *Mental Health and Disorder.* London: Baillière Tindall.

Pavlov, I. (1927) *Conditioned Reflexes.* New York: Oxford University Press.

Reber, A.S. (1987) *The Penguin Dictionary of Psychology*. Harmondsworth: Penguin Books.

Salkovskis, P.M. & Warwick. H.M.C. (1986) Morbid preoccupation, health anxiety and reassurance: a cognitive behavioural approach to hypochondriasis. *Behavioural Research and Therapy*, **24**, 597–602.

Seligman, M.E. (1973) *Helplessness*. New York: Freeman.

Skinner, B.F. (1953) *Science and Human Behaviour*. New York: Macmillan.

SPIRITUAL CARE AND MENTAL HEALTH COMPETENCE

Aru Narayanasamy

AIMS

i) To offer clarification of the meaning of spirituality
ii) To identify the competence required in the provision of spiritual care
iii) To examine the implications for nursing

KEY ISSUES

Mental health and spirituality
Spiritual wellbeing
Spiritual needs
Competences for spiritual care
Putting competence into action through the nursing process

Identify, analyse and assess factors causing distress and illness	Promote health, provide direct care and make interventions	Manage care programmes and services
Be critical, analytical and accountable, continue professional development	Counter discrimination, inequality and individual and institutional racism	Work within and develop policies, laws and safeguards in all settings
Understand influences on mental health and the nature/causes of disorder and illness	Know the effects of distress, disorder, illness on individuals, groups, families	Understand the basis of treatments and interventions

INTRODUCTION

In mental health care a focus on individuals as psychosocial–spiritual beings is gaining recognition, but there is little elaboration on what is meant by spirit. This problem is further compounded by the misuse of the term 'spirituality' in that this word is equated to, or is applied synonymously with, institutional religion. Institutional religions usually refer to Protestantism, Catholicism and Judaism. At the beginning of this chapter the ambiguity concerning spirituality is addressed by clarifying what it really means. Following this and the identification of clients' spiritual needs, readers are introduced to competences required for spiritual care in context of mental health care. In the final section competences of spiritual care are put into action through the nursing process. Several case history scenarios are provided to illuminate understanding through activity-related work.

Spiritual beliefs and practices permeate the life of a person, whether in health or illness. Certain spiritual needs tend to feature during our personal development and growth. The influence of spirituality and religion is commonly seen in the following aspects of a person's life: relationships with others, living style and habits, required and prohibited behaviours, and the general frame of reference for thinking about oneself and the world. Our spirituality features during our development and growth.

WHAT IS SPIRITUALITY?

There is no single authoritative definition of spirituality although a variety of explanations is offered in the emerging literature on this subject. When we talk about holistic approach we mean care for the body, mind and spirit. Holistic care is a popular theme, at least, from a theoretical angle but spirituality as an aspect of nursing care is scarce. We need to understand the concept of spirituality if we are going to offer it as a component of holistic care.

Although there is an overlap between spirituality and other subject disciplines (psychology, sociology, politics and so on), it should be seen as a discipline with developing schools of theories. You will find that religious needs and spirituality are closely connected and sometimes one finds it is difficult to make the distinction between them as one need affects the other.

If you try to think about spirituality for a few minutes, several concepts may arise in your mind:

A belief in God

A belief affecting your life and how it relates to others

Something not necessarily religious

A belief/concept; purpose and meaning

Faith/peace with oneself; a source of strength

Feeling of security/to be loved

Philosophy of life/death/religion

Self esteem/inner self, inner strength

Searching/coping; hope

An idealism, a striving to be good; a trusting relationship

History suggests that since the beginning of humanity, spirituality has always predominated our lives in some way or another. Spirituality is one of the fashionable words in nursing, yet like so many useful and comprehensive terms, it is not easy to define. Spirituality is defined as:

A quality that goes beyond religious affiliation, that strives for inspirations, reverence, awe, meaning and purpose, even in those who do not believe in any god. The spiritual dimension tries to be in harmony with the universe, strives for answers about the infinite, and comes into focus when the person faces emotional stress, physical illness or death.'
Murray and Zentner, 1989

Spirituality equally applies to the needs of believers and non-believers and in contexts where religious beliefs may be varied. It is not uncommon for individuals with no religious allegiance to be able to relate to some spiritual or natural force beyond the physical and self.

Spirituality is seen as an inner thing that is central to the person's being and one that makes a person unique and 'tick over' as an individual. For example, I see it as my being; my inner person. It is who I am—unique and alive. It is expressed through my body, my thinking, my feelings, my judgements and my creativity. My spirituality motivates me to choose meaningful relationships and pursuits. Sometimes we desire for personal quest for meaning and purpose in life; a sense of harmonious relationship (interconnectedness) with self and others, nature, an ultimate other, and other factors which are necessary for our integrity. I would like to illustrate the points that I am making about spirituality in the case of Elsie below:

Elsie looks after her elderly mother who is suffering from senile dementia. She feels that it is her duty to care for her mother who is totally dependent on her. Elsie frequently says to the community psychiatric nurse (CPN) that it has not always been an easy task, but she learnt a lot in the last 10 years, through caring for her mother, she has become more appreciative of the beauty and joy in life. Elsie sees each day as new opportunity to learn and grow. The CPN feels that in Elsie's presence one experiences a sense of peace and who, even in the midst of difficult and trying circumstance, affirms that life is good. Elsie says that she has done some soul-searching over the last 10 years and has come to know herself pretty well. She states to the CPN that when she felt low, she learned to 'go inside myself' and always finds guidance there and achieves a sense of relief and comfort. She also adds that she maintains close relationship with family and friends, with whom she shares love and support. Elsie is a keen gardener and when in her garden she feels close to the earth and to the Creator.

Adapted from Narayanasamy, 1991, p.4

Several of the elements of spirituality can be illustrated in the case of Elsie:

Unfolding mystery—though life's 'ups and downs' and what could be viewed as a burden, she has found meaning as peace and joy.

Inner strength—she has developed a great sense of self awareness, which she has gained by going inside herself (a process also known as introspection) for guidance.

Harmonious interconnectedness—she has loving, supporting relationships with family and friends, a sense of knowing herself.

Source of strength and hope—the garden has become a place where she is able to express a feeling of closeness to nature and to the Creator.

It appears that spirituality is essential to our well-being and is the essence of our existence. It has to do with both solitude and corporate life including the way we think, act and feel in everyday life. In essence, we can now see that it influences the whole of our lives.

Furthermore, through spirituality we give and receive love. One responds to appreciate God, other people, a sunset, a symphony, and spring. Many of us keep our spirits up in spite of adversity and it may well be because something motivates us to do so. This is because of our spirituality. Elsie's situation is a good example of spirituality as it keeps her going in spite of all the odds. We are driven forward, sometimes because of pain, sometimes in spite of pain. Spirituality permits a person to function, motivated and enabled to value, to worship, and to communicate with the holy, the transcendent.

Transcendence is a need as part of our personhood just as is the physiological or psychological. If we take this view, then we as nurses must regard all individuals as spiritual beings and not as a body with just physiological and psychological needs.

SPIRITUAL WELLBEING

Let us now turn our attention to the concept of spiritual wellbeing. Spiritual wellbeing is an important facet of health and is considered as affirmation of our relationship with God/transcendent, self, community and environment that nurtures and keeps us as an integrated whole person. The following are features of our spiritual well-being:

The belief in God that is fostered through communication with Supreme Being

Expression of love, concern, and forgiveness for others

Giving and accepting help

Accepting and valuing self

Expressing life satisfaction

Furthermore, our spiritual wellbeing is usually demonstrated by our ability to find meaning and purpose in present life situations and to search for meaning and purpose in the future. We can attain spiritual wellbeing through a dynamic and integrative growth process which leads to a realization of the ultimate purpose and meaning in life.

MODEL FOR SPIRITUALITY

Several theorists propose that the whole person consists of body, mind and spirit, which are inseparable. Stallwood (1981) developed a conceptual model to illustrate this interrelationship (Fig. 18.1). The outermost circle represents the biological nature of an individual; the middle circle depicts the mind as having four separate components—will, emotion, intellect and moral sense; the smallest, innermost circle represents the spiritual nature. Alteration to any of the three components affects the two other components, and ultimately, the whole person.

Unlike Stallwood, Gorham (1989) suggests a five-component person model. According to this model, a person is made up of five different aspects—the mental, physical, social, emotional, and spiritual. The interaction is so closely related that they are almost inseparable. The spiritual is the most difficult one to be recognized. The inter-

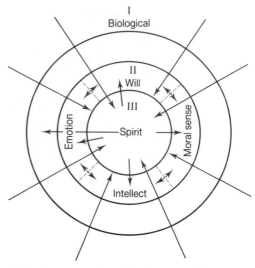

Fig. 18.1 *Conceptual model of nature of person.*

action of these five components is illustrated in Fig. 18.2.

SPIRITUAL NEEDS

As previously seen in mental health care, a holistic view takes into account that we all have needs which are regarded as social, psychological, physical and spiritual. Many of us have no trouble in identifying needs that are described as social, psychological and physical, but we struggle to identify spiritual needs.

Mary, aged 78 years and widowed; lives alone and has a history of depression following the death of her husband. She also suffers from chronic arthritis. Her daughter and two sons visit her regularly and they are her constant source of support. Mary's arthritis gives her a lot of pain and sometimes she wonders why she has to suffer and tries to find meaning in her chronic disability. However, she finds meaning and hope through her prayers as she is a devoted Christian. Mary's daughter takes her to Church whenever possible, where Mary finds the companionship of her fellow church-goers a good source of strength and support.

Her youngest son, John, and his family have just returned to England after a long spell in

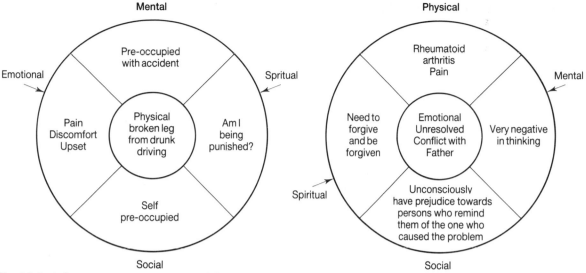

Fig. 18.2 *A five-component person model.*

Australia. He left England for Australia 20 years ago following an argument with his father. Mary feels guilty about the unresolved conflict between her son and husband and feels that reconciliation should have taken place before her husband's death. She tries to seek forgiveness for both through her prayers. Mary is delighted to see her grandchildren from Australia whom she had missed all these years and now finds inspiration, new meaning and hope in her life as a result of this. Mary's renewed hope has given her inspiration to rework her goals and she finds a new purpose in her life. Her arthritis is no longer the dominant feature in her life and is now able to resume painting and finds satisfaction in expressing creative talent through her artistic work.

We express our spiritual needs in a variety of ways and forms. Mary's spiritual needs may include the following:

The need for meaning and purpose

The need for love and harmonious relationship

The need for forgiveness

The need for a source of hope and strength

The need for trust

The need for expression of personal beliefs and values

The need for spiritual practices, expression of concept of God or Deity and creativity

Meaning and purpose

Many people tend to find themselves wrestling with the meaning and purpose in life during crisis, whether in health or illness. In the case illustration Mary tried to find meaning in her suffering. Meaning in this context can be defined as the reason given to a particular life experience by the individual. The search for meaning is a primary force in life. This drives us to search for meaning to life in general and discovering meaning in suffering in particular. We need to find sense out of our life and illness. Mary, in the case illustration above, found new meaning and purpose in her changed circumstances.

There is evidence to suggest that patients struggle with finding a source of meaning and purpose in their lives (Peterson and Nelson, 1987; Burnard, 1990). Mentally ill clients often struggle with finding a source of meaning and purpose in their life. This struggle is illustrated in the following example:

George had been admitted to hospital twice in a state of despair and hopelessness. He shared his despair with staff at the hospital by saying, 'I have lost all hope.' Shortly after his last discharge he went home and killed himself.

It is suggested that people with a sense of meaning and purpose survive more readily in very difficult circumstances and these include illness and suffering. There is some truth in the expression that he who has a 'why' to life can bear with almost any 'how'.

Many of us approach the task of life in a variety of ways and so our ability to cope with a crisis varies. We can find meaning and purpose in the experience of suffering. There is a distinction between the religious and the apparently non-religious person in the way they approach spirituality, that is the religious person experiences his or her existence not merely as a task but as a mission, and is aware of a taskmaster, the source of this mission. That source is God.

In crisis such as bereavement the person experiences meaninglessness, that is, the person expresses a sense of bewilderment and loss of meaning. For example, the person with a diagnosis of HIV infection, the survivor of a traumatic road accident, the death of a child in a family, the patient in a mental health unit, all cry out for help in search of meaning and desperately seek to talk to someone who will give attention and time in their exploration of meaning and purpose. The nurse is very often the nearest person to whom sufferers can reach out (Burnard, 1990).

In a person searching for meaning and purpose there may be a need for exploration of spiritual issues. In some instances the person in search of spirituality may want to talk about religious feelings or lack of them. The person may not be asking for advice or opinions but only for an opportunity to talk about feelings, to express doubts and anguish. Such opportunity for expression can bring about clarity and a renewed sense of meaning and purpose.

People who have strong religious conviction and sense God, still need encouragement to adapt to unexpected changes. They are likely to experience hope even when their usual support systems let them down. Their experiences of God reassure them that God will never fail them. The nurse may have to act as a catalyst in providing the opportunity for finding meaning and purpose in crisis by establishing this relationship with God.

Love and harmonious relationships

Our need for love and harmonious relationships goes hand in hand with a need for meaning and purpose. The need for love is one of the fundamental human needs (Maslow, 1968) which lasts throughout lifetime (from childhood to old age). A spiritually distressed person requires unconditional love, that is love that has no strings attached to it. The spiritually distressed person does not have to earn it by being good or attractive or wealthy. The person is simply loved for the way he or she is, regardless of faults or ignorance or bad habits or deeds.

Many mental health clients seek love and relationships but are unable to establish these with others because of their poorly developed social skills or deterioration of these during illness. For some, their illness, possible institutionalization, stigmatization, and even prolonged medication and its side-effects, are all damaging to their self esteem. Many of them seek out a reason or means to value and respect themselves and thus exhibit a serious spiritual need. Mary in the illustration above met her spiritual need in this area from her family and fellow churchgoers. A further case illustrated below demonstrates this need in another client:

John, a mental health client, while attending a group dealing with feelings shared that the last time he had been hugged by anyone was three years previously. When the group facilitator offered to hug him, he responded enthusiastically and even called on the facilitator the next day to describe his extreme pleasure in being hugged.

The manifestations of the need for love are self pity, depression, insecurity, isolation, and fear. These are indicators of a need for love from oneself, other people and God. The person receiving this kind of love experiences feelings of self worth, joy, security, belonging, hope and courage.

The spiritually distressed person also has a need to give love, which may include, for example, worries about financial status of family during hospitalization/separation from family and worries about separation from others during death.

Forgiveness

The need for forgiveness is commonly seen in mental health clients. Guilt and resentment are products of situations in which forgiveness does not happen. Clients often talk about having done something for which they cannot forgive themselves, or they talk about things that other people have done to them that they cannot forget or leave behind.

We saw in Mary's case the need for forgiveness and this is one of the principal causes of spiritual distress. A person who experiences spiritual distress expresses feelings of guilt and therefore requires the opportunity for forgiveness. Mary sought forgiveness for her son and husband through her prayers. Guilt often emerges when a person experiences the realization that one has failed to live up to one's own expectation or the expectations of others. For example, we may first experience guilt as a child when our behaviour does not measure up to the standards set for us by our parents. We contradict them and do the very things we are told not to do. Guilt breeds in us in the form of regrets not only for the things we have done but for our failure in many things. Unresolved conflicts in relationships can result in feelings of guilt. Another case illustration below provides an example related to guilt feelings:

Leon, who was a war refugee, whilst in hospital as a client was in agony because he believed that he had caused his mother's death. In actuality his mother had been killed while trying to escape from her country. He was ridden with guilt that he was responsible for her death because as a young man he had abandoned the church and indulged in various vices. His guilt prevented him from functioning and caused him to relive horrible, painful experiences.

The feelings of guilt may be expressed as feelings of paranoia, hostility, worthlessness, defensiveness, withdrawal, psychosomatic complaints, rationalizations, criticism of self, others and God and scapegoating. Forgiveness may bring a feeling of joy, peace and elation, and a sense of renewed self worth. It seems that confession of sin is one way in which some people achieve forgiveness from God.

Hope and strength

Hope is seen by psychologists and sociologists as necessary for life and without it we begin to die (Simsen, 1988). For many of us our sense of hope can be a powerful motivator in enabling an open attitude toward new ways of coping. Mary, in the case illustration, achieves new hope and strength from reconciliation with her son and his family. The spiritually distressed person may experience a feeling of hopelessness. The hopeless person may see no way out; there may be no other possibilities other than those dreaded.

Earlier we saw in Mary's situation her new goals and a renewed purpose as result of her son's arrival from Australia. We strive for good relationships with others and this is another facet of our hope. This includes relationships with oneself and the world, where a person believes that what is desired is possible. According to Soeken and Carson (1987): 'Ultimate hope resides in God and belief that the Supreme Being will impart meaning to individual lives and sufferings'. Hope is also necessary for future plans. Further needs of our hope include seeking support, love and the stability provided by important relationships in our life and to put into action future plans. Mary successfully achieved all of these through her loved ones and friends in the case illustration. If the patient believes in God, then hope in God is important. This hoping in God is the ultimate source of strength and supersedes all aspirations that are transitional.

Hope is closely related to our need for a source of strength. A source of hope provides the strength that we may need. A source of strength gives us the courage needed to face innumerable odds in crisis. The main source of hope and strength is found by individuals who pray because of their faith in God/transcendent. Haase's (1987) study found that the subjects concurred that belief in the power of prayer helped them cope with medical interventions and opportunities to express their faith helped them to resolve the situation they described. For some, communication with God and prayer is a source of strength. For most of us a message of hope provides new energy, strength, and courage to preserve or revise goals or plan and these were apparent in Mary's situation.

Trust

We feel secure when we can establish a trusting relationship with others. The spiritually distressed person needs an environment that conveys a trusting relationship. Such an environment is one which demonstrates that carers make themselves accessible to others, both physically and emotionally. Trusting is the ability to place confidence in the trustworthiness of others and this is essential for spiritual health and to total wellbeing. Learning to trust in an environment which is alien could be a daunting task and not an easy skill to accomplish.

Personal beliefs and values

The opportunity to express personal values and beliefs is a known spiritual need. In this sense spirituality refers to anything that a person considers to be of highest value in life. Mary shares her beliefs with her companions at the church and expresses these through her prayers. Her spiritual need in these areas are met easily because she has the opportunity to do so through the support of her family. Personal values which may be highly regarded by an individual include, for example, beliefs of a formalized religious

path, whereas for others it may be, for example, a set of very personal philosophical statements, or perhaps a physical activity.

Spiritual practices, concept of God/Deity, and creativity

The opportunity to express our needs related to spiritual practices, the concept of God or Deity and creativity may present as a feature of spirituality. The concept of God or Deity may be an important function in the personal life of a person. The need to carry out spiritual practices concerning God or Deity may be too daunting for the person if the opportunity is not available or the environment is alien or unreceptive to this need.

Our creative needs may feature in spirituality. Mary achieves spirituality as a creative need through her paintings. A religious minister in a Connecticut Hospice uses the arts as an avenue to the Spirit in which actors, writers, musicians and artists of a university are invited to exhibit their work and give performance (Wald, 1989).

COMPETENCES FOR SPIRITUAL CARE

Although a sufficient knowledge about spiritual needs and problems is necessary, competences of self awareness, communication (such as listening), trust building, giving hope, and enabling spiritual growth need to be developed to equip the nurse to assist in meeting clients' spiritual needs.

Self awareness

Before we instigate effective spiritual care, we must know and understand our level of spiritual awareness. An examination of our personal beliefs and values is a necessary part of spiritual care. The nurse who has a positive attitude to spiritual health is likely to be sensitive to any problem a patient has concerning spirituality. A continuous examination of one's own personal spiritual beliefs enables the nurse to appreciate that everybody does not share the same faith. An awareness of their own prejudices and bias would ensure that nurses do not impose their own values and beliefs on others, especially spiritual doctrines. Self awareness would enable the nurse to adopt a non-judgemental approach and avoid taking any steps that would mount to the accusation that he or she is trying to proselytize. It is likely that a person who has developed self awareness will show more tolerance, acceptance and respect for another person's spirituality.

The benefits of self awareness are stressed here but it is a skill that has to be acquired and continuously developed. In this section self awareness will be explained and a method for developing it will be outlined. Self awareness is an acknowledgement of one's own feeling and behaviours, accepting and understanding or accepting to understand these. Self awareness can be elaborated as an acknowledgement of our:

Values, attitudes, prejudices, beliefs, assumptions and feelings

Personal motives and needs and the extent to which these are being met

Degree of attention to others

Genuineness and investment of self, and how the above might have an effect on others

The intentional and unconscious use of self

It is widely acknowledged that a training in self awareness is a fundamental process before one understands others. According to Burnard (1985), to become aware of, and to have deeper understanding of ourselves is to have a sharper and clearer picture of what is happening to others. Limited awareness of ourselves may mean remaining blind to others. The first step to being self aware is to examine oneself as stressed earlier.

We can develop self awareness by various means. However, the methods used for increasing our awareness must contain the facets of inner search and observations of others.

One simple method of enhancing our self awareness is the process of noticing what we are doing—the process of self monitoring. All that is involved here is staying conscious of what you are doing and what is happening to you. To put it another way, you 'stay awake' and develop the skill of keeping your attention focused on your actions, both verbal and non-verbal.

Assessment of our present understanding of knowledge, skills and the learning of new materials, and techniques will be heavily influenced by our degree of self awareness. We are most likely to lose control of our self development if we remain blind to the need to increase our self awareness. An increase in our self awareness is not only the beginning of wisdom then, but also the growth of our personal and professional effectiveness.

Self awareness can also be developed through the introspection, through experience and through feedback:

Introspection

Meditation and yoga can be a useful way of developing self awareness using the introspection method. Simple breathing and meditation techniques are sufficient for this purpose. Meditation and yoga serve another useful purpose in that these techniques can be useful methods of dealing with job-related stress. Becoming aware of, and consciously noting, experiences are other means of introspection. Complementing these processes the following are useful: identifying past and present prejudices; identifying past and present approaches to personal problem solving.

Experience

Self awareness is also developed through experience. The experiential method is one useful method of learning through experience. Participation in experiential exercises brings the desirable increase in self awareness.

Self awareness through feedback

Self awareness cannot be developed by adhering solely to the introspection and experiential methods alone. Introspection and experiential exercises will give us some understanding of ourselves, but a complete self awareness requires knowledge about behaviour too; for this we require the help of others: it takes two to know one fully.

I am aware of my inner feelings (inner processes) but sometimes I cannot see my behaviour. Another person can see my behaviour, but is not aware of my inner feelings and experience. I can see the other person's behaviour, but not his inner experience. For a complete self awareness, then, we need to strengthen the knowledge gained by introspection with knowledge obtained by feedback from others about our behaviour.

Self disclosure involves the process of revealing information about oneself: own ideas, values, feelings that are similar to the ones experienced by those one is trying to help. There is significant clinical evidence to suggest that a carer's self disclosure increases the likelihood of client's self disclosure (Stuart and Sundeen, 1983). Self disclosure results in successful therapeutic outcome. However, our self disclosure must be handled judiciously, and this is determined by the quality, quantity, and appropriateness of higher disclosures. We must handle our disclosure sensitively so that clients feel comfortable enough to produce their own self disclosure. A limited self disclosure from us may reduce client's willingness to disclose about self and conversely, too many may decrease the time available for client's disclosure or alienate him or her.

Communication skills

Good communication skills are essential for spiritual care. The key communication skill in spiritual care is active listening without being judgemental. The points about self awareness mentioned earlier are necessary for developing non-judgemental attitudes.

Non-judgemental means unconditional acceptance of clients. However, to have faith, trust and respect for another person despite his or her behaviour is often a most difficult quality to achieve, but with increasing self awareness this can be developed. A non-judgemental approach is acceptance of an individual without any kind of judgement, without criticism, and without reservation. This also requires not only unconditional acceptance of a person but to respect him/her without necesssarily knowing what his/her previous behaviour has been.

As pointed out earlier, when providing spiritual care we must reserve or detach from our own personal values, ideals or beliefs. Clients must feel that we are genuinely interested, want to know them, how they think and feel, and still do not judge them. Such a relationship engenders in clients the feeling that if someone else is interested, thinks they are of worth as unique people, and cares, then they too are likely to have a positive image of themselves.

Genuineness is a quality based on the person's ability to be himself or herself. It means being honest and open in expression of one's feelings. Again, self awareness is a means by which this quality can be developed. It demands honesty and courage to be allowed to be seen as a real person.

Active listening is important because its purpose is to enable the client to be at ease and to make use of the listening process in such a way that the listener can help the client deal with spiritual needs and experience further spiritual growth. The active listener acts as a talking mirror, encouraging and reflecting back to the client what the listener hears, sees or senses.

The rudiments of being a good listener

The carer needs to create the right kind of climate in which the individuals requiring spiritual care feel accepted and confident enough to be able to talk about their spiritual thoughts and feelings. Clients need to feel the carer is listening to what they are saying and what they are feeling and not only listening, but accepting and understanding them. All this ties up with responding to people in ways that are helpful. Good listening is really paying close attention to what someone is saying and this is essential, but it is not easy. We need to suspend our thoughts and give the other person our complete attention.

We can demonstrate understanding by reflecting the patient's thoughts back, showing that we are listening hard, that we are making a real effort to understand what the client is thinking and feeling.

Make the clients feel it is alright to go on talking, that their feelings are being accepted. State that you are genuinely interested in what the client is saying, and respond warmly.

Trust building

Trust is necessary because confidence in the nurse–patient relationship is vital in spiritual care and, indeed, to the well-being of the patient. Trust between carer and client develops over time as the client tests the environment, risks self disclosure, and observes the nurse's adherence to commitment. The following approach enhances initial trust:

Listening attentively to client's feelings

Responding to client's feelings

Demonstrating consistency, especially keeping appointments and promises

Viewing situation from the client's perspective

An increasing level of self awareness of personal feelings, along the lines suggested earlier, on the part of the nurse also enhances trust. It enables the client to disclose uncomfortable, even forbidden, feelings in safety. The carer must continue to build on the trust gained earlier and this task can be achieved by being reliable. Reliability is one other factor that strengthens and sustains a trusting relationship. Reliability is measured in terms of the carer's commitment to the spiritual needs of the client and this means promises and adherence to care plans must be carried out promptly and followed through.

Giving hope

Hope is something that we cannot easily give to another, but every effort can be made to support and encourage the hoping abilities of a patient. Mental health carers are often in ideal positions to foster or hinder hope. A caring relationship can be offered that permits, rather than stifles, the efforts of the client to develop hope. The carer can support the person who is testing his or her own beliefs or struggling with questions of fear and faith. Further encouragement can be given to clients to talk about their fears. Helping clients to relive their memory is another way of facilitating hoping. Memories of events when life's needs were met, when despair was overcome and when failure was defeated, can all be used to take on a fresh view and face the future with confidence as part of spiritual recovery.

Herth (1990) identifies hope-fostering strategies which could be used as part of spiritual care. She defines hope-fostering strategies as 'those sources that functioned to instil, support or restore hope by facilitating the hoping process in some way'. The following can be utilized as hope-fostering strategies.

Interpersonal connectedness

A meaningful and shared relationship with close ones and others (including carers) is said to be a feature of interpersonal connectedness. For example, a harmonious and supportive relationship within the family offers the client hope and strength which are fundamental parts of a person's spirituality. The willingness of a carer to share in patient's hopes is a feature of this strategy.

Light heartedness

The features of this are feelings of delight, joy or playfulness that are communicated verbally or non-verbally. The carer can foster lightheartedness among clients. The spirit of lightheartedness can provide a communication link between persons and a way of coping with deteriorations in body function and confused emotions; it can provide a sense of release from the present moment.

Personal attributes

The carer can enable clients to maximize their attributes of determination, courage and serenity. A search for a sense of inner peace, harmony and calm is one way of enabling the client to achieve serenity.

Attainable aims

A characteristic of these is the direction of efforts towards some purpose. The presence of aims often fosters hope. The carer who helps clients to search for meaning and purpose in life actually fosters hope. Helping clients to redefine their aims and channelling their thoughts on to other events or significant others are useful strategies of hope-fostering.

Spiritual base

The presence of active spiritual beliefs (in God or a 'higher being') and spiritual practices is a source of hope. This may enable clients to participate in specific practices and these may include praying, corporate worship, listening to spiritual music and spiritual programmes on the radio or television, religious activities, maintaining specific religious customs, and visiting members and leaders of their spiritual community.

Uplifting memories

Recalling uplifting memories/times is another hope-fostering strategy. The carer can help clients to share happy stories from the past and to reminisce through old picture albums. Reliving positive activities from the past, such as an enjoyable holiday, significant events (birth of child, receipt of a medal) and 'sunset over mountains', can serve to renew the hoping process. It is most likely that memories of past events can serve to enrich the present moment.

Affirmation of worth

Having one's individuality accepted, honoured and acknowledged can foster hope. Carers, family and friends can be party to a client's feeling of self worth as a dignified human being. This can be very uplifting and act as a source of hope.

Enabling spiritual growth

The client needs to grow spiritually to achieve a full status of health. A good health orientation includes body, mind, spirit and additional consideration of cultural background. This can be achieved when a carer creates a relationship in which carer–client education takes place. The client may be educated to develop the hoping strategy. Trusting is another skill that can be learned and the nurse can provide opportunities for the client to develop this aspect of a relationship.

Clients need a learning opportunity to gain insights into their own spiritual awareness. They need an orientation that would help them to search for meaning and purpose. The carer as a teacher can help clients to explore this search for meaning and purpose.

The other aspects of client education may include the identification of the nature of 'right' relationship with others. Morrison (1990) asserts that caring concentration on this particular area can lead to improvements in clients' physical health. Educating clients to face up to defective relationships with others is an important aspect of spiritual care. Examples of defective relationships include the denial of the death of a loved one, a lack of social concern and an inability to accept hostility. The inability to experience the 'right relationship' is a known cause of spiritual distress (Morrison, 1989).

Learning is seen as a two-way process in which the client experiences spiritual growth and the carer achieves a greater spiritual awareness as well. Millison (1988) found in his study that carers experienced heightened spirituality as a result of their work with ill people and that all carers reported that they felt they received more in terms of spirituality than they were able to give. An increasing level of knowledge, insight and coping strategies relating to spirituality can be achieved through the process of sharing as part of learning to cope with spirituality.

PUTTING SPIRITUAL CARE COMPETENCES INTO ACTION (Through the Nursing Process)

The systematic approach of the nursing process can be employed to assist in meeting the spiritual needs of clients. The following four stages are included in the nursing process: assessment, planning, implementation and evaluation.

Assessment

Information obtained on religious needs alone is not enough for spiritual care. Such information does not allow us to go deeper into feelings about meaning and purpose of life, love and relationship, trust, hope and strength, forgiveness, expressions of beliefs and values. Also, this approach may lead to the assumption that a person who does not belong to a formal religion has no spiritual needs. As indicated earlier the unreligious may have spiritual needs. The person who does not express obvious religious beliefs may still struggle with guilt, or lack meaning and purpose, or with need for love and relationships. On the other hand, a person who declares as belonging to a particular religion may not necessarily abide by the beliefs and practices of that religion. Assumptions or conclusions should not be drawn about spiritual needs on the basis of clients' religious status.

The carer must remain sensitive to verbal and non-verbal cues from clients when carrying out spiritual assessment. These cues might indicate a need to talk about spiritual problems.

Assessment of clients' physical functioning may also provide valuable information for understanding their spiritual component. Such obvious status about clients' ability to see, hear, and move are important factors that may later determine the relevance of certain interventions. Also, psychosocial assessment data may serve a useful purpose in determining clients' thought patterns, content of speech, affect (mood), cultural orientation, and social relationships. All of these may provide the basis for identifying a need, or planning appropriate care, in conjunction with spiritual intervention.

George is a 56-year-old client in an acute mental health unit. Prior to his admission he was expressing feelings of despair, hopelessness and eventually became withdrawn and uncommunicative. He has been in the ward for a few weeks and now he is beginning to communicate and expresses that he wants to go to the church. At the initial assessment interview the nurse was unable to carry out a spiritual assessment of George because of his withdrawal and uncommunicativeness. Now the nurse wants to complete George's spiritual assessment.

Stoll (1979) offers a useful guide for spiritual assessment. The guide includes four general areas that can be appraised to derive data about spiritual concerns:

Concept of God or Deity
Is religion or God significant to you?

Is prayer (or meditation) helpful to you?

What happens when you pray (or meditate)?

Does God or Deity function in your personal life?

If yes, can you describe how?

How would you describe your God or what you worship?

Source of strength and hope
Who is the most important person to you?

To whom would you turn when you need help?

Are they available?

In what ways do they help?

What is your source of strength and hope?

What helps you the most when you feel afraid or need special help?

Spiritual practices
Do you feel your faith (or religion) is helpful to you?

If yes, would you tell me how?

Are there any religious practices that are important to you?

Has being sick made any difference to your practice of praying (or meditating) or to your other religious practices?

What religious books or symbols are important to you?

Relation between spiritual beliefs and health
What has bothered you most about being sick (or in what is happening to you)?

What do you think is going to happen to you?

Has being sick (or what has happened to you)

made any difference in your feelings about God or the practice of your faith?

Is there anything that is especially frightening or meaningful to you now?

Tubesing (1980) suggests a spiritual assessment procedure in which there are five questions to assess a person's spiritual outlook. Spiritual outlook embraces a person's goal, faith, value, commitments and ability to let go and to receive forgiveness from self and others. Tubesing's assessment questions for spiritual outlook are:

What is the aim of life?

What beliefs guide me?

What is important to me?

What do I choose to spend myself on?

What am I willing to let go?

The presence of religious literature, for example, the Bible or Koran gives an indication of client's concerns about spiritual matters. Objects like religious medals, pins, or articles of clothing are symbolic of clients' spiritual expressions. Clients may keep a religious statue or Deity to carry out religious rituals.

Patrick, a 60-year-old client, has been readmitted to a Mental Health Unit following disordered thinking and a disruptive life style. Initially he was suspicious and hostile to his carers, but now they have gained his trust as his mental state has improved considerably. A nurse is carrying out Patrick's spiritual assessment in order to plan his spiritual care.

The following observation schedules could be used to carry out spiritual assessment by observations:

Non-verbal behaviour
1 Observe affect. Does the client's affect or attitude convey loneliness, depression, anger, agitation or anxiety?

2 Observe behaviour. Does the client pray during the day? Does the client rely on religious reading material or other literature for solace?

Verbal behaviour
1 Does the client seem to complain out of proportion to his or her illness?

2 Does the client complain of sleeping difficulties?

3 Does the client ask for unusually high doses of sedation?

4 Does the client refer to God in any way?

5 Does the client talk about prayer, faith, hope, or anything of a religious nature?

6 Does the client talk about church functions that are part of his or her life?

7 Does the client express concern over the meaning and direction of life? Does the client express concern over the impact of the illness on the meaning of life?

Interpersonal relationships
1 Does the client have visitors or does he or she spend visiting hours alone?

2 Are the visitors supportive or do they seem to leave the client feeling upset?

3 Does the client have visitors from his or her church?

4 Does the client interact with staff and other clients?

Environment
1 Does the client have a Bible or other religious reading material?

2 Does the client wear religious medals or pins?

3 Does the client use religious articles such as statues in observing religious practices?

4 Has the client received religious get-well cards?

5 Does the client use personal pictures, artwork, or music to keep his or her spirits up?

Observations of the ways in which clients relate with 'significant others' (people close to them, friends, and others who matter to them) may provide clues to the spiritual needs. The quality of interpersonal relationships can be ascertained. Does the client welcome visitors? Does their presence relax the client or cause distress? Do visitors come from the church or religious community? Observations of these factors can lead to conclusions about the client's social support system. The social system enables clients to give and receive love and lack of such support may deprive clients of this need and leave them distressed. The client who has faith in God may feel estranged if cut off from this support network.

Observations of a client's environment and significant objects/symbols related to his religious practice may give evidence of his spirituality.

The other area of spiritual assessment includes attention to the three factors: sense of meaning and purpose, means of forgiveness and source of love and relationship. Observations and routine conversations with clients can lead to valuable information about each of those factors. Questions can be framed to include the following:

What is your source of meaning and purpose in life?

Why do you go on living?

Observations may include how clients deal with other clients, if they ruminate over past behaviours or how they have been treated by other people. How do clients respond to criticism? If clients respond with anger, hostility and blame others, these behaviours may suggest that they are unable to forgive themselves and that consequently are unable to tolerate anything that resembles criticism.

The spiritual assessment must also look at the client's ability to feel loved, valued and respected by other people.

Planning

The planning of spiritual care requires careful attention. The data obtained from assessment must be interpreted in terms of spiritual needs and a care plan should be based on this information.

Dorothy is a 40-year-old anxious client and is undergoing anxiety management therapy. She is a practising Christian (Catholic) and her spiritual care is included in the nursing care plan.

The planning of spiritual care should include respect for the patient's individuality, willingness of the carer to get involved in the spirituality of the client, use of therapeutic self, and the nurturing of the inner person, the spirit.

Assistance to meet spiritual needs should be given according to the indications of the individual, which may be unique and specific. If, for example, clients are part of a church or religious group, and the effect on them appears positive, the nurse can strengthen this contact. A client who is accustomed to practices such as meditating, praying, or reading the Bible or other religious books, should be given time and privacy. A visit by the client's religious agent (pastor, rabbi, or others) can be arranged.

The carer can make it easier for clients to talk about spiritual beliefs and concerns, especially about how these relate to their illness. The carer may need to help clients in their struggle and search for meaning and purpose in life. On the other hand, if clients are trying to find a source of hope and strength, then it can be used in planning care.

The other aspects of the care plan may include comfort, support, warmth, self awareness, empathy, non-judgemental listening and understanding. All these measures are the essence of a therapeutic relationship. An empathetic listener can do much to support a person who is spiritually distressed by being available when needed, especially those clients suffering from loneliness, and expressing doubts, fears and feelings of alienation. The presence of another empathetic person may have a healing effect.

A powerful source of spiritual care and comfort can be prayer, scripture and other religious reading. All of these may alleviate spiritual distress. Prayers as a source of help would help a patient develop a feeling of oneness with the universe or a better relationship with God, comfort the client, and help relieve spiritual distress. A particular prayer should be selected according to the client's own style of comfort and needs. Although carers may not belong to the same faith as the clients, they can still support the clients in carrying out their spiritual beliefs.

Meditation, both religious and secular, can play an important role in enabling clients to relax, clear the mind, achieve a feeling of oneness with a Deity or the universe, promote acceptance of painful memories or decisions, and gather energy and hope that may help them to face spiritual distress.

The use of music gives an inspirational and calming effect. A wide variety of religious, inspirational and secular music may spiritually uplift a client.

Implementation

Implementation of spiritual care is a highly skillful activity. It requires education and experience in spiritual care. In carrying out nursing actions related to spiritual needs, it is imperative that carers:

Do not impose personal beliefs on client or families

Respond to client's expression of need of a correct understanding of their background

Do not allow a detached scene to be used as an occasion to proselytize

Be sensitive to client's signal for spiritual support

It is important that if a carer feels unable to re-spond to a particular situation of spiritual need, then he or she should enlist the services of an appropriate individual.

Nursing intervention should be based on an action which reflects caring for the individual. Caring signifies to clients that they are significant, and are worth someone taking the trouble to be concerned about. Caring requires actions of support and assistance in growing. It means non-judgemental approach and showing sensitivity to clients' cultural values, physical preference and social needs. It demands an attitude of helping, sharing, nurturing and loving. These actions fulfil the requirement of individualized spiritual care.

An understanding of the client's unique beliefs and values or religious views is paramount in spiritual care. The carer must respect and understand the need for the client's beliefs and practices even if these are not in accord with the carer's faith. To allow a better understanding of the client's spiritual needs, the carer must establish a rapport and trust which facilitates the client to share those beliefs. The carer's own self aware-ness of personal limitation in understanding these beliefs is paramount and he or she must seek outside help if necessary.

Nursing intervention should be based on a carer–client relationship that encourages the person to express views, fears, anxieties and new understanding through creative acts, writing, poetry, music or art. Time for quiet reflection and opportunities for religious practices would enable the client to develop a deeper understanding of life and a particular belief system.

The person who has no strong philosophical or religious belief may seek the opportunity to explore feelings, values and an understanding of life with another individual who is willing to give attention and time to discuss those areas of concern and share common human experiences. The carer is the person who is most immediately avail-able and receptive to the client's thoughts and feelings. Certain clients may require close friends, family or a religious person to share those thoughts and feelings. The carer must remain sensitive to these needs and make the necessary arrangements. However, it must be remembered that spiritual growth is a life-long process and the carer who initiates spiritual care would have been a catalyst in the client's goal to achieve eventual spiritual integrity and wellbeing.

Evaluation

Evaluation is an activity that involves the process of making a judgement about outcomes of nursing intervention. There are many indicators of spiritual outcomes, one of which is spiritual integrity. The person who has attained spiritual integrity demonstrates this experience through a reality-based tranquillity or peace, or through the development of meaningful, purposeful behaviour, displaying a restored sense of integrity. O'Brien (1982) comments that the measure of spiritual care should establish the degree to which 'spiritual pain' was relieved. Another view offered by Kim *et al.* (1984) suggests spiritual care may be measured as the disruption in the 'life principle' is restored. The contents of clients' thoughts and feelings may also reflect spiritual growth through a greater understanding of life or an acceptance and creativity within a particular context.

SUMMARY

Clearly, there is no one single authoritative definition of spirituality although some authors have attempted to define it in broader terms. Spirituality refers to a broader dimension which is sometimes beyond the realm of subjective explanation. It is an inspirational expression as a reaction to a religious force or an abstract philosophy as defined by the individual. It is a quality that is present in believers, and even in atheists and agnostics, provided there is the opportunity to feel and express this inspirational experience according to the individual's understanding and meaning attached to this phenomenon.

Spiritual needs include the need for meaning and purpose, the need for love and harmonious relationship, the need for forgiveness, the need for a source of hope and strength, the need for trust, the need for expression of personal beliefs and values, and the need for spiritual practice, expression of concept of God or Deity and creativity. These are by no means exclusive, but it is commonly recognized that it is within the province of mental health nursing to incorporate them into care plans as part of the spiritual care of clients.

Competences such as self awareness, communication (listening), trust building, giving hope and enabling spiritual growth (client education) are important prerequisites for spiritual care. These competences, together with the previous introduction to the knowledge of spirituality, offer a basis for the formulation of care plans related to spiritual care.

Effective spiritual care can be given through the systematic steps of the nursing process. Appropriate assessment strategies and tools should be employed for the purpose of assessing client's spiritual needs. Data obtained from assessment strategies can be used for planning spiritual care. Certain pertinents outlined in this chapter should be considered when implementing spiritual care.

ACKNOWLEDGEMENT

My thanks are due to Quay and BKT Publishers for permission to adapt material from my book, *Spiritual Care: A Practical Guide for Nurses* (1991).

FURTHER READING

Carson, V.B. (1989) *Spiritual Dimensions of Nursing Practice*. London: W.B. Saunders.
The concept of spirituality is adequately treated in Chapter one of this book.

Shelly, J.A. & Fish, S. (1988) *Spiritual Care: The Nurse's Role*. Downers Grove, Illinois: Inter-Varsity Press.
Although written from a Christian perspective readers will find useful sections which explore the concept of spirituality. Chapters one to three are particularly useful and assist the reader to 'grasp' the concept of spirituality. The book also includes a workbook section which contains individual exercises for developing spiritual awareness.

Narayanasamy, A. (1991) *Spiritual Care: A Practical Guide for Nurses*. Lancaster: Quay/BKT.

Readers wishing specific direction on religious needs of clients may find Chapter three of this book useful. Chapter three provides a resource guide to religious faith and needs.

REFERENCES

Burnard, P. (1990) Learning to care for the spirit. *Nursing Standard*, **4** (18), 33–39.

Burnard, P. (1985) *Learning Human Skills*. London: Heinemann Nursing.

Gorham, M. (1989) Spirituality and problem solving with seniors. *Perspectives*, **13** (3), 13–16.

Haase, J.E. (1987) Components of courage in chronically ill adolescents: a phenomenological study. *Advanced Nursing Science*, **9**, 64.

Herth, K. (1990) Fostering hope in terminally ill people. *Journal of Advanced Nursing*, **15**, 1250–1257.

Kim, M.J., McFarland, S.K. & McLane, A.M. (1984) *Pocket Guide to Nursing Diagnosis*. St Louis: C.V. Mosby Company.

Maslow, A.R. (1968) *Toward a Psychology of Being*. New York: Van Nostrand.

Millison, M.B. (1988) Spirituality and caregiver, developing an underutilised facet of care. *American Journal of Hospice Care*, **March/April**, 37–44.

Morrison, R. (1989) Spiritual health care and the nurse. *Nursing Standard*, **4** (13/14), 23–29.

Morrison, R. (1990) Spiritual health care and the nurse. *Nursing Standard*, **5** (5), 34–35.

Murray, R.B. & Zentner, J.B. (1989) *Nursing Concepts for Health Promotion*. London: Prentice Hall.

Narayanasamy, A. (1991) Spiritual Care: A Practical Guide for Nurses. Lancaster: Quay/BKT.

O'Brien, M.E. (1982) Religious faith and adjustment to long-term haemodialysis. *Journal of Religious Health*, **21**, 63.

Peterson, E. & Nelson, K. (1987) How to meet clients' spiritual needs. *Journal of Psychosocial Nursing*, **25** (5), 34–88.

Simsen, B. (1988) Nursing the spirit. *Nursing Times* 14, Vol. 84, No. 37, pp. 31–35.

Soeken, K.G. & Carson, Y.J. (1987) Responding to the spiritual needs of the chronically ill? *Nursing Clinics of North America*, **22** (3), 603–611.

Stallwood, J. (1981) Spiritual dimensions of nursing practice. In Beland, I.L. & Passos, J.Y. (Eds) *Clinical Nursing*. New York: Macmillan.

Stoll, R.G. (1979) Guidelines for spiritual assessment. *American Journal of Nursing*, **79**, 1574–1577.

Stuart, G.W. & Sundeen, S.J. (1983) *Principles and Practice of Psychiatric Nursing*. St. Louis: C.V. Mosby.

Tubesing, D.A. (1980) Stress: spiritual outlook and health. *Specialised Pastoral Care Journal*, **3**, 17.

Wald, F.S. (1989) The widening scope of spiritual care. *American Journal of Hospice Care*, **July/August**, 40–43.

MEETING THE NEEDS OF PEOPLE WITH ENDURING MENTAL HEALTH PROBLEMS

Julie Repper and Paddy Cooney

'The mass provoked mostly irritation, hostility and impatience. Their behaviour affronted, caused uneasiness; they wept and moaned; they quarrelled and complained. They were a nuisance and treated as such. It was forgotten that they too possessed a prized humanity which needed care and love, that a tiny poetic essence could be distilled from their overflowing, squalid truth.'
Janet Frame, Faces in the Water, 1961.

TERMINOLOGY

This chapter is concerned with people who have ongoing problems and multiple needs as a result of mental illness. Such clients are variously referred to as 'chronically mentally ill', 'psychiatrically disabled', 'long-term mentally ill' and 'people with enduring mental health problems'. There is controversy over the use of all these terms, not only does a common identity belie the variation that inevitably exists within the group,

but such titles may unwittingly prove negative, stigmatizing and self-fulfilling. The title of the chapter was chosen as it implies less dependence on a medically orientated model than other commonly used terms, and is felt to be the least negative term in use.

INTRODUCTION

Whilst recognizing the problems associated with labelling a group homogeneously, the overall purpose of this chapter is to raise the profile of all people with enduring mental health problems. It examines their particular needs for care, and the most effective means of providing care and services which best meet their needs.

The need for specialist sections

The nature and severity of the problems faced by people with enduring mental health problems, and the services they require warrant special and specific attention. Bennett and Freeman (1991) suggest that, in the past, services have often failed to be effective because the acute model has been applied uncritically to long-term problems. Indeed, the efficiency of mental health services as a whole is increasingly being judged by their success in meeting the needs of people with long-term problems (Reed, 1990).

The need for specialized services and approaches for people with enduring mental health problems arises from the multiplicity of their needs and the long-term nature of their difficulties. The complex and frustrating nature of their personal experience, and the feelings this engenders in carers and service providers must not only be acknowledged, but also positively addressed by service providers. Traditionally, health care providers work within a philosophy of 'cure' of resolution of problems, a culture that values certainty, seeks causes, and so is perhaps keen to attribute blame. This places extraordinary pressure on clients with recurrent and ongoing problems, and on carers and professionals involved in their care.

Yet in considering the profound needs of this client group, it is all too easy to dismiss their strengths, aspirations and inherent rights as individuals and citizens. It is the responsibility of all concerned with the provision of services for these people to make the client's views paramount in planning and delivering care, to find out and impart information which enables their clients to make choices about their lives, and to work on behalf of clients to challenge positively longstanding misconceptions held about mental illness, which may be particularly negative with regard to this client group (D'Arcy and Brockman, 1977).

The purpose of care is for the client to have maximum independence and optimum quality of life at all times. The skill of the worker lies in assessing the client's potential with regard to both of these factors, and through adopting a client-centred approach offering an individually tailored programme of care that balances the client's needs, wishes and potential.

The structure of the sections

This chapter is divided into three sections, and the concepts introduced in each are shown below. The first chapter is concerned with describing clients with enduring mental health problems, and the challenges they provide for service providers. The need to prioritize people with enduring mental health problems as a distinct population is clarified. Since this is closely related to the provision of care in the community, a brief history of the development of mental health services is given, and the problems associated with community care policy in practice are explored. The various subgroups within this population are described with reference to their social and health care needs.

The second section focuses on recent policy legislation of relevance for people with enduring mental health problems. It traces the problems to be addressed, and the questions to be considered when planning services that are based on clients' needs. An emphasis is put on the role of care management in co-ordinating care and informing the provision and planning of services.

The third section is concerned with providing care for the individual. The location of care is examined in relation to the functions it needs to fulfil. In terms of the role of the service provider a focus is placed on the principles of care which provide the context for therapeutic interventions.

SECTION

1

PEOPLE WITH ENDURING MENTAL HEALTH PROBLEMS

AIMS

i)   To describe clients who experience enduring mental health problems
ii) To establish the need to prioritize people with enduring mental health problems as a distinct population
iii) To explore the problems associated with community care policy in practice

KEY ISSUES

The legacy of community care
Defining people with enduring mental health problems
Social supports
Institutionalization
Users' views
Categories of people with enduring mental health problems
The prevalence of enduring mental health problems
Marginalized groups
Community care problems in practice

Identify, analyse and assess factors causing distress and illness	Promote health, provide direct care and make interventions	Manage care programmes and services
Be critical, analytical and accountable, continue professional development	Counter discrimination, inequality and individual and institutional racism	Work within and develop policies, laws and safeguards in all settings
Understand influences on mental health and the nature/causes of disorder and illness	Know the effects of distress, disorder, illness on individuals, groups, families	Understand the basis of treatments and interventions

THE LEGACY OF 'COMMUNITY CARE'

The delineation of clients with enduring mental health problems has only become a problem with de-institutionalization. Prior to this it was clear that long-term clients were those who had been in hospital longest. With the advent of community care not only are there longstanding inpatients being discharged into the community, but people who would previously have remained in hospital for long periods are being discharged earlier, thus the client group is less discreet. Yet it is in the nature of these changes in service provision that the need to identify the longer-term clients lies; the majority of people with enduring mental health problems now receive care—or not—from various sources within a dispersed community rather than under the single roof of the hospital. Thus, they are less easy to trace, identify and monitor, yet it is increasingly evident that their needs are not adequately being met. Since people with enduring mental health problems of a serious and disabling nature have only become a distinct priority with the advent of community care, the history of the move towards community-based systems of care will briefly be described.

The rise of the asylum

Care of the mentally ill has always taken place in the community and by the community, but since the mid-nineteenth century formal psychiatric care has generally been provided in mental hospitals. Institutional provision has always been available but this was varied and provided arbitrary treatment—or neglect—until the Victorian era, when a series of large institutions was built on the outskirts of cities. These were founded with great optimism and high therapeutic hopes (Jones, 1972). Increasing stories of rape, murder and abuse in the old Madhouses caused alarm, and such people as William Ellis in Wakefield, Gardiner Hill in Lincoln, John Connolly at Hanwell, and Pinel in France pioneered and successfully implemented non-restraint methods and humane treatment of the mentally ill. Thus, the stage was set for major reforms, and the Lunatics Act of 1845 required all counties and major boroughs to make proper provision for the care of lunatics.

Within two years of this act 36 counties had public asylums.

Perkins (1988) describes the three cornerstones of this era of moral enlightenment as:

---

1 *Moral insanity.* Madness was not defined as loss of reason, but as deviance from socially accepted behaviour, and was seen as arising, amongst other things, from social causes, such as domestic grief, unemployment, loss of property, jealousy, and 'over-excitement at the Great Exhibition'.

2 *Moral management.* It was recognized that patients' behaviour might in large part result from the harsh way in which they were treated. The premise of moral management was that by treating patients as rational people, a sense of self esteem could be cultivated that would help the sufferers to exercise will and self control. Treatment consisted of social re-education, work, leisure pursuits, and the encouragement of normal habits and domestic activities. By 1854, 27 of the 30 asylums used no restraint methods.

3 *Moral architecture.* The asylums were planned as therapeutic environments where lunatics could be controlled without the use of force. They were designed along domestic lines as safe, homely refuges.

These principles reflect similar ideas to those held today: respect for the patient, behaviour seen as a function of the way in which people are treated, an emphasis on homely environment, social re-education and occupational activities.

The decline of the asylum

Although in the era of moral treatment, there was a belief in the curability of the mentally ill, many of the inmates in fact failed to get better. The asylums became filled with the most difficult and enduring cases. Hospitals grew and hospital populations grew. The number of inpatients rose from 7,114 in 1850 to 119,659 in 1930 and in 1954 it peaked at 148,000. The average number of patients per asylum was 116 in 1827, 542 by 1870,

961 by 1900 and by 1930 it had risen to 1,221. Standards deteriorated under the pressure of numbers and shortage of staff. Hospitals became unattractive places to work in, staff became demoralized and custodial practices re-emerged. Most patients were admitted under a legal order and the major aim was to achieve quiet behaviour and a minimum of escapes.

However, outside these growing asylums, improvements were being made; several mental hospitals were treating non-certified patients as both inpatients and outpatients, a reflection of growing interest in neurotic conditions and psychiatric treatment. The report of the Poor Law Commission of 1909 stressed the importance of public health measures in preventing illness. In 1921 the mental nursing certificate became nationally approved and recognized (although many attendants in the asylums remained unqualified). The Royal Commission on Lunacy and Mental Disorder of 1924–26 suggested that 'the key-note of the future must be prevention and treatment'. They strongly recommended the development of out-patient and community services, and proposed that future legal intervention should be continued to ensure that clients' liberty was only infringed as long as necessary in their own or the public's interest and in ensuring the receipt of proper treatment.

In 1930, the Mental Health Act made provision for voluntary treatment and officially approved the establishment of out-patient clinics and unlocked wards. It also changed official terminology from asylum to mental hospital and from lunatic to patient or person of unsound mind. The principles of this act were strengthened by the establishment of the National Health Service in 1948. For the mentally ill this provided a single administration which went some way to prevent the two-tier system of care wherein poor people with major psychiatric illness were looked after in hospital and wealthier people were cared for in the community. It also emphasized after-care and prevention and encouraged local authorities to provide for the mentally ill.

The two main themes of early post-war policy were the establishment of therapeutic communities and of open-door policies. These reflected the new generation of radical social psychiatrists influenced by recent memories of concentration camps and war and by the effect of these open regimes on wartime neuroses. The simultaneous introduction of major tranquillizers for the treatment of psychoses is often seen to be the main impetus behind de-institutionalization; in fact it only served to accelerate a movement which had already begun (Murphy, 1991).

These piecemeal improvements in psychiatric treatment and care must be seen in the context of other pressures that were also coming to bear upon the asylums. Goffman (1961), in his classic book *Asylums*, talked of psychiatric hospitals as 'total institutions' segregated communities isolated from general life which developed practices common to other total institutions such as prisons. (Institutionalism is discussed further towards the end of this chapter.) This extreme view was one of a number raised in the late 1950s and 1960s; others questioned the existence of madness in various ways. Antipsychiatrists, for example Szasz (1973), explained madness as a simulation of craziness; Laing (1967) described psychosis as an expression of intellectual fulfilment that may be caused by the 'tyrannical bourgeois family'. Sociologists, for example Scheff (1967), asserted that psychological disorders were nothing more than the consequences of attaching an illness label to various behaviour patterns that deviate from conventional norms.

Thus the concept of institutional care came to have pejorative implications, and there was a desire for more human conditions in institutions. As reports of the conditions inside the long-stay hospitals were publicized (see Martin, 1984), a growing awareness of the need for accountability of public services, and a stronger insistence on the rights of the individual developed.

In 1953 the new climate of opinion was summarized in a World Health Organization report which condemned the 'classical' system in which the mental hospital dominated the service, operating a virtually closed system and controlling the services in the surrounding community. It asserted that this was to be replaced by a modern system in which a variety of services; in-patient, out-patient, day-care, hostels and others operated as 'tools' in the hands of the community, and the hospital became only one tool at the disposal of the medico-social team (Jones, 1972). The Royal Commission on the law relating to mental illness and mental deficiency (1957) confirmed the importance of making 'community care' a reality.

The commitment to community care has been remarkable in view of the lack of evidence that it is an effective means of providing mental health care. This begs the question 'What is community care?' and 'Why does it carry such support?'

What is community care?

The original meaning of community care has never been defined, as pointed out by Titmuss:

'And what of the everlasting garden trailer, "Community Care"? Does it not conjure up a sense of warmth and human kindness, essentially personal and comforting ...? I have tried and failed to discover in any precise form the origins of the term "Community Care"'.
Titmuss, 1968.

Whatever its precise meaning, the word 'community' is accepted positively, probably because it is confused with the quality of 'gemeinschaft' a term used by Tonnes, referring broadly to community of spirit. Yet, merely calling something a 'community'-based facility does not automatically invest it with gemeinschaft. Indeed, the word 'community' is inherent in every definition of de-institutionalization, and has become synonymous with 'non-institution'. So, for the client, the reality of community care may be no more than a change in the physical location of their care.

Ideologically, community care is less about location and more about the style of the care, increasing the emphasis on the positive aspects of clients, providing a less stigmatizing environment and promoting their development as valued members of society. It is in this sense that community care is seen to be socially and morally acceptable. Political acceptability of community care comes from the ambiguity of the term: 'community care' implies care in the community—gaining the support of libertarian radicals, and

care by the community—which appeals to fiscal radicals (Bachrach, 1978).

In the same way as the ambiguity of the meaning of community care has provided it with general support, it has also led to negative connotations which have generated extensive literature. There is great concern over the burden of caring being shifted to informal carers—mainly female relatives. It is questionable whether it is compatible for governments to rely on the unpaid labour of women whilst at the same time being committed to helping women take their full place in society as citizens and as workers.

Some have seen community care as synonymous with expenditure cuts and the decline of the welfare state. It is commonly believed that community care is both cheaper and more effective than was institutional provision for many people; but there is only limited information on precisely when one mode of care is more costly than another, and this is confounded when effectiveness is examined, since there is no consensus over what constitutes effectiveness, nor from whose point of view it should be measured.

Another concern is that community care reflects a cyclical pattern in psychiatry. In the nineteenth century institutions were built to prevent the existing neglect of the mentally ill in the community; in the twentieth century the dismantling of the institutions was partly driven by the apparent neglect of their inmates. There is now increasing legislation to reduce the subsequent neglect of the mentally ill in the community.

Thus, community care might be said to mean different things to different people—it is a versatile concept and can easily be misunderstood. This diversity is captured by Jones (1985) in her oft-quoted paragraph: 'To the politician, community care is a useful piece of rhetoric; to the sociologists it is a stick to beat institutional care with; to the civil servant it is a cheap alternative to institutional care, which can be passed to the local authorities for action or inaction; to the visionary it is the dream of the new society in which people really do care; to the social services departments, it is a nightmare of heightened public expectations and inadequate resources to meet them. We are only beginning to find out what it means to the old, the chronic sick and the handicapped'.

This section is concerned with just what community care can and should mean for people with enduring mental health problems. The focus must be on *how* care is provided rather than *where* it is provided. In order to be clear about the *kind* of care that needs to be provided we need to be clear about *who* we are trying to provide it for.

DEFINING PEOPLE WITH ENDURING MENTAL HEALTH PROBLEMS

It is not possible to discuss the needs and care of people with enduring mental health problems without first defining the population. Whilst we might all have our own ideas about who the term refers to, it is of benefit to explore the reasons why their identification has become a priority, and the problems associated with this process. In describing the characteristics and subgroups of the population, major research findings are drawn upon. It is hoped that this will not only clarify those people that this section is concerned with, but will also serve to demonstrate the relevance of such research to all service providers.

The need to identify people with enduring mental health problems

The lack of a clear definition of those with enduring mental health problems may be indicative of the diversity that exists within the group and the associated difficulties of marking precise boundaries around the group. These people do not suffer from one particular psychiatric disorder, their service-use patterns vary from years of hospitalization to none at all, and they frequently face a wide range of disabilities.

Schinnar *et al.* (1990) examined the definitions of 'severe and persistent mental illness' used in 17 different North American services. They concluded that the large differences in prevalence of this population across services resulted from differences in definitions. They go on to suggest that 'unless consensus can be reached on a framework for defining serious mental illness, treatment will depend more on the community where one resides than on the severity of mental illness'. Similarly, in Britain, *Caring for People* (DH,

1990), not only prioritizes this client group in terms of service provision, but clearly advocates common criteria to identify this group across districts and services.

Diagnosis, duration and disability

Bachrach (1988) describes three dimensions which are increasingly being used to distinguish people with enduring mental health problems: duration of time since the onset of the disorder; level of disability, or impairment in social functioning; and diagnosis. Yet in discussing the problems associated with defining 'chronicity in the mentally ill', she states that:

'First, chronic mental illness is a composite designation in which some elements are more readily ascertained than others. Second, there is no consensus on the specific character or the relative importance of the composite elements. Third, there is no consensus on the interrelationship between the composite elements'.

In short all three factors combine in defining enduring mental health problems so that no single factor is adequate. However, taken separately they provide a useful framework for describing the population.

Diagnosis

Schizophrenia has been found to be the most common diagnosis in all groups of people with enduring mental health problems. This is borne out in the survey results reported in relation to the old long-stay, new long-stay and new long-term groups. (These groups are discussed in detail on pp. 395–6). Whether in hospital, or in the community, the effectiveness of care systems must therefore be judged largely by their effectiveness in the treatment and long-term management of schizophrenia. Indeed Shepherd (1988) asserts that if community services do *not* contain a majority of schizophrenic patients, then they are not providing for those people most effected by the run down of the mental hospital. However, schizophrenia is not the only chronic and disabling condition—invalidism, loss of skills and dependence can be found in all forms of long-term disability. In a survey of long-term patients attending a large urban after clinic in Chicago, Summers and Hersh (1983) found no differences in symptomatology and social functioning between patients suffering from schizophrenia and those with other diagnoses. They conclude that 'once it is known that a patient is chronic, knowledge of living situation or social performance indicates more about a patient's functioning than does a knowledge of their diagnosis'. As Birley (1991) suggests, schizophrenia may lead to more of its sufferers developing a chronic handicap than those with other psychiatric conditions, but the reasons for this may have as much to do with the previous personality and adjustment of the patient as with the particular nature of the neuropsychological disturbance.

The next largest group in terms of diagnosis are those suffering from an affective disorder—depression or manic depressive disorder—and the remaining 25–30% have primary diagnosis of personality disorder or some kind of organic disorder ranging from drug or alcohol abuse to dementias. Many people have multiple impairments: the diagnosis of psychiatric disorder is associated with physical disability, blindness, deafness, epilepsy, brain damage, addiction to alcohol and other drugs, mental retardation or dementia (Wing and Morris, 1981).

Most research attention has focused on long-term patients with a diagnosis of schizophrenia (e.g. Wing and Brown, 1970; Hoult, 1986), although this may serve a high proportion of the population, it has been assumed to provide a model for all people with enduring mental health problems. In fact, it effectively excludes those with other primary diagnoses; in practice, it is those people with a personality disorder who are most disadvantaged through this approach of personality disorder (Showalter, 1987). It is these patients who are becoming recognized as a major problem today; they are in danger of fitting no group in terms of mental health service planning (Wintersteen and Rapp, 1986).

Duration

The most common categorization of the client group is based on their history of contact with hospital. This is usefully viewed in the context of mental illness in the total population, Goldberg and Huxley (1980) describe the filter between primary health care in the community, through psychiatric out-patient clinics to admission to a mental hospital. Two hundred and fifty people in a population of 1,000 each year experience mental health problems, of these 230 refer themselves to their general practitioner, of these 17 are referred to a psychiatrist and six are admitted to specialist psychiatric services. At each level there are different patterns of social correlates; for example more married women consult their GPs with problems of a psychiatric nature than any other group; more single men are seen in psychiatric out-patient clinics and more single people from social class V are admitted. The most important single factor in determining a person's passage through the system is the severity of the original disturbance; at every stage in the system only the more severely disturbed move on, and the most disturbed move from community to hospital very quickly.

Once in hospital further filtering takes place. Most people are discharged within a matter of months (in the US, Bachrach (1988) found 25% discharged within one week, 40% discharged within two weeks). After one year in hospital the prospect of discharge is very slim; in 1976 less than 5% of all discharges from mental hospitals in England and Wales had been in hospital for more than one year (DOH, 1986). Two-thirds of all admissions are re-admissions who find their way into hospital through psychiatric services that have retained contact since their first episode.

Thus people become recognized as having enduring mental health problems, either through repeated admissions or through remaining in hospital over a long period of time. However, attempts to define those with enduring mental health problems in terms of length of stay or frequency of admissions vary between districts and between services. This points to the inadequacy of this single criteria to define this population. Indeed, if specialist services for those with enduring mental health problems depend upon admission history to select appropriate clients, they may effectively deny access to a large group within the targeted population. Hospital-based measures are becoming increasingly irrelevant as services become more community based. Moreover the move towards community care provision is geographically patchy in that admission procedures vary from district to district, and any standardized criteria based on hospital use would include very different patient groups.

Disability

Disability or 'handicap' in the mentally ill refers to physical, social and psychological difficulties. It has been clearly analysed in relation to people with enduring mental health problems by Wing and Morris (1981), who define it as 'the state of an individual who is unable to perform socially up to the standards expected by him or herself, by people important to him or her, or by society in general'. Wing's classification of handicap in terms of its origins is a useful framework for understanding some of the problems that patients experience in terms of disability.

Premorbid handicap refers to disabilities that pre-existed the illness itself. They may be related to the illness, for example characteristics and problems as a child or having a parent with mental illness. Or they may be unrelated, for example physical disability or low intelligence.

Primary handicap refers to those disabilities that arise directly from the illness itself, or the psychiatric symptoms such as anxiety, depression, delusional beliefs, hallucinations, retardation, withdrawal, and poverty of thought and speech. The primary symptoms of people with enduring mental health problems are disturbances of thinking, concentration or emotional response, and problems of lethargy and lack of motivation. Odd or unacceptable behaviours and poor social relationship are frequently present. Often, there is also a vulnerability to being upset by the smallest life events (Brown *et al.*, 1972). The most common syndromes associated with this group and generally seen in chronic schizophrenia are social withdrawal, apathy, slowness, underactivity, flattened affect (or mood) and difficulty in communicating due to poverty of speech and poor non-verbal skills. These inevitably lead to disturbances in relationships both within the family and with the public in general.

Secondary handicap refers to the disabilities that arise from having been mentally ill, currently or in the past. They include both those that may follow treatment, such as dependency and loss of skills as a result of 'institutional' care, lethargy and other effects of drugs; and, the effect of the illness on other people such as relatives, carers and employers. The social consequences of the latter category may result in loss of social status, and restricted access to jobs and housing. Secondary handicaps thus comprise a wide range of physical, psychological and social disadvantages. Because of the stigma of mental illness people often suffer a great deal of secondary handicap with only minimal primary symptoms. In fact, studies of stigma, as felt by psychiatric patients, suggest that it is highly related to continuing disability and its accompanying demoralization (Gove, 1975).

Birley (1991), examines not only the 'origins' of disability, but also the 'mechanisms' or ways in which such handicaps may have developed. He includes:

---

1 *Cognitive disturbance*, where the patient does not filter internal and external information in the normal way, so has a poor attention and concentration, and may withdraw in order to reduce input from the environment.

2 *Cognitive distortion*, which refers to the effect of delusions and hallucinations on the patient's view of the world. These lead to a degree of distortion and misinterpretation of the environment, including the behaviour and language of others.

3 *Failure to recognize social or affective cues*, shyness, difficulties in making friends, and awkwardness in company may be due to difficulty in recognizing social signals such as posture, expression or words. It is not clear whether this is due to a specific problem, or more generally associated with focusing attention.

Birley (1991) suggests that although the mechanisms responsible are not understood, the effects of self neglect, retardation, mood disturbance, vulnerability and sensitivity constitute further handicaps. It is important to acknowledge the importance of the contribution of 'institutionalism' to disability, and this is described below.

Surveys of the long-term, mentally ill indicate that of the population as a whole over half have problems with some aspect of social functioning. In a survey of the long-stay population in five hospitals scheduled for closure, Clifford (1989) found that 40% had moderate or high levels of social functioning; 22% low, and 35% poor or very poor. More than half the population surveyed needed supervision with basic activities of daily living and the 'vast majority' were unable to shop or cook for themselves or use public transport unaided. The new long-stay group reflects even greater levels of problems with high levels of difficulty in most areas of functioning. Of those new long-stay patients not awaiting transfer into a community resource, 80% had problems with self care and 90% had some idiosyncratic problem that was difficult to manage. Less is known of the new long-term group, but studies of young adult chronic patients (18–35-year-olds) report problems in social functioning in over 50% of the subjects studied (Pepper *et al.*, 1981).

INSTITUTIONALIZATION

Any account of the needs and care of people with enduring mental health problems would not be complete without reference to the problems of institutionalization. Despite the increasing proportion of care provided in the community, institutionalism continues to occur. The origin and nature of the problems associated with institutionalism are described.

It was a psychiatrist (Barton, 1959) who first described the behaviour of long-stay patients as 'institutional syndrome'. He characterized this as typically presenting apathy, lack of initiative, loss of interest and apparent inability to plan for the future, submissiveness, deterioration in personal habits and standards generally, and loss of individuality and resigned acceptance that things will go on as they are, unchangingly, inevitably and indefinitely. Barton suggested that this behaviour

was a response to factors in the institutional environment, and represented the most trouble-free way of coping with these. He categorized the factors most commonly found in the environment under eight headings: loss of contact with the outside world; enforced idleness; brutality, browbeating and teasing by the staff; bossiness of staff; loss of personal friends, possessions and personal events; drugs; ward atmosphere and the loss of prospects outside the institution.

However, the concept of institutionalization or institutionalism, is essentially a sociological one, and it was sociologists who identified it with asylums. Most notably Goffman (1961) talked of psychiatric hospitals as a form of 'total institution' a segregated community, isolated from general life which developed practices common to other such vital institutions, for example prisons:

All these institutions are 'total' in that residents work, sleep and play in the same place.

They are segregated from general social life, and residents have restricted contact with life outside.

There are rigid routines guiding every detail of inmates' lives, designed to ensure smooth running of the institution rather than for the benefit of the inmates.

They are regimented and employ block treatment, the same rules and practices apply to everyone irrespective of their individual needs.

They are depersonalizing: patients are not accorded their individual rights and status as people.

There is a large social distance between staff and residents.

Residents have little control over what happens, decisions are made by staff.

Residents are deprived of normal social roles.

In short, mental hospitals like other institutions were considered to be authoritarian, custodial and deadening, they were seen to produce the apathetic, shambling, inactive patients found on long-stay wards.

However, the belief that all long-stay patients' problems were the consequences of prolonged exposure to an institution regime was probably naive. Wing (1962) and Wing and Brown (1970) examined the interaction between premorbid, primary and secondary handicaps and the social environment found in large institutions. Premorbid handicaps such as poor education, physical disability and poor social networks were found to render a person particularly susceptible to the effects of institutions. Primary handicaps are markedly influenced by different social environments: over-stimulation can lead to a breakdown or exacerbation of florid symptoms, whilst under-stimulation can lead to social withdrawal, passivity, inertia and the lack of interest associated with institutionalization. In terms of secondary handicaps (not part of the illness itself, but the effects of being ill), once admitted to hospital people cease to perform normal social roles. The longer they stay in hospital the more likely they are to lose the ability to perform these roles. The expectations of staff within the institute become paramount and the person is unlikely to want to leave.

This social psychiatry position offers a synthesis between the traditional psychiatric view and the extreme sociological position, and is supported by the findings that institutionalization is not associated exclusively with large mental homes. The institutional practices are characteristic of a large institution and can also occur in smaller units, not staffed by professionals (King *et al.*, 1971).

Wing and Brown (1970) showed a relationship between social poverty of the hospital environment and clinical poverty of the residents. One of the critical variables was the amount of time the resident was allowed to spend doing absolutely nothing. However, there is evidence that this kind of social under-stimulation has the same harmful effects on schizophrenic patients in non-hospital settings; Brown *et al* (1966) found evidence of this in some forms of community residential accommodation. This was confirmed by Ryan (1979) who found that group homes can actually promote inactivity.

CATEGORIES OF PEOPLE WITH ENDURING MENTAL HEALTH PROBLEMS

Duration of contact with services, and the nature of this contact, have been used to identify three subgroups of people with enduring mental health problems (Wing and Morris, 1981). These are the 'old long-stay', the 'new long-stay' and the 'new long-term'. These terms are commonly used in practice, although inevitably over simplified. They provide a useful reference to people with clearly differentiated histories and needs.

Old long-stay

These people are generally considered to be those who have been in hospital for over five years. They have often grown old there and are increasingly physically frail. In 1977, Christie-Brown *et al.* surveyed 220 patients who had remained in hospital for a period of over five years. They had an average age of 54 years, were predominantly single, male, and had been in hospital for 21 years on average. The majority had a diagnosis of schizophrenia, and 20% had significant physical disabilities. A more recent survey by Ford *et al.* (1987) found a smaller proportion of patients on the old long-stay group, but an older, frailer population with 30% of patients aged over 75 years. Perhaps the most striking finding in relation to this group is their social isolation. Ford *et al.* (1987) reported that 50% of this old long-stay group were rarely or never visited and 74% seldom went out of the hospital. This reflects a general trend due to the more able patients being discharged earlier, and those with most needs being difficult to place outside the hospital. As Shepherd (1988) comments, in order to survive in the community they will need a great deal of supervision in view of their physical frailty and the duration of their hospitalization, and also appropriate day facilities, extensive rehabilitation and social supports.

New long-stay

These patients have remained in hospital for between one and five years. This group is distinguished from the old long-stay group who were admitted earlier without the benefits of newer treatments and whose clinical disability was, in some part, due to the lack of social stimulation provided by psychiatric institutions (Wing and Morris, 1981). Clifford (1989) suggests that as de-institutionalization and new philosophies continue, this group should be expanded to include patients hospitalized for between one and ten years. Mann and Cree (1976) surveyed 400 patients from 15 different hospitals, all of whom had been in-patients for a period of between one and three years and presented a detailed report of their characteristics. The most common diagnosis was schizophrenia, and 16% had a severe physical disability. Although they constitute less than 7% of all hospital admissions, they are by their very nature the most disabled individuals currently presenting to psychiatric services. Despite their relative youth, they have long psychiatric histories and considerable social and occupational problems. They generally remain in hospital because they have tried to live in a variety of alternative settings unsuccessfully.

As with old long-stay patients, the prevalence of this group varies depending on local demography, the availability of community provision, and local admission and discharge policies. But in all areas where records are kept, there is evidence of their accumulation. Community care provision needs to recognize the need for specialist services to meet the needs of this particular group. They are likely to require intensive, long-term rehabilitation with a highly staffed, multiprofessional team. In accordance with the philosophy of community care, this will ideally be provided in small domestic-scale settings which are integrated with the local community as far as possible.

New long-term

These are people who do not stay in hospital over long periods of time, but make frequent use of a variety of services on a prolonged and repeated basis. Sturt *et al.* (1982) calculated the prevalence of the group to be 139 per 100,000, and in a survey of a well-resourced London Borough found that their average age was 52 years, 60%

were female, and 47% had a diagnosis of schizophrenia.

'Young adult chronic patients'

It is within this group that a new group of patients has been identified who pose particular problems for service providers. In the US they have been termed 'young adult chronic patients', or YACPs. They are generally considered to be aged between 18 and 35 years, and are characterized by a pattern of poor engagement in services, yet they may be dependent on multiple care resources (Prevost, 1982; Bachrach, 1984a). Their compliance with prescribed medication is poor yet alcohol and poly-drug abuse is reported to be exceptionally high (Pepper, 1981; Caton, 1981). They have been found to have 50% more multiple diagnoses than other age groups, are more likely to commit suicide (Pepper *et al.*, 1981) and more likely to have been arrested (Test *et al.*, 1990). They have marked impairment in social functioning, and a frequent but problematic pattern of service use and misuse. They typically are difficult to engage in services, have a high likelihood of forensic history, poor social supports, and homelessness and mobility between district services. They are also more likely than other groups to have a dual diagnosis, often including personality disorder or substance abuse (Bachrach, 1984a; Wintersteen & Rapp, 1986).

Sheets *et al.* (1982) describe the characteristics of this client group in more depth: they suggest that 'young adults with chronic disabilities may have youth and loneliness in common, but that they differ dramatically from one another'. They interviewed 22 direct service providers in various parts of New York and identified three distinct groups of patients with distinct characteristics, service needs and wants. These included a low-energy, low-demand group; a high-energy, high-demand group; and a high-functioning, high-aspiration group. They key features of this hypothcsizcd typology are shown below:

Hypothesized typology of young adult chronic patients
(Sheets *et al.,* 1982)

Low-energy, low-demand group

Well ensconced in the role of the patient

Do not do well, even in remission

Concretely attached to programmes and programme places

Probably entered mental health system in early adolescence

Passive, poorly motivated

Accepting of mental health services

Appear burned out at an early age

High-energy, high-demand group
Able to shop around and get what they want

Fluctuating functional abilities and interests

'Give me what I want or stay out of my life' attitude

Low frustration tolerance, act out, encounters with the law

Frequently evicted, mobile

Expectations of self reliance

Included 'revolving door' patients and street people

High-functioning group
Generally have higher socioeconomic status

Better appearance

New to mental health system

Resist involvement with services on the basis of conviction

May have entered system due to substance abuse

Want to understand their disorder and reduce relapse

Want to blend into local population

Although in the US these three groups have been associated only with clients in younger age groups, they provide a useful profile of the difference between all long-term clients in the community. Certainly anyone working with this client group is likely to encounter people of all ages who share the characteristics of these groups. Indeed, it might be suggested that the characteristics associated with 'young adult chronic patients' are associated less with age than with their history of service use, and may be true of the new long-term group as a whole.

The importance of planning services to meet the needs of this new long-term group cannot be underestimated. An increasing number of people with enduring mental health problems will fall into this group as hospitals close and the duration of admissions becomes shorter. It is likely that at some time these clients will need hospitalization, either during crises, to provide intensive rehabilitation, or to give informal carers respite. But, whereas prior to de-institutionalization they would have spent long periods of time in hospital, their admissions are now likely to be short and repetitive. On the whole they live in the community, in need of a variety of residential, day, and domiciliary care and support from a number of sources.

OPERATIONALIZING 'ENDURING MENTAL HEALTH PROBLEMS'

People with enduring mental health problems are those who show most disability in terms of primary and secondary handicaps, rather than those with a particular type of diagnosis. However, the questions remain as to how long a disability must persist before it qualifies as an enduring mental health problem, and how to deal with the episodic and fluctuating nature of the problems. Once defined as a member of this group, is it possible to lose the label?

In giving priority to people with enduring mental health problems as recommended in the NHS and Community Care Act (1990), all services must find some way of defining the population. The criteria used by the Nottingham Needs Assessment Project (1990) are shown below:

Criteria for defining people with enduring mental health problems (Nottingham Needs Assessment Planning Project, 1990)

1 Three or more admissions in two years

2 Continuous attendance at a day resource for more than a year

3 Two or more years' continuous contact with psychiatric services

4 A continuous stay in hospital of six months or more in the last three years

5 Prescribed major tranquillizers continuously for one year or more

6 Lives in sheltered accommodation as a result of mental health problems

7 Major impairment of functioning/motivation/daily living skills

8 Carer or client makes frequent requests for help

9 Has severe and enduring problems that in opinion of service provider warrants client in need of inclusion in this population

---

(Clients were considered to meet the definition if they fulfilled two or more criteria.) This is a broad list to identify all clients with the needs associated with enduring mental health problems to be identified. The next step is for all these people to be assessed in order to prioritize those in need of more or less intensive service input.

THE PREVALENCE OF ENDURING MENTAL HEALTH PROBLEMS

The numbers of people within the three categories of enduring mental health problems have changed over the past two decades. The short and new long-stay groups have remained stable whereas the old long-stay group has declined. This is due to discharges as the less disturbed old long-stay group are moved into community resources, and to deaths from this ageing population.

The average number of people who remain in hospital for over a year despite resettlement policies is 12–15 per 100,000 per year, a figure that has remained stable since 1976. Wing and Morris (1981) estimated that there were approximately 420 per 100,000 of the population who had been in touch with psychiatric services for more than one year (giving a national estimate of 210,000 people).

In Nottingham, over 1,700 people were identified as meeting the criteria of enduring mental health problems shown above. This is likely to be an underestimate since it did not include those people who had lost contact with services or were only in contact with their general practitioner. It does, however, illustrate the high numbers of people fitting a broad definition of enduring mental health problems, and gives some idea of the size of service required to ensure that even the most minimal needs are met.

USERS' VIEWS

Although the reasons for defining people with enduring mental health problems have been described, it is important to set out the users' views on this categorization, and to take these into account, both in practice, and when reading this section, in order to balance the generalizations that are made and the sometimes negative picture that is painted.

A group of users offering their view on community care, describe the problems they see in delineating 'people with severe long-term mental illness' (Beeforth *et al.*, 1990). They feel that any categorization runs the risk of discounting differences between individuals, and that this particular category conflates the separate issues of severity and longevity. To this group of users, categorizing people into groups takes no account of the different paths that people take through serious problems, nor of their strengths, good periods, personalities or situations, rather it implies hopelessness and uniformity.

'What's more, there is no acknowledgement that the problems originate outside you—the illness becomes part of you, presumably some kind of inherent defect. And that means your views are likely to be discredited—as indeed happens now when users are disbelieved by the police when they are burgled, or by their GP when they are physically ill'.

MARGINALIZED GROUPS

In society as a whole, people with mental health problems are marginalized, stigmatized and accorded low priority in terms of policy and local health and social service planning. Within this much neglected group, those with enduring mental health problems have lower status. Even within this second-class world, women and people from ethnic minorities are likely to be treated as second-class citizens.

Gender issues

Although studies of the long-term mentally ill show little proportional difference between male and female patients, admissions to mental hospitals as a whole show highest numbers of unmarried men and married women. In further analysis of hospital admissions as a whole women have been found to come into contact with psychiatric services later, and are diagnosed later (Test and Berlin, 1981; Bachrach, 1984b; 1985). This may be due to an absence of pathology, later breakdown or a better prognosis, but in discussing the research results, the authors speculate that it is possibly due to society having lower expectations of women, perceiving their role as inferior and more passive.

Research focusing on younger chronic patients has found that the majority are male, generally between 55 and 66% (e.g. Pepper *et al.*, 1981; Bachrach, 1984a). However, findings are rarely analysed by gender and it is unclear whether reported problems of substance abuse, high arrest rates, suicide and irregular service utilization are problematic only for young adult males, or whether young women with serious mental illness also experience problems in these areas.

Bachrach (1984) has argued that de-institutionalization has had 'special effects' on severely disabled women in such areas as sexual exploitation and violence, homelessness, diversion into the criminal justice system and stigmatization. She found that, in the US, programmes for men with enduring mental health problems are likely to be based on higher expectations of performance than are programmes for women (Bachrach, 1985). These expectations are reflected in different patterns of placement in community services and different emphases in treatment planning. A similar picture was found in a long-term care and rehabilitation service in London, by Perkins and Rowland (1991). Whilst the functioning level of men and women did not differ, women were under-represented amongst those receiving a high level of input from the service. Perkins (1991) concludes that the stereotyping of women as passive, emotional and childlike tends to deprive them of access to the care that they need. Service providers need not only to be aware of these issues, but to look at effective ways of ensuring that they do not follow these patterns.

Ethnicity

There is a great variation in health status between ethnic minority groups, and between them and the native population (Townsend, 1980). Taking rates of mental hospital admissions for paranoid schizophrenia, Cochrane (1977) found differences between 80 to 100 admissions per 100,000 population over 15 years of British, Italian, German and American males and 290 admissions of West Indian males for the same population. Harrison *et al.* (1988) found even greater differences in the incidence of schizophrenia in British and second generation West Indian adults in Nottingham. Explanations in terms of different expectations of the role of psychiatry, racial discrimination and different understandings of mental illness have been offered.

However, studies of the long-term mentally ill very rarely analyse the results by ethnic origin, or mention the proportion of the population from ethnic minority groups. It appears that whereas they are over-represented in acute services, they are under-represented in long-term services. This may be due to these groups finding these services unable to meet their needs. Perkins and Rowland (1991) found that although 25% of referrals to the District Services Centre in London were Afro-Caribbean, 58% of those who failed to engage in the service were Afro-Caribbean. As Murphy (1991) recounts, black people find services overwhelmingly dominated by middle class, white professionals who know little of black culture; they naturally resist accepting help from these people they do not trust. They often attend services in crisis, unwillingly; they are more likely to be locked in secure settings, more likely to be treated with drugs and electroconvulsive therapy, and professionals are likely to spend less time with them.

Many of these problems are deeply embedded in cultural differences, and in the current disadvantaged position of ethnic minorities in Britain as a whole. Improving this situation depends upon fundamental changes in educational and employment opportunities within the whole society. Similarly, within mental health services, the aim is for a totally integrated service, responsive to the needs and differences of people from all races and cultures. This can only evolve through service planners and providers actively considering the special needs of their local ethnic populations, consulting users, their families, community leaders and organizations in planning services as a whole, and each individual client.

COMMUNITY CARE PROBLEMS IN PRACTICE

The problems of community care present a difficult reality for clients and their families. The practical difficulties faced by these people and by service planners and providers are explored in this section.

Problems with the system

In 1986 the Audit Commission found that up to 37,000 people had been discharged from long-stay wards in the last 10 years but nobody knew where most of these people were. Griffiths responded to this concern:

'A system involving the assignment of a person in need of support to an individual carer, so as to become his responsibility is rarely made, even when applicable, for example in the case of patients discharged from long-stay hospitals'. *Griffiths, 1988*

The identification of an individual person to take responsibility for people in need is not only applicable to old long-stay patients, it is equally important for those who have spent short periods in hospital, but who remain dependent on psychiatric services. This need has become increasingly visible as people with long-term problems have filled acute beds in general hospital units despite the bulk of their needs being for social care. They are generally unemployed, sometimes homeless, usually unable to survive independently, and in need of intensive support over a long time period.

Whereas traditional institutions provided every aspect of care under the same roof, the effect of community care is to disperse services, workers and clients. The effects of this are increasingly becoming apparent for clients with enduring mental health problems who are often involved with several different parts of the service; for example, they may see their psychiatrist as an out-patient for review of their medication, are visited by a community psychiatric nurse for monitoring and support, attend one or more day centres and drop-in centres, and possibly live in some kind of supported accommodation. Other care staff may be called in when they are needed, for example a social worker may visit to advise on benefits or sort out housing problems, their GP is called on for physical problems, an occupational therapist may assess their self-care skills, or undertake social skills training. On top of all this, if they relapse they may be admitted to an acute ward, introduced to a new care team, and probably discharged to a new set of services and personnel. This host of staff has no identified anchor point. They all work on limited information, and often see their role as specific rather than holistic. They may assume someone else is detailing with particular problems—which allows the client to drop out of the service, or several services to duplicate the same care—giving conflicting messages to the client and managing their own time inefficiently.

For the client it is difficult to know who to turn to with which problems, the system is confusing and some aspect of it is always changing; long-term relationships with care staff are rare. They may well feel they are being shunted around the system rather than taking an active part in it.

The real problem with the system is that it has not been set up with the long-term client group in mind. It is best suited for people who use one service at a time, improve and can be discharged. People with enduring mental health problems are not only likely to be in contact with different parts of the service, they also, by the very nature of their problems, are likely to need help for a very long time. There will be times when they withdraw from services, reject help and lose insight into their needs, putting themselves at risk. Since services generally work on a throughput model, seeing clients move on as they improve, or rejecting clients as they do not attend when scheduled, they are rarely in a position to provide outreach services which can pursue clients who have withdrawn from contact. Also there is no identified person to work with the client in the long term to help them gain insight and understanding into the patterns of their symptoms and the interventions that might help them.

Problems for service providers

People with enduring mental health problems offer particular challenges to direct service providers; their prognosis is on the whole poor, progress is slow and often hampered with setbacks; they may well be difficult to engage in services; they may not be appreciative, and may not cooperate with the ideas of staff. This paints a bleak picture, but it is these factors that lead staff working with this client group to burn out quickly and either leave, or bring a demoralized and negative attitude to their work. This client group is not given high status by nurses undertaking training courses in community psychiatric nursing, and

they rarely choose to specialize in the care of this group (Brooker, 1990). Since it is these nurses who are likely to become the managers and teachers of the future, the low status accorded these clients is likely to be perpetuated. Even those nurses working with this client group, tend to focus their attention in the less disabled; Community psychiatric nurses in Salford were found to concentrate on the administration of medication for clients with schizophrenia, and spent significantly less time with individual psychotic clients than they did with people suffering from neuroses (Wooff and Goldberg, 1988).

It is not only individual staff who move towards less disabled client groups; Sayce *et al.*, 1991 found a general trend 'up-market' among day centres. Although the centres studied were set up for long-term client groups, they progressively specialized and focused on clients who might respond positively to the care offered. The picture in North America is similar, case management systems set up to provide services for the most severely disabled clients have moved away from those most in need, and subsequently more intensive teams have been organized to provide for those no longer served by the original case managers.

Job satisfaction will always be low if people working with these clients pursue a 'cure' philosophy of care, there will be less staff burn out, better job satisfaction, slower staff turnover, and less inclination for the service to move up-market if the guiding philosophy is geared towards maximizing clients' functioning in a variety of roles. This is a key value in the third section of this chapter.

Problems for the client

Service users not only suffer as a result of the problems within the mental health service system, they have wider ranging difficulties in the areas of housing, finance and employment.

Housing

Accommodation is related to personal, financial, social and support issues, all of which are magnified for people with ongoing mental health problems. Obtaining and maintaining suitable housing is increasingly difficult for anyone in view of the national housing shortage. For people with a history of mental illness, often unemployed, it is not only difficult to find landlords willing to consider them as tenants, but the stress resulting from poor housing conditions and homelessness contributes to their vulnerability and the likelihood of further breakdown of their mental health. The nature of the problems that they endure often means that these individuals do not have the persistence and motivation to maintain necessary payments. They often live in less than satisfactory conditions, not through choice but because of the effort involved in the day-to-day running of a reasonable home.

Recent literature reflects increasing concern about the lack of monitoring and evaluation in many types of accommodation used by this client group (for example, board and lodgings, bed and breakfast accommodation and registered homes). Warden *et al.* (1990) also found that clients in registered homes face dire financial problems and that the care provided has no formal monitoring.

Much attention has also been placed on the increasing problems of homelessness. In March 1990 Roger Freeman stated in Parliament that there were up to 3,000 homeless people with mental health problems living on the streets of London. Others have estimated that up to 40% of the homeless population are mentally ill (Timms and Fry, 1989). These numbers are contributed to by the number of new long-term clients who are characteristically itinerant and cross district boundaries becoming lost to services.

MIND, the National Association for Mental Health, points to the limitations of referring solely to those people living on the streets. Homelessness includes those living in squats, bed and breakfast hotels and temporary hostels. These situations place an inevitable strain on people's mental health. MIND suggests that people do not become homeless as a direct result of hospital discharge or community care policies, but that it is due to chronic housing shortages that effect disadvantaged groups disproportionately.

Finance

Wing and Morris (1981) identified poverty as a social disadvantage that maintains or amplifies the social disablement of people with enduring mental health problems. Since the majority of these people are unemployed, the majority live in poverty. As in the case of managing their accommodation, people often find the benefit system impossible to understand. The hours of form filling and waiting in benefits offices places huge demands on people who find social contact difficult, and often have symptoms of anxiety and paranoia.

The level of the benefits available also places severe limitations on the quality of life of these people. Warden *et al.* (1990) suggest that poverty has the effect of 'sentencing these people to live within their sickness'; they found that residents in registered homes generally received only £10 per week to cover all personal expenses: clothes, newspapers, cigarettes, snacks and all the other items beyond food and shelter that allow some quality of life, through involvement in amenities open to the general public.

Employment

Owing to the level of impairment in social functioning within the population with enduring mental health problems, the employment situation as a whole, and to the resistance of employers to employing people with mental health problems, the majority of this group are unemployed. This not only places them in a financially disadvantaged position, they also lack the status that work affords. They do not have a structure to their day, nor do they have the regular social contact that work offers. The lack of work also deprives them of the affirmation and satisfaction of achieving something. Their days may be isolated and unstructured passages of time—they may be required to vacate their accommodation for certain hours of the day, yet they do not have the money to make choices about how they spend this time.

Poor occupational stability is associated with poor educational qualifications. These can be seen as leading to mental illness or as a result of it, as Shepherd (1984) surmises 'The past is often a good guide to the future'. A tendency to need long-term care and difficulty engaging in day care have both been associated with unstable employment prior to admission (Bender and Pilling, 1985).

The problems for carers

It is estimated that relatives and friends provide the bulk of community care for about two million chronically ill and disabled people under the age of 65 years in England and Wales (DH, 1989). This is not surprising when one considers the prognosis of schizophrenia; Wing (1982) found that up to 75% of patients with a diagnosis of schizophrenia have persistent disabilities or recurrent attacks at follow up. Kuipers and Bebbington (1988) found that five years after they were first diagnosed, 90% of sufferers were living in the community and as many as two-thirds lived with relatives. The onus on relatives to meet the needs of these people inevitably leads to the carers themselves having needs. Kuipers and Bebbington found this was due to normal reciprocal arrangements breaking down such that the carer ends up doing more for the client, and consequently the carer's usual activities are restricted.

Many studies have focused on the burden placed on carers through living with a person with mental illness. Wing *et al.* (1964) found that for two-thirds of patients discharged to live with their families, relationships were subsequently 'strained beyond tolerable limits'. The reasons for the hardship on the relationship have been identified as the stigma of mental illness, the fear of social discrimination and subsequent reduction in family friends, and the stress caused by spending up to 60 hours a week in face-to-face contact with the person with mental health problems. An added difficulty is the financial effect of living with someone with enduring mental health problems. The income into the home is reduced either through the breadwinner becoming ill, or because relatives cannot work because they need to care for the patient.

Relatives have difficulties coming to terms with the changes in their role and in their relationship with the identified patient. They suffer grief over the loss of the 'old person'. They feel guilt, rejection, fear, anger and their level of distress appears to increase over time (Kuipers and Bebbington, 1988). Despite their problems, relatives receive little help or advice. An idea of the problems felt by these people is possible when one considers the pleas for help and advice from the National Schizophrenia Fellowship (the main voluntary organization for carers for people with schizophrenia). In 1988, they received more than 5,000 calls, over 3,000 of which were for general advice, others were concerned with community care and treatment, family support, accommodation, social services, obtaining benefits, legal advice and hospital care. As Groves (1990) states, one of the hardest things about caring for a relative with mental health problems is that it is often a forced choice. The alternatives for service user are limited, and for relatives, the guilt of subjecting a member of their family to bed and breakfast or hostel accommodation may appear worse than living with them.

The problems of living with someone with mental health problems are not all one way; the negative symptoms of schizophrenia such as withdrawal and apathy are particularly difficult for carers to cope with. They have been found to view these handicaps critically, as signs of laziness, selfishness and uselessness (Wing and Creer, 1974). Where the emotional atmosphere in the home is critical or over-involved, relapse has been found to be hastened (Leff and Vaughn, 1985). The needs of families are explored further in the final section of this chapter.

Users' views

This section ends with reference to the views of the most important people to consider when planning or providing care, the service users. The views of the users have already been described in relation to categorizing people with enduring mental health problems. This same group explains their views on co-ordinating community care clearly and articulately (Beeforth *et al.*, 1990). They offer a poignant summary of the problems of community care:

'The problem with community care is not just about management. It's about misery, poverty and a style of mental health service that offers no real choice about the type of support available'.

The problems presented by community care have eventually led to policy changes. These are described in the following section, with particular emphasis on case management.

REFERENCES

Bachrach, L.L. (1978) A conceptual approach to deinstitutionalisation. *Hospital and Community Psychiatry*, **29**, 573–578.

Bachrach, L.L. (1984a) The concept of YACPs, questions from a research perspective. *Hospital and Community Psychiatry*, **35**, 537–580.

Bachrach, L.L. (1984b) Deinstitutionalisation and women: assessing the consequences of public policy. *American Psychologist*, **39**, 1171–1177.

Bachrach, L.L. (1985) Chronically mentally ill women: emergence and legitimation. *Hospital and Community Psychiatry*, **36**, 1063–1069.

Bachrach, L.L. (1988) Defining Mental Illness: A Concept Paper. *Hospital and Community Psychiatry*, **38**(4), 383–388.

Barton, R. (1959) *Institutional Neurosis*. Bristol: Wright.

Beeforth, M., Conlon, E., Field, V., Hoser, B. & Sayce, L. (1990) *Whose Service is it Anyway? Users' Views on Co-ordinating Community Care*. London: Research and Development for Psychiatry.

Bender, K. (1981) YACPs: visibility and style of interaction in treatment. *Hospital and Community Psychiatry*, **32**, 475–478.

Bender, M. & Pilling, S. (1985) A study of variables associated with under-attendance at a psychiatric day centre. *Psychological Medicine*, **15**, 395–401.

Bennett, D. & Freeman, H. (1991) Principles and prospect. In Bennett D. & Freeman H. (Eds) *Community Psychiatry*, London: Churchill Livingstone.

Birley, J. (1991) Schizophrenia: the problems of handicap. In Bennett D & Freeman H. (Eds) *Community Psychiatry*, London: Churchill Livingstone.

Brooker, C.G.D. (1990) A description of clients nursed by community psychiatric nurses whilst attending English National Board Course No. 811: clarification of current role. *Journal of Advanced Nursing*, **15**, 155–156.

Brown, G.W. (1966) *Schizophrenia and Social Care*. Oxford: Oxford University Press.

Brown, G.W., Birley, J.L.T. & Wing, J.K. (1972) Influence of family life on the course of schizophrenic disorders: a replication. *British Journal of Psychiatry*, **121**, 241–258.

Caton, C.L.M. (1981) The new chronic patient and the system of community care. *Hospital and Community Psychiatry*, **32**, 479–500.

Christie-Brown, J.R.W., Ebringer, L. & Freedman, K.S. (1977) A survey of long-stay psychiatric populations: implications for community service. *Psychological Medicine*, **7**, 113–126.

Clifford, P. & Webb, Y. (1989) Assessment of needs of long-stay patients in 5 hospitals. National Unit for Psychiatric Research and Development, London.

Cochrane, R. (1977) Mental illness in immigrants to England and Wales. *Social Psychiatry*, **12**, 25–35.

D'Arcy, C. & Brockman, J. (1977) Public rejection of the ex-mental patient: are attitudes changing? *Canadian Review of Sociology and Anthropology*, **14**, 68–80.

Department of Health (DH) (1986) *Mental Health Statistics for England*. Booklet 12. London: HMSO.

Department of Health (DH) (1989) *Caring for People*. London: HMSO.

Department of Health (DH) (1990) *NHS and Community Care Act*. London: HMSO.

Ford, M., Goddard, C. & Lansdall, R. (1987) The dismantling of the mental hospital? Glenside Hospital Surveys 1960–1985. *British Journal of Psychiatry*, **151**, 479–485.

Frame, J. (1980) *Faces in the water*. London. Women's Press.

Goffman, E. (1961) *Asylums*. Harmondsworth: Pelican.

Goldberg, D. & Huxley, P. (1980) *Mental Illness in the Community*. London: Tavistock.

Gove, W.L. (1975) Labelling mental illness: a critique. In Gove W.L. (Ed.) *The Labelling of Deviance*. New York: Wiley.

Groves, T. (1990) What does community care mean now? *British Medical Journal*, **300**, 1060–1062.

Harrison, G., Owens, D., Holton, A., Neilson, D. & Boot, D. (1988) A prospective study of severe mental disorder in Afro-Caribbean patients. *Psychological Medicine*, **18**, 643–657.

Hoult, J. (1986) Community care of the acutely mentally ill. *British Journal of Psychiatry*, **149**, 137–144.

Jones, K. (1972) A History of Mental Health Services. Routledge and Kegan Paul, London.

Jones, K. (1975) *After Hospital: A Study of Long Term Psychiatric Patients in York*. York: Department of Social Policy and Social Work, York University.

King, R., Raynes, N. & Tizard, J. (1971) *Patterns of Residential Care*. London: Routledge & Kegan Paul.

Kuipers, L. & Bebbington, P. (1988) Expressed emotion research in schizophrenia: theoretical and clinical implications. *Psychological Medicine*, **18**, 893–909.

Laing, R.D. (1967) *The Politics of Experience and The Bird of Paradise*. Harmondsworth: Penguin.

Leff, J.P. & Vaughn, C.E. (1985) *Expressed Emotion in Families*. New York: Guildford.

Mann, S. & Cree, W. (1976) 'New' long-stay patients: a national sample of 15 mental hospitals in England and Wales 1972–1973. *Psychological Medicine*, **6**, 603–616.

Martin, J.P. (1984) *Hospitals in Trouble*. London: Basil Blackwell.

MIND (1991) *Mental Health, Housing and Homelessness*. London: MIND Information Unit.

Murphy, E. (1991) *After The Asylums*. London, Faber & Faber.

National Schizophrenia Fellowship (1988) *Slipping Through the Net*. Surbiton, Surrey: National Schizophrenia Fellowship.

Nottingham Needs Assessment Planning Project Survey (1990), Unpublished, Planning Department, Mapperley Hospital, Nottingham.

Pepper, B., Kirschner, M.C. & Rylewicz, H. (1981) The YACP: Overview of a Population. *Hospital and Community Psychiatry*, **32**, 463–469.

Perkins, R. (1988) Institutionalisation. Unpublished Paper, Springfield University Hospital, London.

Perkins, R.E. (1991) Women with long term mental health problems: issues of power and powerlessness. *Feminism and Psychology*, **1**, 1131–1139.

Perkins, R.E. & Rowland, L.A. (1991) Sex differences in long term psychiatric care: Are women adequately served? *British Journal of Psychiatry*, **158**, 75–79.

Prevost, J.A. (1982) Youthful chronicity: paradox of the 1980s. *Hospital and Community Psychiatry*, **33**, 173.

Reed, J. (1991) The future of psychiatry. *Psychiatric Bulletin*, **15**, 396–401.

Ryan, P. (1979) Residential care for the severely mentally disabled. In Wing J.K. & Olsen R. (Eds) *Community Care for the Mentally Disabled*. Oxford: Oxford University Press.

Sayce, L., Craig, T. & Boardman, A. (1991) The development of community mental health centres in the UK. *Social Psychiatry and Psychiatric Epidemiology*, **26**, 14–20.

Scheff, T.J. (1967) (Ed.) *Mental Illness and Social Processes*. New York: Harper & Row.

Schinnar, A.P., Rothbard, A.B., Kanter, R. & Jung, Y.S. (1990) An empirical literature review of definitions of severe and persistent mental illness. *American Journal of Psychiatry*, **147** (12), 1602–1608.

Schwartz, S.R. & Goldfinger, S.M. (1981) The new chronic patient: clinical characteristics of an emerging sub-group. *Hospital and Community Psychiatry*, **32**, 470–475.

Sheets, J.L., Prevost, J.A. & Reihman, J. (1982) Young adult chronic patients: three hypothesised sub-groups. *Hospital and Community Psychiatry*, **3**, 197–202.

Shepherd, G. (1984) *Institutional Care and Rehabilitation*. New York: Longman.

Shepherd, G. (1988) *Current Issues in Community Care*. Report of 2nd Annual Conference on the Rehabilitation of Psychiatric Patients and their Care in the Community, 13.12.88. Leicester: Association of Psychological Therapies.

Showalter, E. (1987) *The Female Malady*. London: Virago.

Sturt, E., Wykes, T. & Creer, C. (1982) Demographic, social and clinical characteristics of the sample. In Wing, J.K. (Ed.) *Long Term Community Care: Experience in a London Borough*. Psychological Medicine Monograph Supplement 2.

Summers, F. & Hersh, S. (1983) Psychiatric chronicity and diagnosis. *Schizophrenia Bulletin*, **9**, 122–132.

Szasz, T.S. (1973) *The Manufacture of Madness*. London: Paladin.

Test, M.A. & Berlin, S.B. (1981) Issues of concern to chronically mentally ill women. *Professional Psychology*, **12**, 136–145.

Timms, P.W. & Fry, A.H. (1989) Homelessness and mental illness. *Health Trends*, **21**, 71–72.

Titmuss, R. (1968) *Commitment to Welfare*. London: Allen & Unwin.

Warden, A., Walsh, A. & Beckers, S. (1990) Sentenced to live within that sickness. Mental health, social security and registered homes. Benefits Research Unit, Nottingham University in Conjunction with Nottingham Welfare Rights Services.

Wing, J.K. (1962) Institutionalism in mental hospitals. *British Journal of Social and Clinical Psychiatry*, **118**, 311–322.

Wing, J.K. & Morris, B. (1981) Clinical basis of rehabilitations. In Wing, J.K. (Ed.) *Handbook of Psychiatric Rehabilitation Practice*. Oxford: Oxford University Press.

Wing, J.K. (1982) Course and prognosis of schizophrenia. In Wing, J.K. & Wing, L. (Eds) *Handbook of Psychiatry, Vol. 3. Psychoses of Uncertain Aetiology*. Cambridge: Cambridge University Press.

Wing, J.K. & Brown, G.W. (1970) *Institutionalism and*

Schizophrenia. Cambridge: Cambridge University Press.

Wing, J.K. & Creer, C. (1980) Schizophrenia at home. In Rollin, H.R. (Ed.) *Coping with Schizophrenia*. London: Burnett/National Schizophrenia Fellowship.

Wing, J.K., Bennett, D. & Denham, J. (1964) *The Industrial Rehabilitation of Long-Stay Schizophrenic Patients*. MRC Memo 42, London.

Wintersteen, R.T. & Rapp, C.A. (1986) The YACP: a dissenting view on an emerging concept. *Psychosocial Rehabilitation Journal*, **9**, 4–13.

Wooff, K. & Goldberg, D.P. (1988) Further observations on the practices of CPNs in Salford: differences between community psychiatric nurses and mental health social workers. *British Journal of Psychiatry*, **153**, 30–37.

SECTION

2

THE POLICY CONTEXT AND ORGANIZATION OF CARE

AIMS

i) To examine the implication of recent policy legislation for people with enduring problems
ii) To identify the problems to be addressed and the questions to be considered when planning services based on clients' needs
iii) To explore the role of care management in co-ordinating care and informing the provision of planning services

KEY ISSUES

Making a reality of community care
The National Health Service and Community Care Act 1990
Care management

Identify, analyse and assess factors causing distress and illness	Promote health, provide direct care and make interventions	Manage care programmes and services
Be critical, analytical and accountable, continue professional development	Counter discrimination, inequality and individual and institutional racism	Work within and develop policies, laws and safeguards in all settings
Understand influences on mental health and the nature/causes of disorder and illness	Know the effects of distress, disorder, illness on individuals, groups, families	Understand the basis of treatments and interventions

INTRODUCTION

As was seen in the previous section, the 1990s represent a period of considerable change in community care in general, and the mental health field in particular. The aim of this section is to examine further the reasons for the change at this point in time and some of the key tenets of that change.

'The objective of any changes should be to create an environment in which locally integrated community care can flourish. The present statutory framework constitutes a

barrier to the necessary changes. The focus is on services, not clients; decisions about different services for the same client are taken in different agencies and may been to be referred upwards through different professional hierarchies …. What is not tenable is to do nothing about the present financial, organizational and staffing arrangement. This will have serious consequences. Progress towards community care will continue to be slow; and the uneven pattern of services will persist. The switch from hospitals to residential care funded through Supplementary Benefits will continue. The opportunity presented by the closure of large psychiatric and mental handicap hospitals and to build community services will pass. A pattern of care based on private residential care will become entrenched. In short, the care provided for some of the most deprived members of society will continue to be neither as economic, efficient nor as effective as it can or should be.
Audit Commission, 1986

MAKING A REALITY OF COMMUNITY CARE

The situation described above by the Audit Commission led in 1990 to the introduction of the National Health Service and Community Care Act (DOH, 1990a). The Commission's report (1986) led to a further review by Sir Roy Griffiths (1988) (who a few years previously reviewed and recommended changes in the way the Health Service was managed). Both reviews pointed to several problems.

Lack of co-ordination of care

The other major factor revealed was the lack of organization behind the delivery of care to vulnerable people. There was little co-operation or clarification of responsibilities between the main service providers, especially health and social services. This was as inefficient as it was wasteful.

This led the Parliamentary Social Services Committee to state that:

'The lack of incentive for any one agency to take the initiative in developing a proper community care-based service has meant that each agency has tended to pass the buck to the other. For example, the NHS has an incentive to reduce its costs by discharging people into the community from long-stay hospitals, but the local authority is then left to respond to the social needs of these discharged people without being given any additional resources, since the cost was previously met by the NHS'.
Social Services Committee, 1990

The need for primary responsibility

Griffiths (1988) confirmed the Audit Commission's view of the situation and recommended changes in the primary responsibility for service provision to the various client groups. Although stressing the need for close co-operation and effective joint planning, he felt that the lack of clarification about who was responsible for what mitigated against a quality service for the clients.

Increased visibility

In the same period there was concern about what was perceived to be a growing number of people with mental health problems who were homeless or in the prisons. Although this was blamed on the closure of the psychiatric hospitals, very few in fact closed, which in itself was a cause for concern. The reasons for the growth will be examined below, but it appeared to be too easy to fall through the net of care that was assumed to be in place for vulnerable people. The greatest gaps appeared to be at the point of overlapping responsibilities whether between health and social services, or between the secondary services of mental health providers and the primary care services of the GPs. Pressures for Government action to address these defects in service came through pressure groups such as MIND and NSF, and the public's response to seeing more people with disturbed behaviour roaming the streets.

The user movement

The 1980s saw the birth and growth of the user movement in this country. At the World Mental Health Conference in Brighton in 1985 both users and professionals were impressed by the presentations of the Patients' Councils and Advocacy Groups from Holland. This led to a further conference in Nottingham and visits by the staff there to Holland, funded by the Health Authority. Social Services agreed to employ a member of the Clients Union for Holland to work in Nottingham for six months. Soon after saw the birth of the Nottingham Patients' Council Support Group and then further such groups developed in other parts of the country. As these groups grew so a National Self-Advocacy Network, Survivors Speak Out, grew with the goal of:

'Facilitating communications between groups throughout the UK and others interested in becoming involved .... Enlightened Health Authorities are realising that participation by, and consultation of, users is the most effective way of ensuring mental health services meet the real needs of their clients. The role of an umbrella organisation of the various self-advocacy groups has been and will continue to be, important in promoting this change.'
Lorraine Bell, 1987

Users began to speak for themselves, rather than rely on other organizations to represent their interests.

This growth of the user movement was followed by the development of Advocacy groups within the Mental Health field. (Prior to this, advocacy work had been developed in the field of learning difficulties.) The aim of advocacy is summed up by Garry Robson of the Nottingham Advocacy Group as:

'Its end result is the realisation of a person's

interests, the methods of achieving this can be through a mixture of the following:

(a) Lay or citizens' advocacy—where skilled volunteers supported by an independent agency, work with individuals on a long-term basis.

(b) Paid advocacy—where skilled workers are paid by an independent agency to represent the interests of individuals, usually in the short term.

(c) Self-advocacy—where, singularly or collectively, individuals work on their own behalf to realise their own interests.'

NATIONAL HEALTH SERVICE AND COMMUNITY CARE ACT 1990

The Griffiths report (1988) was followed by the White Paper *Caring for People* (DH, 1989) and then the NHS and Community Care Act 1990, (DH, 1990) in an effort to address the issues outlined above. Its key objectives were:

To promote the development of domiciliary, day and respite services to enable people to live in their own homes wherever feasible and sensible.

To ensure that service providers make practical support for carers a high priority.

To make proper assessment of need and good care management the cornerstone of high quality care.

To promote the development of a flourishing independent sector alongside good quality public services.

To clarify the responsibilities of agencies and so make it easier to hold them to account for their performance.

To secure better value for taxpayers' money by

introducing a new funding structure for social care.
HMSO, 1990

In pursuit of these objectives, several recommendations were detailed:

Community care plans

Every local authority was required from April 1992 to publish annual community care plans. These plans are to give a timetabled statement of the authorities' strategic objectives for meeting the community care needs of their population. This would include targets by which to measure progress, the scope and arrangement of the services, the resource implications and statements of how they would monitor quality. These plans are to be developed after consultation with users of services, their carers, other voluntary agencies and agreed with health authorities before publication.

Assessment and care management

Local authorities are to be responsible for assessment of needs of individuals within available resources and managing the provision of that care. The process is detailed in Fig. 19.1. While need is a relative concept, an attempt is made to define it in the Department of Health's guidance as:

'the requirements of individuals to enable them to achieve, maintain or restore an acceptable level of social independence or quality of life, as defined by the particular care agency or authority ... No two individuals will perceive or define their needs in exactly the same way. Care management seeks to recognise the individuality of need by challenging practitioners to identify the unique characteristics of each individual's needs and to develop individualised, rather than stereotyped, responses to those needs within the constraints of local policy and resources'.
DH, 1991

Commissioning and purchasing

Key to the reforms was the Government's wish to see a mixed economy of care developed. Until this Act, the local and health authorities were the largest direct provider of services. For the most part they identified the need and then provided the service to meet that need, although the voluntary and private sector did exist and provided not unsubstantial services. In future they were to see themselves 'the enabling authority':

'In practical terms in developing the enabling role authorities will need to distinguish between aspects of work in SSDs concerned with:

1 The assessment of individuals' needs, the arrangement and purchase of services to meet them, and
2 Direct service provision.
   It will be important that this distinction is reflected within the SSD's management structure at both the "macro" level (involving plans to meet strategic priorities as a whole) and at the "micro" level (where services are being arranged for individuals)'.
DOH, 1990a

This movement is reflected in other areas such as the separation between district health authorities and the individual hospitals or units that previously they managed directly, but are now becoming self-governing through trust status. Within housing, local authorities are being restricted in their housing programmes while the housing association movement is being encouraged to fill the gap. Most recently, we have seen this in education where schools are being separated from the education department to become self governing. In other words, the various authorities have a strategic role of assessing needs within the local population, and ensuring that the 'provider units', be they housing associations, hospital units, schools or the voluntary sector, provide services that will meet those needs.

Underpinning these developments is the notion that social services departments cannot be judge and jury; it cannot decide what is necessary and then critical appraise how well those services meet the needs it identified. The danger as the Government saw it was that people would be assessed as needing the services the local authority provides and freeze out the private sector:

> 'The distinction has been described in shorthand as "the purchaser/provider split". It will enable different functions to be effectively monitored and the people involved to be clear about their own role. It will also prevent any potential conflict of interest between commissioners, who must look at all available options from which to obtain optimum service, and providers'.
> *DOH, 1990a*

Transfer of resources

To ensure this link between assessment and purchase of services, the social security benefits for registered homes, board and lodging and other community care grants has been transferred to local authorities from April 1993. This should help gain control of the spiralling costs of residential care, and allow more appropriate use of the monies. For example, if it cost £200 per week to place somebody in a residential home, then that money could be used for a package of care which would keep them in their own home. It would possibly be cheaper and certainly more appropriate. It should be noted that local authorities cannot use this transferred money to support people in the residential establishments that they continue to provide; this is seen as an incentive for them to develop a mixed economy of care.

Inspection units

Registration and inspection of voluntary agency and private homes had long been a responsibility of local authorities. (Health authorities were and remain responsible for nursing homes.) The legislation changed the responsibility in two significant ways. Firstly the reorganized inspection units had to be 'at an arms length distance from the social services department structures'. While they

would probably be a part of the department, they would be directly accountable to the Director of Social Services, who in turn is accountable to the Social Services Committee for duties undertaken by the unit. There was to be no overlap in the management structure between the inspection units and the management of any residential services that the authorities continued to provide.

Secondly, the local authorities own residential services would be subject for the first time to inspection by its own inspection unit. The inspections are concerned with all aspects from the state of the building, the numbers of staff, quality of care, numbers per room, food, privacy, personal possessions, etc. That many authorities' homes have begun to fail these inspections, shows the move to be long overdue.

Complaints procedures

Local authorities are required to establish and publicize procedures for considering representations and complaints regarding the discharge (or failure to discharge) their duties as social service departments. This should have a two-fold effect. It will be seen as an appeal system should clients feel they have been declined a service they feel they are entitled to, or challenge the inadequacies of a service they are receiving. Secondly, if implemented properly they will:

> 'ensure quality and protect individuals when they stem from a recognition of users, needs and rights'.
> *DOH, 1990a*

Mental illness specific grant

The only new monies provided under the Act was a specific grant for the development of social care services for people with a mental illness—the mental illness specific grant (MISG), 30% of which had to be found from the local authorities' own budgets. The use of this grant had to be agreed with health authorities before the money would be released by Department of Health through the regional health authorities. There was also provided a specific grant for making payments to voluntary organizations providing services for alcohol and drug misusers.

Summary of changes

The thrust of the changes was to ensure assessment of every individual to establish what their needs were and then seek the most appropriate way of meeting those needs. The spin off would be to gain some control over the expenditure ensuring the bias to residential care is removed, and all those going into such care being guaranteed that it is the most appropriate form of care. Where it is inappropriate, plans are agreed to ensure good support which allows users of service to remain in their own homes as well as recognizing the support needs of the carers. However, such an ambitious aim would need co-ordinating both for the sake of the client and to inform the planning decisions in the provider agencies. This is perceived to be the role of care management, which will be examined later.

THE USER OF SERVICES

As was seen in the last section, the range of mental health problems is as diverse as those experiencing them, and the needs are not just to do with the individual mental health problems but the experiences resulting from the mental illness whether they be homelessness, lack of job opportunities, loss of skills to manage day-to-day living, opportunities for meaningful daytime activities or loneliness. In planning services, we need to consider who we hold in our mind's eye when thinking about this and all too often it is those people who have been residents of psychiatric hospitals for many years. The constant danger is that the reprovision in the community will be aimed at the residents in hospitals that are closing, that the services which we develop will meet only their needs and nobody else's. In reality we are dealing with two distinct users of service all with their individual needs.

The first is those who have had a long history of institutional care. Their response has been to transfer the distinguishing features of institutionalization from the hospital to the community. This is shown in many cases by an uncritical acceptance of the care arranged for them, attending day centres on the days stated, turning up at outpatient appointments regularly and for the most part being passive recipients of the care or activities offered. They have got used to the routine of being in hospital for many years and accept that routine when they move into the community. Goffman referred to the institutional care as 'Under one roof under one authority'. If everybody could be seen from the nursing station and all the services were provided in the hospital, there was little problem in co-ordinating the care or of losing people in the system. That is not to say that their needs were always being met, but there was little need to think about the management of the care. With that experience behind them, the needs of the service providers to maintain an all-embracing care structure which matched that of the hospital has often been the dominating factor in developing services in the community.

The second group are those who do not have a history of long-term institutionalization although they may have had numerous admissions to hospital. It is this group that are often held up as the example of the failure of community care and it is mistakenly thought that after many years in hospital they are just discharged to fend for themselves. This client group is a younger client group who in the past might have been admitted for long-term care. Within the rehabilitation service in our own area there is a marked reduction in the age of those being referred with over 70% being under the age of 45 years and 50% under the age of 35 years. Comparable figures have been recognized in many other services dealing particularly with those with enduring mental health problems. In other words the first group is maintaining contact with the service but we are failing to engage this younger client group for a sustained period, and that we are failing to engage them is obvious from high dropout rates and the high numbers of homeless or those in prison with mental health problems.

Because too often services have been developed with the first client group in mind, Repper (1991) found that this young client group will not engage with those same services. They go to day centres and fail to identify with the longer-term group they meet there and feel that the centre cannot meet their needs. Because there is often a lack of stability in their own housing circumstances it becomes easier to lose contact with them.

As described in the first section in this chapter, they are a group who are sometimes more articulate and demanding in what they want; they rightly refuse to be passive recipients of the service that professionals feel to be appropriate for them. In the past, this failure to provide appropriate services was too often redefined as a lack of motivation on the part of the clients, but if we are serious about providing real community care they will have to be actively pursued in order to engage them in developing services that truly meet their needs.

Another distinguishing feature of this client group is the role of their carers. In the past carers' expectations of the service were low and they were rarely disappointed. But as a group they have realized that they have rights which have been reinforced by the Community Care Act, and they have become more demanding both as individuals and through pressure groups. If the person for whom they are caring refused to participate in certain care activities, they will no longer unquestioningly accept the view of the professional that it is the individual's problem; they too are pointing to services that do not adequately meet needs and demanding change. However, the role of the carer needs not only to be realized and accepted by the professionals, but must be encouraged further to help them assert their views and needs.

These pressures for change have culminated in the National Health Service and Community Care Act 1990 (DH, 1990). It was not just driven by uncontrolled spending on residential care (even if that was the driving factor for the review of services), but that needs of users of services should be more accurately defined and appropriately met. The Act states that these needs will be best met by improving management of care, and it is this care management we will now turn to.

CARE MANAGEMENT

In developing community care initiatives we need to understand the care management role and the relationship with the client as well as with other agencies in the user's life. The process of care management will be examined and key questions in the organization of a care management service will be addressed. (For the purposes of this chapter 'case' and 'care' management are interpreted as the same. Users of service found the term 'case' demeaning to the individual as it is the care that is being managed not the individual.)

'Case management involves having a single person responsible for maintaining a long-term supportive relationship with the client, regardless of where the client is and regardless of the number of agencies involved. The case manager is a helper, service broker, and advocate for the client...'.
Intagliata, 1982

'The function of case management is to address the overall maintenance of the mentally ill person's physical and social environment with the goals of facilitating his or her physical survival, personal growth, community participation and recovery from, or adaptation to mental illness'.
Kanter, 1989

'Any strategy for managing and co-ordinating and reviewing services for the individual client in a way that provides for continuity of care and accountability to both the client and the managing agency'.
Dept of Health Guidance, 1990

In the White Paper *Caring for People* (DH, 1989) the Government stated that care management and assessment are 'the cornerstones of quality care'. Unlike social work or community nursing which stress only the relationship between the user and the worker, care management must be seen in a wider context. Although the relationship is crucial to effective care management, it includes the user's environment and the agencies that impinge on him or her, the care manager's environment and the agencies that control the service delivery. It is the interlinking of these agencies with the user that is the distinguishing feature of care management.

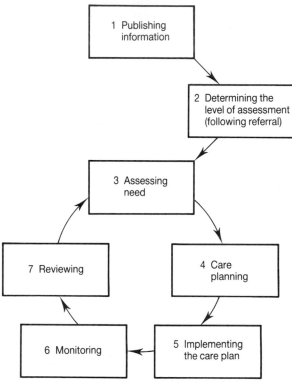

Fig. 19.1 *The process of care management (DH, 1991).*

The process of care management as outlined in the Government's guidance is shown in Fig. 19.1. This process is easily recognizable to many professions as the nursing process or care review. It's significance in terms of care management is the requirement to publish who is entitled to a service as defined by the priority groups. The assessment will determine whether the person falls within the entitled group and it will give a picture of their present circumstances from which needs can be established.

Developing assessment systems

In developing assessment systems there are three particular dangers. The first being that we assess only in the light of the services that are provided by statutory bodies, failing to find out about other possibilities. Secondly, carrying out a 'comprehensive assessment', assessing everything that is assessable about the client, but only using a small part of the information to provide services, the rest being collected 'just in case'. The final danger is following the ethos of most agencies in training workers to assess the user's weaknesses, to measure their lack of skills in relevant areas or their inability to carry out certain tasks. Where skills are identified, they are too often ignored or seen as an area that does not need to be worked on. Some of the most exciting work in care management is looking at the work of Charles Rapp and his development of the strengths model of care management. This challenging approach:

> 'lays primacy on letting the agendas be set by what the client wants, by the uniqueness of each client's circumstances and the uniqueness of the personal resources that the client will have to work towards goals. The strengths model concentrates on wants, desires and aspirations, and not, probably for the umpteenth time in the client's life, primarily focusing on problem or deficit areas'.
> *Prance, 1992*

In summary the assessment should acknowledge strengths, and gather the minimum information necessary to identify a need and plan the delivery of service. A useful guideline is 'If users ask why I am asking a certain question, can I justify the answer and will it be understandable to them?'

Although important, assessment should not be seen as an end in itself. It is a tool which is probably best seen as a kick start to the process whereby all those involved in the care process, crucially the user and the carer, have a shared view of the present circumstances. Thereafter, the review process should take over, with another assessment being completed only if the user drops out of service for a period and then returns or there are major life event changes requiring a fundamental rethink.

Review systems have been notoriously haphazard once a person leaves hospital. They are often reviewed at out-patients by a doctor on rotation, seen in their own homes by a community psychiatric nurse or social worker and reviewed at a day centre. Occasionally there is a review involving all these people, but too often the communication is fleeting and from the user's perspective, the same things come up in review year after year, assuming there is at least an annual review.

The role of the care manager in assessment and review

Integral to care management is the systematic management of reviews involving all of the services that the user is involved with. Once an assessment has been completed, a review involving the service user, carer and other persons involved in the care would be called by the care manager. This would confirm or add to the assessment and provide a forum for agreeing a care plan specifying agreed priorities for action and a clear understanding of who is to undertake what. The care manager's responsibility is to ensure the care plan is being followed by all, and to identify services needed that were not able to be delivered by those present at the review. It is the care manager's responsibility to establish who or what agency would be best able to fill these gaps.

This plan should be the starting point of the next review to identify the successes and problems, determining why it was a success or a problem before updating the care plan. In this way there should be a continuity through each review with a clarity of expectations from all concerned. If this seems obvious, it is but too rarely practised in the community. They have often received little and expect less.

Challenges to practitioners (DH, 1991)

Practitioners will need to:

1 Acquire needs-led attitudes and approaches

2 Develop skills of needs assessment, defining objectives in terms of the outcomes desired by users and carers

3 Promote greater participation by users and carers, building on their strengths

4 Think creatively about service options within and between agencies

5 Adjust to more devolved responsibility for resource allocation and financial management

6 Give higher priority to the specification and monitoring of quality standards

7 Increase their skills in negotiation and co-ordination

The challenges posed to the practitioners by the development of care management systems are detailed. In summary, effective care management places the users at the centre of the care process so that services are determined by his or her needs as opposed to the needs of the service providers.

Care manager's relationship with the client

The care manager is responsible for helping clients identify their needs and then co-ordinating services to meet those needs whether or not they provide the services. This can be seen in Fig. 19.2; the care manager is alongside the service user giving information about the availability of services and the choices to be made. The care manager is also reflecting the needs of the service user back to all the other agencies involved.

Care manager's relationship with service providers

This relationship is outside the normal role boundaries, so not only will care managers need to be aware of the role and services provided by other agencies, they will also need a mandate from other agencies to act in this capacity. This mandate is important in order to avoid conflicts and role boundary disputes. The care manager's role is often seen as powerful by other agencies involved in service delivery to the client; they sometimes feel they are being told what to do. In

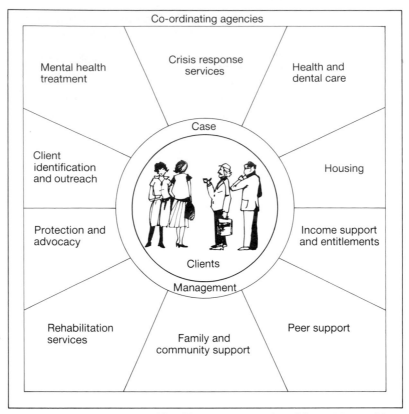

Fig. 19.2 *A client-centred comprehensive mental health system (reproduced from: National Institute of Mental Health, 1987).*

so far as the care manager is alongside clients helping them to identify their needs and allowing users to determine their care package, they are powerful but they are dependent on the service providers to meet those needs. The early research findings from Research and Development for Psychiatry (RDP), who have been undertaking a four-year research project in mental health care management in four centres, showed that a shared understanding of the care management role and the service provider role is crucial to avoid the user becoming the ball that is passed around or jealously guarded by one player.

To examine the care management role in more detail, let us look at the present role of those providing services. The user is involved with a number of individual agencies and members of the care team. These include statutory and non-statutory services with different funding arrangements. One of the agencies such as social worker or community psychiatric nurse may broker on behalf of the user; that is, refer to, negotiate access to, or communicate with these other agencies, but the agencies themselves often have little or no knowledge of the involvement of the client with other services beyond their own. Essentially clients have a direct relationship with each of these and are responsible for organizing their care between these services (see Fig. 19.3). While many would argue with much justification for clients being their own care managers, the users of mental health services not only have a history of disempowerment but are often at crisis points in their own lives and for many it is difficult enough to get the service they want without taking on the role of sorting out the agencies' relationships to each other.

The result of this lack of co-ordination is that users of services do not get access to those things that would enhance the quality of their lives, therefore have unmet needs. In some cases, through a failure to review their care properly,

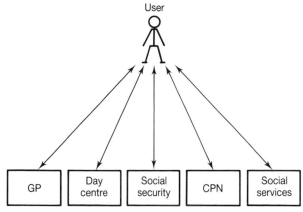

Fig. 19.3 *User's relationship with service providers.*

users may also have what we might call 'met unneeds', that is service inputs that they do not need or want but that leave them with an unwarranted intrusion into their lives. There are many examples of users of services warily asking 'Do I have to go to the day centre five days a week?', the result of cautious planning to ensure somebody is keeping an eye on them even if users would rather occupy themselves on certain days.

Intagliata's definition of care management (1982) stresses the care manager's partnership with the client seeing the world from alongside the client. The care manager is introduced not to be a barrier between the service providers and users, but to help users make sense of the services and their entitlement from each of the services. The care manager is educating users to the choices available so that they can begin to make real choices where this is possible. The definition by Kanter (1989) puts the emphasis on influencing the client's environment both physical and social; the care manager is reflecting back to the agencies the needs of this individual in particular and the user group in general. Thus the care managers can develop their service based on users needs.

When considering these definitions together, we can see a progression from the focus on the relationship between the user and the care manager (Intagliata) to a focus on the relationship between the agencies in the user's environment, the care manager and the user (Kanter). This is seen in Fig. 19.4. This reinforces the need for the care managers to have a mandate.

Care manager's relationship with purchasers of service

There is a wider context which care management has to influence. The Department of Health's definition touches on the new responsibilities of health and social services for purchasing or commissioning services. In accordance with this the care manager needs to utilize the information gained working with the user. This needs to be collected and collated for presenting to the purchasing bodies in order to influence their purchasing decisions. Thus the care manager becomes the direct link between users and purchasers, providing information about the needs of users to inform the contracts that are given to provide new services.

In the post-White Paper world, information is power and it is equally important that there is a systematic collation of data about the activities being undertaken with the user and the outcome of that work. This allows not only the monitoring of the quality of service but also provides hard evidence to argue for more resources or staff if necessary.

Care programme

The *Caring for People* White Paper (DH, 1989) also introduced the care programme approach. Although much of the underlying reasons for introduction of care management and assessment also apply to the introduction of the care programme, the more specific reason was incidents of perceived failure of treatment programmes for people in the community. There had been a number of occurrences of suicide on the part of people recently discharged, or being treated in the community without recourse to admission. There had also been examples of severe risk to others from recently discharged users of service. The key elements of the care programme approach are:

1　Systematic arrangements for assessing the health care needs of patients who could, potentially, be treated in the community, and for regularly reviewing the health care

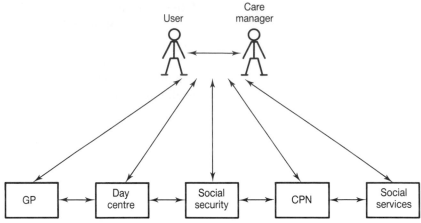

Fig. 19.4 *User's and care manager's relationship with service providers.*

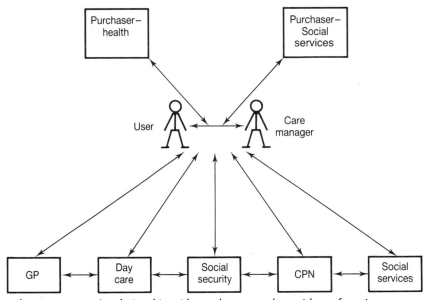

Fig. 19.5 *User's and care manager's relationship with purchasers and providers of services.*

needs of those being treated in the community

2 Systematic arrangements, agreed with appropriate social services authorities, for assessing and regularly reviewing what social care such patients need, to give them the opportunity of benefiting from treatment in the community

3 Effective systems for ensuring that agreed health and, where necessary, social care

services are provided to those patients who can be treated in the community

There has been some confusion over differentiating between care programme and care management and definitions have varied from authority to authority.

Care programme is probably best seen as a narrower concept but on the same continuum as care management. Care programme is most appropriate for those coming into contact with the service, whether being admitted to hospital or not, who will be receiving a service from individual professionals or from a mental health team and whose treatment will be monitored by a key worker agreed by all those involved. Should they remain in contact with the services for a long period of time, have a multiplicity of agencies involved or have a high number of needs, then they would probably be better considered for care management and the high degree of co-ordination that would bring. It is important to note that the criteria for moving from care programme to care management is more than one of duration of contact with the service. There is also a measurement of disability arising from the experience of a mental health problem. In other words, a person may be in contact with the service for a long time, but be happy with their situation and not needing a high degree of intervention. On the other hand, somebody may be in contact with the service for only a short time, but need the high degree of service offered by care management.

Who are the care managers?

The NHS and Community Care Act (DH, 1990) lays great emphasis on the need for social services and health to plan together. Given the history of competitiveness, mistrust and secrecy between the two, this will be no mean feat to achieve. The first question which will be asked by practitioners will be: 'Who will be the care managers?'

There has been an assumption that as care management is a local authority responsibility, care managers will come from the ranks of social workers. Whatever validity there may be to this in other client groups, the profile of social services involvement within the mental health field nationally has been a low one, to say the least. Yet if social workers and community psychiatric nurses sit down to determine what tasks are *exclusive* to their profession, the list is a short one based on the stereotypical, and none the less true for that, view of the role of social workers concerning admission to hospital under the Mental Health Act 1983; and the nursing role in the dispensation of medication. Further delineation of responsibilities relies on differentiating the health needs and the social needs of the user. As seen in the previous chapter, this would be a false divi-

sion in light of the complex and interrelated problems faced by the users of mental health services. The reality is that where both professions are working with those people with enduring mental health problems, there is little difference in their role. It is essentially one of co-ordination whether it be social security benefits, meaningful daytime activities or housing. The Department of Health summarizes it thus:

> 'The skills required of care managers may be found in a number of professions and will vary according to the needs of service users and the model of care management that is adopted'.
> *HMSO, 1990*

Care managers as purchasers or providers

Various models of care management have been put forward from those that see it as an extension of the present provider role to purely brokerage systems. While the relationship with the user is important to both, the former sees co-ordination as a part of service delivery while the latter sees co-ordination as a task in its own right which should be separated from serviced delivery.

> 'A progressive separation of the tasks of assessment from those of service provision in order to focus on needs, where possible having the tasks carried out by different staff ... Care managers should in effect act as brokers for service ... They should not, therefore, be involved in direct service delivery; nor should they normally carry managerial responsibility for the services they arrange. This removes any possible conflict of interest ... The keyworker carries the main service-providing role, so to the extent that assessment and care management have been separated from service provision, it will not be possible for the two roles to be combined in the same practitioner'.
> *HMSO, 1990*

In short if care managers are to act as advocates and brokers with the user, they should not also be delivering services. This would have the effect of making them both judge and jury when reviewing the success of the implementation of care packages.

This change is not as great as may be first assumed. In working with people with enduring mental health problems, up to 90% of the work involves co-ordination of care. Care management formalizes that responsibility; the care manager is responsible for completing an assessment with the client, organizing the review and monitoring the implementation of the review decisions. To be bound up in the service delivery would be to put the care manager on both sides of the fence without the independence required to monitor or broker on the delivery of respective services. This separation is often described as the splitting of the therapy role from the co-ordination role, and although true, is simplistic because of the assumptions made about the co-ordination role. This is not to dismiss the nature of the relationship between the user and the care manager because by definition for the relationship to work, it will be therapeutic. The Department of Health guidance clarifies this position:

'The counselling component of assessment may be carried over into the subsequent monitoring and reviewing phases, but where it shades into a therapeutic intervention in its own right, for example, family therapy, it should be regarded as a service to be provided by a different practitioner ... Care managers are not expected to have any part in service provision'.
HMSO, 1990

SUMMARY

We can see then that care management, rather than being a new profession, in itself is a method of working which draws on the skills of many professionals and agencies. It facilitates communication to enhance the service delivery to users in a systematic and co-ordinated fashion. The problems of community care in the 1980s can be seen to lie in the relationship between clinical issues, management issues and resource issues, and the failure of each of these systems to inform the others. Care management provides the means of linking the three in order to provide services responsive to the needs of service users as individuals and as a prioritized group.

REFERENCES

Audit Commission (1986) *Making a Reality of Community Care*. London: HMSO.

Bell, L. (1987) Survivors speak out. In Barker, I. & Peck, E. (Eds) *Power in Strange Places—User Empowerment in Mental Health Services*. Good Practices in Mental Health.

Department of Health (DH) (1989) *Caring for People*, London: HMSO.

Department of Health (DH) (1990) NHS and Community Care Act. London: HMSO.

Department of Health (DH) (1991) *Care Management and Assessment—Practitioners' Guide*. London: HMSO.

Department of Health (1990a) NHS and Community Care Act: London: HMSO.

Department of Health (1990b) The care programme approach for people with mental illness. London: HMSO.

Ford, R., Repper, J., Cooke, A., Beardsmore, A., Norton, P. & Clarke, C. (1992) *Implementing Case Management: Research Report on the Process of Developing Case Management for those with a Long Term Mental Illness*. London: Research and Development for Psychiatry.

Griffiths, Roy Sir (1988) *Community Care: Agenda for Action*. London: HMSO.

HMSO (1990) *Community Care in the Next Decade and Beyond—Policy Guidance*. London: HMSO.

House of Commons (1990) *Eleventh Report Community Care: Services for People with a Mental Handicap and People with a Mental Illness*. Social Services Committee. Session 1989–90, London: HMSO.

Intagliata, J. (1982) Improving the quality of life for the chronically mentally disabled: the role of case management. *Schizophrenia Bulletin*, **8** (4).

Kanter, J. (1989) Clinical case management—definition, principles, components. *Hospital & Community Psychiatry*, **40**.

Prance, N. (1992) We'll do it your way. Unpublished

paper in *Care Managers Induction Pack*. Nottingham: Rehabilitation and Community Care Services.

Repper, J. (1991) Audit of 1000 Consecutive Referrals to Nottingham's Rehabilitation and Community Care Service. Nottingham. Mental Health Unit.

Social Services Committee (1990) Session 1989–90. Eleventh Report. Community Care: Services for People with a Mental Handicap and People with a Mental Illness. London: HMSO.

SECTION

3

THE PROVISION OF CARE FOR PEOPLE WITH ENDURING MENTAL HEALTH PROBLEMS

AIMS

i)   To explore the location of care in relation to the needs it must fulfil
ii) To examine the role of the service provider
iii) To examine the principles and practice of interventions proven to be effective with the client group

KEY ISSUES

The location of care
Rehabilitation
An overall approach to providing services for this group
Assessment
Planning
Implementation
Evaluation

Identify, analyse and assess factors causing distress and illness	Promote health, provide direct care and make interventions	Manage care programmes and services
Be critical, analytical and accountable, continue professional development	Counter discrimination, inequality and individual and institutional racism	Work within and develop policies, laws and safeguards in all settings
Understand influences on mental health and the nature/causes of disorder and illness	Know the effects of distress, disorder, illness on individuals, groups, families	Understand the basis of treatments and interventions

INTRODUCTION

The focus of this section is on the provision of care for people with enduring mental health problems. The location of care is explored in relation to the needs it must fulfil, before moving on to the role of the service provider. The familiar framework of assessment, planning, implementation and evaluation is used to examine principles, practice and proven interventions with specific reference to this client group.

THE LOCATION OF CARE

The nature of the difficulties, and the degree of disability suffered by people with enduring mental health problems, means that direct care provision is offered in a wide variety of settings. It is useful to look briefly at the types of services offered, the functions they serve and the client group they provide for.

Ideally, services in the community would be developed once the needs of the client group that they are designed to serve have been assessed. Thus, the functions that services need to fulfil would be considered before the service is offered. However, as we saw in the last chapter, the reverse is all to often true; services are set up, and clients are fitted into them. Service provision is limited in both quantity and scope; it is led by the whim of service planners and providers, rather than by the needs of clients. Services for people with enduring mental health problems have further suffered through being low priority in terms of resource allocation.

As described in the previous section, two initiatives laid down in the 1990 NHS and Community Care Act will have an effect on the form of service delivery in the future: the selective purchasing power of case managers, based on the assessed needs and wishes of clients, will ensure that services develop along needs-led lines rather than in an *ad hoc* manner. This effect will be enhanced through more global measures to assess the needs of the population and allocate resources accordingly, giving priority to the elderly, the long-term mentally ill, and people with learning disabilities (DH, 1990).

At present, the types of services required by people with enduring mental health problems can be identified through consideration of the types of functions which they must serve. This takes us back to the needs of different client groups within the population with enduring mental health problems, as explored in the first section in this chapter.

Needs of the old long-stay client group

Many of the old long-stay patients who remain in hospital are there because they need a type of care which fulfils the functions of the old asylum. Although they do not need to be in the old mental hospitals, they need services that offer the same facilities. Shepherd (1988) has compiled a list of basic requirements of a 'quality' service:

---

1 Basic shelter and support

2 A style of care that is responsive to individual needs, that is, provides a level of input that reflects individual levels of functioning, neither offering too much nor too little, care. Encouraging independence, while not denying disability.

3 A service that provides some degree of choice and personal privacy, for example, the availability of personal possessions and privacy when required.

4 An appropriate range of daytime activities—work and leisure—although preferably not in the same place.

5 Opportunities for social contact when required and social withdrawal when needed.

6 Contact (integration) with 'ordinary life' and shelter from it.

7 Medical, nursing and other 'expert' help when required.

These functions may be provided in small units, dispersed throughout the community with close involvement with a number of different agencies. These units are smaller than the old mental hospitals and so potentially offer advantages over the old system of care: they allow greater individualization of care and involvement of a wider range of agencies with a lower proportion of professional staff, reducing the danger of institutional practices; they are also likely to be more integrated with the local community which in the long term may serve to reduce the stigma of mental illness.

Alternatively, the functions of the asylum may

be offered on the existing hospital site, through the development of smaller, domestic-sized units. This offers the advantages of an existing pool of staff and resources on site, but carries the risk of perpetuating both institutional practices and the stigma associated with mental hospitals.

The needs of the new long-stay group

The Department of Health has been encouraging districts to develop a further type of service as an alternative to hospital-based care. This provision is specifically aimed to meet the needs of the new long-stay client group (those admitted continuously for between one and five years). The favoured type of facility is known as a 'ward in a house'. This seeks to combine the functions of a hospital within an ordinary house. It provides intensive, long-term rehabilitation with a highly staffed, multiprofessional team, in a domestic-style setting. This has access to the facilities on the hospital site, but is also integrated with the local community. These settings have proven effective in improving the social functioning and level of negative symptoms in their clients. In the long term, they have also managed to resettle clients into less supervised accommodation outside the hospital (Wing and Furlong, 1986; Garety et al., 1988).

This type of provision should not be seen as an end point in care. Where possible clients need to move into appropriate housing in the community, their need for support to live independently should be assessed and provided separately. Where this has been successfully set up, housing is provided on a long-term basis through housing associations, and professional support is offered on a flexible basis according to the varying needs of the client for up to 24 hours a day. Thus the housing and care needs of the client have been recognized as two distinct needs and dealt with separately.

For some people, these alternatives to hospital do not prove tenable. There are individuals who are too disruptive or run too many risks to live in an open community-orientated setting. For these, quality care in a hospital ward may offer the only safe facility.

In short, the large old mental hospitals had disadvantages, but these have been in danger of overshadowing the essential merits of the system. Some people remain in need of many of the services previously offered by the asylums, yet this needs to be offered in the way that was envisaged when the mental hospitals were originally built. Care providers in these settings need to ensure that the problems associated with institutionalization are not repeated, but that they endeavour to offer a quality service, fulfilling the assessed and individual needs of each client.

The needs of the new long-term group

For the majority of people with enduring mental health problems, care will not be provided in a residential setting. Although they may live in some form of supported accommodation, the focus of care is generally the prevention or minimization of admissions to hospital. Studies of active rehabilitation and care in the community in Australia and the United States (Stein and Test, 1985; Hoult, 1986) have shown that where time spent in hospital is reduced through assertive community intervention there is less disruption of social functioning, and higher levels of patient and carer satisfaction are reported. Although effective community-based treatment may reduce the length of hospital admissions it does not entirely eradicate the need for admission. These are necessary at times of crisis when the risks of staying at home are too high, or when adequate community provision is not available; this often refers to the lack of availability of appropriate housing and social support, rather than purely health-related support.

Adequate provision of care for this group cannot be provided by hospital facilities and professional community workers alone; these need to be set in a context of a network of statutory and non-statutory agencies. These need to provide different types of day care—both work- and leisure-orientated, from informal drop-in facilities to adult education, and sheltered work initiatives; and various types of housing and accommodation to meet the different needs of individuals within the group.

THE ROLE OF THE SERVICE PROVIDER

Attention has been drawn to the variety of settings in which service providers may work with people with enduring mental health problems. There is inevitably a different focus to the care provided in different settings; the following paints a broad picture of the principles that underlie the work with this client group.

Who is the service provider?

Although much of this section applies equally to other members of the care team, the focus is on the role of the nurse. It is not the purpose of this chapter to define the unique role of the nurse, but it is recognized that the nurse plays a pivotal and fundamental role in the care and rehabilitation of people with enduring mental health problems. They usually have a significant amount of face-to-face contact on a daily basis, frequently on a 24-hour basis. They work in many of the points of contact for these people, increasingly being employed by voluntary and private resources, as well as in statutory services. They represent one, if not the largest professional group providing care, working from community centres, day resources, residential settings and as community psychiatric nurses. They may also be employed as case managers, having a provider, co-ordinating and purchasing role. The fundamental role of the service provider with this client group, is portrayed in Sundeen's description of the role of the nurse:

'The nurse evokes the client's perception of his experiences and together they attempt to find solutions to his heath problems. Nursing helps identify and express client needs and incorporates experiences into the person's life situation. Nursing actions are directed towards finding meaning in the client's coping responses, maximising strengths and maintaining integrity'.
Sundeen et al., 1976

The aim of this section is to outline what we regard as good practice, tailored to meet the specific needs of people with enduring mental health problems. In order to achieve this, it is essential that those providing the service have a progressive outlook and are able to embrace the changes in ethos and practice that are occurring as the characteristics and needs of the client group become fully recognized and change with the effects of de-institutionalization. The rapidity of developments in nursing practice with this client group become clear when one considers that only 20 years ago training sessions involved teaching nurses to detect signs of wilfulness and cunning in patients on long-stay wards (Archives, Mapperley Hospital, Nottingham). This section is concerned with inculcating those attitudes that will ensure users of services are exposed to interventions that will best meet their needs. It is set firmly within a context of user empowerment, not just in relation to the services for the individual, but in terms of their place in the wider community.

The multidisciplinary team

As people with enduring mental health problems often have multiple needs, they are usually in contact with several different services and many different professionals. Service providers are therefore all part of a team working with clients to maximize their potential for independent living. This multidisciplinary team is an important context for communication and decision-making in which the different qualities and opinions of different disciplines can be drawn upon.

In order to be effective, this team should not function as a hierarchical group. Psychiatrists have traditionally held a powerful and often leading role in the multidisciplinary team, in reality, their expertise is often confined to that of medical consultants—just another member of a team in which all members have a particular area of expertise and knowledge of lesser or greater relevance to clients who have both social and health care needs. Nor must the team function as a secret society, clients are the focus of concern and the experts in telling their own story and assessing the appropriateness of planned care. Wherever possible they should be involved in multidisciplinary meetings, if this is not to be the case, the advantages and disadvantages of their absence must be considered. The team should comprise not merely people from different professional disciplines, but must work in partnership with all those groups or people whom the clients feel are important in their life, so that the caring team comprises all those able to offer users what they want and need.

Although the team should not be hierarchical, it does need leadership; for many meetings this may be provided by a designated team leader, or where clients are concerned it may be organized on a client basis, so that the care manager or key worker leads the review or meeting. Whatever the system, the team needs to agree on the organization of multidisciplinary meetings. They need a shared vision of goals and a shared value base. In order to prevent disruption and ill-feeling within the team that reflects on team functioning and ultimately on client care, there also needs to be an in-built system to check that the team is working effectively and all members are pulling in the same direction.

The client

The previous sections have given some insights into the various and varying needs of people with enduring mental health problems. Before considering the means by which these needs can be met, it is important to consider the conceptualization of the population by the service providers themselves: the way in which these people and their personal circumstances are viewed will effect the manner in which services are provided, and the satisfaction of both the client and the service provider. The importance of a positive framework within which to work with these people cannot be underestimated and needs further explanation.

The debate on the causation and treatment of severe mental illness has been waged for many years. On the whole it has been dominated by the medical model which is associated with such negative practices and effects as disempowering the client through disregarding the client's views, preferences and social situation, and seeking to apply a label of some kind in order to inform the prescription of physical treatment. In emulating medical practice through such developments as

the introduction of nursing diagnoses, and prescribing specific nursing interventions, it is essential that clients are not reduced to a mere set of numbers who have symptoms, negative traits, poor functioning, lowered skills and faulty genetic structures. For the service provider, the meaning of the illness for individual clients, their hopes and goals or everyday needs, are more important than generalized expectations associated with a given diagnosis. We must never let ourselves run the risk of pathologizing the individual to the extent that their personhood be reduced to insignificance.

> 'To be a mental patient is to be stigmatized, ostracized, socialized, patronized, psychiatrized. To be a mental patient is to be a statistic. And so you become a no-thing, in a no-world, and you are not'.
> *Lawson, 1992*

In acknowledging the centrality of clients, and addressing their care needs on their terms, we have come to understand their personal struggle, and to respect their rights to determine how they feel help can be most effective. Indeed, help must increasingly be perceived as useful in some way by clients in order for them to be willing to accept it. Under-engagement in services, and non-compliance with treatment are real problems amongst the new long-term client group who, rather than being institutionalized and passive, is likely to be young, demanding and articulate.

In essence, the role of the service provider is not to adopt practices that perpetuate the power-coercive model of traditional psychiatry, but rather, to rise above this and become a true collaborator with clients, trying to understand and work within their perspective, acknowledging their individual qualities, and facilitating an improvement in the quality of their life as they see it.

REHABILITATION

Rehabilitation is the commonly used term for services and work with people with enduring mental health problems. The meaning of rehabilitation is discussed, and the implications of working in rehabilitation are briefly introduced. This provides the context for the care process as described in the remainder of this section; that is, assessment, planning, implementation and evaluation.

Services for people with enduring mental health problems, and the type of work undertaken within them, are often referred to as rehabilitative. Literally, rehabilitation means treatment, therapy or cure. However, in practice it refers to the work done once the florid and acute symptoms have subsided and it generally implies concern with the most severely disabled client group, in need of services on an ongoing basis. Rehabilitation services are the complex networks of facilities that are developing to provide for people with enduring mental health problems.

The process of rehabilitation has been variously conceptualized, depending on the ideological viewpoint of the author, the client group to whom it refers, and prevailing social conditions. The problem with many of the definitions put forwards is their negativity and the implied passivity of the client. For the purpose of this section Anthony and his colleagues propose the most appropriate and meaningful description of rehabilitation:

-

'philosophically ... rehabilitation is directed at increasing the strengths of clients so that they can achieve their maximum potential for independent living and meaningful carers'.
Anthony et al., 1981

Whilst avoiding generalized pessimism, service providers must be realistic in order to maintain and sustain motivation in working with this group; many of the psychiatric and social disabilities associated with this client group may show very little change over time. For workers this means that, rather than setting up the client and themselves to fail through holding unrealistic expectations of 'cure' or discharge from services, it may be sufficient to aim simply to keep in contact with the client. It is important for service providers to see their role as working with the

client in the long term, taking small steps together, persevering through setbacks together, and enjoying achievements—however small. This involves getting to understand the client's view and experiences as far as possible, realizing the importance of being flexible, whether this means moving in unfamiliar directions that the client sees as important, or trying strategies repeatedly—what did not work in the past may work if tried again, when the client feels ready.

In any rehabilitation programme, the central point is the individual. The process involves the four stages which are now familiar through their use in nursing and have already been discussed in the previous section in relation to case management: assessment, planning, implementation and evaluation. These four stages are explored in turn through the remainder of this section.

OVERALL APPROACH TO PROVIDING SERVICES FOR PEOPLE WITH ENDURING MENTAL HEALTH PROBLEMS

The way in which clients are assessed, care is provided and relationships with clients and their family are developed depend to a large extent on the value base of the service or the individual worker. This may be a formally stated philosophy or an implicit belief system. Increasingly, nursing services are adopting and modifying models to inform their care delivery. For the purpose of this section, we do not advocate the use of any particular model. In the ever-changing world of health care research and the increasingly challenging views of users, being a theoretical purist may be limiting. It is essential that services utilize a perspective that can evolve and develop in response to changes in practice, knowledge, context, and the needs and demands of clients. Rather than a full philosophical framework, we therefore offer several key values to guide an approach to practice. These are drawn from the theories and models considered to be of most relevance to this client group: social role valorization or normalization theory (Wolfensburger, 1983); the strengths model, developed in the US for case managers working with severely disabled mentally ill (Kisthardt and Rapp, 1989), and family systems theory (Campbell and Draper, 1985).

Rights of the individual

People have a right to live an ordinary life, in which they determine the quality without prejudice from others. They should be free to make choices that can advantage their quality of life and those in regular contact with them. They should also have access to people who can help them make such choices or act on their behalf when they are not able to do so effectively.

Risk management

We do not believe that when people are ill they should be allowed to take a course of action that will disadvantage them or expose them to neglect and potential abuse. However risks must be taken, and clients must be allowed to make informed choices to a point. It is difficult to draw the line between reasonable risk and potential danger, for each client it will be different. A check system within the service, whether through quality review teams, or through client-focused meetings is needed to ensure that self determination is not subverted on the premise and belief that clients cannot reason and make real choices. It must be remembered that clients in the new long-term group are often familiar with the risks involved in living on the margins of society and this experience must be acknowledged when assessing risk.

Research-based practice

The service provider has a responsibility to provide good practice, use good practice from other sources and critically examine relevant research, where possible incorporating findings into practice. They must also be aware of the level of client satisfaction, and the extent to which their service is meeting the needs of the population, being ready to adapt and change their service according to needs if this appears necessary.

Consideration of context

In order to inform a basically humanitarian and respectful non-blaming approach, it is essential to understand that people do not exist or act in isolation of their context. To be human is to live interdependently with others, acknowledging the value and support others can bring. The wider context of the person is therefore both a necessary target for assessment and intervention and a resource for learning and growth. With this in mind, the approach should be sensitive to both the client and his or her family, taking into account their views, expectations, beliefs, and the meaning that the mental health problems have for them. It should respect the way the user and family have developed and adapted to the illness and difficulties that arise, responding to their story and their struggle to come to terms with the problems that have arisen. Within these values lies a belief that individuals and families respond to crisis and ongoing difficulties by utilizing the choices that appear available to them at the time. Sometimes these patterns of behaviour inadvertently impede growth and harmony. Thus the service provider must adopt an approach of uncritical acceptance of ways in which the client's family behaves towards one another.

The philosophical approach

Together, the client and the worker will search for the resources, assets, positive attributes, successes and strengths in and available to the user and his or her family or important others. In understanding the problems presented it should help the user and family begin the process of finding viable solutions, building on their strengths and helping them identify stressors which they need to overcome. This process will encourage self direction and determination in setting goals that build upon the desires and aspirations of the client. This approach is based on recognition of the capacity for all to continue to learn new skills, adapt and change; although at times steps will be small, and there will be setbacks, these must be seen as an essential part of living and learning. Thus the service provider lays open the conditions necessary for achievable goals to be met and is prepared to accompany the user and family in their endeavours.

ASSESSMENT

Assessment refers to the collection of relevant information about the client in order to offer appropriate and effective care. It is not a one off event, but a continuous process running through contacts between the client and the service provider. It can be formal, taking place in interviews, or being conducted with the use of specialized assessment tools; or informal, through observing and talking with the client generally. When selecting an approach to assessing clients, service providers must bear in mind that these clients have often spent many years going from one part of the mental health service to another, repeatedly being assessed for many different purposes. Their experience of disempowerment, alienation, confusion and perceived rejection by services has implications for the current assessment procedure. Assessment was introduced in the last section with particular reference to the care manager. We now need to examine assessment in terms of the direct service provider.

For the service provider, the first question to ask in terms of assessment is, assessment for what? For example, if clients have been referred by their case manager to a work-orientated day centre two mornings a week, the day centre does not need to know about all areas of their life. Some knowledge of certain areas will be essential in order to provide the service required, but clients' right to privacy and respect must be considered. It is likely that new areas of need will become apparent through working with the client and gaining a trusting relationship, but these need not be addressed in the initial assessment. Therefore, although this section offers a comprehensive framework for assessment, it is the responsibility of service providers to limit the amount of information collected to that which is necessary, or which the client wishes to share. Essentially, whatever the chosen method of assessment, it gives both the service provider and the client opportunities to get to know one another. It is a social encounter, the beginning of a relationship

in which respect is demonstrated, and trust developed. Since clients may have difficulty in answering questions and formulating or conveying their ideas and wishes clearly, the key skills at this point are active listening and observation, prompting, facilitating and sustaining conversation. Through the development of a trusting relationship, the worker and the client form a partnership that will lead to a collaborative assessment of the client's present situation, needs, strengths and hopes for the future.

Key points in the assessment process

1 Assessment has to be as collaborative as possible. Thus the service provider does not make decisions on the part of the client which serve to undermine his/her self-determination.

2 The assessment may involve many meetings. Rather than beginning with a formal and potentially threatening interview, the initial meeting should be seen as a conversational opportunity to give some information about the service, and assessment procedures, to ask and answer questions, to get to know each other and begin to foster a rapport.

3 If assessment tools and formal interview schedules are used, their purpose and perceived benefits must be explained. To reduce confusing and alienating the client they must have relevance for the client, or for imminent service developments.

4 Rather than making assumptions about the client, observations and understandings reached by the worker should be checked out with the client. This gives them a chance to give these conclusions more meaning, or to suggest alternative meanings.

It is helpful to see assessment as an evolutionary process; as urgent needs become apparent, service providers can begin to undertake practical tasks to meet these. This helps to prove their value in the eyes of the client, builds up trust, and helps them get to know the client better so that qualities and strengths are recognized and areas of personal difficulty can be identified. Thus assessment becomes part of an engagement process, in which both parties become trusted and valued.

Areas to assess

Every service needs a basic checklist of areas to be covered in assessment. This may include no more than a list of risk factors, or it may demand a full and comprehensive account of the client and his/her social network. Whatever this basic framework for assessment, the reasons for omission, and the relevance of all areas must be clear to those using it. As far as possible the user should be given opportunities to influence the areas of assessment. If it is to be a collaborative relationship a level of equality needs to be established. The skill of service providers lies in their ability to draw out the user's aspirations and seek clarification, introducing ideas and encouraging the client to consider all options, sustaining the assessment so that goals can be agreed.

Many models of practice point to a range of areas to be assessed, often dependent on the conceptual underpinnings of the approach. The starting point for us is gaining an understanding of what users see as pertinent at the time of contact, recognizing that the assessment process is ever evolving, as clients gain insight into further areas that they wish to pursue, and gain the confidence in their worker to entrust this information.

When the user is less able to be involved in directing the assessment, the service provider can draw on the views of the case manager, who may have had more opportunity at this stage to formulate with the user those areas he or she wishes to consider. We stress that any such discussions should be conducted with the client's knowledge, or with them in person.

Where clients have been referred for a general assessment of need, either for case management or for residential service provision, it is not sufficient to allow them to define the areas which are assessed. A more comprehensive assessment of their abilities and difficulties is necessary in order to gain a full picture of their need for services, and their satisfaction with their current lifestyle.

The needs of clients should be understood in the context of their life as a whole. It is all too easy to miss areas of low satisfaction and unmet needs and thereby reduce the opportunities for the users to take control of all areas of their life. Some people find it easier than others to express their needs and identify aspirations for the future. Many people in this client group have been inducted into a system where their low expectations, lack of confidence and poor skills are accepted if not expected. They have not had the encouragement nor the opportunities to appraise their potential and limitations for themselves within a safe, encouraging and informative environment. They do not know what to aim for because they have never considered the possibilities available to them.

A general assessment of all areas of the client's life is not always advocated, but when undertaken appropriately, as for example by the case manager, it provides a useful opportunity to evaluate with the situation globally, and to consider general, as opposed to specific, changes that need to be made. It can also provide an opportunity to give the user feedback on strengths and successes which can be utilized in planning care. The important point here is the need to avoid compiling a demoralizing and long list of deficits or problems; inquiry into these areas should take place through consideration of strengths and must be framed positively. Assessment should encourage expansion in the user's life and not close down possibilities.

Whilst attention needs to be given to the relevance of assessing all areas of a client's life, the broad matters that would need to be covered in a general assessment include:

1 *Mental health*, including symptomatology, although this need not be over-emphasized as the level of symptomatology is often not related to the client's level of functioning. Knowledge of factors which the client perceives as stressful, and of previous admissions is more useful in giving a predictive picture.

2 *Physical health*, including chronic physical illness and disabilities.

3 *Finance*, including benefits received, arrears, regular outgoings.

4 *Housing*, including type of accommodation, adequacy, and if appropriate the type of accommodation that the client would prefer.

5 *Daily living skills*, including self-care skills and ability to use community facilities.

6 *Home management skills*, including cooking, shopping, cleaning, budgeting and simple household maintenance.

7 *Social skills and social support network*; social interaction skills, family relationships members of the client's social network and roles they play.

Each of these areas may be examined in greater or lesser depth depending on the value base and chosen means of assessment within the service, and their meaning to the client.

When working with people with enduring mental health problems, who have multiple, complex and inter-related needs, the process of assessment is informed mainly by the unique needs and wishes of each individual client. Since the mental state of the client is only one of many potential areas of need, this is not the primary focus of the assessment unless identified as such by the client. The aim of assessment is to clarify client's wishes, and to facilitate clients in identifying their goals. In order to identify their needs it may be necessary to explore a wide range of areas of their life, and discuss their views on the appropriateness of alternative options. This necessitates a slow approach based on the development of a trusting relationship with the clients.

PLANNING

Once the nurse and user have fulfilled an initial assessment, and agreed overall goals, all the information will be drawn together in order to plan the steps to be taken to meet the identified needs and goals of the user. Obviously, it may be appropriate for urgent needs to be addressed before a full assessment has been completed. Indeed achieving a few prioritized tasks may, as already suggested, facilitate the development of a relationship between the client and worker which enables a more accurate assessment to be completed in the long term.

In planning the work that needs to take place in order to meet needs and achieve goals, several questions need to be addressed: who will do what, when will progress be reviewed, and how will both parties know whether they have achieved what they set out to achieve?

In formulating a plan that addresses these issues, the worker and the client need to negotiate their roles, and they need to draw on the expertise of others. A review needs to be called with all those involved in the assessment, and those likely to be implementing the plan so that all the information collected can be collated. It is essential that the client is involved at this stage, if not in person then through some form of advocacy. Increasingly care managers are taking an advocacy role—as far as possible within their professional role—as they may have the most comprehensive knowledge of the client and have least vested interest in the service provider unit. As an employee of one of the statutory agencies, they can never be a truly independent advocate as defined in the last section.

In this planning review goals must be set and agreed with the client. These must be achievable, measurable and realistic with timescales for their achievement or review. Working with this client group is by definition a long-term process, so time is available for goals to be split into multiple small stages, each of which is a source of achievement. Any constraints incurred in the plan must be identified at an early stage so that they do not form the stumbling block that deters the client from trying further, for example financial costs and travelling difficulties. Alternatively, it may be necessary to work through psychological barriers before moving on. For example, if a client wants to attend an employment training centre, but has not got out of bed before midday for the last few years, strategies to help the client get up need to be discussed and if the client is willing, these may be rehearsed before their work assessment begins.

Whilst recognizing the limitations on services available, the goals must not be constrained by existing practice; it is important that the review team thinks as broadly as possible, not merely directing the client into mental health services, but drawing on resources that exist in the community, organizing the necessary support in creative and innovative ways.

Essential in this planning process is the maintenance of comprehensive information that will inform future reviews, and form the basis of an ongoing record of progress and events. Along with assessment information including the client's and the case manager's, or service provider's views and goals, the agreed methods for achieving these goals need to be recorded with a method for identifying the role of different people, including the client, in this work. The timing of the next review needs to be set, with an agreed person to co-ordinate this and ensure that all appropriate people and information are prepared.

By ensuring that set goals are written in such a way that they are measurable, evaluation becomes part of the review system. The progress of individuals can be assessed easily provided records are maintained that indicate the extent to which goals are attained, and the circumstances and the support required. On an individual level this informs future action and the formulation of future goals; at a service level it begins to indicate more or less useful methods of achieving goals for clients with similar needs. There also needs to be a built-in system for recording unmet needs and goals and the reasons for the lack of achievement. This should be collated with the same records of other clients to inform future service planning through identification of gaps or insufficiencies in existing services.

At all times the client's views are paramount in assessing the effectiveness and acceptability of the services used and strategies adopted. Their opinions, personal aspirations and informal responses must be integral to the care planning and evaluation process. They must have access to assessment information and to their own care plan and progress notes. The team must discuss the arrangement of a system in which clients are positively encouraged to view their records and able to add their own views to existing records.

IMPLEMENTATION

Following assessment clients will work towards achieving agreed goals with the help identified in the planning process. As they begin to engage in relationships and services their goals may change and more needs and strengths will become apparent. Therefore the care process must be flexible and reflexive according to the clients' wishes and abilities at that time.

The relationship with the client

For many long-term clients, the main intervention may be long-term support and continuous contact with one named service provider. The client and care manager, or service provider, may agree that the focus of their relationship should be based on regular meetings to talk things over, gain information and advice when it is needed. In the absence of a social network, the worker may be their only reliable point of contact. Although this work can be seen as low key and unchallenging, 'being there' is probably the bedrock of rehabilitation. It provides the continuity, familiarity and trust which might be crucial in overcoming stressful life events, coping with increasingly disturbing symptoms, and negotiating everyday complexities such as paying bills, understanding official letters, preparing for and surviving visits from family and managing upsetting encounters. Far from unchallenging, it is demanding work, requiring persistence, high-level interpersonal skills and a high degree of commitment in order to ensure that the client continues to feel valued and understood.

However, this relationship should not be seen as an end point which perpetuates low expectations as self-fulfilling prophecies. It is within this supportive relationship that the service provider can maximize opportunities to enhance the client's self-determination, stimulate learning, redefine problems and needs, and help the client find viable solutions and recognize long suppressed aspirations. One important element in this relationship is the service provider's role in enabling the client to develop effective coping strategies. By working with clients to gain an understanding of their life and their meaning systems, workers can identify with clients how and when distress arises and what they can begin to do to anticipate it and deal more effectively with it when it occurs.

Thus the ground work of rehabilitation is the therapeutic nature of the relationship between client and worker. This is based on empathy, genuineness and warmth, the service provider internalizing a value system that prioritizes and respects the client, and explicitly helps the client maintain a positive equilibrium in health. All other interventions are secondary to this and are likely to be more effective if this relationship exists. It is through the development of this relationship that clients can accept more complex modes of care and treatment so that they can develop, achieve more, manage setbacks, and eventually move away from this relationship as their main support.

Individual interventions

We will now concentrate on some of the valuable approaches the nurse can adopt in meeting the needs and goals of the user. Yet again, the point to stress is the need for the service provider to be acutely aware of the user's own ideas and beliefs and to apply sensitivity when approaching an aspect of the users life or illness. Any intervention must be collaborative, based on working with the client rather than 'doing to' him or her.

The interventions below are not comprehensive, and are only introduced briefly, but, it is hoped that sufficient information is given to increase curiosity and further reading. Those interventions selected emphasize the essential belief that the client lives interdependently in a broader context. This environment and people within it are meaningful in the way the client establishes an identity and role within society, their social network and their family or home. In addition interventions have been explored which enable the client to develop and maintain a position in the wider context of the community. Many of the interventions introduced in other sections of this book are equally useful for this client group, provided the care is provided on a basis of collab-

oration with the client, and is offered to meet needs which the client identifies.

Working with the family

The focus of the individual in providing care often involves separating or estranging clients from their family, whether they are living with them at the point of referral, or in regular contact. Unless the family is involved in the treatment and care of the individual, this aspect of service provision may become a missed opportunity for improving the quality of life for both clients and their relatives.

As discussed in the first section, community care often means family-based care. Relatives are frequently faced with managing the often difficult behaviour of the identified patients and coping with his or her diverse needs. They often have little direct support, and are given little information to help them understand the problems of the client, or on the most useful ways of helping and enhancing the opportunities of the client.

Obtaining basic information about medication, diagnoses and available help is often left to the family. Families frequently do not even know what questions to ask about how to interpret the client's behaviour, what expectations they may reasonably hold, and the means of improving communication within the family. The response of services to their requests can leave them feeling blamed and helpless, as disempowered as the clients themselves, and therefore unable to come forward to express their needs. Although carers' groups are demanding a change in attitude of providers, on an individual level it is all too easy to dismiss or forget their position.

There is growing evidence and opinion to suggest that working with families and considering them in any care package should be a routine part of service delivery (Kuipers and Bebbington, 1985; Smith and Birchwood, 1990). Service providers therefore need both to acquire the appropriate skills for working with families, and shift their working philosophy from working with the individual to involvement of the wider context. Training programmes are being developed for nurses to work with the families and carers of people with enduring mental health problems, and evaluations of these initiatives have demonstrated their effectiveness in reducing relapse and improving difficult behaviour in clients (Smith and Birchwood, 1990; Fallon *et al.*, 1990; Brooker *et al.*, 1991).

The increased interest in working with the family in recent years stems most directly from the research into 'expressed emotion'. Expressed emotion (EE) is a 'global index of particular emotions, behaviours and attitudes expressed by relatives about a family member with schizophrenia. The specific factors that make up the construct of EE are criticism hostility, and emotional over-involvement' (Jenkins and Karno, 1992).

Families that exhibit high levels of EE have been associated with earlier relapse whereas low EE families, characterized as warm, uncritical and sympathetic, are associated with reduced relapse (Brown *et al.*, 1972; Vaughn and Leff, 1976). This effect has been found to be more marked in families where the client is non-compliant with medication. However, this dichotomy has been criticized as it suggests that only those families with high EE require intervention, when EE in fact varies over time, and all families require some form of help. It also effectively labels families as good or bad. Some of these families are now speaking out (Hatfield *et al.*, 1987).

The work on EE has provided a basis for the development of approaches to working with families that are not based on cure but on developing appropriate coping strategies within the family and reducing relapse; these are commonly referred to as 'psychosocial interventions' (see Brooker *et al.*, 1991; Tarrier, 1991). The purpose of this section is not to detail these training programmes but to highlight the need to engage with families and other care givers and prescribe some basic principles, emphasizing the necessary attitudes and skills of the service provider. Many of the values propounded thus far can be seen to overlap with the components of family work.

It is important that the needs of all families are considered; it has been suggested that family work should not be initiated solely with families demonstrating high EE as this may lead to the neglect of those with low EE (Smith and Birchwood, 1990). These families may well have very different needs and there may be a possibility that they condone or make undue allowance for the client's negative behaviour, leading to poor social functioning and decreased opportunities for the user to take control of his or her life situation. Every family has a right to support and help to improve the client's quality of life.

Psychosocial interventions with families are based on behavioural approaches and have a broad systems perspective. They are not purely concerned with deficits but assert the need to examine the strengths and the assets of the people involved. Thus the emotions, beliefs and behaviours of individuals within the family are not seen in isolation, but understood in the way they combine among family members to determine the meaning of their relationships. In addition, this approach is explicit in not attributing blame to any one person or group, rather the way the family behaves is accepted as the current best option for dealing with stress, even if it is not desirable.

Ham (1991) reviews the psychosocial packages of family interventions and suggests that seven commonalities exist among them. These form the basis of the skills which the service provider must develop in order to offer effective care to the family with a member with enduring mental health problems:

1 A positive approach and genuine working relationship that is non-blaming, and stresses positive assets and the potential for change. Attempts are made to understand the view of all the family members and to see each person's behaviour as his or her best attempt at coping. Behaviours which the worker might view as undesirable are reframed in a positive, non-blaming manner. All members' needs are respected, and the stress they are placed under in attempting to support the client is acknowledged.

2 Meetings are arranged on a regular basis, providing structure and stability. A contract may be set up with the family including the availability of outside contacts. The family is given help to set appropriate limits and moderate levels of interpersonal distance.

3 The meetings focus on the here and now, looking at current problems and stresses.

Present coping strategies and previous effective behaviour is identified. There is an emphasis on the way the family interacts and the individual's perceptions about this. The family is introduced to new methods that might be useful in controlling the family atmosphere including the discouragement of criticism, over-involvement and over-permissiveness.

4 Family concepts are used to clarify the family structure and reduce the merging of interpersonal and generational boundaries, and to support subsystems within the family including the marital coalition.

5 Information is given in an educational way to help the family make sense of the behaviours and feelings of the client and relatives.

6 A behavioural approach is used such that viable goals are agreed. Priorities are then set, and the goals broken down into small recognizable steps. Tasks are assigned to individual members and the family as a whole, these are reviewed at each meeting.

7 Attempts are made to improve communication. This involves expressing requests for change in a clear, simple and specific way. Detailed steps are taken to rehearse and offer feedback on useful aspects of communicating.

This is not a comprehensive list and not all studies include all of these in explicit ways. However, it provides an illustration of the range of skills needed and the attitudinal base. Most psychosocial training packages also stress the importance of the acceptance of a disease model in providing information. They also condone medication, and presume that family intervention does not take place in the absence of other service provision.

The importance of engaging families cannot be over-stressed. Where the client is adamant that this is not desirable, the service provider must weigh up the benefits and costs of not doing so. It is likely that the client is living with the family, or will be returning to do so, in which case time must be taken to negotiate a form of contact that is agreeable to both parties. Workers who adopt a stance of protecting the client from the family, in the belief that working with the whole family will betray the trust of the client, must consider their rationale carefully. Does this approach hide an underlying belief that the family is to blame? In the long term, estranging the family may well be to the detriment of both clients and their relatives, both in relation to self-determination and quality of life. Any change that may be fostered in the client away from the family may prove difficult to sustain without reciprocal change in those around them.

It needs to be added that the principles of psychosocial interventions are not only useful with families; they have been applied both by workers in residential settings (Elliot *et al.*, 1991), and to educate workers in private residential homes (Ould, 1991). From the evidence available this appears to have been successful in reducing relapse and improving clients' satisfaction.

Medication

The majority of people with enduring mental health problems are prescribed some form of major psychotropic medication, however there are several areas of controversy over the role of medication with this client group.

The problems.   Firstly, although medication is effective in reducing or eliminating the symptoms of mental illness in the short term (Hirsch, 1982), there are questions regarding its long-term effectiveness. It is reputedly less effective for negative symptoms and social disability, which are often the main problems of this client group (Silverstone and Turner, 1988). In fact, medication has been found to be most effective for people with enduring mental health problems when combined with other treatment interventions, for example family work (Vaughn and Leff, 1976), rather than as the sole mode of treatment.

Secondly, long-term psychotropic medication is often prescribed at a constant level over long periods of time without adequate review procedures. Holloway (1988) reported evidence of over-prescribing of both single and multiple drugs in a study of long-term users of day centres. Although depot administration can lead to a reduction in relapse, the dose, frequency and review of medication needs to be refined on an individual client basis. Lack of attention to medication is particularly neglectful when one considers the side-effects; up to 40% of people prescribed neuroleptics suffer one or more distressing side-effects. The fact that severity and duration of these effects vary from individual to individual, and cannot be predicted, further confirms the need to consider every client separately and review frequently.

Thirdly, and perhaps not surprisingly, non-compliance with medication is probably a common cause of relapse. It is difficult to estimate the level of non-compliance amongst people with enduring mental health problems, but it is those living independently who are most likely to miss medication, or take more than prescribed, either through forgetfulness, a poor routine, over-dependence on medication, or a decision to stop taking medication because of side-effects or perceived improvement in their mental state. The underlying reasons for non-compliance are likely to be a poor understanding of the role of medication and the way that it works; problems in the doctor–patient relationship resulting in the client feeling a lack of control over the prescription; difficulty in obtaining their medication—just not being organized enough to get to the pharmacy or the depot clinic when medication is due; and the meaning that medication holds for the client. This may be based on a belief that being well is dependent on not taking drugs, on bad experiences of medication in the past, or on family attitudes to medication. Again much of this rests on poor information about the prescription.

The service provider's role. Although the prescription of medication is the domain of the psychiatrist, service providers must have a knowledge of psychotropic medication, accepted dosages, the benefits of alternative drugs, and the side-effects. This will enable them to know when it is appropriate to refer to a medical practitioner for a review of medication, or to call on the community pharmacist for information. More importantly, they will be in a position to discuss the role and relevance of medication with clients and where appropriate, their family.

The care manager has a responsibility to ensure that medication is reviewed regularly—frequently if there are particular problems—as part of the care package. It may be necessary to accompany clients in their appointments to the doctor to help them explain their anxieties and to negotiate alternative prescriptions. Where it is known that the client has professional support it may be possible to reduce medication and take the risk of relapse in the knowledge that a safety net is available.

For all clients prescribed medication, an assessment of their prescription, their knowledge, attitudes, side-effects and pattern of administration is essential. This will not only provide an opportunity for workers to provide information and rectify misperceptions, it will also alert them to the need for review of medication, and to the possibility of non-compliance.

Where non-compliance is a problem the service provider has an important role in discovering the reasons for this, and finding a way of resolving the problems. It may be that there is a difference in opinion between the staff and the patient over medication and the client refuses it. The consequences of this decision need to be made clear, and the service provider needs to support and monitor the client through this time. It is the client's right to refuse medication unless he or she is held under a section of the Mental Health Act, but if the client is overall felt to be in need of continuing medication, steps need to be taken to make medication acceptable to him or her. This may take time, and will be facilitated by a close relationship between the service provider and client. The basis of the client agreeing to take medication may well be improved understanding of the positive benefits as against the negative consequences. This may be helped by altering the drug, the means of administration, the times of the day it is taken, negotiating a reduction over time, and teaching clients to build drug-taking into their daily routine.

Essentially clients should be encouraged to take control over their medication, recognizing themselves as the expert in their personal response to their drugs. This involves recognizing their symptoms and related stressors and becoming aware of the effectiveness of medication in relation to these. In this way they can discuss their level of medication in a knowledgeable way with their service provider and it can be prescribed and taken in an effective yet flexible and client-centred manner.

Work or occupation

Work, meaning any purposeful activity directed towards goals beyond the enjoyment of the activity itself (Shepherd, 1988), has held a central position in the care and treatment of people with mental health problems since the initiation of 'moral treatment' (see the first section in this chapter), and it continues to form the mainstay of rehabilitation. As Shepherd (1983) states 'no other single activity is so rich and complex in its psychological, social and material significance'. Despite the current economic recession and correspondingly high levels of unemployment—making it difficult for those without mental health problems to obtain and maintain employment let alone people with long-standing mental health problems—work continues to be the only clear indicator by which society judges wellness and normality. Work not only offers the client a positive role, position and status in society, it offers social contacts and support, a means of structuring time, financial reward and a sense of personal achievement.

Work experience or occupational rehabilitation for people with enduring mental health problems is usually only part of the care package. Thus both the staff at the workplace and other service providers have particular roles to play in facilitating an effective and satisfying work experience. The delivery of services providing work or occupational experience is undertaken by variously trained personnel all of whom need to be alert to changes in the client's condition and able to inform appropriate others. They need to work with other members of the care team to monitor symptomatology, and if necessary, supervise medication. Non-attendance and under-engagement in occupational rehabilitation needs to be investigated and communicated to others where appropriate. Ideally staff from the client's workplace need to be involved with others in the care team on a face-to-face basis so that both formal and informal communication can take place effectively.

The main service provider, or care manager, has a pivotal role in introducing the client to suitable and acceptable work schemes. As Wansbrough (1981) notes, all clients, however disabled, should be given the opportunity to benefit from work. The client's aspirations to work and reasons for wanting to work must therefore be taken seriously. Their previous work experience, interests and skills must be assessed when considering the type of work most suitable. Since there is a shortage of work-orientated day care provision for people with enduring mental health problems (Wansbrough and Cooper, 1980), the service provider must be prepared to look widely at possible opportunities. Indeed where the shortage of a particular type of work is apparent, service providers have a responsibility to draw this to the attention of planners and current work provision units.

Once a client is engaged in some form of work, the main service provider has a key role in communicating with both the client and the work place, offering support and information to both, if necessary negotiating time out or reduced expectations when the client is under pressure. It is this type of intensive support and communication that will make the difference between a successful and unsuccessful work experience.

Social networks

People with enduring mental health problems have very small networks often only consisting of family members (Mueller, 1980). This is due to several factors including the social withdrawal that is often a feature of the illness; estrangement from previous friends as they carry the stigma of mental illness, or behave in a way that others cannot understand; over-protection and segregation by their family and social drift away from their family and childhood peer group as they fail to sustain employment and are forced to live in poverty. Where they claim to have friends, these are often people also in contact with mental health services and at times they may be experiencing stress or crisis. Erickson (1988) coined the term 'truncated' to describe the networks of people with enduring mental health problems. He suggested that adjectives such as small or diminished did not 'adequately convey any true sense of networks that may approach a membership of zero'.

The size of normal networks varies and is often dictated by the choices a person makes about friendship and family ties. The client should also be afforded these choices. Having a number of people around that the client can call friends, and look to for informal support, can also encourage the client to engage in activities outside his or her own setting and create opportunities for 'normal living'.

There is no formal method for improving clients' social networks, but there are means of working that may enable clients to overcome the underlying problems that have led to their isolation. The service provider has to have a knowledge of local resources and a degree of tenacity and assertiveness in exploiting these to the benefit of the client.

If clients identify loneliness, the lack of someone to turn to, or isolation, as a problem, the service provider needs to find ways of helping them develop a social network or make more use of their current network. The starting point is appraisal of the present situation. This involves identifying with clients: the positive attributes they bring to others, their opportunities for increased networking and the constraints they see in developing and using a network. They need to consider what has happened to network size over time and the reasons for it becoming truncated. Moxley (1988) has developed an interview tool to aid the practitioner and client in assessing the social network. It covers four main areas: structure of the overall network; identification of people the client perceives as supportive; description of the interactional qualities of the relationships in the network; and description of the socialization and social support content of the network.

Through examination of these areas the focus of working will become apparent; for example clients may need to improve relationships with their current network, they may need to extend their present network, and they may need to develop skills to overcome the constraints that have prevented them maintaining a network, for example lack of confidence, lost skills in social interaction or high levels of anxiety in social set-

tings. If the client is currently living in a hospital setting, ways of maintaining current contacts need to be facilitated.

The next stage in improving a client's support network involves discussing what he/she wants from other people. This may be friendship, it may be a companion to go out with, or someone to help when in a crisis. The worker can also help the client identify potential situations and people who might meet their needs at the available and effective levels, possibly drawing on their extended network or exploring new contacts.

The service provider and client need to agree their roles in making relevant contacts, for example the worker may accompany the client in social situations, might suggest other clients with similar needs, might explore new contacts and venues with the client, and will inevitably give support to the client in sustaining new or renewed contacts and rehearsing skills or overcoming anxieties.

In some cases clients will not be able to go beyond the networks they build up as a result of long-term contact with services and their available network may consist of other service users. This may be appropriate, as they may feel most comfortable with people who share their experiences and with whom they have regular contact and shared acquaintances. For some people, therefore, this is the group that the service provider will target. Although clients should be encouraged to use community services as a whole, they may not feel able to do this in isolation. In this situation it may be appropriate for service providers to work with a group of clients who can explore community resources together.

Social skills and daily living skills

Skills training is frequently seen to be the focus of rehabilitation with people with enduring mental health problems. It is predominantly carried out using behavioural methods based on an assessment of strengths and weaknesses, identification of priorities, use of rehearsal and feedback and problem-solving techniques. Alternatively, or simultaneously, the worker can use a more cognitive approach by offering opportunities for clients to talk over their social anxieties and fears individually or in a group. (A comprehensive over-view of work in this area is provided by Liberman *et al.* (1986).) It is not within the scope of this section to describe the range of interventions available, many of which have been introduced elsewhere in this book.

Despite the importance attached to skills train-ing, it does not appear to be effective in the long term. Although clients' social skills and social functioning may improve immediately after train-ing, this improvement is not maintained. The problem appears to lie in the difficulty maintain-ing improvement once the intervention has ceased, and in transferring skills learnt in a specific context to the client's every-day living environment.

Several factors may be helpful in improving the effectiveness of training. First, since clients with enduring mental health problems may have mul-tiple problems in this area, it is particularly im-portant that priorities are set and broken into small steps so that the client is not demoralized and over-burdened with the task of changing many different behaviours at the same time.

Secondly, in order to make the skills more meaningful to the client, they can be addressed most effectively in helping the client attain goals which hold meaning for them. For example, if clients are determined to live independently, they will need to acquire basic self-care skills. Further-more, if they do not want staff calling in every day, they will have to show that they are able to maintain a basic level of self care without super-vision. Thus, the client can see the usefulness of the skills, and acquiring them becomes part of regaining an independent and respected identity.

Thirdly, skills are likely to be generalized out-side the training situation if they are taught in diverse situations, diverse reinforcers are used, informal carers are involved in reinforcing skill improvements and self-report and self-monitoring techniques are used.

Finally, the long-term relationship advocated in this section can form a safe and trusted environ-ment for giving clients informal but meaningful feedback on their social skills. They can be made aware of the effects of their behaviour, and learn or relearn more acceptable modes of communi-cation. They can also discuss their difficulties with

daily living skills, and the type of support they find most useful. In this way skills training be-comes an individualized, reflexive and long-term process in pursuit of other goals.

EVALUATION

The importance of continuous evaluation cannot be overstressed. In order to provide flexible and client-centred care, evaluation must occur in all stages of the care process. For this to be useful in the long-term, ongoing records of events, changes and clients' feelings about the services provided must be maintained.

More formal evaluation of individual care occurs in regular multidisciplinary reviews of the client. These must be carefully co-ordinated so that attention is given to the client's views, service provider's views, and if possible repeated measures of an objective assessment can be pre-sented to demonstrate changes in targeted areas. However, outcome studies with this client group demonstrate little long-term change in any area other than client's perceived quality of life and satisfaction with services. Although complacency and under-achievement must not become the norm, expectations must be realistic. For some clients, the processes of maintaining a relation-ship, some form of stability and finding means of coping with the stresses of every-day life are suc-cesses to be celebrated as heartily as measured improvements in social functioning are for other clients.

Evaluation in a review system ensures that strategies are constantly reviewed, which gives the opportunity for the team to pool its ideas and expertise to find alternative interventions. Equally importantly, it provides a check on the quality of service being offered.

Although evaluation might imply hard work ahead and progress is often slow, it is an oppor-tunity for peer support and to share success. In order to maintain the commitment and motiv-ation of both clients and service providers, it is important for them to learn to frame their experi-ences positively as providing opportunities for growth and learning.

SUMMARY

The last two decades have been marked by a general lack of interest in the long-term users of mental health services. They have received neither the priority nor resources that were due to them. The result was in many instances the failure of community care. However, throughout this chapter we have seen the process of the needs of this client group becoming recognized. Simultaneously, a policy framework has been put forward for organizing care. We are now in a position to create services which, in addressing the problems identified, could lead to those services being equally valued by users, staff and the community in which they are located.

We are faced with the challenge and the opportunity to provide services that both prioritize people with enduring mental health problems and are driven by the users' needs. Within this framework, we offer a way of working with individual users that values their strengths and uses these as the basis for attaining the goals important to them.

The development of new community care systems will not occur immediately nor will it be without problems. It is important that the framework laid down in the NHS and Community Care Act (DH, 1990) is seen, like any process of change, as evolutionary. The changes need to develop in a way that recognizes local experiences, needs and resources, and are flexible, responsive and open to the changing characteristics of users and their families and the community in which the care takes place.

Whilst community care has remained the domain of the professionals it has led to the neglect and disempowerment of those using services. Now is the time to give them a say, see them as the experts in their own experiences and aspirations, put them at the centre of planning and to make them the final arbiter on the appropriateness of their own care.

FURTHER READING

Bennett, D. & Freeman, H. (Eds) (1991) *Community Psychiatry*. Edinburgh: Churchill Livingstone.

Lavender, A. & Holloway, F. (1988) *Community Care and Practice: Services for the Continuing Care Client*. Chichester: Wiley.

Murphy, E. (1991) *After the Asylums*. London: Faber & Faber.

Ramon, S. (Ed.) (1991) *Beyond Community Care: Normalisation and Integration Work*. London: MIND Publications/Macmillan.

Shepherd, G. (1984) *Institutional Care and Rehabilitation*. Longman: London.

REFERENCES

Anthony, W.A., Pierce, R.M., Cohen, M.R. & Cannon, J.R. (1981) *The Skills of Diagnostic Planning: Psychiatric Rehabilitation Practice Series*. Baltimore: University Park Press.

Brooker, C., Butterworth, C., Tarrier, N., Barrowclough, C. & Goldberg, D. (1991) The outcome of training community psychiatric nurses to deliver psychosocial intervention: report of a pilot study. *British Journal of Psychiatry*.

Brown, G., Birley, L. & Wing, J.K. (1972) Influence of family life on the course of schizophrenia disorders: a replication. *British Journal of Psychiatry*, **121**, 241–258.

Campbell, D. & Draper, R. (1985) *Applications of Systemic Family Therapy*. London: Grune & Stratton.

Department of Health (1990) *NHS and Community Care Act*. London: HMSO.

Department of Health (1993) The Mental Health Act. London: HMSO.

Elliot, H., Stockwell, C. & Metcalf, M. (1991) Family therapy in a rehabilitation hostel. *Nursing Standard*, **5**, 29–31.

Erickson, G.D. (1984) A framework and themes for social network interventions. *Family Process*, **23**, 187–197.

Fallon, I.R.H., Krekorian, H., Shanahan, W.J., Laporta, M. & McLees, S. (1990) The Buckingham project: a comprehensive mental health service based upon behavioral psychotherapy. *Behavioral Change*, **7**, 51–57.

Garety, P.A., Afele, H.K. & Issacs, D.A. (1988) A hostel ward for new long-stay psychiatric patients: the careers of the first 10 years' residents. *Bulletin of the Royal College of Psychiatrists*, **12**, 183–186.

Hatfield, A.B., Spaniol, L. & Zipple, A.M. (1987) Expressed emotion: a family perspective. *Schizophrenia Bulletin*, **13**, 221–226.

Ham, D.H. (1991) Psychosocial family intervention in

schizophrenia: a review of empirical studies. *Psychological Medicine*, **21**, 423–441.

Hirsch, S.R. (1982) Medication and the physical treatment of schizophrenia. In Wing J.K. & Wing, L. (Eds) *Handbook of Psychiatry, Vol. 3. Psychoses of Uncertain Origin*. Cambridge: Cambridge University Press.

Holloway, F. (1988) Prescribing for the Long-term mentally ill: a study of treatment practices. *British Journal of Psychiatry*, **152**, 511–515.

Hoult, J. (1986) Community care of the acutely mentally ill. *British Journal of Psychiatry*, **149**, 137–144.

Jenkins, J.H. & Karno, M. (1992) The meaning of expressed emotion: theoretical issues raised by cross-cultural research. *American Journal of Psychiatric*, **149**, 9–21.

Kisthardt, W.E. & Rapp, C.A. (1989) *Bridging the Gap Between Principles and Practice: Implementing a Strengths Perspective in Case Management*. Kansas City, Kansas: The University of Kansas Press.

Kuipers, L. & Bebbington, P. (1985) Relatives as a resource in the management of functional illness. *British Journal of Psychiatry*, **147**, 465–470.

Lawson, M. (1991) A recipient's view. In Ramon, S. (Ed.) *Beyond Community Care: Normalisation and Integration Work*. London: MIND.

Liberman, R.P., Mueser, K.T., Wallace, C.J., Jacobs, H.E., Eckman, T. & Mussel, H.K. (1986) Training skills in the psychiatrically disabled: learning competence and coping. *Schizophrenia Bulletin*, **12**, 631–647.

Moxley, D.P. (1988) Measuring the social support networks of persons with psychiatric disabilities: a pilot investigation. *Psychosocial Rehabilitation Journal*, **11**, 19–27.

Mueller, D. (1980) Social networks: a promising direction for research on the relationship of the social environment to psychiatric disorder. *Social Science Medicine*, **14**, 147–161.

Ould, J. (1991) Psychosocial training with workers in psychiatric registered homes. Paper Presented at the Innovations in Schizophrenia Conference. Derbyshire.

Shepherd, G. (1984) *Institutional Care and Rehabilitation*. London: Longman.

Shepherd, G. (1983) The current role of work in the rehabilitation of the psychiatric patient. In Gilhome Herbst, K. (Ed.) *Rehabilitation: the Way Ahead or the End of the Road?* London: The Mental Health Foundation.

Shepherd, G. (1988) *Current Issues in Community Care*. Report of the 2nd Annual Conference on the rehabilitation of psychiatric patients and their care in the community, 13.12.88. Leicester: The Association of Psychological Therapies.

Silverstone, T. & Turner, P. (1988) *Drug Treatments in Psychiatry*. London: Routledge & Kegan Paul.

Smith, J. & Birchwood, M. (1990) Relatives and patients as partners in the management of schizophrenia. *British Journal of Psychiatry*, **156**, 654–660.

Stein, L.I. & Test, M.A. (1985) *The Training in Community Living model: A Decade of Experience*. San Francisco: Jossey Bass.

Sundeen, J.S., Stuart, G.W., Rankin, E.D. & Cohen, S.P. (1976) *Nurse–Client Interaction: Implementing the Nursing Process*. St Louis: C.V. Mosby.

Tarrier, N. (1991) Familiar factors in psychiatry. *Current Opinion in Psychiatry*, **4**, 320–323.

Wing, J.K. & Furlong, R. (1986) A haven for the severely disabled within the context of a comprehensive psychiatric community service. *British Journal of Psychiatry*, **149**, 449–457.

Vaughn, C. & Leff, J.P. (1976) The influence of family and social factors on the course of psychiatric illness. *British Journal of Psychiatry*, **129**, 125–137.

Wansbrough, N. & Cooper, P. (1980) *Open Employment After Mental Illness*. London: Tavistock.

Wolfensburger, W. (1972) *The Principle of Normalisation in Human Services*. Toronto: National Institute on Mental Retardation.

CHAPTER

20

BIOLOGICAL ASPECTS OF TREATMENT AND INTERVENTION

Antoine Farine

AIMS

i) To identify aspects of neurophysiology relevant to treatments and intervention
ii) To consider the main characteristics of schizophrenia, depression, Alzheimer's disease, Parkinson's disease, Huntington's chorea and epileptic seizures and to explore the use of drugs and other biologically-based interventions in each one

KEY ISSUES

Section 1: Aspects of neurophysiology
Section 2: Schizophrenia
Section 3: Depression
Section 4: Dementia of Alzheimer's, Parkinson's and Huntington's chorea
Section 5: Seizures and epilepsy

Identify, analyse and assess factors causing distress and illness	Promote health, provide direct care and make interventions	Manage care programmes and services
Be critical, analytical and accountable, continue professional development	Counter discrimination, inequality and individual and institutional racism	Work within and develop policies, laws and safeguards in all settings
Understand influences on mental health and the nature/causes of disorder and illness	Know the effects of distress, disorder, illness on individuals, groups, families	Understand the basis of treatments and interventions

SECTION

1

ASPECTS OF NEUROPHYSIOLOGY

AIMS

i) To introduce those structures of the brain thought to be involved in the pathophysiology of mental disorders
ii) To consider the role of neurotransmitters

KEY ISSUES

Basal ganglia—structure and function
Limbic system—structure and function
Neurotransmitters

Identify, analyse and assess factors causing distress and illness	Promote health, provide direct care and make interventions	Manage care programmes and services
Be critical, analytical and accountable, continue professional development	Counter discrimination, inequality and individual and institutional racism	Work within and develop policies, laws and safeguards in all settings
Understand influences on mental health and the nature/causes of disorder and illness	Know the effects of distress, disorder, illness on individuals, groups, families	Understand the basis of treatments and interventions

INTRODUCTION

This brief review will focus on: (i) structures which are believed to contribute to the pathophysiology of mental disorder and also of physical disorders which may require psychiatric intervention and (ii) related neurotransmitters and their receptors and pathways. The purpose of the section is to identify aspects of neurophysiology which are relevant to the treatments and interventions explored in later sections of this chapter.

For more in-depth or detailed anatomy and physiology of specific structures in the brain, you may wish to consult appropriate textbooks (see Further Reading). Other chapters in this book, particularly Chapter 8 (Behaviour), also consider biological aspects of health and disorder and refer to basal ganglia, the limbic system and neurotransmitters.

Here the basal ganglia and their connection to other parts of the brain will be discussed, a brief section on the limbic system will be included and some basic properties of neurotransmitters will be considered.

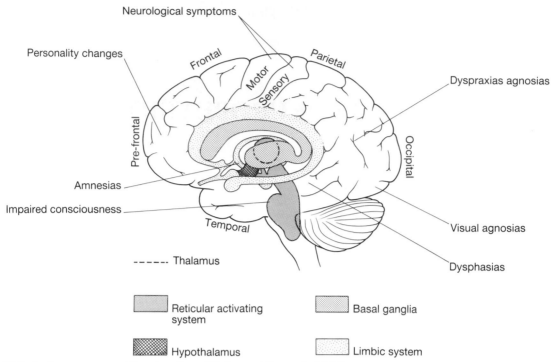

Neurological symptoms

Personality changes

Frontal

Motor

Sensory

Parietal

Dyspraxias agnosias

Pre-frontal

Occipital

Amnesias

Impaired consciousness

Temporal

Visual agnosias

Dysphasias

----- Thalamus

Reticular activating system

Basal ganglia

Hypothalamus

Limbic system

Fig. 20.1 *Brain structure and function (from Weller and Eysenck, 1992).*

BASAL GANGLIA

There is increasing evidence that the basal ganglia are involved in many disorders of the central nervous system, either through the loss of specific groups of neurones affecting the concentration of neurotransmitters or malfunctions which alter the metabolism of neurotransmitters. In order to understand how and why an individual may be affected, a grasp of the essential anatomy and physiology of the basal ganglia is important.

The basal ganglia are found in a core of grey matter deeply seated in each cerebral hemisphere (see Fig. 20.1). They consist of several nuclei which are interconnected—the caudate nucleus, the putamen, globus pallidus, subthalamic nucleus and the substantia nigra. The caudate nucleus and the putamen form what is known as the corpus striatum. The caudate nucleus is C-shaped and lies in proximity to the lateral ventricle. It consists of three parts, the head which is adjacent to the anterior horn of the lateral ventricle in the frontal lobe; the body which runs along the lateral

wall of the lateral ventricle; and the tail which runs in the roof of the inferior horn of the lateral ventricle. The globus pallidus lies medial to the putamen and lateral to the internal capsule. The globus pallidus and putamen are often referred to as the lentiform nucleus.

The nuclei of the basal ganglia, especially the corpus striatum, have an intricate network of neuronal circuits. They receive afferent neurones from the cerebellum, the cerebral cortex (mainly the premotor cortex) the substantia nigra and the thalamus. The basal ganglia do not have direct afferent or efferent connections with the spinal cord. Their motor functions are mediated by the frontal cortex.

Functions of the basal ganglia

The neuronal connections of the basal ganglia are extremely complex and since they are not easily accessible, explanations of their functions have been possible mainly through studying post-mortem brain specimens of patients with specific

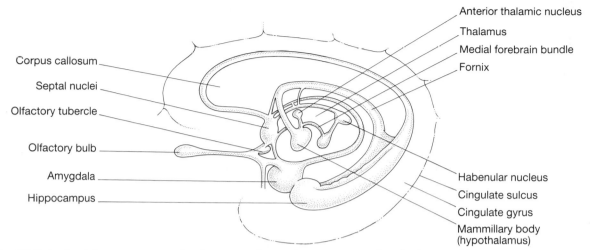

Fig. 20.2 *Limbic lobe connections: the diagram indicates the major cortical and subcortical brain structures implicated in the limbic system (from Hinchliffe and Montague, 1988).*

diseases and also by studying the effects of medications in specific diseases. Since diseases of the basal ganglia produce abnormal motor responses in the form of tremor, athetosis (slow, writhing movements of the fingers and hands), chorea (rapid, flick-like movements of the limbs and facial muscles) and ballism (rapid, flick-like movement), it has been deduced that their normal functions must be associated with co-ordinations of the fine motor movements and these are dependent on specific neurotransmitters.

Neurotransmitters which are important in maintaining a balance between the many neuronal pathways in the basal ganglia and thus contribute to the co-ordination of motor movements are dopamine, gamma aminobutyric acid (GABA), and acetylcholine. Disturbances in their concentration (i.e. a lower concentration) as indicated by post-mortem brain studies may affect movement in a variety of ways (see Chapter 8 and later sections in this chapter).

Neurotransmitters interrelate through their excitatory or inhibitory nature and it is unlikely that a specific neurotransmitter will be the sole agent responsible for a particular function. So, until more elaborate studies are undertaken *in situ* in live patients with specific basal ganglia disease or in healthy volunteers, the precise role of the nuclei in the basal ganglia and their neurotransmitters is likely to remain rather unclear.

LIMBIC SYSTEM

The limbic system is derived from the word limbus which means border. In fact, it forms a circle on the medial side of each hemisphere (see Fig. 20.1). The limbic system is a very complex structure consisting of cortical areas, nuclei and major connecting tracts and connections. The cortical areas consist of the parahippocampal gyrus, the hippocampus of the temporal lobe, and the cingulate gyrus which overlies the corpus callosum. The hippocampus is a C-shaped structure that gives rise to the fornix and mamillary body (Fig. 20.2).

The nuclei-forming parts of the limbic system are the amygdaloid nucleus, which lies deep within the temporal lobe, and the septal and hypothalamic nuclei. The amygdaloid is thought to be involved in the control of emotional behaviour such as fear and rage.

Functions of the limbic system

The extensive interconnections between structures forming the limbic system have made it very difficult for neurophysiologists to identify specific function of this complex system. For example, the exact pathways that control the emotions and motor behaviours are not clearly understood, but it is believed that the limbic system works in association with the autonomic nervous system and the spinal cord. Thus, it allows for co-ordination of blood pressure, heart rate and pupillary size. The limbic system also influences all of the endocrine systems of the body by controlling the release of hypothalamic hormones. The hippocampus is believed to play an important part in the retention of memory.

Stimulation of the septal nucleus can produce aggressive behaviour in animals, while tumours within that area can give rise to irritability and emotional instability in humans. Stimulation of structures such as the amygdala, hypothalamus and cingulate gyrus can also produce behavioural disturbances. In some studies it has been observed that destruction of the cingulate cortex in monkeys increases tameness. There are reports that psychological processes involving the cingulum or the cingulate gyrus can control intractable fears, anxiety, hostility and obsessional states.

The limbic system plays a vital role in the control and modulation of emotion, but it is still difficult to understand abnormal behavioural responses as a result of faulty connections within the limbic system. In terms of psychiatric illness, as long as the pathways forming the limbic system and their functions are not clearly understood, a dilemma will remain as to how best to manage affected individuals and help them choose the most appropriate or effective therapy.

NEUROTRANSMITTERS, RECEPTORS AND PATHWAYS

To appreciate altered physiology and its effects on the brain, it is essential to understand the normal interactions of neurotransmitters and their specific receptors in the nervous system. Through the understanding of these specific physiological functions, it has been possible to produce drugs which either mimic neurotransmitters (agonists) or block the receptors, or release of the transmitters and therefore preventing the neurotransmitter functioning (antagonists). Such drugs have revolutionized the treatment of some mental disorders and have also made it possible

for researchers to begin to understand the possible associated physiological changes.

An increase, reduction or absence of neurotransmitter, will affect brain functions. Neurotransmitters are low molecular weight substances released across the synaptic cleft in response to an action potential passing down the nerve axon. They interact with specific receptor sites on the postsynaptic region of the receiving neurone. Neurotransmitters are distributed throughout the brain but are localized in specific clusters of neurones whose axons project to other highly specific brain regions (see Fig. 20.3). Neurotransmitter receptors are transmembrane glycoproteins and their function is to allow communication between cells. The receptors have parts sticking out above and below the membrane like floating icebergs. The surface of the neurotransmitter receptor is precisely tailored to match the shape and configuration of the transmitter molecule, so that the latter fits into the former with the precision and specificity of a key entering a lock.

Many transmitter receptors have two functional components: (i) a binding site for the transmitter molecule, and (ii) a pore/channel passing through the membrane that is selectively permeable to certain ions.

The binding of the transmitter to the receptor alters its three-dimensional shape so that the pore is opened and ions inside and outside the cell membrane flow down their concentration gradient, resulting in either an excitatory or an inhibitory effect. There are two basic types of transmitter receptor; those reacting rapidly through mediating the transfer of information by controlling the permeability state of an ion pore and those that are long-acting receptors that cause the formation of a second messenger chemical which then triggers a series of physiological events.

There are specific receptors for specific neurotransmitters and some examples are: muscarinic and nicotinic acetylcholine receptors, dopamine D_1, D_2 and D_3 receptors, adrenergic receptors, GABA receptors, serotonin and opioid receptors.

Neurotransmitters which help transmit excitatory impulses in the main include: dopamine, noradrenaline, serotonin and acetylcholine, whereas gamma aminobutyric acid (GABA) has

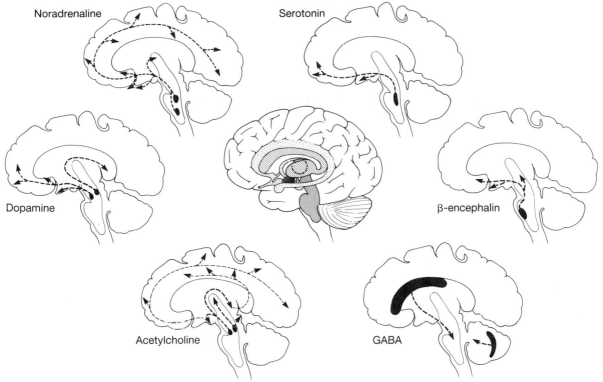

Fig. 20.3 *Principal neurotransmitter pathways (from Weller and Eysenck, 1992).*

an inhibiting effect. Other amino acids and polypeptides may also act as neurotransmitters or in some way affect transmission of impulses. The principal neurotransmitter pathways illustrating how neurotransmitters are localized into clusters of neurones, are shown in Fig. 20.3. The ideas and concepts included in this section will find application in the remaining sections of this chapter.

FURTHER READING

Doane, B.K. & Livingstone, K.F. (Eds) (1986) *The Limbic System: Functional Organisation and Clinical Disorders*. New York: Raven Press.

Hinchliffe, S. & Montague, S. (1988) *Physiology for Nursing Practice*. London: Baillière Tindall.

Holmes, O. (1990) *Human Neurophysiology*. London: Unwin Hyman.

Siegel, G., Bernard, A.E., Albers, R.W. & Molinoff, P. (1989) *Basic Neurochemistry*. Molecular, Cellular and Medical Aspects, 4th edn. New York: Raven Press.

Weller, M. & Eysenck, M. (1992) *The Scientific Basis of Psychiatry*. London: W.B. Saunders.

Wilkinson, S. (1992) *Neuroanatomy for Medical Students*. Oxford: Butterworth/Heinemann.

SECTION

2

SCHIZOPHRENIA

AIMS

i) To summarize the main characteristics of schizophrenia
ii) To examine the use of drugs in the treatment and management of schizophrenia

KEY ISSUES

Characteristics of schizophrenia
Drugs: their action and side-effects

Identify, analyse and assess factors causing distress and illness	Promote health, provide direct care and make interventions	Manage care programmes and services
Be critical, analytical and accountable, continue professional development	Counter discrimination, inequality and individual and institutional racism	Work within and develop policies, laws and safeguards in all settings
Understand influences on mental health and the nature/causes of disorder and illness	Know the effects of distress, disorder, illness on individuals, groups, families	Understand the basis of treatments and interventions

INTRODUCTION

Schizophrenia is one of the commonest psychiatric disorders accounting for approximately one half of first admissions to the psychiatric hospitals. It is classified as one of the functional psychotic disorders and its incidence in the population is approximately 1% (8–10 per 100,000 of the population) (Kallman *et al.*, 1938). This figure is believed to be fairly uniform throughout the world (with the exception of Ireland, North Yugoslavia and parts of Scandinavia which have slightly higher rates) even though different defi-

nitions of schizophrenia are used by clinicians in different countries. The onset is most common in the 15–35 years age group (Kendler *et al.*, 1985).

Since its classical definition by Eugen Bleuler in 1911 in Switzerland, there have been several attempts in the elaboration of definitions and classification of schizophrenia. The current criteria of schizophrenia require that a patient be continually ill for at least six months and that one or more of the following groups of symptoms be present:

Auditory hallucinations (hearing voices)

Bizarre delusions, often of a paranoid nature

Disorder of thought consisting of marked poverty of speech, loss of normal association of ideas

Passivity of feelings (loss of emotional responsiveness)

It is also possible to group symptoms of schizophrenia into catatonic, paranoid, hebephrenic and simple subtypes (Snyder, 1982). Crow (1980) has postulated the existence of two discrete disease syndromes: Type I and Type II. Type I corresponds to acute schizophrenia and is associated with the 'positive' symptoms of hallucinations, thought disorder, delusions with a good prognosis and excellent response to neuroleptics as well as normal cerebral ventricles. Type II is associated with 'negative' symptoms which include affective flattening, poverty of speech and loss of drive. Patients respond less well to neuroleptics and tend to have enlarged ventricles. On the basis of response to treatment Crow suggests that Type I schizophrenia involves neurotransmitter (dopamine) abnormalities whilst Type II schizophrenia is associated with organic brain changes.

The search for the pathophysiology of schizophrenia has been one of the most fascinating areas of study in psychiatric illness. Several lines of investigation have been undertaken and whilst for some there is evidence for the basis of pathology, others clearly lack such evidence. The lines of investigation have focused on (i) chemical neurotransmitter systems in the brain (dopamine hypothesis), (ii) altered functional structures in the brain, (iii) genetics and (iv) infection.

Perhaps the most compelling evidence for the involvement of the neurotransmitter system is that of the introduction of the drug largactil (known to block dopamine receptors) in the 1950s which completely revolutionized the treatment of schizophrenia, and also the discovery that drugs such as mescaline and lysergic diethylamide acid (LSD) can cause hallucinations and other disruptions of normal mental function resembling those in schizophrenia.

With the development of several neuroleptic drugs which could ameliorate the symptoms of acute schizophrenia research has tended to focus on the neurotransmitters.

DRUGS IN THE MANAGEMENT OF SCHIZOPHRENIA

Drugs which are used in the treatment of symptoms of schizophrenia are commonly referred to as neuroleptics or antipsychotics. The very first drug synthesized was chlorpromazine in 1950 by Charpentier. Chlorpromazine was first used in 1951 in the treatment of schizophrenic patients at the Val-de-Grace hospital in Paris (MacKay, 1982).

Neuroleptic drugs can be divided into three main groups: phenothiazines (chlorpromazine, thioridazine, trifluoperazine), butyrophenones (haloperidol) and thioxanthenes (thiothixene).

Pharmacological effects of neuroleptics

There is general agreement that neuroleptics block dopamine D_2 receptors in certain parts of the brain mainly in the nigrostriatal and mesolimbic pathways (Bartolini, 1976; De Belleroche and Neal, 1982). This is in accordance with what is known as the dopamine hypothesis in the causation of schizophrenia.

Neuroleptics have effects on other neurotransmitter systems and can block α-adrenergic, serotonin and cholinergic receptors. Gamma aminobutyric acid (GABA) is also affected. Neuroleptics can produce severe extrapyramidal side effects (to be discussed later) and this is due to their anticholinergic properties. Neuroleptics with the least anticholinergic properties (thioridazine) have the most extrapyramidal effects, whilst those with most anticholinergic properties have the least extrapyramidal side-effects. It would appear that extrapyramidal side-effects occur because the balance mechanism between cholinergic and dopamine neurones in a particular part of the brain (the striatum) is affected when dopamine receptors are blocked.

It would appear that neuroleptics are much more effective in the treatment of the so called 'positive' symptoms of schizophrenia (e.g. delusions, hallucinations).

Side-effects of neuroleptics

Neuroleptics can produce many side-effects, but the most common ones are those involving the extrapyramidal system and they include dystonia, tardive (late) dyskinesia, bradykinesia, akathisia. These side-effects occur as a result of a reduction of dopamine in the extra-pyramidal pathway and they are similar to Parkinsonism.

Dyskinesia

Dyskinesia is a disorder of movement. It is characterized by resting tremor and may present as an acute reaction. Tardive or late dyskinesia involves involuntary movements of the tongue, mouth and face which may present as grimacing or chomping (Weller, 1981). The patient is often largely unaware of these bucca-lingual-masticatory movements. Tardive dyskinesia is more common in older patients who have been treated with high doses of neuroleptics for many months or years. The basic mechanism is thought to be the development of supersensitivity to dopamine in the extra-pyramidal system (especially the nigrostriatal system). The symptoms are made worse by the use of anticholinergic drugs. A neuroleptic such as thioridazine which has greater affinity for the mesolimbic pathway may be less likely to induce tardive dyskinesia.

The management of tardive dyskinesia is difficult and there is much controversy as to the earlier use of anticholinergic drugs, since there is suggestion that anticholinergic drugs may themselves predispose to tardive dyskinesia.

It has even been suggested that tardive dyskinesia may be an aspect of schizophrenia itself and not the result of neuroleptics alone.

Bradykinesia

Bradykinesia leads to symptoms that affect normal spontaneous movements such as the swing of the arms when walking. More severe bradykinetic effects are similar to symptoms in Parkin-son's disease, such as a mask-like, expressionless face and sometimes excessive salivation.

Akathisia

Akathisia is an increased motor restlessness, which prevents the individual from sitting still for more than a few minutes. It takes the form of persistent rocking from one foot to the other, or stamping alternative feet. It is believed that the mechanism of this side-effect is as a result of the involvement of the mesortical dopamine pathway (Marsden and Jenner, 1980).

Dystonia

Dystonia (persistent pathological change in muscle tone) occurs in the first few days of treatment and is more common with the more potent neuroleptics such as haloperidol and piperazine phenothiazines. Symptoms may be expressed as torticollis (affecting neck muscles), trismus (affecting the jaw muscles), contraction of the tongue, opisthotonos (spasm affecting neck, back and legs) and occulogyric crises (affecting eye muscles). Passive movements of the limbs may be prevented by persistent resistance which is referred to as lead-pipe rigidity and later gives rise to the so called 'cogwheel' rigidity.

Other side-effects

Many of the other side-effects of the neuroleptics are due to antimuscarinic activity in the peripheral nervous system. This may produce dry mouth, blurred vision, constipation and difficulty in micturition. Hypotension can occur especially if neuroleptics such as haloperidol or piperidine-type phenothiazines are given intramuscularly. Allergic (contact) dermatitis used to be common in nursing staff handling phenothiazine syrups. Toxic effects such as agranulocytosis can also occur. Agranulocytosis has been associated with chlorpromazine and thioridazine. Patients on maintenance therapy should have differential blood counts every six months.

Patients on chlorpromazine may become sensitized to the effects of sunlight and the use of sun-creams may be helpful. Long-term exposure to neuroleptics sometimes gives rise to abnormal melanin deposits in skin exposed to sunlight and the skin appears metallic-grey. Opacities can occur in the cornea and the lens.

Other uses of neuroleptics

Neuroleptics can be used as sedatives, anxiolytics and some of them (metoclopramide and prochlorperazine) are effective as anti-emetics.

Gilles de la Tourette syndrome and tics respond to neuroleptics.

CONCLUSIONS

Neuroleptics have revolutionized the management of schizophrenia since the 1950s, and the most important benefit has been that of allowing patients to be treated in their own home and their early discharge from psychiatric hospitals.

Despite the introduction of newer neuroleptics, they are in the main prophylactic drugs and therefore reduce symptoms, but they do not offer a cure for schizophrenia.

The obvious severe side-effects of the neuroleptics pose serious concern amongst psychiatrists, as for example whether or not to use anticholinergic drugs (WHO, 1990) to prevent extra-pyramidal side-effects.

It is known that most neuroleptics block dopamine receptors in the mesolimbic and nigrostriatal pathways. The latter is responsible for the extra pyramidal side-effects. Other neurotransmitters are also involved and it is a combination of those other pharmacological effects that obscures the precise efficacy of neuroleptics. Thus, until more specific neuroleptics are developed, and the precise pathways of the various neurotransmitters are mapped out, their physiological functions clearly identified, the treatment for schizophrenia will remain in the *status quo*.

However, such biochemical studies are extremely difficult unless precise techniques are developed which can allow *in vivo* studies to be carried out on the brains of patients. Obviously this poses a very big ethical issue.

FURTHER READING

Crow, T.J. (1982) The biology of schizophrenia. *Experientia*, **38**, 1275–1282.

REFERENCES

Bartolini, G. (1976) Differential effect of neuroleptic drugs on dopamine turnover in extrapyramidal and limbic system. *Journal of Pharmacy and Pharmacology*, **28**, 423–429.

Bleuler, E. (1911) *Dementia praecox or the group of schizophrenics*. New York: International Universities Press. (Translated by Zirkin, J., 1950.)

Crow, T.J. (1980) Molecular pathology of schizophrenia: more than one disease process. *British Medical Journal*, **280**, 66–68.

De Belleroche, J.S. & Neal, M.J. (1982) The contrasting effects of neuroleptics on transmitter release from the nucleus accumbens and corpus striatum. *Neuropharmacology*, **21**, 529–537.

Kallman, F.J. (1938) *The genetics of schizophrenia*. New York: Augustus.

Kendell, R.E. (1985) Schizophrenia: Clinical Features. In Michaels, R. & Cavenar, J.O. (Eds) *Psychiatry*. Philadelphia: Lippincott.

Kendler, K.S., Ernenberg, A.M. & Tsuang Ming, T. (1985) Psychiatric illness in first degree relatives of schizophrenic and surgical control patients. A family study using DSM—III criteria. *Archives of General Psychiatry*, **42**, 770–779.

MacKay, A.V.P. (1982) Antischizophrenic drugs. In Tyrer, P.J. (Eds) *Drugs in Psychiatric Practice*. Sevenoaks, Kent: Butterworth.

Marsden, C.D. & Jenner, P. (1980) The pathophysiology of extrapyramidal side effects of neuroleptic drugs. *Psychological Medicine*, **10**, 55–72.

Snyder, H.S. (1982) Neurotransmitters and CNS disease. Schizophrenia. *The Lancet*, **ii**, 970–973.

Weller, M.P.I. (1981) Schizophrenic neuroleptics and Parkinson's disease. In Rose, F.C.R. & Capildeo, R. (Eds) *Recent Advances in Neurology*. London: Pitman Medical.

WHO (1990) Prophylactic use of anticholinergics to patients on long-term neuroleptic treatment: a concensus statement. *British Journal of Psychiatry*, **156** p. 412.

SECTION

3

DEPRESSION

AIMS

i) To explore the biological basis of depression
ii) To examine the use of drugs in the treatment and management of depression

KEY ISSUES

Types of depression
Drugs:
    Tricyclics
    Monamine oxidase inhibitors
    Electroconvulsive therapy

Identify, analyse and assess factors causing distress and illness	Promote health, provide direct care and make interventions	Manage care programmes and services
Be critical, analytical and accountable, continue professional development	Counter discrimination, inequality and individual and institutional racism	Work within and develop policies, laws and safeguards in all settings
Understand influences on mental health and the nature/causes of disorder and illness	Know the effects of distress, disorder, illness on individuals, groups, families	Understand the basis of treatments and interventions

INTRODUCTION

Depression is a very common psychiatric disorder and may be described as reactive or endogenous. Reactive depression usually occurs as a result of a loss or any other major stressful events in an individual's life, whilst endogenous depression (the most severe form) occurs without any apparent cause. The type of depression to be described here is the endogenous type.

Depression is classified as an affective disorder, marked by distinct symptoms which in its most severe form can lead the patient to commit suicide. Fifteen per cent of depressed patients commit suicide.

Over the last 20 years depression has also been described as unipolar (UP) or bipolar (BP). Unipolar is characterized only by periods of depression whilst bipolar co-exists with episodes of hypomanic mania (less severe than mania) which is manifested as euphoria in which the individual appears elated. This may also be accompanied by hostility, irritability, and sudden irrational decisions. In extreme cases delusions and hallucinations may be present. Women are affected about two to three times more often than men in unipolar depression. In bipolar both sexes are affected equally. Unipolar illness may be endogenous or reactive (Aubelas 1987).

Depression covers a wide spectrum of symptoms such as:

Insomnia, giving rise to morning awakening (3 a.m. is not unusual). Loss of appetite (although as reported by Young et al., 1990, some women have increased appetite and weight gain)

Negative self concept in which there is severe lack of confidence, self worth and the individual may be unable to maintain personal cleanliness

Unresponsiveness to normal stimuli which is preceded by depressed mood

Changes in motor activity, poverty of movement, lack of motivation, restlessness, slowing down of thoughts, difficulty in concentrating, persistent repetition of tasks

---

The pathophysiology of depression is still obscure, although several biochemical theories have been postulated which include changes in neurotransmitter activity, and neuroendocrine abnormalities. There is also perhaps a very strong genetic predisposition for the development of endogenous depression. Some studies also show a link between seasonal variation and depression.

DRUGS IN THE MANAGEMENT OF DEPRESSION

Although various therapies may be used in the management of depression, only drugs (e.g. antidepressants, lithium) and electroconvulsive therapy will be described here.

Antidepressant drugs fall into two main groups, the tricyclics and the monoamine oxidase inhibitors. The precise mechanism by which those two drugs work is not clear, but the result is an increase in postsynaptic neurotransmitter either through blocking the re-uptake of neurotransmitter from the presynaptic bouton or preventing it from being degraded by the enzyme monoamine oxidase. In so doing, more neurotransmitter is available for the postsynaptic bouton and its receptor sites. Thus the levels of noradrenaline and serotonin are raised.

Tricyclics

Tricyclic antidepressants are the most widely prescribed antidepressants and they have been found to be beneficial in about 70% of depressed patients (Klein and Davis, 1969).

It is believed that most tricyclic antidepressants exert their effects by blocking α_2 adrenoceptors (autoreceptors) on the presynaptic bouton (Raisman et al., 1979). In so doing, this causes increased neuronal firing boutons and hence release of neurotransmitter. In the intact system (absence of depression) α_2 adrenoceptors inhibit the release of neurotransmitters. Several studies have suggested that there is an excess of α_2 adrenoceptors during depressive illness.

Another mode of action of tricyclic antidepressants is to cause blockade of re-uptake of neurotransmitters. For example imipramine and amitryptiline, which are tricyclic antidepressants, inhibit the uptake of 5-hydroxytryptamine. Tricyclic antidepressants also act as antagonists at the cholinergic muscarinic receptors and this accounts for some of the side-effects such as dry mouth, urinary retention, constipation, blurred vision and even confusion. Postural hypotension can also occur as a side-effect and this is as a result of adrenergic blockade. Other side-effects which can also occur especially in the elderly are: cardiac arrhythmias, tachycardia, weight gain, sweating, epilepsy, aggravation of glaucoma.

Many drugs belong to the tricyclic antidepressant group, including amytriptyline, nortriptyline, mianserin, trimipramine, oxaprotiline, alaproclate, fluoxetine, citalopram, talsupram, nomifensine, bupropion and maprotiline.

Monoamine oxidase inhibitors (MAOIs)

MAOIs cause irreversible inhibition of the enzyme monoamine oxidase A and thus block deamination of the neurotransmitters, 5-hydroxy-

---

Information card for users of monoamine oxidase inhibitors

MONOAMINE OXIDASE INHIBITOR

What you need to know

Drug ....

Name ....

Carry this card with you always. Show it to any doctor who may treat you, to your dentist if you require dental treatment, and to the pharmacist when you buy any medicine for yourself

Please read carefully

While taking this medicine, and for ten days afterwards, you must follow these instructions

Do not eat or drink anything which contains

- Cheese, Bovril, Oxo, Marmite or similar meat or yeast extracts

- Pickled herrings

- Broad bean pods (the long green envelope which contains the beans, you can eat the beans themselves)

Adapted from Weller and Eysenck, 1992

Avoid

- Chianti wine completely, and drink no more than a little alcohol of any kind

- Game, or meat that has not been well preserved

Other foods cause no problems

Do not take other medicines

(including tablets, capsules, nose drops, inhalations or suppositories) whether bought for you or previously prescribed by your doctor without first consulting him

N.B. Cough and cold cures, pain relievers, tonics and laxatives are medicines

These drugs are safe if the above precautions are observed

- You may use plain Aspirin BP or plain Paracetamol BP if necessary

- If you need something for constipation ask your pharmacist for a bulk laxative

Report any severe symptoms to your doctor and follow any other advice given by him or her

---

tryptamine and noradrenaline, in the nerve terminals. They therefore increase the level of neurotransmitters available to be released from the presynaptic bouton or terminal. MAOIs also act upon the walls of blood vessels.

It is stated that MAOIs may be useful in depression combined with anxiety, including phobic anxiety, hypersomnia (Stewart *et al.*, 1989).

MAOIs can give rise to several side-effects such as urinary retention, dry mouth, blurred vision, failure of ejaculation, liver damage, postural hypotension, and epilepsy. One of the most undesirable side-effects of the MAOIs is the so called 'cheese effect' which gives rise to such symptoms as hypertension, headache, hyperpyrexia and possibly stroke. This occurs because of the accumulation of tyramine, a chemical substance

found in many foods and drinks such as cheese, yeast extracts and Chianti wine. Tyramine is usually metabolized by MAO, but in the absence of the latter, it binds with presynaptic vesicles and causes the release of noradrenaline and since it is also a sympathomimetic agent, this accounts for the symptoms mentioned above.

Patients on MAOIs should carry an information card indicating the foods that they should not drink or eat and foods that they should also avoid. Example of such a card is given above.

Because MAOIs can often cause insomnia, they are usually prescribed to be taken no later than noon. There are several drugs belonging to the MAOIs group:

Generic name	Trade names
Phenelzine	Nardil
ISO Carboxazid	Marplan
Iproniazid	Marsilid
Tranytcypromine	Parnate

Other antidepressants

Over recent years many newer compounds have been used as antidepressants, although their actions are not very clear. Some of these newer compounds are: Mianserin, Anoxapine, Maprotiline and Flupenthixol.

Lithium

Lithium is a drug that has been used successfully to treat manic depressive illness since 1979 (Cade, 1980). It exerts a prophylactic effect (Souza *et al.*, 1990) although its pharmacological action is still unclear. There is a delay of two to three weeks before any clinical improvement is observed, once treatment is started.

Lithium is administered as lithium carbonate and it has a low therapeutic index and thus can give rise to many side-effects on account of toxic concentrations. It is therefore important that serum lithium is monitored regularly following its administration, for example after 7, 14, 21 and 28 days and thereafter at 3–6 weeks. Mild neurological side-effects may occur and they include mild lethargy and fine tremor. More serious side-effects at toxic levels are coarse tremor, drowsiness, vomiting, dysarthria, ataxia and eventually convulsions, coma and death. Long-term side-effects can occur following several months of treatment, for example hypothyroidism, polyuria and polydipsia. Permanent renal glomerular and tubular damage may also occur. It has been reported that lithium toxicity can occur in the presence of diminished renal function. It is also suggested that patients who are on diuretics and thus can lose sodium are more at risk, since the renal tubules cannot distinguish between sodium and lithium. Therefore when the kidneys need to conserve sodium, lithium will also be re-absorbed

which will increase blood lithium levels. But despite toxic effects, lithium continues to play an important role in the management of the bipolar form of depression.

ELECTROCONVULSIVE THERAPY (ECT)

ECT has been used for a very much longer period of time in the treatment of major unipolar and bipolar depression. It can produce full remission or marked improvement in about 90% of patients suffering from severe depression.

Although the mechanism of ECT therapeutic action is still not understood, it is believed that it may well cause changes in aminergic receptor sensitivity. (It should be remembered that changes in amine concentration in the brain is thought to be associated with depression.) ECT is given under anaesthesia with complete muscle relaxation. It induces a generalized seizure. A series of 4–12 treatments is usually administered (average 6–8) at 2-day intervals over a 2–4 week period and this usually produces remission of symptoms.

In the history of psychiatry, ECT is the one treatment that has caused and continues to cause much controversy. Since its application in psychiatry by Laslo Meduna (1935), there have been various modifications, for example the use of anaesthesia and muscle relaxation. ECT is opposed by many advocacy groups and the one issue of concern is the memory impairment which is an adverse effect of ECT.

However, many psychiatrists (Royal College of Psychiatrists, 1987; American Psychiatric Association, 1978 and the recent consensus conference of 1985) recognize the efficacy of ECT in the management of depression and other medication–refractory disorders.

ECT in the management of depression

There is conclusive evidence (Fink and Ottoson, 1980; Abrams, 1988) that ECT is effective in the management of depression. To show that ECT has a therapeutic action, many studies have been undertaken in the United Kingdom (Lambourn and Gill, 1978; Freeman *et al.*, 1978; Johnstone *et al.*, 1980; West, 1981; Brandon *et al.*, 1984;

Table 20.1 *Studies comparing real and simulated ECT*[a]

Study	No. of subjects	Stimulus parameters	Anaesthesia	Outcome
Lambourn and Gill (1978)	Real = 16 Simulated = 16	UL Brief pulse 6 treatments	Methohexital Suxamethonium	No difference
Freeman *et al.* (1978)	Real = 20 2 Simulated + Real = 20	BL Sine wave Treatment no. variable	Pentothal Suxamethonium	Real superior More ECTs in similar group
Johnstone *et al.* (1980)	Real = 31 Simulated = 30	BL Sine wave 8 treatments	Methohexital Suxamethonium	Real superior
West (1981)	Real = 11 Simulated = 11	BL Sine wave 6 treatments (with cross-over)	Althesin Suxamethonium	Real superior
Brandon *et al.* (1984)	Real = 43 Simulated = 34	BL Sine wave 8 treatments	Methohexital Suxamethonium	Real superior
Gregory *et al.* (1985)	Real (UL) = 23 Real (BL) = 23 Simulated = 23	UL or BL Sine wave 6 treatments	Methohexital Suxamethonium	Real UL and BL superior

[a] All treatments administered twice weekly.
UL, unilateral; BL, bilateral.

Gregory *et al.*, 1985) by comparing real and simulated ECT (anaesthesia and muscle relaxant only) in the treatment of depression. All the studies but one, demonstrated that ECT is indeed effective in the treatment of depression (Table 20.1).

The recommended treatment is the administration of moderately suprathreshold (100–150% above initial threshold) which must be adjusted to age and sex (Sackeim *et al.*, 1987).

The technique of ECT involves the use of electrodes which can be applied bilaterally (for bilateral treatment, BL) or unilaterally (for non-dominant treatment, ULND). There is much debate in the choice of ULND versus BL treatment, although it is generally accepted that ULND electrode placement significantly reduces memory impairment (Weiner *et al.*, 1983). It is therefore recommended that ULND ECT be the treatment of choice unless the patient does not respond and therefore BL is then applied.

McAllister *et al.* (1987) suggested that twice and three times weekly schedules of ULND ECT is effective, whilst Lerer *et al.* (1990) believe three times weekly treatment induces a significantly more rapid antidepressant effect, although it is associated with more memory impairment.

Health workers (such as nurses) who are closely involved in the management of patients undergoing ECT therapy must be aware of the emotive issues and should be familiar with the observations that should be undertaken before and after ECT treatment. It is paramount that the patient is given as much information prior to consenting to ECT treatment.

Pharmacological manipulation of seizure duration

There is a significant increase in seizure threshold and reduction in seizure duration when patients are undergoing a series of ECT treatment. To remedy this situation, the clinician usually increases the stimulus intensity, although the latter is associated with increase cognitive adverse effects.

In an attempt at resolving such a problem, Shapira *et al.*, 1985 have demonstrated that the use of intravenously administering caffeine sodium benzoate (500–2000 mg) 10 minutes before ECT did increase seizure duration. Other studies (Coffey *et al.*, 1990) have demonstrated that caffeine administration was equivalent to increased stimulus intensity in maintaining seizure duration.

Mechanism of action

The precise mechanism of action of ECT is not known, but there are suggestions by various authors that it may interact with different neurotransmitters in different syndromes. Thus, ECT may enhance serotoninergic and noradrenergic systems in the alleviation of depression. The adverse side-effect of ECT such as impairment of memory may be attributed to the effect of ECT on the cholinergic system (Lerer, 1987). The anti-Parkinsonian effects of ECT have also been observed (Grahame-Smith *et al.*, 1978) and may be attributed to the enhancement of the dopamine nigro-striatal pathway.

There are suggestions that ECT may perhaps have a direct effect on the hypothalamus and therefore may enhance release of specific hypothalamic peptides which have effective neurophysiological effects, as for example in the control of depression (Fink and Ottoson, 1980). Further studies are needed to establish the precise neurobiological effects of ECT.

ECT remains a controversial issue, but as more research is undertaken to demonstrate the scientific basic of this treatment, it may become universally accepted and may even be applied in other medical fields. Until then, the main reason in support of ECT treatment is that it does alleviate the symptoms of depression and thus can contribute to the quality of life in affected individuals.

SUMMARY

Several theories based on the reduced activity of amines have been put forward as to the aetiology of depression. There is evidence for some of the theories, but many are still unclear. Tricyclic antidepressants and monoamine oxidase inhibitors through their pharmacological actions, either in blocking re-uptake of amine or in reducing their degradation, give some indications of amine involvement in depression. However, the precise nature of the pharmacological actions is still unclear, for it takes two to three weeks from the time of the drug administration for the depressed individual to feel any improvement of the condition. These hypotheses are continuously being reviewed.

Another pitfall in the hypotheses is that administration of drugs such as lithium, and the use of ECT, control depression effectively and yet they do not behave as tricyclic depressants or monoamine oxidase inhibitors.

The search for the precise mechanism for the aetiology of depression will continue, but until then, the best model remains that of the amine involvement.

REFERENCES

Abrams, R. (1988) *Electroconvulsive Therapy*. Oxford: Oxford University Press.

Aubelas, A. (1987) Life-events and mania — a special relationship? *British Journal of Psychiatry*, **150**, 235–240.

Brandon, S., Cowley, P., McDonald, C., Neville, P., Palmer, R. & Wellstood-Eason, S. (1984) Electroconvulsive therapy: Results in depressive illness from the Leicestershire trial. *British Medical Journal*, **228**, 22–25.

Cade, J.F.J. (1980) The story of lithium. In Ayd, E.J. & Blackwell, D. (Eds) *Discoveries in Biological Psychiatry*. Philadelphia: J.B. Lippincott.

Coffey, C.E. *et al.* (1990) Caffeine augmentation of ECT. *American Journal of Psychiatry*, **147**, 579–585.

Fink, M. & Ottoson, J.O. (1980) A therapy of convulsive therapy in endogenous depression. Significance of hypothalamic functions. *Psychiatric Research*, **2**, 49–61.

Freeman, C.P.L. *et al.* (1978) Double blind controlled trial of ECT and simulated ECT in depressive illness. *Lancet*, **i**, 738–740.

Grahame-Smith, D.G. *et al.* (1978) Mechanism of the antidepressant action of ECT. *Lancet*, **i**, 245–256.

Gregory, S. *et al.* (1985) The Nottingham ECT study. A double blind comparison of bilateral, unilateral and simulated ECT in depressive illness. British Medical Journal, **146**, 520–527.

Johnstone, E.C. *et al.* (1980) The Northwick Park ECT trial. *Lancet*, **ii**, 1317–1320.

Klein, D.F. & Davis, J.M. (1969) In Klein, D.F. & Davis, J.M. (Eds) *Diagnosis and Drug Treatment of Psychiatric Disorders: a Review of mood stabilising literature.* Baltimore: Williams & Wilkins.

Lambourn, J. & Gill, D. (1978) A controlled comparison of simulated and real ECT. *British Journal of Psychiatry*, **133**, 154–159.

Lerer, B. (1987) Neurochemical and other neurobiological consequences of ECT. Implications for the pathogenesis and treatment of affective disorders. In Meltzer, H.Y. (Ed.) *Psychopharmacology, The Third Generation of Progress.* New York: Raven Press.

Lerer, B. *et al.* (1990) Optimising ECT schedule—a double blind study. American Psychiatric Association 43rd Annual Meeting, New York.

McAllister, D.A. *et al.* (1987) Effects of ECT given two versus three times weekly. *Psychiatric Research*, **21**, 63–69.

Raisman, R., Briley, M. & Langer, S.F. (1979) Specific tricyclic depressant binding sites in rat brain. *Nature (Lond.)*, **281**, 148–150.

Royal College of Psychiatrists (1987) Memorandum on the use of ECT. *British Journal of Psychiatry*, **131**, 261–272.

Sackeim, H.A. *et al.* (1987) Effects of electrode placement on the efficacy of titrated low-dose. ECT. *American Journal of Psychiatry*, **144**, 1449–1455.

Shapira, B. *et al.* (1985) Potentiation of seizure length and clinical response to ECT by caffeine pretreatment. *Convulsive Therapy*, **1**, 58–60.

Shapira, B. *et al.* (1988) Medication outcome in ECT resistant depression. *Convulsive Therapy*, 192–198.

Souza, F.G.M., Mander, A.J. & Goodwin, G.M. (1990) The efficacy of lithium in prophylaxis of unipolar depression: evidence from its discontinuation. *British Journal of Psychiatry*, **157**, 718–722.

Weiner, R.D. (1984) Does ECT cause brain damage? *Behavioural Brain Science*, **7**, 1–53.

Weiner, R.D. *et al.* (1983) ECT Parameters and electrode placement. In Lerer B. & Weiner K.D. (Eds) *ECT. Basic Mechanisms.* London: John Libbey.

Weller, M. & Eysenck, M. (1992) *The Scientific Basis of Psychiatry*, 2nd ed. London: W.B. Saunders.

West, E.D. (1981) ECT in depression: a double-blind controlled trial. *British Medical Journal*, **282**, 355–357.

Young, M.A., William, A., Scheftner, J.F. & Klerman, G.L. (1990) Gender differences in the clinical features of unipolar major depressive disorder. *Journal of Nervous Mental Disease*, **178** (3), 200–203.

SECTION

4

DEMENTIA OF ALZHEIMER'S, PARKINSON'S AND HUNTINGTON'S CHOREA

AIMS

i) To distinguish between Alzheimer's disease, Parkinson's disease and Huntington's chorea
ii) To explore the biological basis and treatment possibilities for each condition

KEY ISSUES

Dementia—features
Alzheimer's disease
    Cholinergic involvement
    Drugs in the management of
Parkinson's disease
    Key features
    Treatment
Huntington's chorea
    Features
    Treatment

Identify, analyse and assess factors causing distress and illness	Promote health, provide direct care and make interventions	Manage care programmes and services
Be critical, analytical and accountable, continue professional development	Counter discrimination, inequality and individual and institutional racism	Work within and develop policies, laws and safeguards in all settings
Understand influences on mental health and the nature/causes of disorder and illness	Know the effects of distress, disorder, illness on individuals, groups, families	Understand the basis of treatments and interventions

INTRODUCTION

Dementia is one of the most distressing conditions of the nervous system and its prevalence may be as high as 10% in people over 65 years, rising to 20% in those over 80. It is a progressive illness leading to severe mental impairment and physical changes whereby sufferers are unable to lead independent lives and may be a danger to themselves.

Although there are many causes of dementia, for example Alzheimer's disease, Parkinson's disease, Huntington's chorea, vascular disorder of multi-infarcts (accounting for about 25% of patients with dementia), hypothyroidism and alcoholic dementia, only the first three will be described here, since the individuals affected are likely to require admission to psychiatric units at some stage.

Dementia is defined by the diagnostic and statistical manual of mental disorders (*DSM–III–R*; American Psychiatric Association, 1987) as loss of intellectual ability with resulting occupational and social handicaps and is accompanied by one or more of the following: impaired thinking or judgement; aphasia, apraxia, agnosia, constructional difficulties, and changes in personality. Verbal skills may be affected but show least decline. The most common cause of dementia is Alzheimer's disease.

ALZHEIMER'S DISEASE

Alzheimer's disease (AD) was first described by Alois Alzheimer in 1907, a psychiatrist and neuroanatomist, in a woman patient who died following a progressive disorder with loss of memory and language ability.

AD is the most common cause of dementia in the elderly, accounting for almost two thirds of cases of senile dementia. It may be a genetically linked disorder, for example 15–20% of sufferers fall into the category of familial AD, which is an autosomal, dominant, inherited condition (St George Hyslop *et al.*, 1989). Other evidence of genetic linkage is based on the observation that most people with Down's syndrome (trisomy 21) eventually develop features of AD. Studies confirm that proximal chromosome 21 is likely to be the locus.

Several physical changes have been observed in AD, brain atrophy (weight from 1200 g and 1350 g to 1000 g less) enlarged ventricles, and usually symmetrical cortical atrophy especially frontal and temporal lobes. In post-mortem studies using whole temporal lobe of normal elderly and matched demented patients, Bowen *et al.* (1977) found that about one third of nerve cell compo-

nents are lost from the temporal lobe. Histological studies also show loss of large pyramidal cells (up to 60% in the cortex) from the temporal cortex, occipital region as well as from the hippocampus and amygdala.

Pearson *et al.* (1985) observed that AD spreads along projection neurons from the olfactory cortex to association areas but spares the occipital and motor cortex. Talamo *et al.* (1984) confirmed that the olfactory neurons showed pathological changes in AD patients. Neuronal loss, neuritic plaques (NP) and neurofibrillary tangles (NFT) are common pathological changes.

Alzheimer's disease is characterized by loss of neurones in certain areas of the brain and the presence of NFTs and NPs. NFTs and NPs are found in association areas of the cortex, hippocampus, amygdala and within certain subcortical nuclei.

NFTs are abnormal neuronal soma in which the cytoplasm is filled with filamentous structures arranged in a paired helical fashion (Fig. 20.4). In the cortex, tangles are found in clusters in the pyramidal neurones of layers III and V. Other pathological changes found in Alzheimer's brain is accumulation of products derived from the proteolysis of amyloid (Beyreuther *et al.*, 1988) in arterioles, in meninges and cerebral cortex. NPs consist of clusters of degenerating nerve endings, both round and dendritic with a central core (Fig. 20.5) which resemble an amyloid protein (Katzman and Thal, 1984).

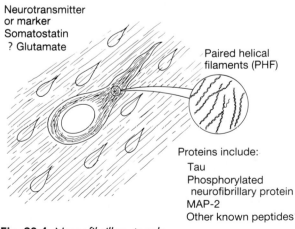

Fig. 20.4 *Neurofibrillary tangle.*

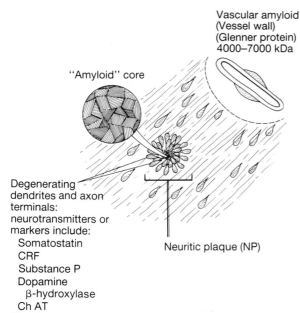

Vascular amyloid
(Vessel wall)
(Glenner protein)
4000–7000 kDa

"Amyloid" core

Degenerating
dendrites and axon
terminals:
neurotransmitters or
markers include:
  Somatostatin
  CRF
  Substance P
  Dopamine
    β-hydroxylase
  Ch AT

Neuritic plaque (NP)

Fig. 20.5 *Neuritic plaque.*

Cholinergic involvement in Alzheimer's disease

It is believed that there is reduced activity of the brain as reflected in studies in which labelled deoxyglucose is used and its utilization measured and shown on positron emission tomography (PET) scans. NPs are easily detected using a fluorescent thioflavine stain. Many plaques are acetylcholine positive. It has been discovered that the degree of dementia in AD patients measured during life is highly correlated with the number of NPs in the cerebral cortex. It has also been found that the number of NPs in the cerebral cortex is correlated with the level of enzyme acetyltransferase.

Several studies on post-mortem AD brain, have confirmed a decrease in the enzyme choline acetyltransferase in the cerebral cortex and hippocampus (Davies and Maloney 1976). Greatest loss of cholinergic activity was in the temporal and parietal cortex, hippocampus and amygdaloid nucleus. Surgical biopsy samples taken from the cerebral cortex of Alzheimer patients in the first year of symptomatology show a reduction in acetyltransferase. Bowen *et al.* (1977) also found a reduction in choline acetyltransferase activity which correlated with the degree of pathological

damage to the temporal lobe. On the other hand, Perry (1980) demonstrated a decrease in acetylcholinesterase activity in parallel with an increase in NP density and pre-mortem intellectual impairment. Sims *et al* (1983) also showed that choline acetyltransferase activity, choline uptake and acetylcholine synthesis were significantly reduced within a year of the onset of the disease.

It is believed that AD may also be associated with loss of muscarinic receptors, but as yet data are sparse and much of the work needs to be confirmed. However, as a result of muscarinic receptors loss, there are claims that there are loss of presynaptic cholinergic terminals (Mash *et al.*, 1985).

Noradrenaline and serotonin in AD

It would appear that there is a reduction in the number of neurons in both the locus coeruleus and raphe nuclei in AD. Post-mortem Alzheimer brain has also revealed reduction in levels of both noradrenaline and serotonin. Bowen *et al.* (1983) also demonstrated reductions in serotonin uptake in brain biopsies.

Glutamate, somatostatin and corticotrophin-releasing factor in AD

There is some evidence that glutamate may be reduced in AD. Hyman *et al.* (1987) demonstrated an 80% reduction of glutamate in some of the cortical pyramidal cells, usually destroyed in AD.

Davies *et al.* (1980) and Beal *et al.* (1986) have shown that the concentration of somatostatin is reduced in the neocortex and hippocampus in an Alzheimer brain. Ferrier *et al.* (1983) also demonstrated that levels of somatostatin were reduced in temporal, frontal and parietal cortex, but increased in the subtantia innominata in AD. It is not clear as to the significance of somatostatin decrease in AD.

It has also been found that corticotrophin-releasing factor is lowered in several brain areas of patients with AD (Bisette *et al.*, 1985). Larger reductions of approximately 80% were found in the occipital cortex.

Nerve growth factor (NGF)

Studies by Seiter and Schwab (1989) suggest that absence of a nerve growth factor (NGF) may be responsible for the degeneration of cholinergic neurones in AD. Evidence for this has been demonstrated by Fischer *et al.* (1987) in their study in which NGF was infused into the brain of aged rats with spatial memory impairment and they recovered spatial memory as observed in a water maze test. It should be remembered that acetylcholine may be responsible for memory storage in the brain.

Drugs in the management of AD

Most of the drugs used in the treatment of AD have so far proved to be ineffective. The search continues in finding a drug that will be able to improve memory of the patient. The approaches to drug therapy have been to:

Increase synthesis and/or release of acetylcholine (use of choline phosphatidylcholine)

Reduce the metabolism of acetylcholine by inhibiting the enzyme acetylcholinesterase (use of physostigmine, tetrahydroamino acridine)

Increase the release of acetylcholine (use of aminopyridine)

Use muscarinic agonists (arecoline)

Increase glucose and oxygen utilization

Use of choline

Choline in the form of lecithin (phosphatidyl choline), which is a natural source of choline found in foods such as eggs and fish, has been administered to patients in many studies in the hope of improving memory (Smith *et al.*, 1978), however the results have been negative.

Sitaram *et al.* (1978) found that a single 10-g oral dose of choline significantly enhanced serial learning of lists of words as compared with subjects on placebos. Mohs and Davis (1982) have also reported that subjects who were given chol-

ine, but had also received physostigmine previously, showed slight improvement in memory.

Anticholinesterases

Kaye *et al.* (1982) have reported that there were small improvements in memory on word recall tests in AD patients who were given the anticholinesterase tetrahydroamino acridine (THA) together with lecithin. Other studies have used the drug physostigmine, but in general the results are still very poor.

Cholinergic agonists

There are reports which indicate that intravenous infusion of arecoline (an agonist at both nicotinic and muscarinic receptors) did improve recognition memory in patients with AD. Use of arecoline has also been shown to enhance learning in both normal young volunteers and elderly monkeys.

Increasing the release of acetylcholine

Since it is known that there is a significant decrease in the level of acetylcholine (Ach) produced in AD, it is reasonable to speculate that any drug that can increase the release of Ach might improve the memory of patients with AD. Drugs like 4-aminopyridine and (THA) have been reported to show improvement in tests of orientation and memory in patients with AD. There was also marked improvements in everyday behaviour in patients who have been taking the drug for approximately 12 months.

Increasing glucose and oxygen utilization

There is some evidence in animal studies that the drug Hydergine can promote glucose metabolism under conditions of ischaemia. Another drug considered to be a metabolic stimulant, Piracetam, has been shown to improve learning in animal studies (Dartus *et al.*, 1983).

Conclusions

It would appear that more studies need to be undertaken to establish the exact pharmacological properties of many of the drugs currently in use. As yet, the evidence for efficacy of the drugs in use is still not very clear. It is reasonable to assume that many drug trials will go on, in the hope of helping existing patients with AD.

In search of the factors that may contribute to AD, it is important to realize that environmental factors may also play a role, for example aluminium (Duckett, 1981). Aluminium has been found in excessive concentrations in the plaques of some patients dying with AD.

PARKINSON'S DISEASE

Parkinson's disease (PD) is one of the commonest progressive degenerative conditions of the central nervous system. It occurs predominantly in those over 55 years, affecting at least 1% of the population. Forty per cent of those suffering from PD progress to dementia.

James Parkinson, a GP from Shoreditch described some of the signs and symptoms of Parkinson's (Parkinson, 1817):

Slowness and poverty of all movements (bradykinesia, akinesia)

Muscle stiffness which is referred to as 'cogwheel' rigidity

Tremor of the limbs mainly at rest

Dementia/depression

Another feature of the disease is the shuffling gait that is observed in all of the patients.

The breakthrough as to the pathophysiology of Parkinson's disease came about in 1960, when Enhringer and Horniewicz reported that there was a decrease in concentration of dopamine in the basal ganglia of post-mortem brains of PD sufferers. This is now universally accepted, but the aetiology is still obscure.

However, there is some speculations that PD may be the result of a viral infection or a particular toxic substance that affects the basal ganglia. This is based on the evidence that many people developed PD following a worldwide pandemic of encephalitis around 1920. Also an outbreak of Parkinsonism occurred amongst Californian heroin addicts in 1982. Research has indicated that

1-methyl-4-phenyl-1,2,3,6 tetrahydro-pyridine (MPTP) can actually induce symptoms identified as PD, if injected cutaneously or through inhalation. It has also been reported (Langston *et al.*, 1983) that in an attempt to synthesize heroin illegally, MPTP was present in the chemical used.

Other distinct pathology in PD is the absence of the dark pigment in the substantia nigra (SN). Cell bodies of neurons that project from SN to the corpus striatum contain melanin granules pigment. It is not known why the pigments are lost, but MPTP does show selective toxicity for the nigro-striatal neurons. Are there perhaps other toxic substances that may be the causation of PD? Studies by Hornykiewicz (1982) also show that many types of neurones are lost.

There is general agreement that patients with PD lack dopamine in the basal ganglia, for patients treated with neuroleptic drugs, which reduce dopamine level, develop symptoms analogous to PD. It is therefore not surprising that patients with PD respond to drugs which raise the level of dopamine.

Treatment of PD

L-*dopa or levodopa*
Treatment has focused mainly on the use of dopamine precursors such as L-dopa, which is a naturally occurring amino acid. But because the drug is absorbed mainly in the duodenum and jejunum, thus causing dopamine formation in the circulation, it gives rise to many unwanted side-effects: postural hypotension, nausea, vomiting and involuntary movements. L-dopa is decarboxylated to dopa in the circulation but not in the brain. Less than 1% reaches the brain unchanged. Side-effects such as vomiting can be reduced if levodopa is combined with benserazide or carbidopa. (Sinemet). Other effects of levodopa in advanced state of PD are mild visual hallucinations, toxic confusional states, and frank paranoid psychosis. Patients on long-term treatment can also develop the so called 'on–off effects' (patients alternately freezes and goes hypotonic) and also end of dose akinesia (in which stiffness towards the end of the dose becomes a problem). Some patients can also develop severe orofacial dyski-

nesia, which occurs as a result of over stimulation of dopaminergic receptors.

Bromocriptine

Bromocriptine, a dopamine receptor agonist, has also been used in the treatment of PD. It is often given in association with levodopa. It has been reported that patients treated with bromocriptine do not experience the abnormal involuntary movements, as seen in those treated only with levodopa.

Selegiline

Selegiline is a selective inhibitor of the mono-amine oxidase isoenzyme type B (MAO_B) found in platelets and also in the striatum. It can be given with levodopa, and there is no need for diet restriction. Its function is to increase dopamine concentration by preventing their breakdown via MAO_B. Side-effects such as euphoria, insomnia and hallucinations may occur.

In conclusion, evidence still strongly suggests that lack of dopamine is responsible for the symptoms of PD, but as yet it is unclear as to the aetiology. Drugs currently in use may arrest the progression of the disease and reduce symptoms short term, but are not effective long term.

Recent studies indicate that treatment may be successful by grafting foetal tissue in the affected area of the substantia nigra. There have been some positive reports from Mexico of clinical trials (surgical foetal tissue transplants) on patients with PD. This could well be the preferred choice of treatment in the future, but there are moral issues and dilemmas.

HUNTINGTON'S DISEASE

Huntington's disease (HD), first described by George Huntington in 1872, is an autosomal dominant disorder, affecting approximately 6,000 individuals in the UK. It is also speculated that 50,000 individuals are at risk of developing the disease. Men and women are affected with equal frequency—about 5 per 100,000 population. The onset of the disease occurs in most cases in the fourth to fifth decade of life. Each child of an affected parent has a 50% chance of inheriting the disease. The disease gene is believed to be close to the top of the short arm on chromosome 4 (Gunsella et al., 1983).

George Huntington observed four characteristics of this disease:

Its heritability

The presence of chorea

The development of dementia

The occurrence of death after 15 or 20 years

The signs and symptoms are many, and they include irritability, depression, fidgeting, clumsiness, sudden falls and absentmindedness. The prominent feature of the disease are uncontrolled involuntary choreiform movements. Involuntary movements disappear during sleep.

Speech is also affected. It is slurred at first, but later becomes incomprehensible and finally it ceases altogether as facial expression becomes disturbed and grotesque. Mental functions deteriorate. The whole body may also be affected by exhausting dyskinesia. Some individuals may have outbursts of excitement or temper and suicide tendencies.

The pathophysiology of HD as revealed through post-mortem studies and also by CT scan shows atrophy and shrinkage of the basal ganglia and loss of cortical neurones. There is loss of a specific set of cholinergic neurones and neurones that synthesize gamma aminobutyric acid (GABA) in the striatum. There is also a marked decrease of both cholineacetyltransferase and the enzyme glutamic acid decarboxylase required for GABA. Some peptides such as substance P, methionine enkephalin and dynorphin are also reduced. The degree of loss of cortical neurones is associated with the severity of the dementia that can occur.

The mechanism by which neurones are lost is unknown, but an animal model in which kainic acid is injected in the striatum, created symptoms similar to those in HD. Because of the striatal involvement in HD, it is postulated that an endogenous neurotoxin like kainic acid might be involved in the pathophysiology of HD.

Treatment

Most drugs used in the treatment of HD are to alleviate symptoms, thus helping the individuals to cope with life. Drugs which can increase GABA concentration, such as the GABA agonist baclofen have given satisfactory results in clinical trials.

Until the pathophysiology of HD is clearly understood, specific drugs for the management of HD remain in the distant future.

FURTHER READING

Sanger, D.J. & Blackmore, D.E. (Eds) (1984) *Aspects of Psychopharmacology*, London: Methuen.

Siegel, G.J. (Ed.) (1982) *Basic Neurochemistry*, 3rd edn. Little, Brown.

REFERENCES

American Psychiatric Association (1987). *Diagnostic and Statistical Manual*. Washington DC: American Psychiatric Association.

Beal, M.F. *et al.* (1986) Somatostatin: alterations in the CNS in neurological diseases. In Martin, J.B. and Barchas, J.D. (Eds) *Neuroleptics in neurologic and psychiatric disease* (Association for Research in Nervous and Mental Disease, Vol. 64), pp. 215–258. New York: Raven Press.

Beal, M., Kowall, N.W., Ellison, D.W., Mazurek, M.F., Swartz, K.J. & Martin, J.B. (1986) Replication of the neurochemical characteristics of Huntington's disease by quinolinic acid. *Nature*, **321**, 168–171.

Beyreuther, K. *et al.* (1988) Molecular pathology of amyloid deposition in Alzheimer's disease. In Henderson, A.S. & Hendersin, J.H. (Eds) *Aetiology of Dementia of Alzheimer's Type*. Chichester: Wiley.

Bisette, G. *et al.* (1985) Corticotrophin releasing factor-like immunoreactivity in senile dementia of the Alzheimer's type. Reduced cortical and striated concentration. *Journal of the American Medical Association*, **254**, 3067–3069.

Bowen, D.M. *et al.* (1983) Biochemical assessment of neurotransmitter and metabolic dysfunction and cerebral atrophy in Alzheimer's disease. In Katzman, R. (Ed.) *Banbury Report 15: Biological Aspects of Alzheimer's Disease*. New York: Cold Spring Harbour Laboratory, pp. 219–223.

Bowen, D.M. *et al.* (1977) Chemical pathology of the organic dementias. II. Quantitative estimation of cellular changes in post-mortem brains. *Brain*, **100**, 427–453.

Davies, P., Katzman, R. & Terry, R.D. (1980) Reduced somatostatin-like immunoreactivity in cerebral cortex from cases of Alzheimer's disease and Alzheimer's senile dementia. *Nature*, **288**, 279–280.

Davis, P. & Maloney, A.T.F. (1976) Selective loss of central cholinergic neurons in Alzheimer's disease. *Lancet*, **ii**, 1403.

Duckett, S. (1981) Aluminium and Alzheimer's disease. *Archives Neurology*, **133**, 730–731.

Duckett, S., Galle, P., Crapper, D.R., Krishnan, S.S. & Quittkat, S. (1976) Letter to the editor. *Archives of Neurology*, **33**, 730–731.

Ferrier, I.N. *et al.* (1983) Neuropeptides in Alzheimer's type dementia. *Journal of Neurological Science*, **62**, 159–170.

Gunsella, J.F. *et al.* (1983) A polymorphic DNA marker genetically linked to Huntington's disease. *Nature*, **306**, 234–238.

Hornykiewicz, O. (1966) Metabolism of brain dopamine in human Parkinsonism. Neurochemical and clinical aspects. In Costa, E., Côté, L.J. & Yahr, M.D. (Eds) *Biochemistry and Pharmacology of the Basal Ganglia*. New York: Raven Press.

Hornykiewicz, O. (1982) Brain neurotransmitter changes in Parkinson's disease. In Marsden, C.D. & Fahn, S. (Eds) *Movement Disorders*. Butterworth.

Hornykiewicz, O. & Kish, S.J. (1987) Biochemical pathophysiology of Parkinson's disease. *Advances in Neurology*, **45**, 19–34.

Hyman, B.T., Van Hoeson, G.W. & Damasio, A.R. (1987) Alzheimer's disease: Glutamate depletion in the hippocampal perforant pathway zone. *Annu. Neurol.*, **22**, 37–40.

Katzman, R. & Thal, L. (1989) Neurochemistry of Alzheimer's disease. In Siegel, G.J. *et al. A Basic Neurochemistry*. New York: Raven Press.

Kaye, W.H. *et al.* (1982) Modest facilitation of memory in dementia with combined lecithin and anticholinersterase treatment. *Biol. Psych.*, **17**, 275–280.

Langston, J.W. *et al.* (1983) Chronic Parkinsonism in humans due to a product of meperidine—Analog. Synthesis. *Science* 219, 979–80.

Mash, D.C., Flynn, D.D. & Potter, L.T. (1985) *Science*, **228**, 1115–1118.

Mohs, R.C. & Davis, K.L. (1982) A signal detectability analysis of the effect of physostigmine on memory in patients with Alzheimer's disease. *Neurobiology of Aging*, **3**, 105–110.

Pearson, R.C.A. *et al.* (1985) Anatomical correlates of the distribution of the pathological changes in the neocortex in Alzheimer's disease. Proceedings of the National Academy of Science USA, **82**, 1–4.

Perry, E.K. & Perry, R.H. (1980) The cholinergic system in Alzheimer's disease. In Roberts, P.J. (Ed.) *Biochemistry of dementia*, Chichester: Wiley.

Perry, E.K. *et al.* (1977) Neurotransmitter enzyme abnormalities in senile dementia—choline acetyl transferase and glutanic acid decarboxylase in necropsy brain tissue. *Journal of Neurology and Science*, **34**, 247–265.

Perry, E.K. *et al.* (1987) Correlation of cholinergic abnormalities with senile plaques and mental test scores in senile dementia. *British Medical Journal 2*, 1457–1459.

Sims, M.R., Bowen, D.M., Allen, S.J., Smith, C.C.T., Neary, D., Thomas, D.J. & Davison, A.N. (1983).

Presynaptic cholinergic dysfunction in patients with dementia. *Journal of Neurochemistry*, **40**, 503–509.

Sitaram, M. *et al.* (1978) Human serial learning: Enhancement with arecoline and choline and impairment with scopolamine. *Science*, **201**, 274–276.

Smith, *et al.* (1978) Choline in Alzheimer's disease. *Lancet*, **ii**, 318.

St George-Hyslop, P. *et al.* (1989) Familial Alzheimer's disease: Progress and problems. *Neurobiology of Aging*, **10**, 417–426.

St George-Hyslop, P. *et al.* (1989) The genetic defect causing familial Alzheimer's disease maps on chromosome 21. *Science*, **235**, 885–890.

Talamo, B.R. *et al.* (1989) Pathological changes in olfactory neurons in patients with Alzheimer's disease. *Nature*, **337**, 736–739.

SECTION

5

SEIZURES AND EPILEPSY

AIMS

i) To describe the main features and characteristics of epileptic seizures
ii) To identify drugs that can be used in the management of epileptic seizures

KEY ISSUES

Characteristics
Pathophysiology
Drug treatment

Identify, analyse and assess factors causing distress and illness	Promote health, provide direct care and make interventions	Manage care programmes and services
Be critical, analytical and accountable, continue professional development	Counter discrimination, inequality and individual and institutional racism	Work within and develop policies, laws and safeguards in all settings
Understand influences on mental health and the nature/causes of disorder and illness	Know the effects of distress, disorder, illness on individuals, groups, families	Understand the basis of treatments and interventions

INTRODUCTION

Epileptic seizures can occur in many diseases which may directly or indirectly involve the brain and these may include disorders of carbohydrates, amino acid, lipid metabolism, ionic and electrolyte imbalance, infections, brain tumours, brain trauma, and fever in the young when no known causes are identified—a type referred to as idiopathic.

Symptoms of epileptic seizures vary in individuals according to the type of seizure (discussed below), but they include a prodrome, which is a gradual build up of change in emotions, behaviour or alertness for several hours or days before a seizure; and an aura or warning sign which is experienced at the beginning of a seizure and may be a motor or sensory sensation depending on the part of the brain where the abnormal electrical seizure begins. If electrical activity continues or spreads, the seizure attack or ictus occurs. During the ictus period the individual may exert a degree of disturbed consciousness which may be followed by stiffness and jerking of the limbs or engagement of purposeless movements called automatism. Ictus is followed by the postictal or recovery, when the patient quickly regains normal function or may be confused, irritable or may fall into a deep sleep.

PATHOPHYSIOLOGY—METABOLIC HOMEOSTASIS

There has been much debate as to the causes and altered physiological processes that take place in epilepsy, but so far no specific factors have been identified. However, there are indications that abnormal neurotransmitter function or abnormal neuronal membrane properties may be major factors in the production of seizure. Both can alter ionic concentration of various ions such as calcium and potassium. For example, it is known that at the onset of the hypersynchronous discharge, extracellular calcium concentration falls and then rises later. Repetitive neuronal firing may cause the release of large amounts of excitatory neurotransmitters at synapses and thus promote seizures. Membrane properties may be altered in the presence of hypoxia, alkalosis, hypoglycaemia, and respiratory poisons affecting adenosine triphosphate (ATP) production. All these may give rise to seizures.

The neurotransmitter gamma aminobutyric acid (GABA) (an inhibitory transmitter) has been implicated in the causation of seizure. The normal physiological function of GABA is the opening of membrane ion channels permeable to chloride. The influx of chloride ions in the neuronal membrane causes hyperpolarization, thereby producing an inhibitory postsynaptic potential. Thus GABA plays an important role in controlling neuronal excitation, and when there is a decrease or absence of GABA, neuronal excitation can increase and hence lead to seizures.

There are many lines of evidence for the involvement of GABA in seizures. For example a deficiency of pyridoxine (vitamin B_6), a substance that is essential for the functioning of the enzyme glutamate decarboxylase (GAD) in the synthesis of GABA, may give rise to seizures. The concentration of GABA in the cerebrospinal fluid of epileptic individuals was found to be at a lower level. Other evidence is the reduction of GAD

which has been observed in human temporal lobe cortex removed during neurosurgery for focal seizure. It has also been observed that drugs that impair the synthesis of postsynaptic action on GABA can also cause seizures (Meldrum, 1975, 1979).

Physiological disturbances that occur during seizure are (i) increase in cerebral blood flow; (ii) increase in cerebral metabolic rate for glucose and oxygen in all regions that participate in seizures (Baldy-Moulinier *et al.*, 1983); and (iii) changes in the lipid composition of membranes in the brain.

CLASSIFICATION OF SEIZURES

Owing to the variations in the types of seizures and the way in which they affect individuals, it has been necessary to classify seizure according to electroencephalography (see below). Generally the classification of seizure falls into two groups: partial (local) seizure (where seizure begins in a specific localized area) and generalized seizure (bilaterally symmetrical and without local onset). Both groups are further divided into subgroups. Partial seizures are described as elementary (simple) with motor, somatosensory or autonomic symptoms in which there is no impairment of consciousness, and partial seizures are described as complex and consciousness is impaired.

International classification of epileptic seizures

I Partial seizures (seizures beginning locally)

   A Partial seizures with elementary symptomatology (generally without impairment of consciousness)
      1 With motor symptoms (includes Jacksonian seizures)
      2 With special sensory or somatosensory symptoms
      3 With autonomic symptoms
      4 Compound forms

   B Partial seizures with complex symptomatology (generally with impairment

of consciousness) (temporal lobe or psychomotor seizures)
1 With impairment of consciousness only
2 With cognitive symptomatology
3 With affective symptomatology
4 With 'psychosensory' symptomatology
5 With 'psychomotor' symptomatology (automatisms)
6 Compound forms

C Partial seizures secondarily generalized

II Generalized seizures (bilaterally symmetrical and without local onset)
A Absences (*petit mal*)
B Bilateral massive epileptic myoclonus
C Infantile spasms
D Clonic seizures
E Tonic seizures
F Tonic–clonic seizures (*grand mal*)
G Atonic seizures
H Akinetic seizures

III Unilateral seizures (or predominantly)

IV Unclassified epileptic seizures (due to incomplete data)
From Gastaut, 1970

Partial seizures

Partial seizure (elementary) with motor symptoms

This type of seizure is characterized by clonic or tonic movements that occur in one extremity or on one side of the face. The seizure often starts in the thumb and mouth, on account of the large representation of the hand and the mouth in the motor area (homunculus as described by Penfield). When the seizure starts focally and sequentially involves body parts, it is called a Jacksonian seizure. A focal seizure can be followed by a temporary paralysis (Todd's paralysis) of the involved part and may last minutes or hours but does not exceed 24 hours. In adults, but not in children, the presence of Todd's paralysis is indicative of a structural lesion.

Partial seizure (elementary) somatosensory symptoms

The symptoms depend on the location of the seizure focus in the brain. For example if the seizure focus is in the parietal lobe the symptoms may range from vague to specific sensations such as warmth or numbness. If the seizure focus is in the occipital or temporal lobe, senses of sight, hearing, smell or taste may be affected. Feeling of dizziness may also be experienced.

Partial seizure (elementary) with autonomic symptoms

Symptoms that affect the autonomic system arise from deep in the brain cortex and the upper part of the brain. Individuals may therefore experience sweating, palpitations, dilation of pupils, pallor or flushing, excessive salivation and nausea.

Partial seizure (complex) with impaired consciousness only

All the partial complex seizures are associated with impaired consciousness and amnesia for the event. However, this type of complex seizure can be distinguished from *petit mal* as it lasts for much longer and there is postictal confusion, and the EEG does not show a primary three per second spike and wave pattern.

Partial seizures with cognitive and affective symptoms

The cognitive and affective seizure symptoms are thought to arise from the limbic system of the brain, in part of the frontal lobe and anterior and medial parts of the temporal lobes (Svoboda, 1979). The cognitive symptoms are as a result of disturbances in thought or memory. Individuals may experience the so called '*jamais vu*' situations these situations may seem new, although, in fact, they are familiar.

The affective symptoms are associated with brief episodes of emotions and/or behaviour unrelated to the patient's immediate environment. Sensations may be those of pleasure, fear, anger, anxiety or displeasure. In cases where individuals break into meaningless laughter, this is referred to as gelastic seizure (Gascon and Lombroso, 1971; Chen and Forster, 1973).

Partial seizure (complex with psychomotor and psychosensory symptoms)

This group comprises one of the commonest type of seizure which is also referred to as psychomotor or temporal lobe seizures. These seizures usually last one to two minutes and are often preceded by an aura. Patients frequently exhibit automatisms (repetitive, purposeless behaviour) such as scratching, chewing or lip smacking. The affected individual may stare blankly and is not responsive to verbal stimulation and often not aware of surroundings. Confusion can occur postictally as can amnesia for event prior to the seizure. The EEG during the ictus may show spikes, sharp waves or rhythmic temporal waves.

Psychosensory seizure symptoms are not as common as psychomotor symptoms. Individuals affected usually experience hallucinations, illusions, unpleasant taste or smell, or dizziness.

Generalized seizures

In comparison to partial seizure, generalized seizure affects the whole body and many body functions at once. There is marked impairment of consciousness during all types of generalized seizures. It is believed that the seizure activity arises from areas beneath the cortex and in deep centres of the brain. EEG patterns are bilaterally synchronous and symmetrical.

This type of seizure is rarely preceded by an aura. Affected individuals fall at the onset of the seizure if they are standing. Some of the manifestations of generalized seizure are abnormal body movements, no movement, loss of muscle tone, and staring. Postictal symptoms may vary.

Absence seizure (previous known as petit mal)

This is one of the most commonest types of seizure occurring in children usually between 4 and 13 years of age (Currier *et al.*, 1963; Livingston *et al.*, 1965). This seizure is not preceded by an aura and usually lasts 10–30 seconds, but the individual may suffer from a brief lapse of consciousness which is associated with staring, eye fluttering and sometimes twitching of the hands and mouth. The individual may not be aware of the seizure and usually resumes his or her activity before the seizure. The frequency of seizure ranges from several a day to as many as 200 per day. Some individuals may exhibit automatism and some degree of confusion.

The EEG shows a bilateral synchronus symmetrical 3–3.5 spike per second and wave pattern. The EEG and seizure can be precipitated by hyperventilation for three minutes.

Myoclonic seizure and infantile spasms

Myoclonic seizure is similar to infantile spasm, but the latter occurs more frequently in male babies between three and eight months of age. The typical myoclonic seizure in adults and young children is sudden, and without warning, brief, involuntary movements of the trunk and extremities.

Babies with infantile spasms may show marked intellectual and motor development (Millichap *et al.*, 1962; Jeavons *et al.*, 1970). Infantile spasm may last no more than a few seconds and is preceded by a cry or colour change followed by a flexion spasm which varies from only involving nodding of the head to doubling up of the entire body.

The EEG shows hypsarrhythmia which is a specific wave pattern denoted by high voltage slow waves and multifocal spikes. After a few years an affected child will develop myoclonic-type seizure where the EEG will show multiple spike foci, single foci spike and wave complexes 2–2.5 per second.

Clonic, tonic, tonic–clonic seizures

According to specific symptoms, individuals can be grouped either under clonic or tonic seizure or both. A clonic seizure occurs when there are only rhythmic repeated jerking movements. A tonic seizure is said to exist when there is stiffness of the extremities and arching of the back.

In the tonic–clonic seizure, the so-called *grand mal* seizure, which lasts from one to a few minutes, the individual may cry or yell at the beginning of the seizure and loses consciousness and falls to the ground. In the tonic phase, the body becomes rigid with the back arched and the extremities extended. There may be apnoea and cyanosis. This phase is followed by the clonic phase when there is rhythmic contraction and relaxation of the trunk and extremities. The individual may be incontinent of urine, faeces or both, may vomit, bite the tongue and have excessive salivation. After the seizure the individual may be quite confused and sleep deeply for several hours and may complain of headache upon awakening.

EEG tracings during seizure show bilaterally synchronous spiking.

Atonic and akinetic seizures

Atonic or 'drop attack' can often be observed in children with absence seizures. This type of seizure occurs frequently in drowsy states when the child has just woken up in the morning. There is momentary loss of consciousness, movement is arrested and the individual falls as normal muscle tone and tension are lost.

Akinetic seizure differs from atonic seizure in that there is no loss of muscle tone and the individual does not fall.

DIAGNOSIS

Apart from the history and a thorough physical examination of the affected individual, several non-specific tests may have to be carried out to detect any abnormality responsible for the seizure, for example blood and urine tests may reveal kidney and liver malfunction. Various tests for detection of infection should also be carried out.

Specific tests on the nervous system in the diagnosis of epilepsy include electroencephalography, skull radiography, echoencephalography and computerized axial tomography.

Electroencephalography

Electroencephalography (EEG) is very useful in detecting abnormal spikes and waves which could help to locate a seizure focus in particular areas of the brain. If possible, an EEG should be recorded during a seizure. The patient can also be monitored by EEG over a 24-hour period.

Skull radiography

Radiographs of the skull may be useful in the detection of a tumour, congenital defects, raised intracranial pressure, calcification or abnormal blood vessels. All of these abnormalities may give rise to seizures.

Echoencephalography

The use of high frequency sound waves to produce a picture of the individual's head may reveal such abnormality as asymmetrical shifting of the midline of the ventricles, which can occur as a result of a haemorrhage, a tumour or atrophy of the brain.

Computerized axial tomography (CAT)

CAT scans may show abnormal brain structures, thus indicating the possible reason for epilepsy.

DRUG TREATMENT IN THE MANAGEMENT OF EPILEPTIC SEIZURES

Although there are other approaches in the management of epileptic seizures (e.g. stress reduction, behavioural strategies and neurosurgery) only drug therapy will be discussed here. An overview of drug reactions will be discussed first and examples of various drugs will be referred to.

Once diagnosed, individuals with epileptic seizures must be treated promptly so as to prevent the development of status epilepticus.

The objective in management is to find the most effective way of controlling or stopping the seizures (reducing frequency and severity) through the use of antiepileptic or anticonvulsant drugs, minimizing the risk of side-effects so that patients are able to function at optimal levels. Because of the long-term treatment some patients may develop adverse drug reactions which can be classified as dose-dependent adverse reactions, non-dose-dependent adverse reactions, and drug interactions.

The dose-dependent adverse reactions occur as a result of the rapid accumulation of the drug in the body. The reactions, mostly related to the central nervous system, are drowsiness, irritability, vertigo, diplopia and dysarthria. The non-dose-dependent adverse reactions may give rise to minor skin rashes which may be localized or widespread. The symptoms may appear immediately or within hours or days of the drug administration. Drug interactions result when two or more drugs are administered.

Drugs used in treatment are known as antiepileptic or anticonvulsants. There are different types of antiepileptics and their usage depends on the specific type of seizure. Examples of some antiepileptic drugs are:

Phenytoin (Epanutin)

Phenobarbitone

Primidone (Mysoline)

Carbamazepine (Tegretol)

Ethosuximide (Zarontin)

Sodium valproate (Depakene)

Clonazepam (Clonoprin)

Although the precise mechanism of action of anticonvulsant drugs is not known, it is postulated that they enhance GABA neuronal system (increasing inhibitory actions) through promoting opening of chloride channels at postsynaptic neurones. They may also promote cationic movements, for example sodium and potassium which may have an effect on both the pre- and post-synaptic membranes.

Phenytoin (Epanutin)

Phenytoin was first synthesized by Biltz in 1908 and was first used as an anticonvulsant by Merritt and Putman in 1938. It is one of the most common drugs used in epileptic treatment. It belongs to the group hydantoins. The daily dose administration is approximate 4–6 mg/kg. Peak plasma level is reached in 8–12 hours. The biological half life of the drug varies from 4 to 72 hours. Initially a loading dose is given as peak level is not reached until 5–7 days.

Side-effects of phenytoin include nystagmus, ataxia, drowsiness, diplopia, blurred vision, dizziness, dermatitis, measle-like rash, and lupus erythematosus. Blood complications can also occur and they may include thrombocytopoenia, leucopoenia, granulocytopoenia, agranulocytosis, and different types of anaemia. Gingival hyperplasia may occur, so good oral hygiene is essential.

Phenobarbital

Phenobarbital is a long-acting barbiturate and is used especially in the generalized tonic–clonic seizure. Adults may require 2–3 mg/kg. It has a long half life. When administered intramuscularly, it should be given deeply into a large muscle to reduce tissue necrosis. Intravenous administration may give rise to respiratory depression, apnoea, laryngospasm, and vasodilatation leading to a fall in blood pressure.

The side-effects include lack of concentration, or inability to perform selected motor skills, slowness, ataxia and decreased level of consciousness. Various allergic reactions may occur in the form of urticaria, fever, rash, and Stevens–Johnson syndrome.

Primidone (Mysoline)

Primidone is a structural analogue of phenobarbital and therefore behaves similarly. It is used for generalized tonic–clonic seizures and complex partial seizures.

Side-effects are similar to phenobarbital, although psychiatric or psychological problems may occur in individuals who are so predisposed (Hughes, 1980).

Carbamazepine (Tegretol)

Carbamazepine has been used especially in individuals with temporal lobe epilepsy. Hughes (1980) reported that 85% of patients with temporal lobe epilepsy would benefit from this drug. It can also be used in patients with generalized seizures.

Side-effects include blurred vision, nystagmus,

dizziness, nausea and vomiting. Aplastic anaemia may also occur occasionally.

Ethosuximide

Ethosuximide is the drug of choice in absence seizures. The dose is approximately 20–30 mg/kg/day. Peak value is reached three hours following oral administration. Side-effects include nausea, anorexia, vomiting and dizziness. Systemic lupus erythematosus can occur.

Sodium valproate (Depakene)

Sodium valproate is used in individuals who have bilaterally synchronous and symmetrical three per second spike and wave complexes in their EEG with absence attacks. It has also been found useful in patients with atonic, akinetic and myoclonic seizure.

Administration is every six to eight hours. Side-effects are few and may include weight loss, weight gain and temporary hair loss. If taken with meals, nausea and vomiting may be prevented.

Clonazepam

Clonazepam belongs to the group benzodiazepine. It is often used in treating individuals with myoclonic, akinetic types of seizures. Clonazepam is a very powerful drug amongst the anticonvulsants. Side-effects may include drowsiness on account of its sedative action. Clonazepam may give rise to the development of tolerance.

Diamox (acetazolamide)

This drug is used frequently for women whose seizures increase prior to or during their menstrual cycles. It is believed that the excess water that is present during the menstrual cycle is responsible for the change in frequency of seizures. Acetazolamide assists in the removal of excess water and it also appears to have direct anticonvulsant effect.

When caring for individuals who experience epileptic seizures, any health worker should be able to observe for any symptoms that may occur as a result of side-effects of the drug being used. They should be able to give advice with regards to the importance of drug compliance in the affected individuals. They should also promote education with regards to self care so that the individual can lead and enjoy a full active life.

FURTHER READING

Porter, R.J. (1989) *Epilepsy: One Hundred Elementary Principles*, 2nd edn. London: Baillière Tindall.

Scambler, G. (1989) *Epilepsy*. London: Routledge.

REFERENCES

Baldy-Moulinier, M., Ingvar, D.H. & Meldrum, B.S. (1983) *Current Problems in Epilepsy: Cerebral Blood Flow, Metabolism and Epilepsy*. London: John Libbey.

Chen, R.C. & Forster, F.M. (1973) Cursive epilepsy and gelastic epilepsy. *Neurology*, **23**, 1019.

Currier, R.D., Koci, D.A. & Saidman, L.J. (1963) Prognosis of 'pure' petit mal. A follow-up study. *Neurology*, **13**, 959.

Gascon, G.G. & Lombroso, C.T. (1971) Epileptic (gelastic) laughter. *Epilepsia*, **12**, 63.

Gastaut, H. (1970) Clinical electroencephalographical classification of epileptic seizures. *Epilepsia*, **26**, 103–113.

Hughes, J.R. (1980) Medical aspects of epilepsy: An overview. In Hermann, B.P. (Ed.) *A Multidisciplinary Handbook of Epilepsy*. Springfield, III.: Charles, C. Thomas.

Jeavons, P.M., Harper, J.R. & Bower, B.D. (1970). Long-term prognosis in infantile spasms: A follow-up report on 112 cases. *Dev. Med. Child Neurol.*, **12**, 413.

Livingston, S., Torres, I., Pauli, L.L. & Rider, R.V. (1965) Petit mal epilepsy: Results of a prolonged follow-up 117 patients. *JAMA*, **194**, 227.

Meldrum, B.S. (1975) Epilepsy and GABA-mediated inhibition. *Int. Rev. Neurobiol.*, **17**, 1–36.

Meldrum, B. (1979) Convulsant drugs, anticonvulsants and GABA-mediated neuronal inhibition. In Krogsgaard-Laresen, P., Scheel-Kruger, J. & Kofod,

H. (Eds) *GABA-Neurotransmitters*. Copenhagen: Munksgaard.

Millichap, J.G., Bickford, R.C., Klass, D.W. & Bakus, R.E. (1962) Infantile spasms, hypsarrhythmia and mental retardation: A study of etiologic factors in 61 patients. *Epilepsia*, **3**, 188.

Svoboda, W.B. (1979) *Learning about Epilepsy*. Baltimore: University Park Press.

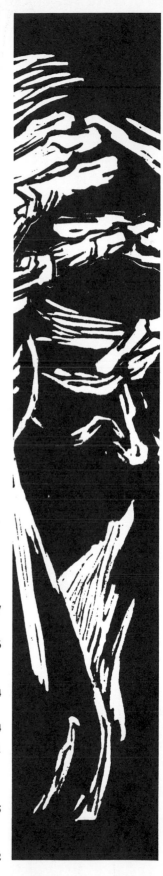

PART

IV

THE ORGANIZATION AND PROVISION OF CARE

This part develops and illustrates the arguments made in Part I. Nurses may work in a variety of settings in a multi-cultural society, and therefore must understand how their particular contribution, in combination with others, can make services more effective. The part examines a sequence from primary care, through community provision to secure forensic settings and analyses some of the characteristics of team-working in interdisciplinary settings. Practitioners must recognize the importance of flexibility while maintaining confidence in their knowledge and skills and providing the highest standards of care.

We aim to extend patient choice, to delegate responsibility to where the services are provided and to secure the best value for money.

Margaret Thatcher, Foreword to Working for Patients, 1989

A CHALLENGE TO PRIMARY HEALTH CARE

Tony Thompson and Peter Mathias

AIMS

i) To analyse the role which is played by the primary care services in mental health provision
ii) To examine the implications for nursing

KEY ISSUES

Legislation
Integrating mental health care into primary care services
Identifying mental health priorities within primary health care
Mental health nursing and the promotion of health
Towards comprehensive policy statements

Identify, analyse and assess factors causing distress and illness	Promote health, provide direct care and make interventions	Manage care programmes and services
Be critical, analytical and accountable, continue professional development	Counter discrimination, inequality and individual and institutional racism	Work within and develop policies, laws and safeguards in all settings
Understand influences on mental health and the nature/causes of disorder and illness	Know the effects of distress, disorder, illness on individuals, groups, families	Understand the basis of treatments and interventions

LEGISLATION

As legislation brought about by the NHS and Community Care Act (DH, 1990) together with Government guidance becomes fully operational, organizations involved with delivering primary health care will need to adapt their practices to ensure a user- or needs-led approach to the delivery. It will become essential that the boundaries which form the present distinction between primary health care and social care do not become an impenetrable barrier for the user of the service. In other words, what is commonly referred to as a 'seamless service' should become a major aim incorporating a statement of mission for those contributing services who wish to achieve high quality goals. It is against this background, which is effected by international considerations as well as national ones, that the workers in the mental health field will have to increase their competence and ability to adapt their practice in the future. It will become increasingly important that workers understand each other's professional language and methods of operation. The impact of the new patterns of service development will be profound and the traditional bodies associated with delivering care will be expected to consult and co-operate in a way in which they have never had to do before. For those working in mental health, it is worth remembering that such agencies as those associated with housing, together with voluntary bodies who will be major providers of services and represent both users and carers, will need to be consulted during the preparation of community care plans. Provision of services tend to cluster into four main groups:

People with physical and sensory disabilities

People who are elderly

People with learning disabilities

People with problems associated with mental health

The pressure on services to respond appropriately will be felt during the remainder of this decade, particularly with the length of the hospital stay being reduced, the long-stay provision of health care being closed, with consequent demand for support for an increasingly vulnerable population being increased. The worker in these fields will notice the numbers of users of services in the local authority sectors rising sharply when the transfer of social security funds begins to be implemented. New skills will emerge as being essential to ensure competent practice. Amongst those skills will be those of accurate budgeting, management of resources, accounting and costing methods applied to particular groups of service users. Health and care economics will form a major component of primary health care systems and whilst the proportion of income support finance that will be identified as the 'care element' to be transferred to the local authorities has yet to be determined, it can be expected that social services budgets for services for adults will rise considerably as the community care services become implemented. Health economics is often associated in people's minds as being finance associated with cost savings, whereas cost benefits feature amongst the standards for monitoring outcomes of cost effectiveness of future mental health services. Of course, any benefits will have to be based upon decisions taken regarding priorities and dependency levels serviced by the care management process described in other chapters of this book.

Although many problems will remain, the legislation being introduced in the UK and its proposed transfer of income support are intended to go someway towards addressing the issues that have been raised with regard to effective primary health care services in the past. The encouragement of the growth of care in people's own homes is an intention of legislative changes associated with transferring the care element of income support to local authorities. It is known that most people with mental health problems also prefer to live in their own homes within the community. People who have been carefully resettled from long-stay hospital provision usually do not wish to return. Of course, a lot of emphasis has to be placed upon such community alternatives being properly resourced and well co-ordinated.

Health authorities are being required to develop care programmes for everyone who is to be discharged from the traditional psychiatric hospital, and this is intended to ensure that a suitable package of care is provided by the health, the local authority and other agencies with someone having clear responsibility for monitoring the circumstances of individuals considered to be vulnerable.

INTEGRATING MENTAL HEALTH CARE INTO PRIMARY CARE SERVICES

For many years the World Health Organization (WHO) has reinforced the need for mental health care to be de-centralized and fully integrated into the primary health care field. This aim has not been without a degree of controversy as it would expect the necessary tasks associated with delivering the services to be carried out where possible by the general health worker. It is not the intention of the World Health Organization to de-skill the specialist in mental health, rather to reserve their skills for the more urgent and priority patterns which emerge when new services are being introduced. In its publication, which sets out practical steps necessary to introduce a mental health component into primary health care (WHO, 1990), the pattern for recent developments in community care can be clearly seen.

Other chapters in this book indicate that member states associated with the WHO have agreed that the key to achieving the goal of health for all is tied to the notion of primary health care. This is because it is recognized that existing systems for the delivery of health care which includes mental health and disorder have often failed to meet the needs of the greater part of the world population. Nurses and other personnel on contemporary training courses are being made aware that the emphasis is now on the promotion of health. The necessity for people to take responsibility for their own health is seen as an important aspect of development of individuals and their communities.

The WHO recognize that care based on the needs of the population rather than on the needs of health organizations and structures, together with bureaucratic or centralized specialist facilities, needs to occur. Such a service, when it is fully implemented, will be de-centralized, will require active participation of the community and family, will be undertaken by health workers and others who may not be specialized workers and will require collaboration amongst personnel in various agencies. The present push in the UK to increase the vocational competence of general health workers in effective techniques that are applicable to the promotion of health is also being seen to have particular application and relevance to mental health. The type of competence which will be recognized includes mobilizing action in the community, encouraging self help and group work, and providing health education which emphasizes promotion of health and disease prevention.

Of course, to sustain such levels of competence it will be necessary for health and social services to be structured in such a way that they can support de-centralized activities. It would appear that in order to ensure that the goals of primary health care systems based upon health for all are realized, then specialist health care personnel, particularly those with skills in nursing and social care, will assume roles of leadership which will enhance the real function and status of the professions but at the same time demand different work patterns than that required in the past. High level competence will be required in the following areas:

Teamwork

Organization

Roles and relationships

Legislation

Intervention

Evaluation of services

Educational skills

Interpersonal skills

Skills of persuasion

All the above may be seen to demand a new approach to the vocational preparation of the new worker in the evolving services. It will become important that key personnel within present services have a vision of the role which will be required of them in effecting these changes rather than a feeling of loss of power and status which often sets off defensive systems which impede progress in a very critical area. More detailed considerations have been identified by the WHO (1987) which point to the difficulties likely to be encountered as conventional work patterns change. Most people working within the mental health services today will agree that social well-being and the emotional aspects of care within the community have been neglected for far too long in the training of health workers and those associated with delivering effective care both of a health and social nature in the community.

The future emphasis on activities that will be undertaken by workers at community level will challenge the assumptions that mental health problems are of lesser importance. Rather than dismissing psychological and social problems as being irrelevant which occurs in most so-called civilized societies at the moment, there will be increasing sensitivity to these problems. The implementation of proper treatment programmes will have to be given priority if the preventative and health promotion ideals are to be realized.

There will be no clear distinction between what is a health and what is a social care problem in the future. Most community nurses will recognize that if patients are seen as people in their home or workplace environment then all the dimensions of a person's make-up are taken into consideration. It becomes completely inappropriate to see a person with a disorder or a mental health problem as an isolated person or the disorder the condition of a single problem.

Attention to mental health is essential if primary health care is to be useful (WHO, 1990).

Many of the chapters contained within this present text reinforce the notion that physical features are often a way of expressing psychosocial distress and the failure to recognize this in the general community leads to a massive wastage of health and social service resources.

Of course, human behaviour is an all important feature in the generation and maintenance of disorder and effective prevention and treatment should rightly concentrate on changing these aspects of behaviour. It is at this level where the skilful application of principles associated with psychological care, biological, spiritual and social care principles are of extreme importance in the preparation of primary health practitioners.

IDENTIFYING MENTAL HEALTH PRIORITIES WITHIN PRIMARY HEALTH CARE

The contemporary preparation of nurses pursuing the mental health branch speciality who have undertaken a foundation programme means that the nurse has been exposed to the main categories of need for people wishing to receive care within a primary setting. It is to be expected that this practitioner will require further information about how services are to be developed which can tackle the variety of health needs and how the overall organization of services can produce the correct balance of the different forms of help. First, organizations can be encouraged to take a pragmatic view of the relevance of psychological, social and behavioural science components of health care. It is important that nurses and other workers contribute particular skills in this area; they are necessary for the identification of service requirements and priorities for primary care. They include:

The enhancement of the quality of life

The improvement of overall functioning of the health and social service

Supporting the health of the nation and its socioeconomic development

The active promotion of mental health

These areas are often overlooked when existing

services consider their input into the primary health settings. Where these areas are considered then it does beg questions in relation to the types of skills and competencies that need to be available to an organization in order to guarantee services to a particular standard. In terms of vocational preparation of future workers it means an emphasis on what people can do as opposed to what they say or write. What they can do becomes of particular importance; in other words, there will be an increasing emphasis upon the health workers function as opposed to previously defined roles.

The other area to consider is that of the control of mental disorder and neurological disease patterns. Although this has been a consideration of health professionals in the general community, it has at the same time been perceived as highly specialized work and often ignored by those at the point of contact within the health and social service areas.

In the future two particular aspects will require effort by all workers due to the changes in demography and personal circumstances of those requiring health service. This includes:

1 Diagnosis and therapeutic input which includes rehabilitation and resettlement.

2 Prevention of mental and neurological disorders. There is increasing evidence that problems associated with mental health feature highly in those problems of a general health nature for which assistance is sought by individuals within the community but they are often unnoticed or ignored. The future demands a highly competent worker who can achieve a standard of skill associated with function within the community which will be aimed at reducing mental health problems and thereby reducing wastage of effort within generic services in order to achieve health care which is effective, efficient and economic. If the practitioner has not been exposed to rigorous training and education then the neglect of the psychological and social components in health together with the behavioural aspects of illnesses will remain a fundamen-

tal deficiency of the existing health and social care systems.

MENTAL HEALTH NURSING AND THE PROMOTION OF HEALTH

Simple skills can improve life (WHO, 1990)

An appropriately educated and trained psychiatric nurse has always made an impact on the quality of life of people with mental disorders. The new arrangements for services which are emerging throughout the UK can potentially both increase and enhance their future role. As part of a primary health care team the psychiatric nurse will promote the idea that whilst the general community can seem free from recognizable disorder or disease, this is not necessarily the same as the community achieving its optimum physical, mental and social wellbeing. Their contemporary techniques will include the use of education in methods of combating stress, effective use of recreational and leisure time and knowledge of forming networks in order to maintain social support systems. For these laudable inputs to be made, nurses and others rely upon programmes pursuing, sharing and collaboration between all those responsible for planning and development of services. A general awareness of social economic development is promoted by the contemporary trained nurse particularly. Experience will have been gained which will allow them to recognize impairment being exacerbated by problems such as drug, alcohol and substance use, breakdown of traditional family life, and the effects of public and societal violence. The management of these problems represents very difficult organizational strategies which have to be effectively implemented if health interventions are to be made effective and the development of the community more productive. A particular attribute of psychiatric nurses is the ability to promote human skills in personnel of all ages who also have to function in the developing community.

Successful community care will require that people place a very high value on mental health. However, it is unlikely to feature high on the agenda of priorities as perceived by the community itself. A high level of competency needs to be gained by the health worker in order to lead the community to an understanding of the importance of mental health in improving the quality of their lives. An emerging skill for all workers in primary care is in assisting communities to develop their own responses to mental health needs by using existing resources including human resources, and the strength within the community itself. New partnerships are being forged between health worker, social care agencies, voluntary and independent sectors.

These will prove to be a vital ingredient to psychiatric nurses in particular who are striving to increase their awareness of the importance of emotional wellbeing and the value systems of the community they will serve. These values may be expressed in different ways and certainly are unlikely to be expressed in terms of mental health by the community at large. This is because the prefix 'mental' is stigmatized and open to misinterpretation. However, they will look to seek respite from distress and unhappiness and altered psychosocial functioning. It is somewhat of a remarkable indictment that the neglect of mental health services within the primary care sector has gone on for so long, when it is considered that the population is more concerned with their quality of life, their morale and their relationships with other people than they are with aspects of physical health alone.

Nowhere are the cultural and social values of society and the evolution of good mental health of the community more apparent than in the consideration of mental health care of women. Our own experience of observing the effects of overwhelming psychosocial distress in societies associated with former eastern bloc countries, bears witness to the particular plight of women in societies that are not able to achieve full social or educational and psychological development. This is often because of cultural attitudes towards their own role in society.

One of the first observations is the poor physical state associated with the plight of these women, but an experienced psychiatric nurse could soon judge the result of their mental and emotional traumas. Whilst women in this position cannot be described in any way to be mentally ill in what has become the traditional sense of the term, there can be little doubt that their problems relate to a failure to achieve and to enjoy what has become identified as optimum mental health. Their position illustrates extremely well the difference between concerns about mental illness on the one hand and the idea of promoting good mental health on the other.

A mental health nurse has a particularly strong role in the prevention of mental and neurological disorders and can provide timely useful information to all disciplines in order to give a composite site picture of both individual and community needs associated with these disorders. The nurse can give leadership to much of the preventative work which can be done within general primary health care services and by promoting the intervention of other agencies, the truly specialized nature of the mental health profession can be seen to be an important one in terms of enhancing the work of other colleagues. The chapters contained in this book reinforce the notion that mental health issues play a most vital contribution to the social and psychological development of community and society as a whole and they have to be recognized as a necessary component in general health promotion. Psychiatric nurses who have been trained and educated from a broad foundation should see an increasing role being formed in improving health education and practice, particularly in developing countries which have tended to neglect the broader aspects of mental health. As the global concept of a healthy state becomes recognized, higher priority for mental health will be seen in the integrated national health programmes.

TOWARDS COMPREHENSIVE POLICY STATEMENTS

The individual philosophies of states and nations naturally reflect the history and current socio-economic status. However, the WHO (1992) identifies certain features which prove to be valuable in ensuring that commitments to mental health policy are reflected in major statements including:

Mental health services should be integrated at all levels as far as possible with general health services.

Comprehensive coverage of populations demands that delivery of mental health care be established in the primary health care setting and promoted by those who are not mental health specialists.

Appropriate training in mental health and psychosocial skills is essential for all health personnel, and also for many working in other sectors, for example, education, community development, social welfare agencies and police forces.

Steps should be taken to promote health attitudes in young people that will prevent behaviour with adverse consequences for health.

Management of health problems associated with alcohol, drug and substance abuse should be an integral component of national mental health policy.

Individuals suffering from mental disorders should have the same rights, treatments and support as those with physical disorders.

Individuals suffering from mental disorders should be treated within or as close as possible to their own communities, using local resources.

It can be seen from the above that a highly educated, proficient and competent mental health worker can greatly assist in the implementation of mental health programmes that are responsive to what people within the community feel their needs to be.

The current preparation of the nurse pursuing the mental health branch programme within the UK is intended to ensure that the provision of care and therapeutic input to disordered functioning does not alienate the community from which the service user is drawn. This has not always been the case and because mental illness can be incomprehensible and perceived as frightening, history has shown that the following outcomes of training must be achieved:

Workers should be an integrated part of the community which they are serving.

The mental health worker requires an accurate understanding of what the community itself regards as priority areas.

The worker within mental health requires to be seen as an understanding, empathetic, and supportive professional by the individual, family, carer and the community as a whole.

When implementing care, the contemporary prepared mental health worker seeks to enhance the wellbeing of the individual and the cohesion of the family, together with making a valuable contribution to the socioeconomic development of the local community.

All of these issues are currently being addressed in the UK by a major mental health working group under the chairmanship of Professor Anthony Butterworth.

This Government-sponsored working group will expect key personnel to consider jointly the problems of achieving the aims of current policies, the outcomes of educational preparation and hopefully arrive at joint solutions to the major challenges facing mental health workers today. Hopefully it will have been identified in this chapter that the local community constitutes the primary level at which health care operates and this includes the provision of mental health services. In a global sense the common denominator of primary services tends to fall into the primary and secondary levels of provision and the primary tasks of health workers in most societies who are looking towards decentralizing services and establishing comprehensive mental health care, apply the following principles:

Primary input

The recognition and provision of basic health services which includes mental health.

The identification of mental disorders which are seen as priority conditions to include epilepsy, chronic psychotic states, dependence on drugs or alcohol and emotional and psychological crises.

Accurate collection of data and identification of patients who should be seen by specialized mental health personnel or referred to higher level authority.

Accurately responding to people in whom physical symptoms are an indication of an underlying psychological problem.

Comprehensive provision of education and training with regard to the maintenance of good mental health to include collaboration with others concerned on an interagency basis.

The compilation of a register of people who are referred back to the community from specialized services with the intention of maintaining them on long-term medication thereby insuring continuity and review of treatment.

The implementation of simple programmes aimed at personal development, to include training and relaxation techniques, the promotion of sound recreational activity and exercise, sensitive counselling and involvement in community activities.

Furthering the use of skills aimed at mobilizing and motivating self help groups and agencies of support which include volunteers in community activities.

The accurate identification of people whose mental health may place them under threat for a variety of reasons. These include family stress, poverty, physical hardship, adverse working and safety conditions.

In populations of circa 500,000 the secondary level of health care is usually represented by district hospitals or large specialized health centres. It has become vitally important for the co-ordination of services at this level and this has to be achieved by the promotion of close co-operation between secondary services and those within the primary health areas. The provision of competent services which are capable of functioning and providing specialized psychiatric skills includes the following:

Secondary input

Accurate diagnosis, treatment and follow up of patients, including those who have been referred from the primary system.

Provision of in-patient and out-patient facilities with specialized mental health skills of a mental health nurse who can act in a consultative capacity to other hospital departments who may have to implement treatment programmes for people suffering from disorders which are essentially psychological rather than physical in their origin.

Providing skilled input into the continued professional development, support and supervision of the primary health care worker, and of other personnel from agencies concerned with mental health.

Initiating and promoting mental health, raising the awareness of mental health issues both within and across appropriate agencies, together with fostering mental health skills within all hospital or health centre departments.

The skilled application of various therapies concerned with mental disorder including medication, electrotherapy, psychotherapeutic counselling and associated regimes.

Initiating and maintaining comprehensive documentation and record keeping, particularly in relation to follow up and continued treatment of long-term patients who return to their communities with the intention of being cared for in the primary health system.

It is at this level that the mental health nurse particularly forms a valuable member of a team which deals with complex problems of diagnosis and treatment referred from the secondary and primary levels of care. Nurses can adopt supervisory responsibilities as well as undertake research and evaluative work within the entire mental health care system.

It can be seen that the division of responsibilities and the need to recognize the distinct needs of individuals or organizations together with potential conflicts in undertaking the above tasks at different levels has to be well managed. Four groups of activities have been identified by Smith (1991) which can help overcome the potential conflict within the division of duties, roles, function and tasks.

The context of Smith's suggestions are that different models of case management may allocate four groups of tasks in different ways. These tasks are used here to demonstrate the need for integrating the concept of the mental health workers' skills within the overall provision of primary care and to illustrate many of the former points as applied to the organization of this care:

---

1 Assessment, initial identification, screening, individual service plan, ongoing monitoring of individual's progress.

2 Administration, negotiating a care package with users and carers against a set budget, linking user to relevant services, evaluation of service quality.

3 Care purchasing, identification and development of providers, developing a contractual relationship, budgetary management ensuring value for money against needs and resources, ensuring contract compliance.

4 Advocacy on behalf of the user to obtain resources and to ensure services meet individual needs.

The potential for multifunctional input into the process can be identified and when a nurse is being educated to be professionally accountable to the public, the above processes will help ensure that minimum professional standards are met.

FURTHER READING

Beck, C.M. & Rawlins, R.P. (1993) *Mental Health Psychiatric Nursing*. Mosby—Year Book, US.

Brooker, C. & White, E. (1993) *Community Psychiatric Nursing*. London: Chapman & Hall.

Marks, I.M. & Scott, R.A. (1990) *Mental Health Care Delivery: Innovations, Impediments and Implementation*. Cambridge: Cambridge University Press.

Shepard, M. (1986) *Mental Illness in Primary Care Settings*. London: Tavistock.

REFERENCES

Department of Health (DH) (1990) *The NHS and Community Care Act*. London: HMSO.

Smith, H. (1991) In McAusland, T. & Wistow, G. (Eds) *Psychiatric Services Beyond the White Papers. A Guide to Key Organization and Staff Development Issues*. NHS Training Authority in collaboration with Nuffield Institute for Health Service Studies.

World Health Organization (WHO) (1987) *Community Based Education of Health Personnel: Report of a WHO Study Group*. Technical Report Series, No. 746. Geneva: WHO.

World Health Organization (WHO) (1990) *The Introduction of a Mental Health Component into Primary Health Care*. Geneva: WHO.

ESTABLISHING A COMMUNITY SERVICE

Mary Headley and Rosaleen Moore

AIMS

i) To describe the development of a community mental health service
ii) To review and analyse the workings of community mental health teams

KEY ISSUES

Community-based consumer-led initiatives in the USA and Europe
Northern Ireland context
Towards community care
Developing community mental health teams
Types of team
Teams working

Identify, analyse and assess factors causing distress and illness	Promote health, provide direct care and make interventions	Manage care programmes and services
Be critical, analytical and accountable, continue professional development	Counter discrimination, inequality and individual and institutional racism	Work within and develop policies, laws and safeguards in all settings
Understand influences on mental health and the nature/causes of disorder and illness	Know the effects of distress, disorder, illness on individuals, groups, families	Understand the basis of treatments and interventions

INTRODUCTION

Since the mid 1970s there has been a concentrated move both in the USA and across Europe towards a process of deinstitutionalization in psychiatric care, and thereby put in place community-based consumer-led initiatives with the opportunity to offer treatment, care, accommodation and work opportunities for recovering mental ill persons in as close an approximation to normalization as possible.

INITIATIVES IN THE USA AND EUROPE

The experience in USA, Europe and the UK displays similarities and contradictions. In America there exists a resistance to state intervention and a redistributive concept of welfare provision. The tension is evident in the attempts to move from a medical hospital-orientated model of care to a community-based one, with the attendant contentious issues of income support and mass urban regeneration when the major consumers of community-based mental health programmes are proved to be drawn from the poorest sections of the community. In Europe different countries have produced varying models. In Italy, with a strong tradition of collectivism and state intervention, direct action by the Government on the number of permitted hospital admissions has had an influence on the development of community care reforms.

Shulamot Ramon (1989, 1991) outlines factors which contributed to the process of change in Italy:

Heavy and unchanging reliance on segregated institutions.

The existence of a number of psychiatrists prepared to act politically.

The autonomous nature of the region's enthusiastic reform being associated with socialist areas and the wide acceptance of the positive value of collective action to mobilize community support.

In the wider European context there is much variation but with a standard focus on community-based approaches with which we can identify. In the Netherlands, long seen as being in the forefront of mental health care delivery with the provision of community treatment in general practice, the provision of psychosocial centres and an emphasis on crisis intervention, there now appears to be a move to halt the trend in hospital bed reduction. This could in part be related to the type of insurance-related financing which only provides cover for hospital-type treatments and care and a reluctance to cover non-hospital alternatives.

France has developed an approach based on 'adaptation and humanization'—not massed closure of psychiatric hospitals. France's policy of sectorization ensures that funding for services is found from both central and local funding arrangements and in France, as in the general European context, the absence of votes from consumers in the area of mental health ensures that these issues are on the lower rungs of the ladder of political priorities.

INITIATIVES IN THE UK

In Britain as a whole there has been no overall, overt Government-initiated hospital closure policy and programme although some would argue that has been the net result. There has been a steady recognition that relevant local services have to be in place first, and long-stay facilities can only close when community services can cope with the increased workload.

In the UK the concept of introducing a bridging finance programme to enable local and health authorities to put such resources in place is a good one, but sufficient new monies were not made available to develop a realistic community programme.

The tenets embraced in the various White Papers on community care reforms indicate that proposed closures have not stemmed primarily from unobjective economic rationalization but because the large outmoded centralized facility had outlived its original social function.

In the UK the problem to be faced was the fact

that whilst devolved national health services would replace the longstay hospital, social work and the ancillary services such as day care, home support, diversional or vocational therapy were provided by local authorities who would be required to take on a long-term support role for the newly rehabilitated chronically mentally ill on transfer from hospital. 'Making a Reality of Community Care' (1986) a report by the Audit Commission for local authorities in England and Wales prepared the ground for a large-scale programme of reintegration and allowed regional health authorities to grant fund local authorities for resettlement programmes.

In 1986 Roy Griffiths was appointed by the Government of the day to carry out an enquiry into community care. The concerns of central Government were focused mainly on the largely unplanned and rapid growth in the residential and nursing home care sector funded almost wholly from the social security budget and from fears that the trends in homelessness among mentally ill people, so visible in the American situation, were becoming the norm in Britain. Griffiths also concerned himself with wider issues around the provision of health and welfare. The idea of privatized informal care free from state intervention was gaining ground under the prevailing economic and political system (Griffiths, 1986).

Knapp (1988) identified the following areas of importance in the community care scene:

Dehospitalization

Joint working (NHS and local authority)

Cost effectiveness

Consumerism and mixing the economy

The move towards consumerism has resulted in individualized systems of care planning as in care management and client advocacy systems. Mixing the economy is the most significant in terms of shifting health and local authorities from direct provision to purchasing and commissioning from a range of private and voluntary sources.

The economic and political climate of the 1980s in the UK focused on the market and the belief

that health and welfare should be treated as a commodity to be bought and sold accordingly. In the move towards decentralization, decontrol and opting out, the market imposes the requirement of competition—competition implies winners and by definition losers. It is arguable that the health and welfare of our population and especially vulnerable people in psychological distress is not best served in such a climate.

For consumers in the mental health arena, a mental illness invariably means a loss of status in employment terms, and a descent in the social and occupational structure. In a period of unemployment and instability, such as we are witnessing, opportunities for meaningful life experiences for persons with a mental illness are minimal.

THE NORTHERN IRELAND CONTEXT

In Northern Ireland we have had an integrated health and social services model of services delivery following the reorganization of local government and the formation of the four health and social services boards in 1973 (Macrory, 1971; and NIHPSS, 1972).

There was an acknowledged need to reform local government and to prevent known abuses. There was a complementary need to bring all allied services together under one administrative umbrella. This resulted in a centralization of control and brought health and social services beyond the field of local accountability far in advance of the rest of the UK.

Theoretically, this should have resulted in an exemplary model of multidisciplinary service delivery, with the foundations laid in the early 1970s. However, health and social care delivery remained, in the main, unidisciplinary. Joint planning remained sporadic, primary care developed on its own and where good multidisciplinary relationships existed they sometimes owed more to individual interests than to any overall plan.

The majority of the finance was, and still is, concentrated in the acute hospital sector. There was no overall strategy for the implementation and delivery of integrated mental health services enhancing community and institutional settings.

The various professions, for example, nursing,

social work and medicine, remained firmly within their own fields and were managed on unidisciplinary lines. With the advent of general management, opportunities were afforded for the first time to stand back and take a hard look at the current state of care and treatment and decide on future directions.

TOWARDS COMMUNITY CARE

The debate generated regarding concerns at the closure of the long-stay psychiatric hospitals and the design of future care and treatment in the community has sometimes failed to take into account that most people suffering from a mental illness are already treated at home with the combined efforts of the GP and community-based staff. Approximately 7% of people suffering from severe mental illness are treated in a hospital setting. Therefore community care has always existed, if in reality it may have meant mentally disordered people being cared for by their families or living alone and managing with a minimum of support systems.

There has been understandable concern both in the public mind and amongst professionals in the field that the run down and closure of large psychiatric hospitals will take place before the requisite finance is provided to ensure that the alternative community services are in place well in advance of retraction. In Northern Ireland we are better placed to make progress and learn from our colleagues. In the UK closures in the late 1970s and early 1980s were not well planned. This led to the philosophy underlying the policies being questioned. As a result there has been less than whole-hearted support from central Government for 'community care'. Legislators, whilst not reversing the policy, nevertheless never wholeheartedly committed sufficient in terms of finance and other resources. Opponents of the closure policy point to the deficiencies in the 'community'—the fictional ideal. The reality they say is that community equals overburdened families with little choice and therefore we should reassess the asylums as being better than no service at all. They have pointed to highly visible signs of 'failure' for community care—the homeless, the destitute on the street, the numbers discharged to inadequate bed and breakfast arrangements and the pressure on in-patient beds resulting in premature discharge from hospital to make room for even more urgent cases.

Community care can work if the programme is properly funded with adequate organizational structures and the commitment of professionals, coupled with a public better educated to understand mental health problems. The majority of finance in the mental health arena is still tied up in hospital facilities. No matter how much money is spent on upgrading to make these Victorian buildings welcoming and less institutional the fact nevertheless remains that the history of the large mental hospital is the main drawback to acceptability by the general public. Every large mental hospital carries the same legacy of its past. There is evidence to suggest that given the choice, people suffering from long-term mental disorder wish to live in their own homes and take part in ordinary community life. The purpose of community care is to help individuals achieve and sustain a fulfilling and rewarding normal life when this has become difficult through mental disorder. Community care must take up the challenge and provide an integrated network of services including physical facilities, adequate trained personnel and appropriate organizational structures to enable the system to work effectively for every individual requiring assistance.

Dispersing the mentally ill within the community places more challenges on those delivering their care. The institution not only provided safety and asylum for the patient, but in many ways fulfilled the same function for staff. It was a readily identifiable centre of excellence for professional skills. It provided a base for peer support when difficulties arose. There was indeed safety in numbers. With staff and patients now more often geographically dispersed it is important that scarce resources are used to their optimum effect. Staff can be professionally exposed and called upon to make individual decisions and take responsibilities in a much more obvious way than ever occurred within the confines of a psychiatric hospital. These developments have required increased interdisciplinary collaboration to ensure co-ordination of specialist skills.

DEVELOPING COMMUNITY MENTAL HEALTH TEAMS

In moving towards a community mental health team model of care and treatment it is very important for the overall organization to have a clear idea of the task in hand and to have conducted a survey of client/patient need and reviewed the current services.

Multidisciplinary teams have been advocated as the most appropriate methods of delivery of community mental health care (Furnell *et al.*, 1987; Ramon, 1989). Multidisciplinary working has been the norm in many psychiatric settings during the last 20 years, but true multidisciplinary *team work* is a rarer phenomenon.

How do these teams work? Who should they comprise? Who should have responsibility for their management? What are their relationships between the individuals within the team? What are their dynamics to determine their success or failure? Finally how do we evaluate their effectiveness in terms of client welfare?

Our Area Mental Health Unit (AMHU) came into existence against a background of general acceptance that services hitherto were unfocused and without a broad community base and generally community services provision was under resourced. The newly formed unit was of the opinion that to deliver services within a multidisciplinary model was the most efficient and effective use of professional skills and expertise.

True multidisciplinary teamwork models were difficult to observe in action. In Northern Ireland various co-operative co-working arrangements have existed and produced good work but there were deficiencies as the different professional models involved were individually line managed.

Ovretveit (1986) has claimed many advantages for multidisciplinary teamwork. Working on the axiom that the sum of the whole is greater than its constituent parts, it would appear that the pulling together of a wide range of professional skills should result in better co-ordination of the different disciplines, less duplication of input and greater understanding and use of specialist skills held by each worker. The end result should be a more comprehensive treatment plan and a quality outcome for the patient.

These aspirations are often difficult to realize, as people from different professional backgrounds often find it difficult to surrender individual autonomy in the interest of the team.

Ovretveit (1986) describes four types of teams:

The managed team. One individual (the manager) is fully accountable for all casework decisions within the team.

The democratic team. There is no leader who has formally agreed accountability.

The co-ordinated team. One member assumes the role of team co-ordinator who can assume responsibility to organize case work and negotiate.

Core teams. These are fully managed by a team leader in particular cases where there is considerable overlap in the roles of the individuals.

In fact the final *modus operandi* may well be a hybrid of any of the above models. The essential ingredient is that team members have *clarity* about how their own model operates and crucially they know who is the team leader and who carries accountability for the performance of the team.

Who should be team leader?

The typical multidisciplinary team will consist of nurses, social workers, doctors and, to a greater or lesser extent, psychologists and occupational therapists (depending on availability). All too often tension arises as to who should be team leader and this raises the next question of whether there should be clinical responsibility, line management responsibility or medical responsibility. Is there a difference between these functions and if so are they mutually incompatible? At first glance clinical and medical responsibility may seem to a doctor to be the same. The Royal College of Psychiatrists (1977) stated that the consultant has a direct responsibility to co-ordinate the various disciplines in order to ensure the best treatment for the individual—which implies clinical leadership—but is it clinical or medical leadership? McKeown (1979) has identified five tasks of clinical medicine—reassurance, treatment of the acute emergency, cure, care and attention. The inclusion of the term 'care' is interesting as it can be provided by a range of professions and in particular social workers see themselves as providing social care *par excellence*. Birley (1987) a psychiatrist himself, clearly identified clinical responsibility as belonging to many other professions and not the preserve of physicians.

Since the 1960s there has been a steady rise in the standards of basic and professional education and training of social workers, nurses and occupational therapists, as well as improved training for psychiatrists. With these increased skills has come increased expectation from the professions of their role in the planning and decision-making of patient care rather than just in its execution. There often appears to be considerable ignorance within the professions about each other. There is very little reciprocal teaching of one profession by the other and therefore little understanding of what each person does. The result can be that although everybody might claim to work in a multidisciplinary team what in fact is happening is that they share the same room whilst someone, usually a consultant, discusses the case, makes decisions about the case management, and allocates duties to each of the professions in turn according to his or her perceptions of what their skills might be.

Apart from the ignorance of each other's roles, tensions can arise within a team as a result of rivalry between professions, particularly if it is perceived that skills are shared or indeed practised by one person to a higher degree of proficiency than the other. On the other hand many people would voice an anxiety about the dilution of skills within a multidisciplinary team. There is often a fear that by consenting to work together within a team environment in some sense implies a readiness to set aside one's own professional skills and become a generic 'mental health worker' whose skills must be reduced to the lowest common denominator.

Finally a source of on-going difficulties is that of dual management loyalties. The health service is still largely within professional line management structure. Having the individuals within a multidisciplinary team reporting to a number of different line managers makes it almost impossible for that team to work effectively. Staff may be appointed, transferred, denied or given access to training without reference to the needs of the team. Most multidisciplinary teams have no control over resources which are normally administered by line managers hence the team itself is not in a position to make best use of its resources. Whilst undoubtedly all staff in teams need professional guidance and support from senior members of their profession it is essential that the overall service provided by that team is managed by one individual. To enable a multidisciplinary team to function properly we must 'free it from the stranglehold of the managerial octopus of line management' (Murphy, 1990).

An alternative community team model

Our model is a variation on the core and extended team model as exemplified by Ovretveit (1986) and takes into account our responsibilities of health and social care. It hinges on the role of the locality manager—multidisciplinary management was seen as a key issue. A single manager with clear responsibility for service delivery on a patch base system is responsible to the director of community services. The community team model in our unit has been evolutionary and has developed at a different pace in each locality.

As the locality teams were being brought into being, considerable time and energy was involved in bringing together the main groups of fieldwork staff, community nurses and social workers. Team building programmes were instigated and progress was made on multidisciplinary training and case co-ordination. This had the net effect of building up trust and confidence in individual professional expertise and skills, and enabling the teams to identify particular gaps in training or skills mix. A considerable amount of work has been expended on the development of back-up systems and procedures to service the teams, for example adequate clerical back-up and information systems, development of quality standards and a move towards a system of outcome measurement.

In our community team models, locality managers from nursing and social work backgrounds have clear responsibility for all directly managed staff and for co-ordinating service delivery within their patch. The role of the senior social worker and senior nurse has been clearly defined and strengthened as team leaders 'from their own profession'. These two staff manage the day-to-day operational issues with regard to social work and nursing and work jointly to provide professional support and guidance to the locality managers on such areas as (i) training and staff development, for example Approved Social Work Training, Practice Teaching and training for Community Psychiatric Nurses and Social Workers which is increasingly multidisciplinary in application; and (ii) developing co-working arrangements, case load management and case location.

In conjunction with the locality manager they spearhead community initiatives with local voluntary organizations and primary health care agencies. The psychology and paramedic component on the team is sessional. These groups of staff receive professional support and guidance within their respective staff groupings but will take the full part in clinical teamwork.

The second phase of the community team development was facilitated by the consultant psychiatrists organizing their sectors to be co-terminus with localities and encompassing groups of GP practices. Consultant psychiatrists on the team have clinical leadership on all cases within their ambit.

The multidisciplinary team under clinical leadership determines the tasks required and the treatment and care of the individual and the relevant therapist is allocated the case on the basis of 'match' of specific skills. Sometimes these particular skill areas are best determined by the respective team leader. Community nursing and social work staff traditionally have received referrals from a wide variety of sources. Increasingly these referrals have been made to the team as a whole and referees are aware that a service will be provided not necessarily by their traditional choice of professional. The continuing interest in GP fundholding and the necessity to adjust to this new culture has ensured healthy primary care links, with closer collaboration on assessment and care management and an awareness by GPs of the range of therapies and other services on offer from the community teams.

Therefore what makes teams fail? Multidisciplinary teams fail because:

1 They do not know who is in charge.
2 There is poor communication between the professions.
3 There is lack of understanding of each other's roles.
4 There is undue interference by line managers.
5 The team is not involved in the selection and recruitment of its individual members.
6 Training is all too often directed at *individual* professional development as distinct from professional development which feeds the needs of the team as well.

How does a good multidisciplinary team work?

A successful multidisciplinary team has the following ingredients:

The team members are constant and therefore able to identify with, and exhibit loyalty to the team rather than their own discipline.

Members within the team openly acknowledge and are confident of each other's individual skills.

Members of the team are also able to acknowledge that in some instance there is blurring and overlapping of roles.

The team is able to meet to discuss general management issues, their own group dynamics, as well as the cases with which they deal.

Whilst there is a clearly identified clinical leader of the team, each client is assigned a key worker who has prime responsibility for the day-to-day management of the case. Key workers will be allocated on the basis of their particular skills and the particular needs of the patient at that time.

FURTHER READING

Coote, A. (Ed.) (1992) *The Welfare of Citizens. Devolving New Social Rights*. Institute for Public Policy Research/Rivers. London: Oram Press.

Olsen, M.R. (Ed.) (1984) *Social Work and Mental Health: A Guide for the Approved Social Worker*. London: Tavistock.

Onyett, S. (1992) *Case Management in Mental Health*. London: Chapman & Hall.

Ramon, S. (Ed.) (1991) *Beyond Community Care. Normalisation and Integration Work*. London: Macmillan/MIND.

REFERENCES

Birley, J.L.T. (1987) Psychiatrists and psychologists working together for planning services in the post-Griffiths era. *Bulletin of Psychiatrists*, **11**, 210–211.

Furnell, J., Fletts, S. & Clark, D.F. (1987) *Multidisciplinary Teams—Some issues in Establishment and Function*: Hospital & Health Service Journal, Jan., 15–18.

Goldberg, D. (1987) *Psychiatrists and psychologists working together for planning services in the post Griffiths era. Bulletin of Psychiatrists* II & II, Birley DLT.

Griffiths, Sir Roy (1986) *Community Care—Agenda for Action*: London: HMSO.

Knapp, P. (1988) *Demonstrating Successful Care in the Community*: Kent: University of Kent Personal Social Services Unit.

Macrory, D. (1971) *Report on Local Government Reforms (NI)*. Review Body on Local Government in Northern Ireland 1970: Report, 1970. Belfast: HMSO.

McKeown, T. (1979) *The Role of Medicine*. Oxford: Blackwell.

Murphy, E. (1990) *Psychiatric Bulletin*, April, 14: 237.

Northern Ireland Health & Personal Social Services Order (HMSO) (1972).

Ovretveit, J. (1986) *Organisation of Multi-disciplinary Community Teams*: Brunel University Health Services Centre. Working Paper. Middlesex: Brunel Institute of Organisation and Social Studies.

Ramon, S. (1989) *Mental health social work—the state of the art: Social Work Today*, **16** June, 16–17.

Ramon, S. (1991) *Psychiatry in Transition—The British Italian Experience*. London: Pluto Press.

The Royal College of Psychiatrists (1977) The responsibilities of consultants in psychiatry within the National Health Service: *News & Notes*, **4**.

Working for Patients 'People First' (1989). London: HMSO.

PROVIDING SERVICES IN A MULTIRACIAL SOCIETY

BLACK PERSPECTIVES

Kamlesh Patel and Gerard Rice

AIMS

i) To identify the experience of black people using mental health services in Britain
ii) To describe the work of a drugs agency in Bradford and its attempts to provide an effective service to the black communities
iii) To suggest ways in which services to black communities can be made more effective

KEY ISSUES

Unequal treatment
Racism as an explanation of unequal treatment
The Bridge Project
   Issues and problems to solve
   Findings
Ways forward

Identify, analyse and assess factors causing distress and illness	Promote health, provide direct care and make interventions	Manage care programmes and services
Be critical, analytical and accountable, continue professional development	Counter discrimination, inequality and individual and institutional racism	Work within and develop policies, laws and safeguards in all settings
Understand influences on mental health and the nature/causes of disorder and illness	Know the effects of distress, disorder, illness on individuals, groups, families	Understand the basis of treatments and interventions

INTRODUCTION

It is evident even to the casual observer that Britain is not only a multiracial society, but is quite overtly polyethnic. Despite this fact it is only in recent years that social, health and welfare services have begun to give serious consideration to the implications for service development and delivery. This lack of development of services can be directly attributable to many issues including racism, power, inequality, inadequate and inappropriate staffing and training and lack of resources. This is clearly evidenced in the provision of mental health services to black people in this country (Brent Community Health Council, 1981). (The term black refers to people of both African and Asian heritage. The term also represents as an extreme the other categories which are also discriminated against on similar grounds of origin, e.g. Jewish people, the Irish, Cypriots, travellers, etc.)

We are conscious that there are many other forms of discrimination that exist with respect to social, health and welfare provision, such as gender, class, disability, age and sexuality. However, these are not within the domain of the present chapter.

UNEQUAL EXPERIENCES OF HEALTH

The differing of standards in the provision of services experienced by black and white people using health (and other) resources in Britain warrants further description, analysis and remedy. Black people receive unequal treatment from the National Health Service in a number of ways:

Lack of provision for such special needs as sickle cell anaemia in terms of research, screening and treatment.

Failure to provide professional interpreters for those people whose first language is not English.

Discrimination in terms of employment and promotion prospect. Though a large proportion of NHS staff are black, they are heavily concentrated at the lower levels of employment in unpopular jobs and are seriously under represented in prestigious, highly paid posts (Brent Community Health Council, 1981; London Association of Community Relation Councils, 1985).

Black people are twice as likely as white people to be compulsory admitted to psychiatric hospitals and once there to receive such physical treatments as drugs and ECT.

Black people are twice as likely as whites to be classified as suffering from schizophrenia.

Black youths are particularly liable to be classified as not only mentally ill, but also dangerous (Burke, 1988).

The above are only some examples of the inequalities that exist in the health service. These inequalities are mirrored in every dimension of social, health, housing, education, employment, legal and welfare provision. Thus creating a situation whereby:

'Britain is now two entirely different worlds, and the one you inherit is determined by the colour of your skin'.
Salman Rushdie, 1982

Therefore the only explanation that can sustain scrutiny is racism, both on an individual and institutional level. When examining any aspect of service delivery to black people, one cannot isolate a particular problem from the general contextual framework of racism. We cannot move forward unless people are willing to accept that we live in a racist society and that racism underpins many of the problems faced by black people in Britain today.

RACISM AND POWER IN PSYCHIATRY

Racism is a system of unequal power where one group has greater access to the power structures and institutions within society, so that other racial groups are systematically discriminated against and consequently are treated less favourably. It must also be acknowledged that individuals who are not themselves racist in their beliefs can, and often do, represent racist institutions and perpetuate inequality. A prime example of this is a practitioner operating within mental health services—services that, as we will demonstrate throughout this chapter, have a history of discrimination against black people.

In acknowledging that power is one of the central themes in racism, it is crucial that we begin our examination of mental health services with a critique of the power that exists in this field. Historically and currently, psychiatry occupies the dominant role within mental health provision, and uses this dominance to define what is 'normal' and 'abnormal' behaviour, workers who are struggling to develop anti-racist practice need a theoretical and practical appreciation of the power of psychiatry. There have been critiques written about the power which psychiatry holds (e.g. Ingleby, 1981; Sedgewick, 1982; Miller and Rose, 1986).

Even black psychiatrists, who by profession are a member of the dominant group, but by race and culture are not, will find it difficult to influence the environment they work in as they are forced to work within dominant structures and are constrained by traditional theories and practices.

The relationship between psychiatry and black people is problematic in a number of respects. For example, the high rate of diagnosis of schizophrenia in certain sections of the black community (a point which we return to later), especially among people of Afro-Caribbean origin and the way in which psychiatry functions as a form of social control. Though often denied, racism is a major force within psychiatric decision-making and treatment and is central to any understanding of black people's experience of psychiatry.

Many psychiatrists fail to recognize or question their role in controlling behaviour which has been defined as deviant. Moreover, they fail to ask why certain groups are controlled more than others. Rather than address this in any positive way, they pathologize and react by diagnosis and treatment which fails to acknowledge the context within which people live. Failure to recognize the impact of a person's gender, race, culture, emotional, physical, social and economic status can lead to increased misdiagnosis and mistreatment.

Impact on research

Racism, both covert and overt has also played a significant part in the nature of the research that has been undertaken, especially with respect to the incidence of mental illness and black people. This has involved the extremes of total exclusion of race as evidenced in Brown and Harris's otherwise excellent study undertaken in (Brown and Harris, 1978) to review depression in women, as opposed to the study by Harrison *et al.* (1988) which claimed to find prevalence rates for schizophrenia 12 times greater amongst the Afro-Caribbean communities studied than the white population.

As a result of the criticisms levelled at these research projects and the differences in the results, it is clear that research is not a value-free activity and therefore it must be viewed in its wider political and social context. Even the most comprehensive and sensitive studies inevitably reflect the values and attitudes of the researcher.

Many of the studies that have been undertaken clearly highlight a high rate of compulsory admissions under the Mental Health Act (1983) of Afro-Caribbeans to psychiatric institutions following a diagnosis of schizophrenia. Surely we should ask what is schizophrenia and why do Afro-Caribbean people have this label so readily thrust upon them, with such dire consequences?

Since the early 1950s psychiatrists have claimed to have found higher rates of schizophrenia amongst Afro-Caribbean people, as high as 12 times the national average. This is in direct contrast to statistics gleaned during a visit by one of the authors to Belle View Hospital (the largest psychiatric hospital in the Caribbean) which show that the incidence of schizophrenia is two cases in every 10,000 people per year. This is identical to the rates of schizophrenia in the white population in Britain.

The problem with schizophrenia is that it can only be diagnosed through an individual's personal history. It cannot be found at the bottom of a microscope. Therefore the label schizophrenia may turn out to be a range of mental illnesses with different causes and different outcomes. It may even be more appropriate to use a combination of names rather than continue to use the overall term of schizophrenia. We must ask, therefore, are they simply measuring the consequences of prejudices, by either a process of misdiagnosis or by highlighting a schizophrenic illness which has been precipitated by racism?

Given the high rate of schizophrenia that is 'diagnosed' in the Afro-Caribbean population, especially young men, it is important that we look at these issues, even if within the limitations of this chapter it will be a brief view.

WHAT ARE THE REASONS?

Below we have outlined some of the explanations put forward by a range of academic and welfare professionals to account for the apparent higher incidence of mental health problems among Afro-Caribbean people and the significant under-representation of people of Asian heritage:

Racism (both individual and institutional)—the stresses and the pathologizing nature of racism are a major contributory factor to mental illness among black people.

Poverty—this, linked with the above, and the resulting deprivation, is a major causal effect on the mental health status of black people.

Misdiagnosis—the consequence of Eurocentric assessments, the predominance of white practitioners, language difficulties coupled with untrained (if any) interpreters, and poor cultural information.

Culture—major issues of culture shock due to migration, generational conflict based on custom and expectation and misunderstanding of aspects of behaviours that are confused with symptoms of mental illness. (For a discussion and critique of trans-cultural work see Mercer (1986).)

Biological—the view that certain ethnic groups,

living in metropolitan countries are vulnerable to mental illness as a result of organic vulnerability.

Social control—police attitude to young blacks, the nature of the control element of psychiatry, the power and use of the Mental Health Act, 1983, coupled with the unwillingness of professionals to accept this issue.

The above all contribute to the debate of the apparent higher incidents of mental health problems among black people. However, there are also a number of valid criticisms to each of the above arguments, considered in detail in Fernando (1988), Francis *et al.* (1989), Sashidharan (1989) and Rogers and Pilgrim (1989).

We feel the areas outlined above, with the exception of biological factors, have an important part to play in helping us to understand the position of black people within mental health services. However, we cannot stress enough that to take these factors in isolation is not only simplistic, but ignores the complex nature of multiple oppression. These and *other* factors can, and do combine in varying degrees to create the interface between black people and the mental health services. The extent to which each factor determines the relationship between the individual and the mental health service varies, and should not be generalized, pathologized or viewed in isolation.

THE ROLE OF SOCIAL WORKERS

It is important to remember the Mental Health Act, 1983 allows the compulsory detention of people in hospital against their will and it is not psychiatrists, but social workers, who have the main responsibility for its operation. Psychiatry as a profession offers a limited critique of its role in this process, and in respect of black people has done little to reverse the process whereby black people feel oppressed by the implementation of this Act. Social workers have at least acknowledged some of their shortcomings in recognizing the importance of an understanding of race. However, this area remains problematic for many reasons. One example of this is the study by Shah (1990), which looked at the attitudes and experiences of approved social workers (ASWs) in Rochdale. This showed that workers themselves identified that current resources were wholly inadequate and that ASWs were operating within a Eurocentric model of care and working with limited resources in an environment of frustration and confusion. They lacked relevant knowledge, training and skills in anti-racist practice. The consequence was that workers inevitably made wrong judgements and users suffered.

As practitioners we feel that a factor that underpins both the 'problem' and the potential solution is based in the provision of services, at a preventative and treatment level both within the psychiatric and wider social work sphere. The works by Rooney (1987), Browne (1988) and Connelly (1989) amongst others clearly highlight the chronic shortfall in resources that are accessible and relevant to the black community.

Barnes *et al.* (1990) looked at the provision of services for black people by social service departments. They focused on the use of compulsory powers within 10 local authorities with significant black communities. Many concerns were raised, two being the appropriateness and quality of services that were offered and the employment of suitably qualified black staff. The study found that the high rates of compulsory admissions of Afro-Caribbean people came as a result in part of the lack of preventative services available, resulting in people being referred at too late a stage to avoid hospitalization:

Adult population	Afro-Caribbean	White	Asian
Compulsory Admissions Population per 100,000	204	116.7	54.3

Although not specifically studied, the same proportions would also apply to informal admission. The low rate of admissions for people of Asian origin might mean that they are not gaining sufficient access to services. The relatively low rate of referral of Asian people was considered to be in part due to a lack of cultural sensitivity by social workers and others in recognizing the presence of mental distress in people from the Indian subcontinent. There was a clear shortage of black professional staff at all levels, especially ASWs coupled with the lack of ethnically sensitive day care and residential services.

Despite the weight of the above evidence, we still face a situation where professionals from a range of disciplines refuse to acknowledge that the services they provide are not relevant or accessible to black people and pose a major contributory factor to under use of services. Instead, we often face blanket excuses such as 'black people do not need our services, they never use them' or 'they look after themselves—anyway they have extended family systems' to explain the poor take up of services by black people. Even those workers who are committed to non-oppressive practice often use the excuse of lack of resources, knowledge, training or appropriate staff. This is both wrong and misleading. We will use the example of the Bridge Project to show how positive steps can and should be taken to tackle this issue.

THE BRIDGE PROJECT

The Bridge Project is a 'street' drugs agency situated in the city centre of Bradford in West Yorkshire. It offers a confidential counselling, advice and information service to anyone experiencing problems with drug use, the families and friends of drug users and other professional workers. It also has a specialist drugs rehabilitation hostel and employs a number of outreach and detached workers. The Project deals with all drugs ranging from heroin, glues and gases to tranquillizers, with the exception of alcohol, and employs a total of 24 staff.

In the first three years of operation the Bridge Project, on average, was seeing well over 1,000 clients a year. However, we quickly realized that only a minute proportion, well under 1% of the people using our services, was from the black community. Given that almost 20% of Bradford's total population of approximately 500,000 people is non-white we were clearly not offering a service to a large section of the community.

Over recent years there has been a growing recognition that drug services have mainly met the needs of the white male community and that they have been failing to meet adequately the needs of all sections of the population, especially black people.

It is difficult to assess the context of any drug-related problems. It is even more difficult to assess the nature and extent of drug-related problems within the black community. We can clearly see the difficulties that arise in terms of appointment of one or two black staff specifically to work with black communities, even in a small city like Bradford.

In 1989, the Project initiated a two-year research study to look into the service needs of the black community in Bradford. It was clear that we would be unable to target and work with every section of the black community within the limited time. After community and client consultation, a worker was employed to conduct research/outreach work with young Pakistani men as this was the largest and most easily accessible client group. We will briefly outline some of the findings of our original research and then discuss how the findings of the research are being implemented.

Issues that were encountered

People were suspicious of being involved with yet another study pathologizing black people. What was important to communicate to everyone was that the research was a qualitative piece of work and designed not only to identify the number of Asian drug users and the type of drugs used, but also for the development of service provision.

Not all black people were keen to talk to the Project about developing services for drug users. It became very clear that the majority of black people had other more worrying concerns including high unemployment, extremely high infant mortality rate, racist attacks, poor housing and education.

Real concern was expressed about confidentiality—people were suspicious of the research and the links between illegal drugs, the Bridge Project and the police. Who is to be told and why? There was a lack of resources at all levels, not enough black staff, a shortage of money, time-limited research and no translated literature. Since the discussions concerned a highly sensitive area, it is understandable that Asian people were reluctant to talk to the research/outreach worker.

The general perception of Asian users was that services were usually run by white people and were for white people. This perception tended to be based on experience. Very little trust or confidence existed in any agencies. Black people found 'white-run' agencies unsympathetic and unhelpful. White-run agencies did not want to admit that they were racist in the presentation and delivery of their services. Racism and the implementation of services rather than policies were the key issues here.

Findings in brief

It is unnecessary for us to expand further on the problems of institutional racism associated with living in inner city areas and the racism that exists for black people coupled with poor housing, education, health services and the problems with policing. Problems, which many agencies and Government bodies, including the Advisory Council on the Misuse of Drugs, have stated are often associated with the problematic misuse of drugs.

As we have maintained throughout this chapter, compared to white people, black people are prone to both similar and at times, more difficult, upheavals in their lives. The physical, emotional, sociological and psychological problems faced by black people, through racism, deprivation, poverty, class discrimination and poor service delivery does create a vast dilemma from which problematic drug use can be seen as a viable source of escape for a young black person. Therefore if a black person is just as vulnerable to using drugs as a white person then why were so few black people using the services of the Bridge Project?

There were two possible answers: (i) black people did not use drugs or, if they did, they were able to sort out their own problems; (ii) the Bridge Project was failing to provide a service that was accessible or relevant to this client group. What was clear was that in order to find the answers to such questions, and to avoid making massive generalizations and assumptions, the Project needed to undertake extensive research and outreach work into the drug-related needs of the black community in Bradford.

Given that the largest section of the 'black' population in Bradford is grouped under the umbrella term Asian—almost 70,000–80,000, approximately 65,000 being of Pakistani origin alone. One needed to examine this term carefully and the implications it had for service development. We have outlined briefly the various groups, religions and cultures that are encompassed under this term in Bradford alone:

Pakistanis (Pathans/Punjabi Muslims/Sindi/Bluchi)

Bengalis (Slyet)

Gujeratis (Gujerati Hindu/Gujerati Muslim)

Sikhs (Indian Punjabi)

Many of whom have different cultures, religions, languages, the main ones being:

Religions:
  Islam

  Hinduism

  Sikhism

Languages:
Urdu	Bengali
Hindi	Hinku
Punjabi	Bluchi
Gujerati	Sindi
Pashto	

Added to the wide variety of different cultures, religions and languages, it is important to acknowledge the many-faceted needs of each individual generation. In addition we have to consider the very important different gender-related needs. This clearly highlights the difficulty that has been around for agencies who employ 'one Asian' worker to help within the community and provide an appropriate service in terms of advice, information, training, counselling and future development.

There were many misconceptions about drug use within the Asian community, especially amongst parents. Education in many forms was seen as a necessity. A point of concern was the disproportionate number of tranquillizers that were taken without question, as they were prescribed by a GP and were legal.

Cannabis was the most commonly used drug by Asian users (though this use was no more or less in proportion to the size of the community). It was not considered to be a major problem except for legal reasons.

Contact was made with a number of Asian heroin users, though the substance was generally shunned by the majority of the Asian community. It was previously assumed Asian and black people did not use heroin intravenously but only smoked. However, the research clearly showed that of the minority of Asian people who used heroin a percentage did inject. Evidently there was a danger that because they did not use the services offered by Bridge and other agencies, they shared needles thus were at risk of contracting HIV. This was compounded by a lack of culturally sensitive information on the dangers of drug use.

The majority of the problems associated and experienced by Asian drug users were similar to those of white people—though there were some cultural and race issues which compounded the problems. What was certain through the research was that drug use did cause problems for some Asian drug users and their families. However, people did not use services on offer because:

---

1 They did not know of the existence of the Bridge Project.
2 Those that did know of the existence of the Project did not use it as they assumed it to be a white-run agency for white drug users. This assumption was based on their dealings with other health and welfare services. The Bridge Project had done nothing to dispel this.

A large number of users expressed a preference

to talk to an Asian counsellor as they felt that they would be understood better because of an approved cultural understanding. Conversely, some Asian users wanted to speak only to a white counsellor as they were afraid that the issues of confidentiality would be difficult to maintain in a close-knit Asian community like Bradford.

The Project found that many Asian users only visited their GP for help as they felt more confident of receiving some form of practical help, that is, medicine and advice. At the same time they were unsure about what the Bridge Project could give them. It was found that posters and leaflets in other languages on their own were not effective and they did not necessarily attract people to a service.

The general perception of services was that they were for white people and were run by white people—the issues of racism and discrimination were the expected factors. Therefore, the popular use of a service by Asian people would not necessarily mean that they were satisfied with that service but only that they used it out of necessity and desperation. Asian people told us that agencies did very little to make their services inviting to them, both in terms of physical appearance and service provision.

THE WAY FORWARD

Recently, especially with the onset of HIV/AIDS, agencies have developed an awareness that they have to consult with people, plan, review, think through, adapt and change policies and practices to attract and accommodate new client groups. we have to use the same methods to attract and work with the black communities.

In order to gain credibility and trust and to attract black people to a service, it is evident that you need, wherever possible, to employ black workers. However, they should not necessarily be employed only to work with black clients but should be employed as generic workers who possess specialist skills and not be merely tokenistic staff who are regarded as 'experts'. It is important to remember that just because someone is black it does not make them an expert on issues of race

and racism. It is unrealistic and damaging to assume that one black worker could research, develop and provide more relevant services on his or her own. Such an expectation is all too apparent in many agencies, and merely reflects tokenistic attitudes to anti-racist service delivery or employment practice.

The make-up of a staff team should reflect the cultural diversity of the local population, and it is vital to recognize the importance of training all workers in the organization to work with their black clients. This should be an ongoing process rather than a series of one-off 'race awareness' courses.

In order to develop services to the black community it is important to consult and liaise with them constantly. It is therefore necessary to employ appropriate outreach workers to undertake these tasks. If black workers are appointed in these posts (and surely they should be) it is important to provide appropriate formal support and supervision by black managers. This must be backed up by the employment of black staff to undertake the work once clients are attracted.

It is clearly important to employ black staff at all levels of the organization as well as to seek adequate representation on management committees. It is equally important that black people are involved at a policy-making level to ensure that policies are racially and culturally sensitive and that black people do have the opportunity to effect change at management level.

Coupled with the employment of black staff, the organization will need to ensure that its environment, that is, its office, is culturally sensitive and receptive and meets the expectations of black clients. It needs to 'advertise' its services to the black community via various media. However, the translation of existing information which is not culturally sensitive can be harmful. Even appropriate literature is not the answer if there are not appropriate staff available to undertake work with the client. Provision, where necessary, should be made for workers/services to hold counselling, advice and information days at local medical centres, GP surgeries and local black community centres, etc.

In terms of those black users who inject, it is important that agencies concerned with raising awareness and education on HIV/AIDS and related issues, those involved in health promotion and safer injecting practices, and those operating needle exchange schemes, make services known and accessible to Asian users.

A drugs agency by itself cannot be effective in offering a service to a black drug user. The response must be a district-wide service. An agency cannot, in isolation, provide or develop an anti-racist service. It needs the help, co-operation and commitment of all other statutory and voluntary drug and alcohol services. This work should be co-ordinated through the local district drugs advisory committee (DDAC) and it should adopt a clear anti-racist strategy.

All these agencies must adopt an individually tailored 'working' equal opportunities policy (EOP) in consultation with staff and where possible various client groups and combine these policies with the development of anti-racist strategies. The participation of the entire workforce in any such development and implementation is vital. Failure to develop an appropriate Equal Opportunities Policy that can be 'owned' and implemented by the entire workforce will lead to piecemeal implementation, tokenism and ultimately failure.

SUMMARY

If agencies, Government bodies and all those involved with working with people do not accept that major changes have to be made, then we cannot move further and black clients will continue to receive second rate and poor services which continue to pathologize drug use by black people.

We recognize that some of the examples of service development and provision outlined above are unique to Bradford, drug services and the Bridge Project. However, it is naïve and complacent to believe that some of the broader issues are not mirrored by agencies and services nationwide.

FURTHER READING

Ahmed, B. (1990) *Black Perspectives in Social Work*. Venture Press/R.E.U. National Institute of Social Work.

Allen & Masey (1988) *Race and Social Policy*.

Awiah, J. *et al.* (1992) *Race, Gender and Drug Services*, ISDD.

Fernando, S. (1988) *Race and Culture in Psychiatry*. London: Croom Helm.

Littlewood, R. & Lipsedge, M. (1982) *Aliens and Alienists*. Harmondsworth: Penguin.

Mercer, K. (1986) Racism and transcultural psychiatry. In Miller & Rose (Eds) *The Power of Psychiatry*. Polity Press.

Rodgers, A. & Pilgrim, D. Mental Health and Citizenship. *Critical Social Policy*, **26**, 44–55.

Webb-Johnson, A. (1991) *A Cry for Change: An Asian Perspective on Developing Quality Mental Health Act*. Confederation of Indian Organizations (UK).

We would like to make special reference to the Antiracist Social Work Education Training Manual published by the Northern Curriculum Development Project, *Improving Mental Health Practice*, 1993, and to thank them for the inspiration and support (CCETSW, 1993).

REFERENCES

Barnes, Bowes & Fisher (1990) *Approved Social Worker Assessments, Race and Racism: Local Authority Policy and Practice*. Social Services Research Group.

Brent Community Health Council (1981) *Black People and the Health Service*. London: CHC.

Brown & Harris (1978) *Social Origins of Depression: a Study of Psychiatric Disorder in Women*. Tavistock.

Browne (1988) *Care in the Multi-racial Community*. Policy Studies Institute.

Burke (1988) Psychic function and mental illness: the ethnic minority population. In Allen & Macey (Eds) *Race and Social Policy*. ESRC.

Connelly (1989) *Care in the Multi-racial Community*. Policy Studies Institute.

Fernando (1988) *Race and Culture in Psychiatry*. London: Croom Helm.

Francis *et al*. (1989) Black people and psychiatry in the UK: an alternative to institutional care. *Psychiatric Bulletin*, **13**, 482–485.

Harrison *et al.* (1988) A Prospective study of severe mental disorder in Afro-Caribbean patients. *Psychological Medicine*, **18**, 643–657.

Ingleby (1981) *Critical Psychiatry: The Politics of Mental Health*. Penguin.

London Association of Community Relation Councils (1985) *In a Critical Condition: A Survey of Equal Opportunities in Employment in London's Health Authorities* London: LACRC.

Miller & Rose (1986) *The Power of Psychiatry*. Polity Press.

Rogers & Pilgrim (1989) Mental health and citizenship. *Critical Social Policy*, **26**, 44–54.

Rooney (1987) *Racism and Resistance to Change.* Merseyside Area Profile Group, Dept of Sociology, University of Liverpool.

Rushdie, S. (1983) quoted in Klug, & Gordon, (Eds) *Different Worlds: Racism and Discrimination in Britain*. London: Runnymede Trust & The London Borough of Lewisham.

Sashidharan (1989) *Schizophrenic—or Just Black?* Community Care.

Sedgewick (1982) *Psychopolitics*. Pluto Press.

Shah (1990) A study of approved social workers assessments under the 1983 Mental Health Act. Unpublished paper.

24

DEVELOPING A SUPPORTIVE SERVICE

A CASE EXAMPLE

Christine A. Kirk

AIMS

i) To decide how one health district is implementing the plans to provide an effective service for elderly mentally ill people and their carers

ii) To highlight pitfalls, lessons learned and successes

KEY ISSUES

Legislation
Values and policies
Style of service
Devising a strategy
Community mental health team for the elderly
Assessment services
Treatment and rehabilitation
Continuing care
Staffing innovations and community units for the elderly
Training issues
Evaluation

Identify, analyse and assess factors causing distress and illness	Promote health, provide direct care and make interventions	Manage care programmes and services
Be critical, analytical and accountable, continue professional development	Counter discrimination, inequality and individual and institutional racism	Work within and develop policies, laws and safeguards in all settings
Understand influences on mental health and the nature/causes of disorder and illness	Know the effects of distress, disorder, illness on individuals, groups, families	Understand the basis of treatments and interventions

INTRODUCTION

Even before the Griffiths report in 1988, which was generally welcomed by those working with elderly mentally ill people and their carers, there was recognition that good practice required the provision of comprehensive, flexible, caring, reliable, locally-based services for this client group, to enable people to live independently for as long as they were able in the community. The Joint Report of the Royal College of Physicians and the Royal College of Psychiatrists (1989) summarized the components necessary for comprehensive psychiatric services for elderly people developing the guidelines of the important Health Advisory Service document, *The Rising Tide* (1982).

The White Paper *Caring for People* (1989) and the National Health Service and Community Care Act (1990) set the Government's policy framework for community care in the next decade and beyond for implementation by April 1993. The key objectives are:

To promote the development of domiciliary, day and respite services to enable people to live in their own homes wherever feasible and sensible.

To ensure that service providers make practical support for carers a high priority.

To make proper assessment of need and good care management the cornerstone of high quality care.

To promote the development of a flourishing independent sector alongside good quality public services.

To clarify the responsibilities of agencies and so make it easier to hold them to account for their performance.

To secure better value for taxpayers' money by introducing a new funding structure for social care.

The policy guidance sets out *what* is expected to meet the proposals on community care but *how* it is done is left for innovation and flexibility at local level.

The Care Programme Approach (Department of Health, 1990) formalizes previous good practice with people with mental health problems in emphasizing the need for an identified care manager (agreed between health and social services) to work with clients and their carers to plan, review and follow-up a care programme.

In addition to the pressures from central Government to provide a co-ordinated, comprehensive, integrated service for elderly mentally ill people and their carers, the increasing consumer voice of users of the service and voluntary organizations representing older people and their carers raises expectations of high standards of care and consumer choice. These are increasingly difficult to provide in a climate of cost-conscious competition and at a time of reorganization of both health and local authority services.

In this chapter I will describe how one health district is implementing its plans to provide a good local service for elderly mentally ill people and their carers in collaboration with other agencies and will highlight some of the pitfalls, lessons learned and the successes attained.

VALUES AND POLICY

The health authority adopted a statement of shared values via the planning partnership group for mental health (health, social services, voluntary sector, housing):

Mental health partnership group
Statement of shared values

The partnership group for mental health recognizes the importance of sharing common values when planning mental health services between agencies. To foster collaboration and commitment, the agencies represented on the partnership group have agreed this statement of shared values, including the principles on which future plans and policies can be measured against.

Aim

To provide a local accessible and

comprehensive mental health service, which is user centred and designed to promote the most acceptable quality of life geared to the individual's rights and needs.

Principles
Mental health services will be based on the following principles:

1   Services should be clearly defined in terms of rights. They should be local, accessible and non-stigmatizing.

2   Services should be supportive without encouraging unnecessary dependence. Information should be readily available and clearly presented so that meaningful choices can be made about the range of services available.

3   Services should be integrated to make the best use of existing resources, provide continuity and be sufficiently flexible to respond to changing need.

4   Services should cater for the needs and interests of families and carers.

5   Services must make clear statements to the community about priority and maintain effective services through regular reviews.

6   Services must take account of the ethnic, religious and cultural needs of service users.

7   Services should be participative by developing the involvement of service users.

The workers within the mental health service for elderly people work with all local statutory and voluntary agencies to plan the care with and for an individual and their carer. They involve the patient, the carers, and significant others in producing the individual management plan, taking into account confidentiality issues.

STYLE OF SERVICE

Our health district serves approximately 40,000 elderly people who are resident in the four sectors of the mental health service. Providing a *sector-*

ized community service means that the specialist mental health workers can get to know and be known by the local community workers, be more easily accessible, be more sensitive to the needs of the community and have earlier contact with patients than if all were hospital based. Our system is similar to the hive system of psychiatric care described by Tyrer (1985), with the central hospital as a parallel to a honey bee hive and the workers coming to and from the hospital to secondary 'units' close to the area of greater psychiatric morbidity. Psychiatric workers spend much of their time in the community, but like the bee have regular contact with the base hospital (hive), discussing the identified need and deploying resources within the community and statutory services' system to meet that need (Fig. 24.1).

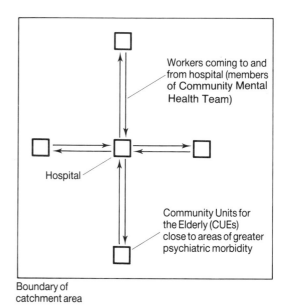

Fig. 24.1 *The hive system of psychiatric care.*

DEVISING A STRATEGY

It is difficult to be sure of the exact prevalence of the commonest psychiatric disorders in elderly people (chronic organic brain syndromes—the dementias, affective disorders and paranoid disorders) because of difficulties in precise case identification, dependent on which instruments are used and whether appropriate cut off scores are used (when does a case become 'a case'?) However, it is known that the prevalence increases with age and with an ageing (particularly very old) population, there will be more pressure undoubtedly on the statutory and voluntary services for this client group.

Very few places have the advantage of co-terminosity between health and local authority boundaries, which increases the complexity for most planners in determining the expected need for specialist services. It is important, nevertheless, for some assessment to be made of the population need, by putting together expected changes in demography with the estimated prevalence of the commonest disorders. Our health district checked out prevalence of dementia (as identified by a validated instrument—the Clifton Assessment Procedures for the Elderly (CAPE)) in a local general practice sample of elderly people (Pattie and Moxon, 1987) and we were relieved to discover that there was no more dementia than elsewhere. The rule of thumb which I use in thinking of our likely local need is that for the population over 65 years, 5% are likely to have a significant degree of dementia (with an increase with increasing age of the population, for example for the over 80s about 20% will have dementia); and up to 20% depression. However, those with depression may not be so easily identified unless sought out, compared with those with dementia. In work with colleagues in social services, it must be remembered that in 'special' places such as residential homes (compared with people in their own homes) there is likely to be a very much higher prevalence of psychiatric disorders (the client's mental state having determined the need for care in the residential home in the first place).

As well as knowing approximately how much psychiatric morbidity there is in the area, it is important to know who else is doing what in terms of dealing with this client group. No agency has resources to waste by duplicating what someone else is providing, and from the client's perspective a single access point to provide for a specific need is required. For example, in our area, social services have little specialist residential or day care for the elderly mentally infirm, but they have developed an intensive domiciliary care scheme working alongside the community mental health team for the elderly. The private sector similarly, has not developed specialist residential or nursing home care for this client group and so it has fallen upon the health services to fill this particular gap which historically, in our area, has been filled by the provision of continuing care beds in mental hospitals.

Our hypothesis was that if we could be involved with patients and their carers early in the course of their illness, we would be able to provide a good, comprehensive, integrated, supportive community-based service with fewer long-stay beds and still be able to cope with the demographic changes, with the increasing elderly (especially very elderly), population and the expected increased prevalence of psychiatric morbidity.

COMMUNITY MENTAL HEALTH TEAM FOR THE ELDERLY

Setting up a community mental health team for the elderly demands a great deal of time, effort and thought, with commitment to this style of working obtained from the multidisciplinary team of workers, their professional line managers and the general manager of the mental health services. Issues relating to this and the continuing running of psychogeriatric teams are described in Lindesay (1991). The success of our team has been helped by the use of several 'time-out' sessions where, with an outside facilitator, we have clarified our operational policy, aims and objectives, and worked out roles and functions, both as individuals and as team managers. Having clear objectives and priorities for work has meant we can evaluate more easily what we are doing and tell other people who need to know (e.g. managers, other community workers) more readily, what we are about. It is important for other workers with this client group to know how to gain access to our specialist skills, what they can and cannot expect from us and to spread the word of what is available via us to their clients and colleagues. If other workers do not know of our existence then our aim of early involvement with patients and their carers cannot be achieved; if they do not know the limits of our capabilities then their expectations will be unrealistically raised, clients will be disappointed and our team will be swamped with inappropriate referrals with the resulting demoralization of all concerned.

The core community mental health team (for 20,000 elderly people) consists of a secretary, four community psychiatric nurses, a social worker, a clinical psychologist, a consultant psychiatrist and junior doctor, an occupational therapist, part-time physiotherapist, community unit for the elderly managers, and ward managers for the main assessment ward and day hospital. Special home care assistants and their home care manager (employed by social services) are also part of the team, but only come to the team meetings serving their particular geographical area. Team members follow the professional ethics and codes of practice of their own profession.

The weekly clinical team meetings act as an information exchange, an opportunity for report giving (assessment and progress), care plan changing, trouble shooting (seeking advice of team members at times of crisis) and the giving and receiving of support. The secretary notes significant information for the case records and data are collected for an audit of team activity. In addition, relevant (to the geographical area) members of the team meet in different areas on a monthly basis with other community workers (district nurse, social worker, voluntary sector workers, home care manager and special home care assistants) to exchange information about 'shared' clients in that particular area. Business meetings of the community mental health team are held every two months and there is a regular time-out meeting for team development every six months.

Referrals to our team can come from any source to any member, but we always ask the referrer to make sure that the general practitioner is aware of the referral. This gets around any difficulties produced by the reluctance of certain individuals to refer on for specialist psychiatric services, produced by the attitude of the 'non-referring' professional of 'what do you expect at her age?' and 'nothing can be done, so why bother busy people'. We hope that by demon-

strating just what we can do to help, we will 'educate' that person, changing inappropriate, ageist views. The majority of referrals do in fact, come from GPs to the consultant, which is the traditional way of team working, but this ratio of consultant versus other team member referral is changing. Traditionally there is concern, if a person is referred to anyone in the team other than a doctor, that a potentially treatable medical condition will be missed, but statistically it is far more likely that a doctor to doctor referral will miss social or functional disabilities, better assessed by other members of the multidisciplinary team.

Team members use their professional skills to decide whether or not to bring each referral to them to the team meeting. The person to whom the referral is made is responsible for the initial assessment, referring on to other team members for additional assessments if appropriate, and informing the referrer and the client of what is happening. A care co-ordinator is then identified who is responsible for devising, recording and reviewing the care plan. The roles of team members are:

Community psychiatric nurse (CPN)
Assessment of nursing needs, provision and evaluation of care plan
Advice to other professional workers in the community
Support for carers and relatives
Specific specialist treatment, e.g. giving injections, different therapies according to skill and expertise of individual CPN
Referring agent for different assessments and care
Education of others about mental disorders in elderly people

Medical staff
Assessment of physical and psychiatric disorders by history taking, physical and psychiatric examination, and organization of appropriate investigations
Involvement in psychiatric treatments, e.g. medication, ECT, psychotherapy
Treatment and management of physical dis-

orders, involving the appropriate specialists as necessary

Accepting medical responsibility for the patient referred by GP

Occupational therapist

Assessment of daily living skills

Assessment of support systems, accommodation, social activities

Treatments including dressing practice, domestic work, relaxation, provision of appropriate aids and equipment to increase independence

Organization of activity/social groups

Physiotherapist

Assessment of patient's physical condition, e.g. posture, co-ordination, mobility

Specific physiotherapy treatments

Advice on appropriate aids and appliances, e.g. seating, walking aids

Work with families, carers and other disciplines on physical aspects, e.g. mobility, lifting techniques

Group work particularly aimed at physical stimulation

Psychologist

Assessment of cognitive, behavioural and emotional functioning

Specialist psychological treatments, e.g. anxiety management, cognitive therapy, behavioural therapy, hypnosis

Counselling and advice to carers and relatives on behavioural management

Advice and support to other disciplines, using psychological assessments and therapeutic approaches

Secretary

Secretarial work for team

Liaising with relatives, carers and patients and putting them in touch with the right team member at the right time

Liaising with community-based organizations and other medical teams

Co-ordinating clinical information for relevant team members

Organizing trainee placements with different team members

All team members are expected to 'educate' other team members about their specific specialist skills and experience.

ASSESSMENT SERVICES

Central to the provision of any specialist service is the good quality assessment of need. The issue of needs-led assessment within the care management process cannot be dealt with here in detail. However, the specialist mental health assessment for elderly people and their carers and how this has been planned in our service will be described.

A multidisciplinary approach is employed to produce a comprehensive assessment of the physical, psychological and social needs and strengths of the individual. Each professional's individual assessment is integrated with information provided by other members of the extended team, that is patient, family, home carers, district nurses, etc. It is most important to work out a sensible, realistic management plan with the patient and relatives (or other carers), involving all the key players in the community care 'package'. Often the interplay of physical, psychological, social and financial factors is so complex that if everyone is not 'signed up' to what is being attempted and why, then the management plan is doomed to failure.

Information must be provided to the patient and carers about the illness, its possible treatment, its likely course and the facilities and help that can be provided. It is sensible to provide this information in written form if possible, often in pamphlets, so that the individuals can take these away to ponder and discuss with, for example, other members of the family and come back and ask further questions if they do not understand it all, or some aspect of the care is not clear. We know from experience and research work in other areas that if relatives and other carers do not agree with, and cannot be persuaded about, a particular management scheme then it is unlikely to be successful for long. Information from carers about their views of things can be sought at formal case reviews or conferences, informally in the community by team members or at relative support groups. Sensitivity to the needs of carers is paramount in producing a long-lasting, effective supportive plan.

Individual carers (and individual patients) need individual opportunities to voice their opinions. Some people are quite happy meeting with a full multidisciplinary team to discuss their relative (client), whilst others prefer a quiet, informal discussion with one key member of the team, perhaps in the relative security of their own home, where they can display openly their feelings of, for example, grief at the illness of their relative. Helping them to be prepared for the future and what it may hold is a critical function of the team members. The aim is to avert potential crises before they occur. Even if this cannot be totally averted, at least the carer knows where to summon help and the team member knows the situation in considerable detail and can make a timely, appropriate response when the call for help comes.

It seems impossible to think of 'assessment' without thinking of management and treatment and the process of assessment is, of course, ongoing with review and evaluation of the management plan.

Up to a point, it does not matter where assessment takes place, but ideally it starts where the patient is living, whether it be their own home, that of a relative, a residential or a nursing home. If sufficient information is available from the patient and an independent informant, a physical and mental state examination and appropriate investigations have been carried out already and it seems after appropriate multidisciplinary discussion that no further assessment is needed, then a management plan can be devised immediately. However, further assessment may be necessary, for example by other professionals, which may take place in the patient's home, or different aspects may need to be assessed in different settings, for example the day hospital or hospital ward.

Such separate specialist assessments have different indications. For example, a patient with a chronic organic brain syndrome (dementia), with a fluctuating course, who lives at home with little support, can be assessed in the day hospital. The advantages of this are that the patient (who is already confused) is not uprooted totally, attendance for two or three days a week gives the multidisciplinary team a chance to see different aspects of the same patient in different settings—at home and in a communal environment—and over a period of time. It then becomes possible to tease out which behaviours occur in which places and to look at possible influence of other people on the patient and his/her behaviour and illness.

After attendance for a reasonable period of time, for example, two days a week for three weeks, a review meeting is held with all concerned and a plan of action drawn up. Specific professionals of the community mental health team will be involved in this assessment process alongside day hospital staff, carers (formal and informal) and the patients themselves. Treatment and rehabilitation are provided as appropriate for patients with both organic brain syndromes and with functional illness. Other advantages of day hospital assessment are that it can test out the feasibility of day care as part of the care package; and relatives and the patient experience what it is like having support organized while the patient remains at home and is not removed to the unfamiliar, artificial surroundings of the hospital ward.

However, it may be necessary to arrange inpatient assessment if the situation has broken down at home; if it seems that alternative residential accommodation is needed and assessment is to include what type of accommodation is required, for example residential home or nursing home; if 24-hour assessment is indicated because of problems, for example, during the night. Inpatient facilities vary from place to place but generally are either in a psychiatric hospital or a general hospital. Obviously for elderly people who are likely to have both physical and psychiatric illness co-incidentally, or interacting, it is ideal to have easy access to the investigative facilities and the specialist staff of a general hospital.

Our service has assessment beds for elderly mentally ill people in both the acute psychiatric hospital adjacent to the general hospital site and in a joint geriatric/psychogeriatric assessment ward in the district general hospital. Our facilities shown below seem to be a reasonable model for this type of service:

District general hospital	22 beds—joint geriatric/ psychogeriatric assessment ward
Mental hospital	34 beds—organic illness assessment Beds in sector wards for functional illness assessment

Approximately one bed per 1,000 elderly people for organic assessment

Few places have successful joint geriatric/ psychogeriatric in-patient units. However, geriatric/psychogeriatric liaison works increasingly well throughout the UK using different models of collaborative links, for example joint out-patient clinics and joint whole departments of medicine and psychiatry for elderly people. Our joint ward developed as a response to local general practitioners who felt that this would help fill a gap in the provision of services for elderly people with both psychiatric and physical illness. Factors influencing its success include having a multidisciplinary team dedicated to the ward; having all the beds designated as 'joint' beds and not a certain number of geriatric and separate psychogeriatric which could lead to dispute; and the fact that the two consultants (one physician for the elderly and one psychiatrist for the elderly) involved in the ward get on well together and have a shared philosophy of how it should work.

Some places have opted to have psychiatric wards for elderly people where people with organic and functional illnesses are assessed alongside each other in the same ward. There are advantages in this for people who have mixed (organic and functional) disorders as they are correctly placed for the best specialist skills, as well as for all elderly people, as the staff have developed expertise in and interest in working with older people (compared with services where older people with functional illness are assessed with those of younger age and where frail, elderly depressed people may have to contend with, for example, young difficult-to-manage schizophrenics on the same ward). Staff are geared up to the slower treatment response and rehabilitation of older people, and some elderly functionally ill people in the rehabilitation phase of their in-patient stay seem to benefit from and enjoy helping other more disabled, demented people.

However, some people with functional illness are undoubtedly upset if they are nursed alongside severely demented people, with possibly deteriorated personal habits. So, if older people for assessment are in a common assessment ward there must be physical space and separate activities, as appropriate, for segregating those with dementia from those with functional illness, but with possibilities of integration for joint social activities.

As can be seen above our service has beds for elderly people with functional illness in the wards serving the sector for general psychiatric practice. In a service that is increasingly community orientated, it is helpful for the staff in the assessment ward to get to know the people involved in the community networks so that discharge planning and the care management process can be facilitated.

We have, on several occasions, attempted to find a way of creating a separate elderly functionally ill assessment ward to serve the whole district but have been unsuccessful given the physical constraints of the hospital building and the requirements also of the general psychiatric service.

Why continue to do our assessments in a central hospital facility at all? It certainly is helpful in terms of communication with key staff, access to appropriate investigative facilities and the efficient economic use of highly trained specialist staff. However, we are assessing and treating patients increasingly in their own homes and in community day facilities, especially in the community units for the elderly (CUEs). This means we and the patient are nearer to, or are part of, the informal community network; there is no stigma of being a psychiatric in-patient which many patients and families prefer; and members of the primary care team can continue to be involved.

Different places have evolved different assessment procedures and documentation but, overall, the aim must be to produce a comprehensive assessment of the person's physical, psychological and social strengths and needs. This must be multidisciplinary but not all cases will require involvement of all disciplines. The type of assessment, rehabilitation and treatment work which each discipline within the team carries out is shown above. Devising the documentation to be used and defining operational details of the assessment process forms part of the team building process.

TREATMENT AND REHABILITATION

Treatment and rehabilitation are provided, as appropriate, for patients with both organic brain syndromes and functional illness. Any member of the community mental health team may be drawn in, as appropriate, to fulfil a specific specialist role and will work with the patient (and other formal and informal carers) wherever the patient is. These therapeutic endeavours will be continued as necessary when the patient moves from one setting to another, for example home to hospital and vice versa. Therefore it is very important that there is close liaison and co-ordination between hospital-based and community-based staff, which emphasizes the importance of a care manager being identified to guide the patient through the intricacies of the care system.

Specific therapies are dealt with elsewhere in this book. However, it is important to realize that elderly people with the loss of adaptability that old age brings, often take longer to respond to specific treatments than younger people. Developing an understanding of and expertise in this is yet another reason why specialist elderly care services have evolved to provide a high quality service for this client group.

CONTINUING CARE SERVICES

A decision had been taken to close one of the three mental hospitals in our area, with one remaining as the acute assessment hospital. One option would have been to pour money into the existing continuing care hospital to upgrade facilities and keep the Victorian buildings in a reasonable state of repair. However, the creative decision was made to involve local providers of specialist EMI services in the planning of an innovative model of continuing care. The concept of community units for the elderly (CUEs) gradually emerged, the objectives of which are:

To provide a locally-based unit with a comprehensive range of services

To maintain people in their own homes through flexible use of resources as long as it is appropriate

To be responsive to local needs and actively encourage local people to participate in the unit

To encourage joint participation between health, social services and voluntary agencies

To encourage co-operation between CUE staff, local GPs, primary care teams, community mental health team, hospital services, social services and voluntary agencies

The facilities to be available for use by the local community and others, e.g. DSS, citizens' advice bureau, health education

---

Each CUE services a population of 4,500–5,000 elderly people (with the health district eventually needing eight such units) to replace the continuing care beds which would gradually reduce and eventually cease to exist with the closure of the Victorian mental hospital. Because of the lack of other specialist EMI residential accommodation in the area, it was important to reprovide continuing care beds for people with severe dementia requiring 24-hour specialist psychiatric care but aiming to provide them near to the patient's home (or that of the relatives) instead of in a central hospital, and of a more homely nature. With 14 residential beds in each unit we would eventually have continuing care bed numbers in line with the Health Advisory Service (1982) suggested figures (2.5–3 per 1,000 elderly people). Of the 14 beds usually 10–12 are continuing care, with the remainder being used for flexible respite care—either regular holiday relief or night care, or respite admissions when required to give carers a break or in a social crisis. Obviously, there has to be very careful management of the bed usage—a very precious and expensive resource. Priorities for bed usage must be established and clear, otherwise every elderly person in the vicinity may be signing on to such an attractive, free facility. Only the most disabled, psychiatrically disturbed people with dementia who cannot be coped with in any other settings can be offered a place in the CUEs for residential continuing care.

Community units for the elderly: model

For 4500—5000 elderly people:
    14 residential beds
    20 day places
    Resource centre
    Domiciliary outreach work
    Team members' base

In addition to the beds, there are 20 day places, seven days a week, for assessment and continuing care of people who live in the vicinity. These places and times are used flexibly to build up the appropriate care package for any individual person and their carer. The advantage of having day places available in the same building as a residential facility is that times of the day service do not have to be rigid and if, for example, it suits a particular day visitor to come at mid-day for lunch and stay until after tea, or mid-evening, there is no problem with this. Equally, if carers occasionally wish to leave a day visitor just for an evening, when they go to the theatre or a football match, it can easily be done and the patients are visiting somewhere which is familiar and with people they know. However, it is important to make sure that the design of the building is suitable for day visitors and residents to be separate from each other if they so wish (e.g. day visitors with some functional illness could be very disturbed if they had to remain all the time with a person with severe dementia with deteriorated

personal habits). We have taken care in the design of our buildings to be sure that there are sufficient 'day' rooms available for several different activities to be going on at the same time, and there still be a place where someone can go just to relax and be quiet. The programme for each person is individually tailored and will include aspects of assessment and social and recreational activities, both in the unit and in the local community, with appropriate members of staff and/or volunteers, and other clients of the service.

The design and function of the resource centre varies from CUE to CUE depending on what the local community requires of it. This is the interface between the NHS facility (definitely *not* a hospital) and the community. Voluntary organizations can use the resource centre for whatever they wish; information is available about elderly care services in the widest sense; trained volunteers are available to provide information and if they do not know the answer to the question they can seek help from the staff in the unit who will, we hope, be able to point the person in the right direction. The volunteers in the resource centre can work with day visitors or visit and befriend the residents, and in the first CUE the volunteers run a coffee shop in the resource centre, which attracts a large number of people from the local community, the nearby shops and health centre. Thus, the community is brought to the CUE!

A 'side-effect' of this is the raising of funds for the unit and the 'Friends of . . . CUE' have bought wonderful 'extras' for the CUE, for example, provide weekly fresh flowers for the unit and pay for holiday activities for the residents and day visitors. The resource facilities are used on a regular basis by, for example, the Department of Social Security, to provide information and advice in the locality; to supply hearing aid batteries for elderly people in the area; and for informal social activities for local elderly people. Young people from local schools come into the unit on a regular basis, which not only stimulates the residents and day visitors but also 'educates' the young people about what we are doing, so reducing the stigma of psychiatric illness in old age and possibly the fear of the unknown for the young people.

Elderly people themselves, and their carers,

frequently say that what they really want is help in their own homes to assist them in being as independent as possible. We have attempted to provide some of this care at home by the workers from the CUE going to people's homes to help with necessary tasks, for example, bathing, getting ready to go to the day centre, going to appointments elsewhere. There are advantages in the outreach worker from the CUE assisting the person with these tasks. The number of people a confused person has to deal with is reduced and they will often be more co-operative with someone they know and trust than with a relative stranger coming to the house. However, there rests a great deal of responsibility on the outreach worker working in a person's home and the type of work is different from that in a hospital with its readily available support from other staff members.

The detailed planning of each CUE is done by a task group, consisting of a local general practitioner, a planning and operational services manager from the hospital, a consultant psychiatrist for the elderly, a social services manager, a senior nurse (elderly), a voluntary sector person and/or carer, an administrator, and the CUE manager when he/she is appointed, and as necessary, a housing department representative and the unit management accountant (with whom we worked on bed reduction targets for the base mental hospital). A separate planning group devises, with the architect, the details of the actual building but there must be crossover of individuals and ideas from both groups. We have learned a great deal as we have gone on through the CUE strategy programme and we have always said that each CUE would be different because of different local requirements and that the first CUE, although good, will be the worst, because we will have learned so many lessons as we have developed.

Whilst we were planning the CUEs, various other developments were taking place:

1 Community, general practice random sample, checking out the *prevalence of dementia* in our area.
2 Establishing *interim day facilities* in already existing local venues. We based this on the concept of *travelling day hospitals* where the specialist psychiatric staff travel to local places, for example church halls, and run specialist day care in different localities different days of the week, so that clients do not have to travel far from their homes and go to places familiar to them with no stigma of mental illness attached to them. This is a relatively cheap way of providing local day care and can be of an extremely high quality with high satisfaction for staff, clients and carers alike. However, the ground work needing to be done to set this up is considerable. For example, finding the right place with suitable toilet facilities for caring for elderly people who are disabled; organizing catering; negotiating the lease; developing working relationships with, for example, the mother and toddler group who may use the facility on another day; and with the hosts who, in the case of church buildings, may also be able to facilitate care by organizing volunteers to work with us, is time consuming and requires considerable diplomacy and expertise. The benefits of such a scheme, as a first phase of a CUE service include giving the staff an opportunity to 'try out' working in that particular community, getting established in the existing networks of support, and emphasizing the CUE service and its philosophy rather than just the building which will eventually take its place in the community. Our experience has been that a great deal of enthusiasm for such schemes is generated amongst all concerned and an amazing amount of the highest quality work is able to be done in such limited facilities. Having to pack everything up at the end of the day is a chore, but one which people gladly do.
3 Planning and implementating a *special home care scheme* (initially called the special home helps), intensive domiciliary care, with our local social services department which gave us some experience in what it would be like working in people's homes, the forerunner of the domiciliary outreach work for the CUE. For the pilot

scheme, a self-selected group of home helps was interviewed and four selected to undergo a two-week training programme, working alongside staff involved with elderly people with mental health problems in different parts of the health and social service provision, to understand the range of problems and how they can be dealt with. These special home helps are managed by their usual domiciliary care manager (social services) and work alongside the community mental health team, especially the community psychiatric nurses, in the day-to-day management of clients. They also attend community mental health team meetings on rotation and their contribution at these meetings is highly valued, as they are often the people most intimately in contact with our clients. They value attending the meetings as it provides them with helpful support.

The initial evaluation of this scheme showed it to be effective in supporting people in their own homes and helping to keep them out of institutional care. The amount of time spent with clients was not out of the range of care given previously to existing clients of the home care schemes. However, the special home helps were able to be more flexible in what they did with and for their clients and, within limits, could organize their time with people more flexibly than previously. Their roles include befriending; accompanying clients to appointments; introducing them to luncheon clubs, day centres, etc; taking them to other social activities and staying with them if necessary; helping with personal care and finances; helping with looking after pets and almost anything else a family carer might do. Although it is difficult to prove, it is my impression that it is this sort of scheme that has made community care possible.

4   We held a *seminar with carers* to check out whether what we were planning was in line with what they felt was necessary. Conclusions from this day were that we should go ahead with what we were doing but that we should pay attention to how people access the service (carers felt that the service they got was good once they got into it, but some had experienced difficulty getting to the right place at the right time); we should not forget the needs of younger people with pre-senile dementia; and should make sure that continence help was available. To run such a seminar successfully, one needs to make sure that transport is available for the carer to the seminar, that it is at a time when carers are likely to be able to come, and that if necessary, some form of 'sitting service' is available to care for their 'sufferer' reliably whilst the carer is at the seminar.

Since the CUE service has been developing, we have taken the opportunity to ask carers how they see this working via the CUE evaluation process (see below).

5   We undertook a *community survey* to find out what services were already in the locality the CUE was to serve, to find out how we would fit into the community and to develop local interest. This involved, for example, schools, churches, voluntary groups and general practitioners. The name of the first CUE, Acomb Gables, was the result of a competition run in one of the local schools. Before Acomb Gables opened, we held two open days for anyone who wished to visit and we were very pleasantly surprised to have over 700 visitors, mostly from the local community. This local interest has continued and we feel we have established a place for ourselves in the community. At first, we were almost too successful in 'selling' ourselves in that people's expectations of what we were able to provide were unrealistic and it felt, at one time as if everybody's granny wanted to come and live with us!

6   We were building up *links with the existing voluntary sector*, for example Age Concern and Alzheimer's Disease Society and helping to establish new groups. The voluntary sector, as well as producing pressure on statutory services to close gaps in provision of services, can act in an advocacy role on behalf of a particular client group; can be in touch closely with sufferers and carers to

provide directly or indirectly for their needs; and can work in partnership with the statutory services to produce good, relatively cheap care—better than the statutory or independent sector can provide separately. Through the voluntary sector, relative support groups, a day care and a sitting service have been established which complement the health and social services provision. The local Alzheimer's Disease Society Branch, in which some of the local health and social services staff are involved, also provides an information and small counselling service. At times, it is difficult to know whether a particular community psychiatric nurse, for example, is wearing a CPN or a voluntary-sector hat in their dealings with a particular client and that is not a bad thing, contributing to a 'seamless' service.

7   *Utilizing existing community facilities* has become part of the development of the service, for example pubs, clubs and an afternoon session providing a social facility in a local cricket club. Many carers, particularly of people with dementia, gradually lose their normal social lives and getting together with other carers in a social (not a formal support group) setting is important to them. They also like to continue a previous life style which may have become impossible for them with their 'sufferer' whose personal habits may have deteriorated to an embarrassing point. By going out for a pub lunch on a regular basis with new friends who are in a similar position to themselves and supported by, for example, community psychiatric nurses and special home carers, they have something to look forward to and a means of continuing something which they have previously enjoyed, and which is fun. This also acts, very often, as a starting point for someone with dementia to recommence social outings which may eventually persuade them to accept some form of day care giving the carer some respite, but which inevitably depends on a separation from their carer which previously they may have found difficult. The carer also learns that they can trust the people who will be looking after their loved one, to care for them well and not to cause distress to them.

The cricket club group arose from the need for some form of low-key, informal social 'club' for people in an early stage of dementia who may have lost confidence for joining in local 'normal' social activities, but who had fairly well-preserved social fronts and who would be distressed by day centres specifically for people with severe dementia. Their carers can go along with them and join in the activities or just chat with others there, or can use the few hours of 'freedom' to get on with whatever they wish; or just put their feet up. Some carers find that this acts as an introduction to a relative support group and they suddenly find, unexpectedly, that they benefit from talking with another carer about the problems and solutions of caring for someone with dementia.

These activities, therefore, are part of a spectrum of 'facilities' available for elderly people with mental health problems and their carers, which form part of an individual tailor-made package of support, available for their needs at that time.

8   We were learning about *managing the closure of the continuing care mental hospital*. Issues there included keeping people informed of what was happening and when and whether we were on target; identifying with staff what the future held for them; organizing training programmes for the transition from hospital to community work; managing the reduction of beds in the hospital to coincide with the opening of the new CUE beds; keeping relatives up-to-date with what the future held for their loved ones; making sure that the financial resources were transferred from one budget to another as planned; keeping up morale in the closing hospital; and making sure that the more distant managers who were involved in the eventual sale of the hospital site were aware that the priority for the site at that time was good-quality patient care.

Staffing innovations relating to the CUEs

Even before the advent of health care assistants, we had decided to create *generic support workers* to assist the multidisciplinary staff in the CUEs. The idea was to make it less confusing for an (already) confused person by reducing the number of people relating to them in assisting them with their every-day care. Each person would have a key worker (one of the professionally trained staff) and a few support workers who would work with them wherever they were—in their own homes, in the day centre, or in the residential part of the unit. The tasks of these workers included physiotherapy and occupational therapy aide, nursing assistant, cleaning, housekeeper and catering duties and they were recruited from existing staff in the hospital service, for example porters, nursing assistants and domestic services staff.

Adjustment to working in a different way and different setting was aided by the training programme arranged, and as time has gone on and with new cohorts of support workers as the CUE strategy progresses, the training has evolved. Nevertheless the transition is stressful, undoubtedly, and considerable support is necessary. Details of the support worker role, training and conclusions about the concept are included in the Acomb Gables evaluation (Pattie and Moxon, 1991).

Developing from the idea of people living in their own local community despite needing long-term continuing psychiatric care as a result of their, for example, dementia, came the notion of asking the *general practitioners* if they would continue to look after their patients when they were involved with the CUE service. To implement this required considerable discussion with and 'education' of the GPs often on an individual basis, about the CUE concept and philosophy and was in line with their 'cradle to the grave' care. Obviously, some GPs were more enthusiastic about this than others, but the majority have remained involved with their patients, providing useful information to the staff of the CUE about the patient and her/his relatives from the GP knowing them for many years, giving a good 'normal' general practice to people in the care of the unit, and allowing the GPs to 'use' the unit staff as a resource when they visit, which they can utilize with others amongst their patients who may not be in contact with the CUE. In the evaluation of the first CUE (Pattie and Moxon, 1991), most of the responding general practitioners were pleased with the retention of general practice responsibility and the staff of the unit felt reasonably supported by the local GPs.

Training issues relating to the CUEs

Some of the training issues identified by the evaluation of the first CUE are:

1   Blocks of training are better than day release.

2   There needs to be ongoing training once the service is established—both formally and informally by knowledge-sharing amongst individual staff.

3   Shared events for qualified and support staff help team building but cannot meet their differing needs which require separate opportunities.

4   Clarification of roles, the extent of sharing tasks and role blurring need to be understood clearly to avoid unrealistic expectations of each other.

5   Specific training needs for transition from hospital (institutional) to community work must be addressed.

6   An understanding of the organization and procedures of other services for the elderly in the area facilitates integration into the local community and services.

7   Transition from temporary premises for day care to the permanent CUE building is stressful for staff. Preparation for, support and recognition of their change of status is required.

8   Specific individual staff have specific training and development needs in providing a flexible, local service, e.g. dealing with bereavement; dealing with unexpected events

in a self-supporting unit; career development specific to a new style of service.

9 The need for training and support should not be underestimated.

Evaluation of the CUE

An evaluation of the first CUE, Acomb Gables, was completed by Pattie and Moxon (1991) and a summary of the report is also available. Topics covered in this are:

1 Dependency/disability of elderly people in the care of mental health and other services

2 Change in dependency, location and type of care over a six-month period of study

3 Elderly people transferred from hospital care to Acomb Gables residential care and the perceptions of relatives and staff in relation to this move

4 Use of residential places, length of stay, mortality

5 The 'before and after' and transitional aspects of the old and new style services

6 Client and carer perceptions

7 Staff perceptions, training, expectations and morale

8 Management issues, in relation to planning, setting up and running the service

9 Impact on and contribution from a variety of professionals and services

10 Architectural and use of the building issues

11 Aspects of quality: the environment, care, atmosphere and subjective views

12 The resource centre

13 Volunteer input

A variety of qualitative and quantitative methods were used; dependency measures, interviews, questionnaires, rating scales and routine data collection involving staff, patients, carers and other service providers in the area.

An ongoing evaluative study monitors the progress of the CUE strategy now that four purpose-built CUEs are in existence and others being planned.

The full details of the first evaluation cannot be included here but in summary:

1 The level of care reflected the dependency and was appropriate to the needs of the individual.

2 Very few very highly dependent people were able to remain in their own homes but some could if they had full-time carers and supportive services.

3 The service was enjoyed and appreciated by elderly people and their carers.

4 The generic support worker role seemed successful and the staff enjoyed working in the service.

5 There needed to be an adjustment in attitude and way of working for all staff in the transition to the new service.

6 The building and location were successful in use and function and the assessment of quality of service was very satisfactory.

7 It was difficult to get adequate data re the comparative costs but the service seemed no more expensive than the traditional service and waiting lists were no longer.

8 The strategy should continue.

An illustrative case of the work of a CUE

Mrs A was a 75-year-old married woman, living with her husband, near to our CUE when she was first referred to the service by her GP as she had become unmanageable for her husband at home since they had come back from a recent holiday visiting a member of the family in the south. Their daughter and son who lived locally were very concerned for both of them and were demanding of the GP that 'something must be done'.

The consultant psychiatrist for the elderly saw Mr and Mrs A at home and she and the GP confirmed by physical examination and routine blood and urine investigations that Mrs A was physically well apart from a urinary tract infection. However, detailed history taking revealed that she had become increasingly forgetful over the past two years and had been able to do less and less at home to deal with her personal hygiene and the day-to-day domestic tasks. Her husband had willingly and increasingly taken those on but found it difficult to cope with her increasing confusion, constant packing and unpacking of clothes into a suitcase and a wardrobe since they had returned home, and her deteriorating standards of personal hygiene and recent occasional urinary incontinence.

Her urinary tract infection was treated with appropriate antibiotics which solved the urinary incontinence problem and although he accepted the idea of day visitor assessment and respite at the CUE, she did not! She clung to him and was verbally aggressive to anyone suggesting she should go anywhere. The family were greatly relieved that a staff member from the CUE would visit the house on a regular basis to assist Mr A with his wife's care, to support him, and gradually get him used to the idea of her dementia and what it meant. Eventually, she agreed to come to the CUE to some social activities with the support worker whom she had got to know in her home. At a later date she came as a regular day visitor and subsequently for respite residential care on a flexible basis when her husband wanted this and was able to persuade her to accept it. By this stage, she was requiring a great deal of assistance with personal care but was reluctant to accept it, was wandering aimlessly unless busy and supervised all the time, was irritable and could become aggressive if she were thwarted or anyone tried to persuade her to do something she did not wish to do.

Her family, for their own reasons, were unable to provide any further practical support but continued to be very concerned about their father's wellbeing. He found it very difficult to come to terms with his grief about her illness and loss of their previously happy relationship but derived some support from meeting with other carers at the carers' group at the CUE. He certainly enjoyed the social opportunities for activities at the CUE which he took part in with his wife and with other people in similar situations.

Eventually he accepted that he could not manage with Mrs A at home much longer, and we, at a meeting with all the family, decided that no facility in the area other than the CUE would be able to cope with Mrs A with her present behaviour. Her name was placed on the waiting list for a continuing care bed and after a short time when it became apparent that Mr A needed the bed to be available quickly, with a bit of juggling, that bed was found. He was helped with dealing with his powerful emotions at that time by the staff of the CUE whom he had got to know well and trust.

A few months later, we were all saddened when Mr A was discovered to have cancer, deteriorated physically very rapidly and died. The family were not sure how to approach Mrs A during his illness and death and asked the staff at the CUE (her new family) to take decisions about whether and how she should be involved in the process of his final illness. Although she was severely demented and appeared to have little language function remaining by this time, she seemed to understand that something important and sad was happening and was helped by the staff in her grief. To the surprise of her family, she coped with going to the funeral and behaved appropriately there and afterwards.

We all felt that it would have been hard to have given her, her husband, and her family the same quality of support without the existence of the CUE service.

CONCLUSIONS

There are still many issues we are learning about and challenges for training, some of which are dealt with in other chapters. We have not solved all the legal and ethical dilemmas relating to the care of elderly mentally ill people and we continue to debate how to get the right balance relating to elderly people's rights, responsibilities, restraint and the taking of risks. We continue to work with families and other carers but would like to do more. We are well aware of the wider issues relating to elder abuse including financial, physical and psychological abuse, and use and abuse of medications in this very vulnerable group of people. All of these issues have implications for the type of training which is evolving and which increasingly should be on a multidisciplinary, multiagency basis.

We are attempting to meet the key objectives of *Community Care in the Next Decade and Beyond*, but it is an extremely complex task and will only be possible with this client group if the different agencies, various professionals and carers work together.

FURTHER READING

Murphy, E. (1986) *Dementia and Mental Illness in the Old: A Practical Guide: Understanding the Problems—How to Manage—Surviving Yourself*. London: Papermac.

Murphy, E. (1991) *After the Asylums. Community Care for People with Mental Illness*. London: Faber & Faber.

Wattis, J. & Church, M. (1986) *Practical Psychiatry of Old Age*. London: Croom Helm.

REFERENCES

Audit Commission (1986) *Making a Reality of Community Care*. A Report by the Audit Commission for England and Wales.

Department of Health (1989) *Caring for People*. London: HMSO.

Department of Health (1990) *The Care Programme Approach*. London: HMSO.

Griffiths, R. (1988) *Community Care: Agenda for Action*. London: HMSO.

Health Advisory Service (1982) *The Rising Tide. Developing Services for Mental Illness in Old Age*. Sutton: NHS Health Advisory Service.

Joint Report of the Royal College of Physicians and the Royal College of Psychiatrists. The Royal College of Physicians of London and The Royal College of Psychiatrists (1989) *Care of Elderly People with Mental Illness*.

Lindesay, J. (1991) Working Out. *Setting Up and Running Community Psychogeriatric Teams*. London: Research and Development for Psychiatry.

Pattie, A.H. & Moxon, S. (1987) *Prevalence of Dementia in York Health District*. A report for Yorkshire Regional Health Authority.

Pattie, A.H. & Moxon, S. (1991) *Community Units for the Elderly in York Health District. An Evaluation of the First CUE: Acomb Gables*. York Health Authority.

Tyrer, P. (1985) The hive system. A model for a psychiatric service. *British Journal of Psychiatry*, **146**, 571.

CHAPTER
25

CARE PROVISION

F.C. Johnson and L.D. Smith

AIMS

i)   To examine the historical perspective of provision for the mentally ill
ii) To itemize the growth of care provision during the last 200 years
iii) To examine the decline of institutions
iv) To discuss the principle of care provision, past, present and future
v)   To examine factors in the environment that affect the human response

KEY ISSUES

Institution
Institutionalization
Dehumanizing factors
Psychiatric units
Environmental factors
Colour and light

Identify, analyse and assess factors causing distress and illness	Promote health, provide direct care and make interventions	Manage care programmes and services
Be critical, analytical and accountable, continue professional development	Counter discrimination, inequality and individual and institutional racism	Work within and develop policies, laws and safeguards in all settings
Understand influences on mental health and the nature/causes of disorder and illness	Know the effects of distress, disorder, illness on individuals, groups, families	Understand the basis of treatments and interventions

A prayer for workhouses and asylums:

'Pour thy blessing, O Lord, upon all institutions designed for the care of the destitute, the lunatic, and the aged. Be thyself the portion of those from who thou has withdrawn the comforts and enjoyments of the world: reconcile them to their position that they may be content therein to abide thy gracious pleasure, and to learn such submission to thy holy will as shall enable them hereafter to rejoice in thy glory'.
Sursum Corda, 1898

INTRODUCTION

Any study of the environment provided for the mentally ill must inevitably draw its comparison with the historical picture presented to the public by the media. If you have seen the film 'Amadeus', which dramatizes the story of Wolfgang Amadeus Mozart (1756–1791) and his conflict with Antonio Salieri, a fellow composer, you will have noticed the opening and closing sequences depicting life in the madhouse at Vienna in the early nineteenth century. Presented to the viewer are all the features of containment and control that is possible for the imagination to conceive. Chains, cages, and restraint boxes abound with keepers wielding whips and clubs to keep the madhouse in order. Although designed to shock, how near to the truth is the picture displayed?

THE HISTORICAL CONTEXT

In England little attention was paid to the standard of provision for the mentally ill prior to 1774. At that date 'lunatics' were to be found in prisons, workhouses, private madhouses and a few public hospitals such as Bethlem (1377). Numbers are not known but it is estimated that no more than two to three thousand were contained within the private madhouses that had sprung up during the eighteenth century (Brockington, 1966).

The Act for Regulating Private Madhouses (1774) presents as the first milestone in improving facilities by a system of inspection. Commissioners were appointed for the London area and for the rest of the country this was done by the Justices of the Peace. The limited terms of reference applied only to madhouses and excluded private hospitals and paupers in workhouses and other institutions and for this reason it is doubtful if the Act had any effect on the raising of standards, apart from the occasional prosecution of a madhouse keeper if conditions were found to be exceptionally undesirable.

By the beginning of the nineteenth century, the conditions available to lunatics contained within workhouses could no longer be tolerated and an alternative was sought. Certain institutions such as The Retreat at York and St Luke's in London had demonstrated a way forward and the County Asylums Act (1808) required Justices of the Peace in every county in England to provide proper accommodation for the reception of such lunatics as were chargeable on the parish rates. Thus began the County asylum building programme and some such as Chester (1816) and Lancaster (1828) still exist today although in a greatly changed form.

But what of conditions in these institutions? Brockington quotes from the report of a visit to Bethlem Hospital in 1814:

'One of the siderooms contained about 10 patients each chained by one leg to the wall; the chain allowing them to stand up by the bench or form fixed to the wall or to sit down on it. The nakedness of each patient was covered by a blanket gown only'.
Brockington, 1966

---

or again of a visit to the York Asylum in 1814:

'Having suspicions in my mind that there were some parts of that Asylum which had not been seen I went early in the morning determined to examine every place. After ordering a great

many doors to be opened, I came to one which was in a retired situation in the kitchen apartments, and which was almost hid by the opening of a door in the passage. I ordered this door to be opened; the keepers hesitated and said that the apartment belonged to the women and they had not the key. I ordered them to get the key; but it was said to be mislaid and not to be found at the moment. Upon this, I grew angry and told them I insisted upon its being found and that if they would not find it I could find a key at the kitchen fireside, namely the poker; upon that the key was immediately brought. When the door was opened I went into the passage and found four cells I think of about 8 ft square in a very horrid and filthy situation; the straw appeared to be almost saturated with urine and excrement; there was some bedding laid upon the straw in one cell, in the others only loose straw. A man (a keeper) was in the passage doing something, but what I do not know. The walls were daubed with excrement; the air holes of which there was one in each cell, were partly filled with it. In one cell there were two pewter chamber pots, loose. I asked the keeper if these cells were inhabited by the patients and was told that they were at night. I then desired him to take me upstairs and show me the place of the women who came out of those cells that morning; I then went upstairs, and he showed me into a room which I caused him to measure and the size of which he told me was 12 ft by 7 ft 10 ins: and in which there were 13 women who he told me had all come out of those cells that morning'.
Brockington, 1966

or again of a visit to a private madhouse in Bethnel Green in 1815:

'Some pauper men were chained upon straw beds with only a rug over them and not in any way defended from the external world'.
Brockington, 1966

It is a grim picture and you may consider that the film 'Amadeus' has a firm grounding in the truth. However, the signs of change were evident, namely the work of Pinel at the Bicetre Hospital in Paris and William Tuke at The Retreat in York. You may also wish to examine the work of Drs Charlesworth and Gardiner Hill at the Lincoln Asylum and Dr John Conolly at the Hanwell Asylum. Legislation continued by way of a number of Government Acts to establish a spate of institution building and inspection measures and note must be taken of the leading role played by Lord Ashley (later the Earl of Shaftsbury) during his long public life from 1828 to his death in 1884.

THE SOCIAL CONTEXT

We would suggest that whilst the considerable effort that went into creating a national network of asylums has received a great deal of adverse publicity in recent years by such writers as Goffman (1961), any such development must be placed with the social context and social conditions of the day. The creation of asylums within each county in England was paved with good intent and it must be stated that considerable effort and money went into establishing self-contained institutions to a standard that were in line with the views held by Victorian society.

Jones (1991) makes this point when discussing the development of asylums from 1808 to 1890. Constructed at a time when building land was cheap and labour costs cheaper they were placed in country areas outside towns and away from endemic and epidemic disease due to the need for sanitary reform. Note must also be taken of the standard of living available to the general public at the middle of the nineteenth century. In his important treatise Chadwick (1842) had brought to the attention of Government the appalling state of poverty and degradation in which the working classes lived and as Jones states:

'The great Report on the Sanitary Condition of the Labouring Classes (Chadwick, 1842) with its accounts of damp and disease ridden hovels without light or sanitation, the piles of refuse, the filthy and stinking gutters, the people 'worse off than wild animals' suggests that those who were admitted to the asylums were relatively fortunate. Asylums provided better care than prisons or workhouses: patients were fed and clothed, housed in dry wards, looked after, and given medical treatment and this was more than many of them could hope for outside. The asylums were not democratic institutions; they were paternalistic and class-conscious, but so was Victorian society'.

'Where else can one find those long drives, imposing facades, mosaic floored entrance halls and endless echoing corridors. These were stately homes for the lower classes'.
Jones, 1991

The number of asylums, later to be called mental hospitals, continued to increase up to the early twentieth century. So of course did the numbers contained as efforts were made to transfer patients from workhouses and prisons. Although total figures are difficult to establish, the figures below compiled from various sources may indicate the rapid growth:

In-patient population

1844	20,611
1859	35,922
1876	64,916
1900	74,000
1930	140,000
1959	155,700

However, we must not be led into thinking that the number of hospitals continued to increase, although extra buildings were constructed on the hospital sites, for example, the villa units provided for the more easily 'maintained' long stay population after the 1939–1945 war. Rather the problem of population increase was compounded by simply cramming more beds into the available space with little thought being given to the long-term effect. Beds in dormitories contained little or no room between, beds appeared in the corridors, and beds invaded the dayrooms. Wards constructed to contain 30 or 40 patients often contained double that number and wards were re-designed to reduce day space and increase the dormitory provision to create large wards of over 100 beds to the extent that it became normal and acceptable practice that continued into the latter half of this century. We consider the report of the Whittingham Inquiry (DHSS, 1972) to be telling in this respect. Comment is made on certain care practices investigated in Ward 16 which provided for 125 chronic and psychogeriatric patients, many doubly incontinent, on three floors with never more than five staff. Whilst uncaring practices could never be condoned, how would you cope with routine physical care let alone any stimulating activities? However, the report is quiet on the point of a ward containing 125 patients! We are also mindful of a ward visited in 1978 containing 165 beds and other examples exist.

Small wonder therefore that the Victorian ideal of asylum degenerated into containment, depersonalization, and with a risk of abuse. The description of the total effect of such a regime was well described by Barton (1959) and stimulated considerable activity to rehabilitate these unfortunate individuals back into society. Barton (1976) is more forceful in his views on causation and lists violence, brutality, browbeating, harshness, teasing and tormenting as important factors in the state he calls institutional neurosis.

It is no surprise that criticism of such a situation arose. A number of inquiries into cruelty and neglect followed and all have hastened the decline of the mental hospital and the establishing of an alternative service. The figures below led on from the previous figures:

In-patient population

1959	155,700
1970	114,200
1980	79,200
1990	Below 60,000

THE WAY FORWARD

Responsibility for the mentally ill became part of the comprehensive health service for England and Wales established under the National Health Service Act 1946. On the appointed day (5 July, 1948) the existing provision, except for hospitals or institutions designated as teaching hospitals, were placed within the fourteen regional hospital boards established to administer the service via hospital management committees (Ministry of Health, 1948). It is interesting to note that in fact this infant health service was originally intended to exclude mental health and it was only pressure from the psychiatrists through the Royal Medico-Psychological Association, arguing that psychiatry should be treated as other branches of medicine, that induced a change of heart in the Government.

It was obviously necessary for the law relating to mental health to be kept in line with changes taking place in the care of the mentally ill both as regards the place of treatment, due to the continued changes in facilities and the numbers contained, and also as the result of advances in medical science. The main piece of legislation was still the Lunacy Act of 1890 followed by the Mental Treatment Act of 1930 which allowed for voluntary treatment and the facility for patients to discharge themselves. Prior to that Act patients were subjected to an order of a magistrate or court at some stage of admission or discharge with the resultant stigma being attached.

Following precedent a Royal Commission was raised to study the need for changes in legislation and reported in 1957. From this 'The Mental Health Act 1959' came onto the statute book and placed emphasis on the informality of treatment, the provision of community care, and the safeguard of mental health tribunals to examine cases when detention had been decreed. The Minister of Health was pleased to announce the new law which placed on the mental hospitals the opportunity to take on a new active, liberal and therapeutic task in the care of the mentally ill.

Such legislation requires change and development as the way forward. During the post-war period a gradual move towards general medicine had been seen by the introduction of psychiatric units on general hospital sites and such a development had been fully supported by Government guidelines issued in various documents. Something of a bombshell came in 1962 with the White Paper on the future of Mental Hospitals which envisaged a number of closures within 10 years. Although this was not achieved, its effect was significant both on the staff of hospitals and the hastening of the development of alternative services.

In 1971 the relevant Government department (the Department of Health and Social Security) issued an important guideline on future services and stated quite clearly:

> 'The objective should be to establish a department for the mentally ill in each district general hospital or group of hospitals providing a district service with the ultimate aim of replacing the large mental hospitals'.
> *DHSS, 1971*

The guidelines also envisage a comprehensive service for the mentally ill including in-patient, day patient, out-patient, general practitioner and local authority services and sets out the principle of the 'therapeutic team' as follows:

> 'The setting up of "therapeutic teams" is an important element in providing a comprehensive service. Each team should include a consultant psychiatrist, medical staff, nurses, occupational therapists and social workers'.
> *DHSS, 1971*

Thus was laid down the way forward and the demise of the mental hospital. The figures overleaf demonstrate the move away from hospitals and the gradual run down of the large institutions:

The move in location of services continues up to the present day. The emphasis on 'community care' (Griffiths, 1988) so many years after the 1959 Act, gathers apace. Many of the old hospitals have now closed and stand as monuments to their Victorian ancestry. Psychiatric units are an integral part of the general hospital site although

	1966	1969	1972	1975	1976
Number of hospitals with over:					
1500 beds	30	28	21	7	5
1000 beds	61	55	46	34	31
750 beds	82	81	70	54	50
500 beds	91	92	89	83	83
250 beds	99	99	100	99	100
Number of mental illness units in general hospitals	103	111	114	126	137
Total places in day hospitals attached to units in general hospitals		967	2039	3350	3650
Total places in day hospitals		5472	7350	10206	11073
DHSS, 1980					

planning for the future may have second thoughts on this and establish units in more convivial surroundings. Community psychiatric services have increased beyond expectation and will continue to do so. A whole spectrum of specialist services now exists to provide for client groups requiring expert advice and care. A radical change indeed over the last half century. In addition, the Mental Health Act 1983 has replaced the previous legislation but has already been criticized as being a 'close-textured' prescriptive law nearer to the 1890 Act than an enlightened way forward and not concerned with 95% of the patient population (Jones, 1991).

Within all this change we suggest a few questions to consider:

What has happened to the Victorian ideal of asylum?

What provision has been made for those less able or psychologically damaged members of society who find the stresses of modern life to be beyond their ability to manage?

Why are people living in doorways and under rail arches in the cities?

Why, as a result of Government policy, is little or no provision made for those needing long-term care?

INSIDE THE INSTITUTION

This section will examine provision available for the mentally ill as regards care facilities within the accommodation in use over the last 100 years.

Mention has already been made of the massive building programme undertaken by the Victorians. Huge institutions constructed mainly in country areas dominated the skyline. You can still see today the massive chimney or gigantic water storage tower and although often now contained within the urban sprawl, they are unmistakable.

Our time is the early part of this century. Our institution has already stood for 50 years. Solid and untouchable.

Note how quiet it is. How safe and secure it feels with its solid timber doors, shining brasswork and ornate tiles. There is a murmuring of voices from the large room on the left that contains an enormous oak table and leather chairs with a fire roaring away in the large fireplace. The Board of Governors is meeting as it does each month. The Chairman is the local squire (we did notice the mounting stone outside the main door for use when he rides over from his country seat) and members come from the trade and professional classes. Membership appears to be very much a status symbol.

On the right is a large office for the Medical Superintendent and next to it a smaller office for the Hospital Steward. An annexe contains desks for two secretaries. Not much paperwork in those days we note.

The Medical Superintendent is an all-powerful patriarch. Absolutely nothing escapes his notice and it is said he knows every one of the 2,000 inmates in his care and the names of every staff member and their family. His large house is connected to the institution by a private corridor and six inmates work in his house and garden. Being unmarried, his meals are provided directly from the main kitchen.

Let us continue our tour. We shall need a bunch of keys before we can go any further because all the doors are locked.

Keys play an important part in the life of the institution. Any staff member losing a key faces immediate disciplinary action and possible dismissal. Staff therefore take great care and are forever jangling them in pocket or in hand. The effect on the inmates must be intimidating.

The first thing we notice upon leaving the entrance area is that the building is divided into three sections. Ahead we have all the central facilities such as the main hall, for dances, films and sports—the main kitchens and the stores and engineering departments. We also notice the workshops that allow the institution to function as a self-contained provision. The upholstery shop, tailor, shoemaker, sewing room and carpenters function to provide for everything and everyone—dresses and suits, boots and shoes, furniture and uniforms all to standard patterns, sizes and colours. A small shop provides for those inmates who wish to purchase tobacco, sweets and other small items but no money changes hands. The Steward issues metal tokens in lieu of cash because money may be stolen or 'lost'.

The picture is one of a total institution. Everything is provided and everything is regulated; individuality does not exist and would probably not be tolerated.

We decide to take the door to the right into the male side of the institution. A similar door to the left would take us into the female side and the two sides only meet on common ground such as the dance and film evenings (but still seated in separate halves of the hall), church services (but still seated in separate halves of the church) and sporting events (but still seated in separate halves of the ground). Woe betide any members of the staff found in the wrong half of the institution and different keys are needed for each side.

Our walk along the seemingly endless male side corridor towards the ward we have elected to visit seems to dampen our spirits a little. It seems darker with naked light bulbs within metal shades, a monotonous standard cream paint on the walls and ceiling and dark woodwork. Strange noises and raised voices are heard behind a number of doors.

We arrive at the entrance for Ward 2 and knock to request admission. Keys rattle and the lock is turned (twice we think; is the door double locked?).

We are faced with a corridor with doors off to various rooms, one for boots and shoes (solid black leather all to the same design with buckles instead of laces), one for overcoats (all the same dark tweed colour), a clothing store containing a full range of clothing from shirts to socks to suits, and a small room for cleaning materials such as floor polish, brasso, and black lead for the grates. Further along is a kitchen for the ward with a large sink for washing cutlery and crockery but no means of heating water for beverages or heating for food (later we learn that tea comes from the central kitchen in large urns and already contains sugar and milk). Cutlery is kept in a locked box with the number of each item marked on the outside and these are checked at each mealtime. Losses have to be reported to the Medical Superintendent.

We are already beginning to have some disturbing thoughts on the way inmates contained within our institution are regarded. The most significant factor concerns the complete absence of any thought being given towards the inmate as regards personal preference and individuality. No personal clothing appears to be allowed and there are no choices in the clothing provided. We also ask the question 'Do all take milk and sugar?'.

Considering these points we wonder if the effect will be to 'de-humanize' the individual and instil conformity to a regime. Barton (1976) discussed this within 'institutionalization'.

Moving into the main ward area we look at the provision in the dayroom. The same cream paint and dark woodwork prevails with a complete lack of any colour to catch one's attention. No curtains to the windows or cushions to the chairs. Heavy furniture built to last. No pictures on the walls and naked light bulbs high up on the Victorian ceiling.

There are obviously some important pointers here as regards the effect of the environment on the individual and that does not exclude the staff. Such factors as colour, light and texture must be addressed in our analysis of the visit.

The dormitory requires special mention. Rows of cast iron beds with little room between. White counterpanes, pillows all in line (one per bed). Lights for ordinary use are clear but a green shade has been placed over one for night use. We also note that here the walls have been painted a strong shade of green. Seventy-five men sleep in this large open dormitory and a few individual rooms at the end. We step into one of them and the attendant taking us round closes the doors to show how quickly that can be done.

They are double doors, the inner one lined with a strong padded canvas which also covers the walls and floor. A shutter over the small window high up the wall can be closed and locked and will exclude all light. The padding absorbs

sound and the effect is to instil a feeling of the removal of all external stimulation.

More environmental factors must now be added to our list. We note in the dormitory the complete lack of individual space and provision for personal belongings of any sort. Overcrowding is very evident and there is no opportunity to withdraw from the company of so many men. The separate rooms themselves would not offer much comfort due to the complete deprivation from contact or sensory stimulation.

Many of the men are outside the ward in the garden and we step through a door to view. The air is certainly fresher. To our dismay our first impression has been wrong and this is not the general idea of a garden but an enclosed area within high cast iron railings where the inmates can exercise twice daily—weather permitting. Groups and individuals walk round and round the pathways or lie on the grass.

Few men on this ward are employed and little else is available for them. They thus spend their time either in the ward doing little except ward tasks, such as cleaning, or walking as an escorted group within the hospital grounds. Little chance therefore of a return to home and the community.

Those who are employed all work in the artisan departments of the hospital including the farms and horticultural gardens. We wonder to ourselves what has changed since Munday toured the county asylums in 1861 and stated that in his view the main aim seemed to be to keep the asylum self-sufficient and preferably profitable (Nolan, 1993).

But our visiting time is running out. We walk back through the grounds noting the well-kept gardens and greenhouses, the farm, sports fields and church. Everything seems to be provided although we wonder if the Victorians who created our building really intended their concept of asylum to concentrate upon containment and control to such an extent. Or is this an anticipated feature of institutions?

Looking back we speculate if ours which looks so permanent, will continue long into the future. Or indeed should it continue?

Are there other ways of providing for the mentally ill that would allow greater opportunity for the individual to return to the family and community?

If we move forward in time to 1985 in our institution, many things have happened to society, medical therapeutics, and the law since our last visit.

To our surprise most of the building (now called a hospital) has closed and one wing has been demolished. We understand that despite enormous sums of money spent on the old building, total closure is planned.

You will recall that Government policy since 1971 has been to close the old hospitals and build up services in psychiatric units at district general hospitals and within the community. This policy is now taking effect.

Entering the building we can see how the money has been spent. All the old woodwork has been painted in subdued colours; wallpaper of various patterns and textures has covered all the old painted walls, and lighting has been modernized and increased.

Emphasis has been placed on producing a living environment conducive to the privacy and individuality of the patients. Far and away the majority of the patients now wear their own clothes and indeed the hospital makes little provision for anything else. Private space has been created in the dormitories by way of curtains and partitions and the padded rooms have long been removed. Furniture is modern and indeed some patients have their own favourite pieces of furniture to use. Other major changes include the recognition that men and women have

mutually beneficial effects on each other and some wards, after structural alterations, are providing for both sexes.

We note that our analysis already includes some of these changes and others are now added. Many factors have come into play over the past 30 years which have brought about this change. Some would argue that the major factor was the introduction from the 1950s of a whole range of drugs designed to control or change behaviour. Others would consider the emphasis on rehabilitation and the need to reconsider the approach to containment and the ever-increasing in-patient population to have been an important trigger. The truth probably lies between the two.

What is certain is that, as our figures have shown above, a remarkable decrease in the number of in-patients has been achieved and alternative provision made. For those who are admitted, or asked to attend a day patient facility, the emphasis is on a short stay with referral on to the community or GP service.

We receive information on the patient population currently in the hospital. The majority are elderly and range from those more recently admitted for assessment or long-term care, to an ageing long-stay population which has grown old in hospital and is considered too difficult to place in alternative provision.

All work with the acutely ill is now provided at the psychiatric unit some miles away and we ask to visit and view the facility.

Leaving, we ask ourselves about the effects on staff providing for long-term care only. You may wish to examine this subject which was highlighted in two documents: *Report of the Committee of Inquiry into Whittingham Hospital* (HMSO, 1972) and *Organisational and Management Problems of Mental Illness Hospitals* (DHSS, 1980).

The psychiatric unit is situated within the multi-storey block of the district general hospital and is close to the town centre. Two wards are designated for acute mental illness and are situated on the fourth floor. A new purpose-built unit is under construction.

The two wards are identical and are of 'race-track' design, that is, all facilities are central and dormitory/sitting areas are around the periphery. This compares with the traditional 'Nightingale' design of older general hospital wards when beds were situated down each side of a large dormitory and facilities are at the side and ends.

The unit is integrated into the main hospital in line with Government guidelines of the time (Hospital Building Notes, 1963). These were conceived in the spirit of the Hospital Plan of 1962 which saw the future of psychiatry as being within district general hospitals.

This policy has been amended over the years as the result of experience. It was realized as long ago as 1973 that whilst it was desirable to provide all services on the one site and a 'psychiatric department is an essential part of the district general hospital', there are advantages in planning it separately linked to, rather than incorporated within, the main hospital block (Hospital Building Notes, 1973).

The staff have already discussed with us the difficulties encountered in caring for acute mental illness in the current facility. The race-track design presents problems with observation and an inadequate provision of day and activity space. Comment was also made on the siting of the unit on the fourth floor of the hospital with occupational departments some distance away and no recreation or relaxation space on site. Owing to its situation there is no opportunity to enjoy and obtain benefit from a garden.

It has been shown (Ulrich, 1984) that a view of the outside world influences the speed of recovery from surgical procedures and Barefoot (1992) has argued that usable outdoor space will help with the recovery of psychiatric patients. In his view 'the racetrack ward is a failure' and much more attention should be paid to the design and location of psychiatric units, colours and the colour of light, and a background of reassurance and comfort.

Change and development is however taking place. A later Health Building Note (1988) provides further guidance on the subject and has generated a number of data packs for use with particular requirements. For example, Pack 31 describes in great detail a number of options for the provision of units for the elderly mentally ill (DH, 1989).

It would appear from personal experience that a great deal of freedom now exists to provide purpose-built and purpose-designed units for the mentally ill that place a much greater emphasis on service principles, such as the rights and needs of individuals for dignity, privacy and self-determination. Such experiments as the Worcester Project (Rooney and Mathews, 1982) have been carefully evaluated and smaller units in various parts of the country have received a great deal of attention from the design stage onwards. Much closer co-operation between the designer and the user group now takes place to ensure that care is provided in a facility that allows a high standard to be achieved to the mutual benefit of all concerned. As Kelly (1991) states in his review of proposed psychiatric provision in Canterbury/Thanet and East Birmingham:

'Buildings are often neglected in the commitment to a value driven mental health service because they are seen as the responsibility of professional groups who may not share these values'.

In his postscript to the document, Paul Rooney, Manager of Mental Health Services, East Birmingham concludes:

'We have attempted to ensure that we did not just pay lip service to our philosophy of care criteria but rather that we accepted or rejected proposals on their ability to fulfil such criteria.

This is an exercise that has to be completed thoroughly and locally before any reference to building guidance'.

We would support this view and anticipate that increasingly greater attention will be paid towards the architect and builder providing for the domiciled care group. Certainly the new units provided for acute illness and the elderly show marked improvements in the quality of the provision.

We must, however, as the result of our findings, return to the questions posed at the end of the first section of this chapter. All we have seen and examined appears to be concerned with those requiring in-patient provision and within an acute illness or in an elderly category. Bearing in mind that our hospitals have in the past provided for a group requiring long-term care, to a greater or lesser extent, our examination would be incomplete without a view of the current position regarding this section of our client population.

Mention has already been made of the policy to reduce the hospital population, the efforts placed on rehabilitating the longer stay element and the emphasis placed on community care. It was also anticipated going back as far as the 1962 Hospital Plan (MH, 1962) that in view of advances in medical science, little provision needed to be made for a group requiring long-term supervised accommodation. Thus as the older hospitals continue on the run-down phase, anything available for this group is removed from the accommodation list.

However, it has become increasingly apparent that demand for places, although reduced, continues; a certain percentage of those who enter the medical health system will either fail to respond to medication or therapies, or be stabilized at a debilitated level of functioning and be unable either to return home or provide for themselves. Thus, as we cannot fail to recognize, we are faced with obviously ill people attempting to survive in the cities; community services and voluntary organizations cannot provide for this increase. It should also be noted that a considerable number of hostels supported by Government money have closed in recent years.

Hence our questions and the deliberate reference to the Victorian ideal of asylum as a haven from the stresses and inequalities of modern life. Concern has been expressed in many quarters and the Government has recently announced the provision of finance for short-term and long-term accommodation (DH, 1993) to be provided by voluntary organization, charities and local social services in an attempt to remedy the problem. Time alone will tell; meanwhile the street population continues to increase.

At this stage we conclude our visit to the facilities provided for the mentally ill over the past 100 years. We have viewed the rise of the great institutions, how they provided for the inmates contained, the changes that took place in later years and the decline in favour of alternative provision and services.

We have also considered the early attempts at provision on a general hospital site and the attention now being given towards newer provisions determined by service requirements; although increasingly affected by costs. The concept of community services and the therapeutic team has been examined with its emphasis on community care.

The next stage in this saga is, in our view, the great unknown. In 1993 responsibility for many clients in the mental health services passes to local authorities under the Community Care Act and with transfer of funding from the National Health Service. We also have increasingly to consider the effect of NHS trusts as virtually self-determining entities. The question of the purchasers and providers of services and the standards to be achieved have been out with the scope of this chapter but will become increasingly important. You should, however, be aware of these developments. The changes have only started.

ENVIRONMENTAL FACTORS—INTO THE FUTURE

In the concluding section we wish to examine in greater detail some of the environmental factors within psychiatric provision we identified in our visits to the various facilities, and to speculate on their importance.

We noted in our early visits to the facilities factors such as light, colour and texture, overcrowding and lack of private space. We have touched on the concept of an institution and the condition of institutionalization, and have speculated on the dehumanizing effect of the old buildings and regimes and the absence of dignity and privacy. The questions of containment and control also arose.

In our later visits we were pleased to see that many of these issues had been addressed and we would not expect any of those elements that have an adverse effect upon the individual to arise in the future. Sufficient checks by management within the arena of 'standards of care' should, or will soon, exist to preclude such a possibility and we have already mentioned that sufficient flexibility now exists within planning to allow for care philosophies to be fulfilled and developed.

From our list therefore we shall select two environmental factors for further examination and discuss the effect on the individual; namely *light* and *colour*.

You will recall the effect on our emotions during our first visit to the old institution due to the dark monotonous colours and naked light bulbs. You will also recall how much better we felt during our second visit due to the upgrading that had taken place. There are clear indications today that light and colour, when intelligently utilized, can go far as definite therapeutic and psychotherapeutic agents.

This fact has already been utilized within therapeutic approaches to the care of those with a learning difficulty. The Snoezelen project, originally developed in Holland, has been taken up in this country and within its provision contains a sound and light room which enable the user to produce visual displays as a means of stimulation (Haggar and Hutchinson, 1991).

Within our care provision, modern architecture usually allows for an adequacy of natural sunlight. Such a source is essential for wellbeing and deprivation can lead to a number of medical conditions such as rickets, and a loss of calcium in the bones of the elderly with resultant increase in the risk of

fractures. Such effects are due to a loss of the invisible end of the light spectrum; namely ultra-violet. It would appear therefore that some ultra-violet light should be available within psychiatric facilities, particularly in areas for long-stay elderly patients and sources are available.

Work has also been undertaken on the use of artificial light sources. Birren (1973) has examined extensively the effect of light upon many living things and with particular reference to psychiatric facilities states:

'As to visible light in an environment, pinkish illumination has been known to produce aggression and bursts of temper. In a similar way, where blue light has been used to counteract jaundice in infants, attending nurses have been known to complain of nausea and discomfort. It would seem that artificial light is best when it emits a balanced spectrum and when perhaps it has a slightly warm tone'.

The use of colour and its effect on the individual is a much wider subject. We all know phrases in common use such as 'seeing red', 'feeling blue' and 'in the pink'. Chromatics, the study of colour, has been practised for many years and chromotherapy, the use of colour in healing, has been practised since ancient times. However, much controversy remains on the physiological effects of various colours and research has shown that the effect of colour is not constant and that people adapt. An example is the 'bubble gum pink' rooms tried in America as an attempt to pacify disturbed children; an experiment first tried in San Bernardino County, California in 1981. The children were placed in a room painted in this rather unusual shade of pink and relaxed quickly. The experiment caused a number of institutions to provide what became known as 'passive pink' rooms but results have not been constant and in the view of experts more factors than colour come into effect.

Other experiments, as indicated by Graham (1990) have shown that colour alone has healing properties and that colour does not necessarily have to be seen to be effective. The interesting phenomenon of people being able to 'feel' colours, whilst amply demonstrated, remains an enigma.

In summary, you may wish to consider the following points. First, as already stated, artificial light should be neutral and preferably slightly warm in quality and should, if at all possible, contain some ultra-violet. The spectrum emitted should, according to Birren (1973) contain and be well balanced in the red, yellow, green, blue and violet bands. It is important to note here that not all sources of artificial light do in fact cover these bands and any deficiency may distort the picture of the environment. As regards brightness, it should not be necessary to use high levels of illumination. Nor should a white colour be used on walls because of the 'glare' factor but it is acceptable for ceilings which are normally out of eyeline.

Secondly, despite all the work undertaken on the effect of colour, substantive guidelines do not exist on the use of colour in our care environment. Certainly the use of overall bland effects is not supported and indeed is not recommended in view of the effect of sensory deprivation. Over the years various experiments have been tried on the use of colours in various rooms, for example, the red room or blue room, but all have been discounted because of the ability of the eye and brain to adapt and negate the colour effect.

What is, however, clear is that to gain the best effect from colour a constant change is required and this certainly counteracts any feeling of sensory deprivation. In planning, therefore, it should be possible to provide colour schemes to match the various activities undertaken in rooms, such as reds and yellows for creative activities, bright colours for the elderly who may suffer from failing eyesight, and cool colours in provision for agitated, anxious individuals.

It is not unusual nowadays for colour consultants to be involved in the decor of our buildings. Talk to them about their colour palette and what they are trying to create.

SUMMARY

We have set out in this chapter to identify and establish two perspectives relating to care pro-

vision. First, everything stems from history and the chapter indicates the background to our current provision for the mentally ill and the way services are changing and moving forward.

Secondly, and more importantly, the chapter intends to indicate areas for further study. We have not set out to provide a definitive work but to highlight areas of change and development that we should bear in mind when we are working within care environments. All too often we hear complaints about design faults and difficulties identified. If staff find problems with an environment, what about the effect on clients brought from home and placed in a strange environment?

FURTHER READING

Berrios, G.E. & Freeman, H. (1991) *150 Years of British Psychiatry*. London: Gaskell.

Faylor, J. (1991) *Hospital and Asylum Architecture in England, 1840–1914: Building for Health Care*. New York: Mansell.

James, P. & Noakes, T. (1993) *Hospital Architecture*. London: Longman.

Malkin, J. (1992) *Hospital Interior Architecture: Creating Healing Environments for Special Patient Populations*. London: Van Norstrad Reinhold.

REFERENCES

Barefoot, P. (1992) Psychiatric wards in DGHs? An architect's comments. *Psychiatric Bulletin*, **16**, 99–100.

Barton, R. (1959) *Institutional Neurosis*. Bristol: Wright.

Barton, R. (1976) *Institutional Neurosis*, 3rd edn. Briston: Wright.

Birren, F. (1973) *A colourful environment for the mentally disturbed. Art Psychotherapy*, **1**, 255–259.

Brockington, C.F. (1966) *A Short History of Public Health*.

Chadwick, E. (1842) *The Sanitary Condition of the Labouring Population of Great Britain*. Poor Law Commission Report to the House of Lords.

Department of Health (DH) (1989) *Planning Principles and Design Description: Nucleus Data Pack 31: Assessment and Short Term Treatment Unit for Elderly People with Mental Illness*. London: Department of Health.

Department of Health (DH) (1993) *Move on Accommodation Needed for the Homeless Mentally Ill says Virginia Bottomley*. Press Release H93/522. Department of Health.

DHSS (1971) *Hospital Services for the Mentally Ill*. London: HMSO.

DHSS (1972) *Report of the Committee of Inquiry into Whittingham Hospital*. London: HMSO.

DHSS (1980) *Organisational and Management Problems of Mental Illness Hospitals*. London: DHSS.

Goffman, E. (1961) Asylums: *Essays on the Social Situation of Mental Patients and Other Inmates*. New York: Doubleday.

Graham, H. (1990) *Time, Energy and the Psychology of Healing*. London: Jessica Kingsley.

Griffiths, R. (1988) *Community Care: Agenda for Action*. London: HMSO.

Haggar, L. & Hutchinson, R. (1991) Snoezelen: an approach to the provision of a leisure resource for people with profound and multiple handicaps. *Mental Handicap*, **19**.

Health Building Note 35 (1988) *Accommodation for People with Acute Mental Illness*. London: HMSO.

Hospital Building Notes 5 and 30 (1963) *Provision for Psychiatry in District General Hospitals*. London: HMSO.

Hospital Building Note 35 (1973) *Department of Psychiatry (Mental Illness) for a District General Hospital*. London: HMSO.

Jones, K. (1991) The culture of the mental hospital. In Berrios, G. & Freeman, H. (Eds) *Years of British Psychiatry 1841–1991*. London: Gaskell.

Jones, K. (1991) Law and mental health: sticks or carrots? In Berrios, G. & Freeman, H. (Eds) *150 Years of British Psychiatry 1841–1991*. London: Gaskell.

Kelly, J. (1991) *Building for Mental Health: Stick to Your Principles*. Medical Architecture Research Unit, PNL Press.

Ministry of Health (MH) (1948) *Provisions relating to the Mental Health services*. London: HMSO.

Ministry of Health (MH) (1962) *A Hospital Plan for England and Wales*. London: HMSO.

Mundy, J. (1861) Five cardinal questions on administrative psychiatry. In Nolan, P. (1993) *A History of Mental Health Nursing*. London: Chapman & Hall.

Nolan, P. (1993) *A History of Mental Health Nursing*. London: Chapman & Hall.

Rooney, P. & Matthews, R. (1982) *Worcester Development Project*. London: DHSS.

Royal Commission Report (1957) *Report by the Royal Commission on the Law Relating to Mental Illness and Mental Deficiency*. London: HMSO.

Sursum Corda (1898) *A Handbook of Intercession and Thanksgiving*. London: A.R. Mowbray.

Ulrich, R.S. (1984) *View Through a Window May Influence Recovery from Surgery*. Science Magazine, USA.

26

A JOURNEY WITHOUT END
CREATING A DEVELOPMENT STRATEGY FOR STAFF IN SECURE FORENSIC SETTINGS

Colin Beacock

AIMS

i) To examine the development of caring cultures in secure psychiatric services
ii) To examine the place of nursing within that culture
iii) To suggest an alternative set of principles for the organization of services within secure psychiatric hospitals
iv) To provide a framework for developing expertise in nursing within the context of secure forensic psychiatry

KEY ISSUES

Dependent/independent learning
Educational prescriptionism
Ownership in education
Therapeutic communities
Community education
Nurses' use of power
Adult learning
Competence-based education and training
Strategy for developing forensic nursing

Identify, analyse and assess factors causing distress and illness	Promote health, provide direct care and make interventions	Manage care programmes and services
Be critical, analytical and accountable, continue professional development	Counter discrimination, inequality and individual and institutional racism	Work within and develop policies, laws and safeguards in all settings
Understand influences on mental health and the nature/causes of disorder and illness	Know the effects of distress, disorder, illness on individuals, groups, families	Understand the basis of treatments and interventions

MEDICAL ORIENTATION—'FOLLOW MY LEADER' IN FORENSIC CARE

Institutional care for the mentally disordered and mentally impaired offender has, and will continue to, attract attention from both professional and social critics. As focal points for concern, such institutions have set standards against which all aspects of therapeutic activity for this client group may be judged. That such standards have tended to reflect negatively upon the institutions themselves, as well as the carers who practise within them, should be of no surprise to anyone. Neither should the fact that, as a result of decades of scrutiny and criticism, the prevailing culture within such establishments has tended to value a defensive and introspective form of educational provision for the majority of its practitioners.

The accountability of the responsible medical officer (RMO), established and reinforced by successive Mental Health Acts in 1959 and 1983, has ensured a continuation of their dominance of management and care regimes within all such institutions. The ability of such a group, therefore, to influence and shape the systems of education and development for fellow professionals is obvious. As a consequence historically there has been a tendancy for educational systems to focus their students towards medical rather than developmental concepts of therapy and rehabilitation. This chapter will seek to address methods of education and training which will enable members of multidisciplinary teams to fulfil their role as 'partners' in care management and practice, whilst meeting the needs of socially dependent individuals whose behaviours and perceptions consistently challenge our previous understandings, practices and beliefs.

ROLES AND RESPONSIBILITIES

Given the traditional domination of the 'medical model' in all aspects of psychiatric care, role performance on the part of professionals whose function is described as 'ancillary to medicine' has logically tended to support the medical function. Opportunities for members of professional groups outwith medicine to examine their potential for practitioner status, whilst proliferating in mainstream psychiatry, have been limited within the field of forensic psychiatry, especially within areas of secure provision. Equally, access to 'alternative therapies' for a person whose treatment is dominated by a single professional is bound to be limited, even more so if the use of such therapies provides a serious challenge to the status and professional logic of that individual. Increasing opportunities for professional and practice development must therefore be viewed in tandem with maximizing patient choice. By virtue of the fact that many practitioners are described as having functions that are 'ancillary' to medicine, they have tended to serve their own interests best by adopting subservient roles. Developments in practice and research have therefore been orientated towards the prevailing model.

The inherent conflict between the role of nurse as therapist and nurse as gaoler has been readily rationalized by the logic that the patient is compulsorily detained and that the prime role of nurses has been to enact the priorities of their medical treatment plan. In such circumstances the prime function of the institution has been to ensure the continued detention of the patient, without which no therapeutic activity could be undertaken. The easiest option for the nurse, or other professional, has been to ensure the patient's continued 'secure' status. Responsibility upon the professionals involved to assure a 'recovery' on the part of the patient has been seen as a secondary issue.

EVOLUTION OF THE EDUCATIONAL CLIMATE AND CULTURE

By virtue of the relationship between the compulsorily detained patient and their RMO, an imbalanced power continuum has developed. As the system of monitoring patient progress and development derives considerably from the observations and comments of those professionals who are responsible for providing residential and day care services, as well as those who provide more scientific systems of treatment and measurement by way of psychological and educational services, subjective comment continues to exert a considerable influence on the life of the patient. Is the nurse or professional allied to medicine equipped with the skills to exert such awesome influence, ensuring that their obligations to the patient are balanced against their responsibilities to society at large? Is a code of professional conduct (UKCC, 1983) alone sufficiently influential to ensure that practitioners will continue to act in an appropriate, patient-orientated manner when the basic tenet of their ethic is called into question each time they pick up their 'pass keys'?

Whilst these conflicts create considerable tension and debate, it is the very nature of the resultant personal and interpersonal conflicts that contributes most to the prevailing educational and caring culture. The manner and means by which the individual practitioner is able or enabled to reconcile these particular issues form the fundamental medium for the educational process of the institution. Whether or not the system of educational provision can assist these groups of staff in achieving positive self-perceptions and maximizing their potential role in patient care is crucial. Without effective systems of education and training how will they overcome the more negative and easily assumed 'professional' mannerisms of the prison officer or 'ancillary' staff?

It appears reasonable to assume that both patients and staff exist within an ordered and interdependent form of culture. In this culture 'knowing where one stands' is an essential component of a skills repertoire which is principally geared towards maintenance and survival rather than development and challenge.

The hierarchical nature of institutional life has tended to create a dependency level amongst care staff which is seldom matched in more open systems of service provision. The larger the institution, the more intense the level of dependency has become. Consequently, distance between management and carers is often more ideological than geographical. In such circumstances antipathy towards the direction of management initiative is commonplace. Without it, however, there is little likelihood of the workforce generating alternative perspectives of their own and the outcome would be a total inertia. Indeed, such a situation existed within special hospitals particularly until recent times.

Try to obtain a copy of the *Report of the Review of Rampton Hospital* (HMSO, 1980) which describes the prevailing culture of a special hospital in the 1970s.

The need to provide professional education has been met by the provision of specialist educationists. These individuals are almost exclusively nurses who have completed an initial training and a supplementary professional teaching qualification.

As a result of previous systems this group has worked from a static base; the 'training school' or 'education centre'. The dependence of potential students is therefore further reinforced by the replication of hierarchical systems within the educational facility and by establishing distance between the educational providers and the practitioners. This is further consolidated by the use of systems of access and needs measurement which are determined by managers. Unless patients' needs are included in the equation the training and educational programme will only reflect the perceived needs of managers. Without a baseline profile of individual skills repertoire against which patient needs may be reflected, the further development of care staff will be subjective and ill-directed. In this situation the care staff have little option but to become dependent upon the in-house specialists. The 'school' assumes a classical pedagogic position within the hospital's culture. The practitioner is perceived as a passive recipient of predetermined sets of information and knowledge and has little or no involvement in determining the content of the educational programme.

OVERCOMING DEPENDENCE: THE ALTERNATIVE TO EDUCATIONAL PRESCRIPTIONISM

The geographical and professional isolation of those 'ancillary' staff who provide care for the mentally disordered offender has led them to become the poor relations within the hierarchical structure of institutional care, despite the fact that considerable resources may have been invested in providing an educational service for them. It is the purpose of such educational services, rather than their specific content, that may need to be brought into question. Illich (1973) described what school and schooling meant to the poor peoples within any society:

'Many students, especially those who are poor, intuitively know what the schools do for them. They school them to confuse process and substance. Once these become blurred, a new logic is assumed: the more treatment there is the better are the results; or, escalation leads to success. The pupil is thereby "schooled" to confuse teaching with learning, grade advancement with education, a diploma with competence and fluency with the ability to say something new. His imagination is "schooled" to accept service in place of value. Medical treatment is mistaken for health care, social work for the improvement of community life, police protection for safety, military poise for national security, the rat race for productive work. Health, learning, dignity, independence and creative endeavour are defined as little more than the performance of institutions which claim to serve these ends, and their improvement is made to depend on allocating more resources to the management of hospitals, schools and other agencies in question'.

You may find it interesting to consider your own experiences of school-based education, in the light of Illich's points. Does your experience of adult education (androgogy) vary greatly from primary and secondary school (pedagogy)?

Illich's point (Illich, 1973) regarding the allocation of resources as a means of improving the performance of institutions is well reflected in services for the mentally disordered offender. The recent history of such establishments has been built around successive enquiries and recommendations. Almost invariably this has resulted in increased resource allocation as a means of overcoming perceived deficiencies.

Equally, the suggestion that 'schooling' (Illich, 1973) serves to confuse process and substance can be substantiated by the fact that traditional curricula within this field of professional education have seldom sought to address the particular specialism to any great depth. Pre-qualifying training has failed to focus with any specificity upon the care of aberrant individuals. The learning outcomes which relate to practice placements in forensic care areas tend to be process orientated and the system of allocation seldom allows students to form meaningful, long-term relationships as a basis for therapeutic individualized care.

An opportunity to address this deficit at pre-registration level now seems more remote than ever. The advent of a more academically substantial form of education for student nurses did offer some cause for optimism but with the common foundation programme of Project 2000 (UKCC, 1986) schemes taking up 50% of the course curriculum planners have a limited number of options in designing the branch programmes. As a result both the mentally disordered patient and their carers are becoming even more distant from mainstream psychiatric care.

At post-qualifying level, the programmes that have been offered have been principally derived from the syllabi of the National Boards for Nursing. These courses have been mainly superficial and have been almost exclusively based in the school setting. Reinforcement of theory through a system of practice-based consolidation has only latterly emerged as a feature of course design. Previous systems were based upon attendance principals and had little if any summative evaluation of learning outcomes. Products, in terms of refined practice, are therefore difficult to identify in the care regime. Traditional methods of care delivery and management have been perpetuated beyond their period of usefulness or contemporary value.

Illich (1973) described how the student is convinced that service, rather than value, is the more acceptable. Such a myopic view of educational strategy has only served to reinforce that situation. A failure to address the need for a more sophisticated academic base and body of specialist knowledge has left the 'ancillary to medicine' groups in a perilously insecure position. By focusing their activities upon mundane, task-oriented approaches which build upon the preoccupation with security, nurses in particular have almost disenfranchised themselves from the more forward-thinking social and educational models of care.

In citing these deficiencies, an opportunity for overcoming the previously dependent learning culture emerges. The medical model encouraged paternalistic approaches towards the development of both patients and carers. Reward systems were linked to the more highly valued characteristics of conformity and obedience. Predictability and consistency were the order of the day. In order to establish profession-specific bodies of knowledge and expertise, non-medical staff must challenge this concept. The prevailing educational culture must enable, rather than restrict, the testing of previous boundaries of practice and responsibility. If patient care is to be based upon the principles of mutidisciplinary working and if assessment and treatment programmes are to capitalize on the total spectrum or available therapies and interventions, the prevailing educational culture must reinforce such concepts. As such there would appear to be no place for singular prescriptive models of treatment, therapy or care in a multiprofessional environment where the focus of activity is the needs of patients both as individuals and as a cohort.

WHOSE SERVICE IS IT? A RATIONALE FOR REORIENTATION OF PROFESSIONAL EDUCATION

If one is able to accept that the basis of the process of professional education is dependent upon a relationship between the needs of the patient and the practice of the carer, then the social organization of the institution is crucial in that it can enhance or detract from the development of a positive educational culture. Fletcher (1980)

offers an analysis of this concept and considers the rationale for the allocation of resources:

> 'If, then, the social organization is put to work at the fulcrum of the reflexive process it is to be situated at the point where individuals are making culture—where they are improving their own conditions together. Culture is only produced, as distinct from reproduced, when different efforts with the same problems or the same efforts with different problems emerge. Education then has the choice to be part of the solution or part of the problem. The question, in relation to the articulation of common causes, is, "whose resources are they"?'

This notion of individuals making culture rather than reproducing it holds significant potential for the development of professional education in those institutions being considered. As Fletcher (1980) argues, the opportunity exists for education to become part of the solution rather than a part of the problem. If professional education is to accept such an opportunity, as surely it must, then a significant part can be played in assisting the development of the necessary knowledge base that will underpin increasingly autonomous function. The system of educational provision can foster this considerably through a reorientation of teaching and learning methodology. Whilst distant from the areas of practice, such methodology has little if any chance of achieving this goal. Where the theory and practice can be brought closer together, the educational process has a greater opportunity of achieving a worthwhile credibility with the practitioners, management and patients. The nature of such an approach allows individual students to reflect principles in practice, especially where the student is utilizing an individualized care planning system. Should such a care planning system be based around the principals of 'shared action planning', the opportunity exists for the process of learning to be extended to all participants involved. Where patient advocacy is practised, an opportunity for carer and patient to learn together arises.

Such a situation gives added impetus to

Fletcher's point regarding resources; 'whose resources are they?'. The concept of patients benefiting directly from the professional education of their carers is surely not absurd given that investment in such programmes is intended to augment the quality of patient care. If one accepts the principles:

Systems of professional education/curricula → Refined and enhanced practice

Systematic appraisal of individual patient need ← Increased quality of individualized care

(↑ connecting bottom-left to top-left, ↓ connecting top-right to bottom-right)

then an opportunity exists for education to intervene and instigate improved quality of care. Where the individual patient is enabled to participate actively, rather than passively, in this process an even greater opportunity exists for further consolidation of learning through joint analysis and interpretation of the care planning process. The point raised by Fletcher (1980) regarding the ownership of resources is extended further by such an approach. Hereby lies an argument that educational resources are being utilized to achieve a learning process in which several parties can achieve personal growth. At the same time the patient involvement in the process of professional education moves from a passive to an active role. Fletcher (1980) continues his analysis regarding the ownership of resources by stating that:

'... The theory does not appear to anticipate conflict with the community but implies that if resources are not currently dedicated it must be because an employer does not wish it to be so. ... This, of course, is not a problem in respect of whether the education will "work" but of whether it will be allowed to work and at this point we must observe that there are liberal and liberating interpretations ... liberal assumes that the person is "free" and should be yet freer and more enlightened whilst liberating assumes bondage and the setting free of whole classes of people'.

Fletcher's comments appear to be of direct relevance, once more, to the institutions in question. The principals involved in shared learning appear to offer scope for maximizing learning within the care team. Yet experience within the special hospitals, has shown a reluctance amongst a variety of professionals to even examine the likely benefits of such approaches. It can only be assumed that as Fletcher (1980) states, it is the failure to allow such education to work that is the fundamental problem within such establishments rather than the lack of any suitable model.

LEARNING AS A COMMUNITY: A MODEL FOR CULTURAL DEVELOPMENT

When in 1989 the Special Hospitals Service Authority (SHSA) was established it heralded a further attempt at achieving major reform in services for mentally disordered offenders in secure systems of care. As the first of the new-style health authorities established following the publication of the Government's White Paper *Working for Patients* (DH, 1990) the authority faced considerable challenges. In its first annual review (SHSA, 1991) the SHSA examined the aims set for the new authority by the Government. One of these was that they were:

'To develop the hospitals as centres of excellence for training staff of all disciplines in forensic and other branches of psychiatry, psychiatric care and treatment'.

In order to achieve this the Authority would have to pay tremendous detail to the prevailing culture within the special hospitals. In describing the challenges faced by the Authority the review stated that:

'The greatest of all perhaps is the need to continue to generate a change of culture within the service. The Authority must put patients first and engender pride and enthusiasm among staff. ... Modern attitudes, progressive ideas and new ways of doing things are essential if the special hospitals are to play their full part in the development of psychiatric care'.

The SHSA review made this statement as part of a section headed 'Changing the Context'. In order to shift the context previously described in this text, and to achieve a more comprehensive and appropriate system of educational provision which encourages the concept of putting 'patients first', the use of an alternative model against which to judge the principals and functions of the overall regime is essential. If the medical model is to be replaced by a developmental, socially derived approach in which the education of all parties is to be crucial, what form might it take? How should the prevailing culture be developed?

Given that the institutions described constitute communities within their own right, Fletcher (1980) once more offers a concept for consideration. He suggests three premises in respect of 'community education'. The first premise he suggests is that:

'The community has its needs and common causes and is a maker of its own culture. This is a new premise, one that stands in opposition to the Rennaisance view of knowledge. In the latter ideas exist independently of and outside people. The more ideas they have the more knowledgeable they are and the civilizing process is that of putting the ignorant sufficiently close to the knowledgeable'.

Such a premise says that culture is an active, shared component of life. It does not exist independently of its creators and its creation depends very much upon the problems people face and their celebration of their causes. Fletcher's second premise is that:

'Educational resources are to be dedicated to the articulation of needs and common causes. Articulation does not mean mobilization or publicity; it means the making of clear, distinct connections. It means joining ideas and analysis and being disposed to seek for needs rather

---

than wait for demands. The resources are those of capital, plant, land, equipment and people ... it is held that the theory of community education is rather more than a prescription for good professional practice'.

Fletcher's third premise is that:

'Education is an activity in which we alternate between the roles of student, teacher and person. The roles are not occupied separately but in interdependence; this means being sympathetic to the other person, playing another part and believing in the purpose and principal of alteration. This means not wanting to be distant and absorbed in oneself, not believing that some types of people will never be able to lead and other types will never be able to follow. This implies trust, co-operation, joint achievement, a mature and equal relationship'.

On analysis, these premises appear to have relevance in what have come to be known as 'forensic' settings. That such closed institutions are makers of their own culture is surely without question. Successive reports into the management and organization of special hospitals (e.g. Elliott, 1972; DHSS, 1980) have criticized their remoteness and tendency to develop valuing systems which are not in keeping with their contemporaries. This chapter supports that fact and seeks to analyse the main reasons behind how such a culture has developed.

A CULTURAL CONTEXT FOR COMMUNITY EDUCATION

Identifying the fact that such institutions already have an active, if inappropriate, culture is not difficult. In seeking to reorientate that culture the use of a coherent educational strategy is a major priority. Any such strategy must recognize Fletcher's (1980) point regarding resources. Having stated a commitment to putting patients first, the SHSA showed that there was indeed a focus for common needs and causes. The deployment of resources must be central to the creation of an appropriate developmental culture. If community education is of relevance to systems of forensic care it must offer 'more than a prescription for good professional practice' (Fletcher, 1980). The civilizing of a system that has been found repeatedly to dehumanize both patients and staff depends on more than 'putting the ignorant sufficiently close to the knowledgeable' (Fletcher, 1980). How can these premises offer guidance for educational planners in forensic settings?

Part of the answer might lie in the last of Fletcher's statements. The concept of interdependence between student and teacher and believing in the purpose and principles of alteration are fundamental to achieving the cultural shift sought by management groups such as the SHSA. The other points raised by Fletcher are recognized as aspects of unconditional positive regard, an essential component in the communication repertoire of the practitioner in psychiatric settings. How then should such positive developmental features be incorporated into the educational climate and caring culture in institutional settings? Are such issues not being addressed already?

That such issues are being addressed already is without doubt. The continued efforts of managers and educationists in forensic settings had led to the development of meaningful, multidisciplinary programmes of post-basic education and an increasing awareness of the need to confront negative culture norms. Models of care provided within regional secure units in the UK and elsewhere are recognized as a potential template for the design of services for the twenty-first century (DH, 1992).

The simple replication of systems will not in itself produce success. What is required is a system in which humane principles and philosophies inform the daily function of the practitioner—a system in which the concept of responsibility and accountability is shared across the care team. Such systems must enable clients to accept responsibility for their actions and to have opportunities to contribute to the planning and monitoring of their own regime of care. Issues of scale, geography, legislation and so forth, whilst important, should not be viewed as imperatives. The system must be based upon the inherent resources of people and their personal strengths. The concept of community education can only be of benefit if the community has positive contributions to make to each of its members and each member has the opportunity to make positive contributions to the common and personal good.

If such a community were to exist might it have application within the existing institutions provided for mentally disordered offenders? If community education is of value what principles might promote its viability?

FEATURES OF THE POSITIVE DEVELOPMENTAL COMMUNITY

The description of a community as being positive and developmental implies a dynamic environment and one in which personal growth is not only valued, but actively encouraged. This further implies a community in which all individuals are valued for the positive contributions they bring to every-day life. The very act of living within such a community would appear to hold positive potential for any mentally disordered person. For the mentally disordered offender such a community would offer a complete opposite to the alternative custodial regime of a prison.

The concept of the 'therapeutic community' has been established over many years. Institutional care in the UK has evolved from the ideal of the self-reliant colony, in which the mentally disordered and their carers were able to establish their own quite independent community. The great misfortune is that the very people for whom the institutions were established—the mentally disordered themselves—have had so little opportunity to make active contributions to the management and development of these communities. Almost invariably, these establishments became little more than the vehicle for the self-advancement of their various staff. The well-intended designs of mainstream society were structured around ideals of Protestant work ethic and self-determination. Treatment and therapy were seen as one and the same thing in the care of most of those resident in such institutions. What then differentiates between these Victorian concepts and the role played by the modern concept of the 'therapeutic community'? Moreover, if the existing large-scale hospitals which treat the mentally disordered offenders are offering a medically dominated model of care which is inappropriate for the treatment of most of their patients, how might the systems of a therapeutic community assist in developing a more appropriate culture?

Kennard (1983) described certain common attributes associated with therapeutic communities. First, he described how such communities enjoy an informal and communal atmosphere. Such an atmosphere is characterized by a lack of uniforms or formal dress. In such circumstances it is quite the norm to be unable to differentiate at first glance between patients and their carers. Such informality should not imply a purposeless atmosphere where relaxation is the only significant therapy. Rather, the informality assists in developing relationships which allow for confrontation and challenge to be offered within the context of a developmental lifestyle. Equally, laughter and personal expression of all forms is encouraged. The stereotyped boundaries associated with the nurse/patient relationship in existing secure hospitals are substantially challenged by such an approach.

The second characteristic described by Kennard (1983) is the place of group meetings within the life patterns of a therapeutic community. Such meetings have a variety of purposes but involve the whole of the community and vary in their sophistication from one community to another. The purpose of such meetings is to assist in the management and development of the community as a whole. Information sharing, team building, decision-making, the offering of personal feedback and the facilitation of group and consumer pressure are all achieved through such meetings. Such systems would draw into question many of the fundamental practices of secure hospital-based provision. In such settings, information is a very valuable asset and decision-making of a critical nature lies in the hands of the few. The ability to receive feedback and the use of consumer pressure is not readily developed in existing hospital settings.

The sharing of work in running and maintaining community life is cited by Kennard (1983) as a third feature of life within therapeutic environments. Such work involves patients in the administrative as well as routine maintenance tasks of the community. Paid staff would undertake tasks on an equal basis with patients fulfilling chores as a means of freeing patients so that they might participate in the most meaningful and relevant work at hand. Hierarchical roles common in secure hospitals would be of no value in attempting to achieve such ideals. Task allocation is justified by its relevance to the development of the individual and community, rather than any socially conferred rank.

A fourth common characteristic suggested by Kennard (1983) is the recognition of the therapeutic role which can be fulfilled by the patient or client within such communities. The value of such people as contributors to the overall therapeutic regime is often an accepted yet informal feature. The benefits of giving and receiving comments regarding behaviours, attitudes and beliefs should not be the domain of the staff members alone. At the same time the utilization of the patient or client as a therapist within the team must be recognized and valued.

That evidence of each of these features is not already available in all of the existing services for the mentally disordered offender in the UK is not in question. However, what does need to be challenged is the lack of strategic planning in the provision of such services which has culminated in the development of sporadic services with substantial variation in quality. To suggest that the benefits of approaches such as those illustrated by Kennard would have benefit to secure hospital-based provision alone would be facile. However, it is within such hospital provision that these concepts offer their biggest challenge to existing practice and consequently offer a potential for achieving their most notable benefits.

ROLE CONFLICT: THE PLACE OF NURSING IN THE SECURE THERAPEUTIC COMMUNITY

Having previously described the dilemma faced by nurses when they are expected to fill the dual role of carer and gaoler, would this not be further compromised by their role as an enabler within the context of a therapeutic community? Where such a community had the conflicting purposes of restricting the patient's access to mainstream society and at the same time acting as the medium for their treatment, therapy and development the nurse's role would appear to be even further compromised.

The status and function of any nurse is dictated by a large but finite number of social constructs. Cultural norms, practice setting, role specification and hierarchical systems are just some examples. The given commonality is that each individual must have completed a prescribed form of training and education and demonstrated a degree of competence which is commensurate with their level of registration on the UKCC Professional Register (UKCC, 1983). The content of the syllabus of study determined the part of the register that each nurse will enter. Beyond these common factors nurses will be principally influenced by the social norms of the organization within which they function. As yet, there is no requirement for the nurse to demonstrate ongoing competence beyond initial registration. The pressures brought to bear by the cultural norms of the practice settings are of immediate effect upon the practitioner. The pressures of professional legislation are seen to emanate from a more distant, bureaucratic level with little or no effect upon the daily role performance of the individual practitioner in the institutional setting. Within existing secure settings the role performance of the nurse is influenced far more by local than national norms.

Rushing (1964) examined this phenomena with particular reference to the way in which various professionals utilized power strategies within psychiatric settings. Rushing utilized a form of referential framework that considered the role performance of professionals in terms of 'costs'. By this he implied that the stategy employed by any professional to elicit required outcomes from a given patient required a degree of effort which might be spent in other, more desirable activity.

Rushing (1964) described three main forms of power strategy which were common to all psychiatric settings. 'Cost-inducing' strategies were those that would require the practitioner to forego other, more valued, activities. Another strategy might create embarrassment, anxiety or some other form of psychosocial discomfort; the practitioner may have to make an effort to achieve patient outcomes that they feel should be given automatically, in view of their status or reputation. Such approaches may be considered as threats to the dignity of the practitioner suggesting that the imposition of rules is an example of how power can be utilized by the professional as a form of 'cost-reducing' strategy. The use of relationships between professional and client has a 'cost-preventing' connotation. By this, Rushing suggests that as a result of interpersonal relationships, the professional may be able to elicit desired outcomes from the patient without incurring any immediate 'costs' in the form of inconvenience or distraction from more valued activities.

The predominance of differing forms of power strategy is directly attributable, Rushing believes, to the cultural norms of the given institution.

You can probably think of examples in your own experience of behaviours which might be considered cost-inducing, cost-reducing and cost-preventing.

TOWARDS ENABLEMENT: CREATING THE ADULT LEARNER

As health care and education policies have developed over the last 10 years, so the institutions of each have been increasingly exposed to the influences of market forces. A degree of interdependence has developed as a result of the consequent dilemmas faced by each. The crux of market-led management systems in the new-look NHS is quality and systems of information. An essential prerequisite for such a system is reliable, quantitive and qualitative data. The drive towards research in respect of such data has led many health care organizations to the door of institutes of higher education, most notably to universities and polytechnics.

As reforms in higher education have affected such establishments, the colleges and universities of the UK have seen an ever-increasing market for research and consultation in health care establishments. Consequently, collaboration between educational services in the NHS and the institutes of higher education has resulted in the production of courses of study that are jointly validated by professional bodies and institutes of higher education. The standard and content of programmes of post-basic studies has evolved dramatically. Perhaps most importantly, educational managers in the NHS have less dependence upon centralized systems of accreditation and an increasing opportunity to develop multidisciplinary schemes of education and training.

As the relationships between the NHS and higher education are evolving, many functional issues arise. The need to create a more substantial academic base for nursing in particular, has been a major issue. Nursing's professional body, the UKCC, has chosen to take the route of creating a whole new structure for pre-registration training. The terminal nursing qualification will have a diploma status, conferred and validated by a suitable institute of higher education following a three-year period of practitioner preparation. The overall aim is to create a more independent and insightful practitioner, who can cope more ably with the responsibilities of autonomous practice.

Such a strategy can only have medium- to long-term benefits for health care organizations and the consumers for whom they provide services. This is especially true in the existing secure hospitals within the UK. Low staff turnover and a decreasing need for registered nurses has led to a situation of stasis in many areas of these institutions. This has left a large residual group of nursing staff with skills that are at best outmoded and, too frequently, inappropriate to specific patient needs. Furthermore, as patient mix has changed both in terms of gender and diagnostic category, many nurses now find themselves having completed initial trainings that are no longer relevant. Whilst the professional bodies have placed so much emphasis on the pre-registration student, this group have become increasingly disenfranchised.

Significant developments in the field of higher education can assist greatly however in providing this group with meaningful, post-basic study programmes. At the 1987 Annual Conference of the Society for Research in Higher Education, Percy (1988) addressed the issues affecting the recruitment of adult learners to courses based in the modern university. Percy felt that there were no clear principles regarding the place of adult learning in his own university but did feel that there were certain hypotheses that were relevant in all such institutions where this group of students were concerned.

These hypotheses he summarized as being, first, participation in courses or classes. The traditional university view of education did not, he felt, sufficiently recognize that systematic adult learning may well take place outwith such a structured format. Secondly, Percy felt that adult learners did not necessarily express their areas of interest and academic concern in a manner that was easily recognized by the establishment of professional educators. Many such students may find concepts of education and learning to be totally alienating, yet fulfil a role as both learner and teacher in their every-day life. The predominating modes of access to courses of higher education were suggested by Percy as a third factor. Many adult learners felt such establishments were intimidating and the structure of full-time courses was such that attendance for study would be wholly impracticable. Fourthly, he considered that accessing courses was an issue that might well deter potential adult learners. The structure of study programmes should be such that adult learners could share in schemes of university study which recognized their variable levels of motivation and commitment. In so doing, the universities might well nurture the individual's interest and confidence as a 'university learner'.

Whilst accepting that many universities were beginning to address such issues, Percy (1988) did not feel that the motivation of many such institutions could be brought into question. He felt that:

'It does seem, however, that the current rhetoric about access to higher education is concerned with securing adult students to institutions rather than adapting institutions for adult students. The emphasis is upon institutional survival rather than upon the circumstances of adult learning. ... There is nothing wrong with this rhetoric but it seems to follow from the evidence of this paper that it is only partial rhetoric.

Pragmatically, the indicators of success and performance for universities in access provision will continue to relate to the increased admission of non-traditional students to degree courses and to their nurturing to a good degree performance. But the indicators ought also to measure a university's performance in being a community educational resource ...'.

Perhaps Percy's comments appear justified and there is some question about the morality of universities being forced by the influences of economic, rather than educational factors, to encourage adult learners into their fold. None the less, it does mean that educational planners who have responsibility for the development of the 'ancillary to medicine' groups have an opportunity not only to create an academically credible pathway for such practitioners, but also to negotiate from a position of some strength. Percy's final point regarding the value of the university as a community resource has relevance in respect of Fletcher's earlier remarks. The community as a facility for the development and education of all its members needs sufficient resources to be able to meet all individual needs. Here lies an opportunity for mentally disordered offenders and their carers to share in programmes of higher education, as equitable adult learners.

At the same annual conference in 1987, Clark (1988) considered the problem of accessing course in higher education and the need to accredit non-academic learning. He argued the obvious point that institutions which recognized both employer and learner needs through the development of accreditation of competence as an alternative form of entry criteria to academic qualifications could make significant financial gains. He also argued that this was not, in itself, sufficient to enable adult learners to maximize their learning opportunities. Clark suggested that

diverse modes of study, credit transfer and studying on a stop–start basis were other relevant features and that:

'The key to curriculum reform in higher education may be modularization. This would facilitate a swing towards more task-based learning, which will suit the less academic sorts of learner and those who have developed, from their life experiences as much as from their education, an appetite for solving problems and getting practical results and skills in working with others'.

COMPETENCE-BASED EDUCATION AND TRAINING: OPENING DOORS

Clark's (1988) mention of the value of life experience and learning through practical experience, raises the issue of vocational learning and the recent rise of vocational training and education as a credible alternative to academic achievement. The recognition of levels of achievement, based upon vocational training and learning from experience are beginning to offer options to potential candidates as a means of accessing courses in higher education. How then might such a system have application within a structure geared to meeting the needs of the mentally disordered offender through enabling their carers?

The largest group of 'ancillary to medicine' professionals within the existing service is nursing. As already indicated this group is deemed on registration to be competent in performing specific functions. These competencies are enshrined within the rules and regulations of the UKCC. As such, however, these are statements of minimum levels of achievement and do not represent the further development of the individual nurse, nor do they allow for any differentiation between the higher achiever and those candidates who have demonstrated no more than the basic level of achievement at the moment of qualification. Can these issues be addressed within the context of an educational framework for forensic care? If so, how can groups such as nurses be assisted to overcome the deficiencies of their existing system? How can other 'ancillary' groups be assisted to overcome the fact that many of them require no formal qualification to practise and are, therefore, seriously disadvantaged when seeking access to any organizational system of development?

Within the context of a strategic approach, the consistency brought through having a flexible structure for planning and providing a system of development is invaluable. The purpose of such a structure should be to ensure that all developmental provision is focused, directed and relevant to the mission of the organization. In promoting the principles of the 'therapeutic community' and 'community education', any such framework must offer the adult learner all those facilities available from contemporary educational systems. If vocational approaches are to work to the advantage of potential learners in the field of forensic services we must first consider some of the principles upon which they are built.

Tuxworth (1989), in considering the origins and background of vocational education and training, suggested that a fundamental concept was that the competence of any given individual must be determined by some form of performance-based assessment. The implication is that work-based assessment is an approach that would need to become an essential feature of the caring and educational culture. Also implied is the need to ensure that work-based learning is provided through an appropriate system of practice supervision and mentorship. Tuxworth (1989) suggests that the most appropriate terminology for such an approach is 'competence-based education and training' (CBET) and recognizes that it holds a considerable threat to established concepts of achievement and learning. As a guide to developing systems of competence-based education and training, Tuxworth suggests several points for consideration. These include:

'CBET does not diminish the importance of knowledge and understanding; it does, however, change the grounds for its justification.

Methods of occupational/professional analysis

should be sophisticated enough to give a multi-dimensional view of competence.

CBET has great potential in continuing professional development, particularly where it is necessary to ensure that professionals maintain and adapt their competencies to new conditions. Licensed occupations need to maintain competence through continuing professional development and regular performance review.

The notion of "minimum competence levels" is useful for certification purpose but carries some risks if these are the only standards available. Many organizations depend upon high-level performers for their success. We should be looking for ways of cultivating excellence in occupational competence and the recognition of enhanced performance.

The providers of education and training have a great deal to do to improve access, to extend opportunity to a wide range of learners and to develop more flexible learning resources. We can make more use of experimental learning, credit accumulation and transfer; these changes are not dependent upon CBET but may be greatly assisted through it'.

Tuxworth is offering CBET as a means of broadening the scope of professional and occupational development. If CBET changes the ground for justifying knowledge and understanding it would appear to be compatible with creating a skills' base which is more related to the needs of a specific client group within a specialized environment, in the same way that research and academic rigour can assist in establishing a robust, specialist body of knowledge. The multidimensional view of competence and its application in extending minimum competence levels also appear to have application in a multiprofessional organization. Here the adaptability of the practitioners has relevance to the maintenance and development of individualized systems of care planning and therapy. The idea of internal 'licensing' of the practitioner, by the employing authority, may well assist in overcoming the deficits of nationalized or profession-specific form of regulation of standards of performance. If such an approach were to be aligned to a system of professional/occupational education, the resulting motivational factor may well assist in overcoming any detrimental cultural values attached to the pursuit of excellence in practice.

Tuxworth's mention of credit accumulation and transfer and the use of experiential learning highlight the need to harness contemporary systems of educational management in providing a structure to guide strategic planning. Whilst CBET does appear to have application in respect of offering a means of overcoming existing deficits in professional and occupational education and training, Tuxworth highlights the need to consider issues in respect of access. These can be considered not only in respect of access to CBET courses, but also as to how the outcomes of these courses can be accredited towards further and higher educational activities.

Part of the answer to the issues surrounding access to higher education and further education lies in the role CBET has to play in assisting in the overall development of the understanding of the specialist nature of forensic care. Oates (1989) sees considerable scope for CBET in that:

'... the scope of competency-based learning is not limited to a problem of staff development. In responding to the challenge of individualizing learning, linking learning to the work role, new modes of assessment, new content, new patterns of attendance and new client groups, higher education institutions will need to adopt responses within curriculum development, staff development and institutional development.

The current diversity of curriculum development processes in higher education will continue, but the developments in competence-based learning may mean that greater pressure is placed on institutions to establish the function of their provision with a level of specificity which higher education has never contemplated previously'.

From these comments there appears to be a significant role for CBET to play in enhancing the content and methodology of higher education curricula. The case against recognizing both vocational qualifications and experiential learning is weakened considerably by this argument. As previously stated the need to develop all areas of practise skills is essential in overcoming prescriptive forms of education. If the use of CBET can assist in focusing upon the specificity of the skills base in forensic care, especially where it derives from high-order rather than minimum standards of competence, than its contribution to a structure for strategic planning can be significant. As a means of access, therefore, CBET has much of offer as a stepping stone to academic study within the structure. It also has virtue as a means to guiding individual development in the form of a developmental profile. The application of techniques such as 'assessment of prior experience and learning' and 'credit accumulation and transfer', utilizing such a profile, will assist in developing the value of on-going personal and professional development, thereby addressing previous negative norms and perceptions.

THE GRAND DESIGN: GIVING SHAPE TO THE STRUCTURE

For professional/occupational education and training to contribute fully to the development of services to the mentally disordered offender, it must have a credible and relevant structure. The structure must encompass and build upon contemporary features of further and higher education. Having suggested vocational approaches as a basis for such a structure, there is a case for saying that, in order to fulfil a purposeful role in the specialist areas of secure therapeutic environments all staff, and indeed many patients, need to establish pre-vocational skills and knowledge.

Pre-vocational knowledge and skill can be described as that which each individual needs to be able to survive and function in their every-day working environment and to ensure a minimum standard of health, safety and welfare for all who live within the caring environment. Much of the material content for delivering the educational programme in support of pre-vocational studies is covered by mandatory courses, such as fire prevention, health and safety awareness, first aid and security training. Within the secure, forensic setting each of these elements have specific, as well as general, application. Too frequently, however, the main source of information and knowledge at pre-vocational level emanates from informal, culturally derived systems based in the workplace setting. Consequently, what is valued in the classroom, the traditional place for providing such programmes, often as part of 'induction' or 'orientation' schemes, is never reinforced in the work-setting. Any model or structure must recognize this as an opportunity to overcome negative cultural norms and reinforce quality practice. Principals of adult learning can be established at this early stage by providing a format and system of delivery that encourages the individual to reflect on the relative value of the content of such programmes, whilst reinforcing theory—practice integration. Work-based assessment of outcome skills can also be offered as a precursor to vocational studies. This stage of education and training would be characterized by high levels of practice-based learning and reinforcement.

From this level, the learner may progress through to a stage of preparation for practice. Characterized by an increasing sophistication of learning and assessment techniques, this stage would enable the individual to develop progressively towards becoming a practitioner in a specific occupational function. This may involve a period of professional preparation, for example, nursing, occupational therapy. The outcome should be geared towards providing a suitably skilled workforce with a complementary body of knowledge and attitude. It may be necessary for the employing authority to provide a system of accreditation for an award which is more in keeping with its purpose as a therapeutic service. To this end, it may be appropriate to develop complementary qualifications which have direct relevance to the care of this particular client group, for example, developmental therapist.

As a consequence of the need for the practitioner to demonstrate on-going academic achievement and the furtherance of levels of competence, a post-qualifying programme of training

and development will need to be provided. The current systems, as offered by the respective professional bodies do not build into a cohesive system with logical points of qualification. Whereas the *Framework and Higher Award* (ENB, 1991) is geared to the needs of nurses, up to and including undergraduate studies, it does little to address the needs of a broader multidisciplinary care regime. What is needed is a structure that builds on the benefits of credit accumulation and transfer and accreditation of prior experience and learning, whereby a learner can follow a modular form of study with terminal qualification points at certificate, diploma and degree levels. The further development of the knowledge base for forensic care would require a higher level of achievement in the form of a Master's degree to ensure further research and analysis within the speciality.

What would be achieved, therefore, is a structure that would allow the individual to progress from pre-vocational studies, via a relevant system of practitioner preparation, to under- and postgraduate studies. The systems of validation and confirmation would be overseen through an associate college arrangement with a relevant institute of higher education. All quality assurance mechanisms would be covered by such an agreement as a means of ensuring academic standards. The accreditation of modules of learning at pre-certificate level could be validated both academically and vocationally.

As a structure a five-tier model would appear:

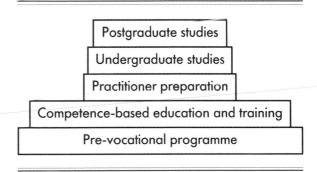

Although appearing as a hierarchy, the structure indicates that each element is interdependent and interrelated. At a functional level the structure allows individuals to achieve any of the indicated levels. It would allow any member of staff to progress through to a suitable level of academic or vocational achievement. In ensuring the ethos of the therapeutic community and community education the structure should also be made available to patients within secure forensic settings.

As the structure progresses vertically the proportion of subject-specific study should increase in relation to the course content. At the same time as the amount of research-led learning increases the need to ensure consolidation of learning through practice-based reinforcement diminishes.

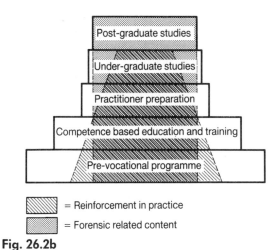

Fig. 26.2b

By ensuring that patient needs are reflected in the content of all levels of education and training, the structure is able to overcome areas of perceived deficit. Shortfalls in skills-mix can be addressed at varying levels of function.

SUMMARY

Clearly issues of educational methodology, especially in areas of assesment, teaching style and access, are crucial if such an approach is to achieve any impact. As with the content itself, the structure must reflect and build upon the resources of the organization. Expenditure on education and training in the special hospitals and elsewhere has for too long been ill-directed and often irrelevant to the needs of the mentally disordered offender. If patient needs are to be met through the training and education of their carers and if a more appropriate system of care can only be achieved through a major orientation of services, then this must be underpinned by a sophisticated articulation of the specialist nature of forensic care. Assessment of needs as a basis for designing content and systems of educational provision is an especially difficult task. Furthermore, when the culture upon which such educational approaches are built is tarnished by a legacy of industrial unrest, consistent accusations of cruelty by professional practitioners, victimization of propagators of change and antagonism towards therapeutic activity, the task can appear even more daunting. Without a structure upon which to base strategic educational planning the task will not be successfully completed. All journeys pose problems. To travel an unfamiliar route without a map has led educational planners into many a dead end. Fellow pilgrims may well be willing to journey into the brave new world. If we are to recruit them with confidence we must be able to indicate where it is we plan to go. The route by which we travel may well lead us into pockets of resistance. With the aid of strategy and a structure against which we can judge our progress and more appropriately direct our educational efforts, the benefits can be more readily achieved and the journey be made a great deal more fulfilling.

FURTHER READING

Bean, P. (1986) *Mental Disorder and Social Control*. Cambridge: Cambridge University Press.

Bines, H. & Watson, D. (1992) *Developing Professional Education*. Milton Keynes: Open University Press.

Collins, J. & Collins, M. (1992) *Social Skills Training and the Professional Helper*. Chichester: Wiley.

Department of Health/Home Office (1992) *Review of Health and Social Services Mentally Disordered Offenders and Others Requiring Similar Services*. London: HMSO.

Department of Health (1989) *A Strategy for Nursing*. London: HMSO.

Department of Health (1990) *Working for Patients*. London: HMSO.

Department of Health (1990) *Caring for People—Community Care in the Next Decade and Beyond*. London: HMSO.

Eggins, H. (1988) *Restructuring Higher Education*. Milton Keynes: Open University Press.

Elliott, J. (1972) *A Survey of Rampton Hospital*. London: DHSS.

Griffiths, Sir R. (1988) *Care in the Community—Agenda for Action*. London: DHSS.

Kennard, D. (1983) *An Introduction to Therapeutic Communities*. London: Routledge & Kegan Paul.

Kerruish, A. & Reardon, C. (1990) *Power Sharing: The Health Service Journal*, **102** (5299), 26.

Menzies-Lyth, I. (1988) *Containing Anxiety in Institutions*. London: Free Association Books.

Report of the Committee of Inquiry into Complaints about Ashworth Hospital (1992). London: HMSO.

Rushing, W. (1964) *The Psychiatric Professions*. Raleigh: University of North Carolina.

Thompson, J. (1980) *Adult Education for a Change*. London: Hutchinson.

REFERENCES

Clark, E. (1988) Opening access to higher education by recognising capability. In Eggins, H. (Ed.) *Restructuring Higher Education*. Milton Keynes: Open University Press.

Department of Health and Social Security (1959) *Mental Health Act*. London: HMSO.

Department of Health and Social Security (1983) *Mental Health Act*. London: HMSO.

Department of Health (DH) (1990) *Working for Patients*. London: HMSO.

Department of Health (1992) *Report of the Committee of Inquiry into Complaints about Ashworth Hospital*. London: HMSO.

Department of Health and Social Security (DHSS) (1980) *Report of the Review of Rampton Hospital*. London: HMSO.

Elliott, J. (1972) *A Survey of Rampton Hospital*. London: DHSS.

English National Board (ENB) for Nurses and Midwives (1991) *Framework and Higher Award*. London: ENB.

Fletcher, C. (1980) The theory of community education and its relation to adult education. In Thompson, J. (Ed.) *Adult Education for a Change*. London: Hutchinson.

Illich, I. (1973) *Deschooling Society*. London: Penguin.

Kennard, D. (1983) *An Introduction to Therapeutic Communities*, London: Routledge & Kegan Paul.

Oates, T. (1989) Emerging issues: the response of HE to competency based approaches. In Burke, J. (Ed.) *Competency Based Education and Training*. London: Falmer Press.

Percy, K. (1988) Opening access to a modern university. In Eggins, E. (Ed.) *Restructuring Higher Education*. Milton Keynes: Open University Press.

Rushing, W. (1964) *The Psychiatric Professions*. Raleigh: University of North Carolina.

Special Hospitals Service Authority (1991) *SHSA Review*. London.

Tuxworth, E. (1989) Competence-based education and training: background and origins. In Burke, J. (Ed.) *Competency Based Education and Training*. London: Falmer Press.

United Kingdom Central Council (UKCC) for Nurses, Midwives and Health Visitors (1983) *Statutory Instruments, Rules and Regulations*. London: UKCC.

United Kingdom Central Council (UKCC) for Nurses, Midwives and Health Visitors (1986) *Project 2000—A New Preparation for Practice*. London: UKCC.

THE THERAPEUTIC USE OF SECURITY
A MODEL FOR FORENSIC NURSING

Paul Tarbuck

AIMS

i) To develop a practical model for nursing patients in controlled and secure settings

KEY ISSUES

Adopting a therapeutic model in secure settings
Historical and current context
Person-centred views
Individuals receiving forensic nursing
Human society and the human security context
Mental health and the forensic nursing context
Dangerousness and forensic nursing
Forensic nursing
Process of forensic nursing
Standards of care
Assessment

Identify, analyse and assess factors causing distress and illness	Promote health, provide direct care and make interventions	Manage care programmes and services
Be critical, analytical and accountable, continue professional development	Counter discrimination, inequality and individual and institutional racism	Work within and develop policies, laws and safeguards in all settings
Understand influences on mental health and the nature/causes of disorder and illness	Know the effects of distress, disorder, illness on individuals, groups, families	Understand the basis of treatments and interventions

'Mental health problems do not affect three or four out of every five persons but one out of one'.
William Menninger

INTRODUCTION

This chapter represents the first attempt by one purporting to call himself a 'forensic nurse' to construct a meaningful and practical model by which the nursing of patients within a controlled environment may be depicted. As such, this theory joins the many that have been propounded since Nightingale's seminal works, for as George (1989) appositely comments:

'As an emerging profession, nursing continues to be deeply involved in identifying its own unique knowledge base. In identifying this base of knowledge, various concepts, models and theories specific to nursing are being recognised, refined and developed'.

The model proposed is offered at the 'recognition' phase—the author is content to be judged by his peers—some of whom may care to discard this approach, others of whom may care to refine and develop it.

Nursing in controlled environments has occurred since the time of Bedlam, yet it has consistently failed to distance itself from penal and moralistic overtones. And whilst some have attempted to utilize existing theoretical constructs when nursing forensic patients (Rix, 1988; Mason and Patterson, 1990) no one has yet described and tested a dedicated forensic nursing model.

The high security English special hospitals—rescued from the hands of the Home Office by the Department of Health, who more latterly have passed the torch to the Special Hospitals Service Authority (SHSA)—are now joined by a family of medium-secure units based in the English and Welsh regions. Indeed some would argue that the time has now arrived for the SHSA to hand on the torch yet again to the regionally-based units (Bynoe, 1992), a debate which is shortly to occur within a ministerial review group commonly known as 'Reed Two' (DH, 1992). Consequent upon the demise of the large psychiatric institutions the smaller district general hospital psychiatric facilities are finding it necessary to create secure or intensive therapy units for the care of those persons whose behaviours are unmanageable within open wards and units. The model proposed in this chapter is directed at forensic nurses working within the high security, medium security and intensive therapy units.

My hope is that as a community of carers forensic nurses will adopt a therapeutic model in concord and thereby forever distance themselves from the institutional custodialism of the past which is still evident in some parts of the secure health care system. Consequently the processes of clinical practice, education and research—often so tortuously slow in development—will accelerate in evolution with the advent of a clearer focus for contemplation, analysis and critical evaluation.

WHERE FORENSIC NURSING IS COMING FROM

Fawcett (1989) states that 'considerable agreement now exists that the central concepts of the discipline of nursing are: person, environment, health and nursing', and further labels these abstractions as 'metaparadigms'. Torres (1989) agrees with Fawcett concerning the four metaparadigms though asserts that the 'core of nursing practice is the individual. It is from the patient that other nursing concepts arise'.

Accepting the propositions of Fawcett and Torres, contemporary thought would suggest that nursing has, at its theoretical core, a quadrilateral or pyramidal model (Fig. 27.1a and b). We exist in an age when the collectivist systems of the world are crumbling, and when the ideological world view of the primacy of market forces is being vigorously asserted—the consumer is king. Setting aside the political context of these global shifts (and their ramifications for the health care

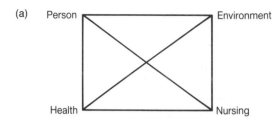

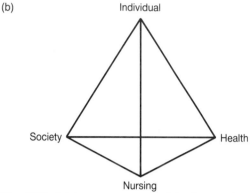

Fig. 27.1 *(a) Current conceptual thinking within nursing: Fawcett's metaparadigms. (b) Current conceptual thinking within nursing: Torres' concepts.*

of nations) one would hope that the rights associated with citizenship in an individualistic consumerist society will endure, for although the application of market principles to healthcare in the UK is painful to accommodate for those who actually deliver care, it is undeniably beginning to yield rights to the majority of consumers to which they were not entitled in the past. *The Patient's Charter* (DH, 1991a) represents the first attempt to codify those rights in a unified document in the UK. Further enhancement of the position of the consumer, or 'service user', is also occurring via the Mental Health Act Commissions' Code of Practice, which gives guidance on aspects of human rights and humane care and treatment (DH, 1991b).

Against the present global political climate, Torres' conceptual framework offers a more accurate representation of what is happening on the ground in the UK at the moment than does Fawcett's, and certainly more accurately echoes the strength of the service users' voice in terms of the advocacy movement both within the UK and within European mental health services in the 1990s.

THE CONCEPTUAL DINOSAUR—A SECURITY WORLD VIEW

Many of the problems encountered whilst attempting to care for persons within controlled environments have arisen because the profession has not sufficiently considered the relationship between the concepts fundamental to nursing, as identified by Torres, and the concept central to the forensic enterprise—security. The traditional world view has been one of the requirements for over-arching security above all else—so much so that Torres' framework, in order to depict reality, would have to acquire a fourth elevation and would have the concept of security at its vertex (Fig. 27.2), thus displacing the individual. This is the position in most penal establishments and within many areas of the special hospitals.

This model has some occasional advantages and utility, and indeed might be particularly important at times of heightened vigilance, though its incompatibility with contemporary thinking in mental health care is undeniable in that one cannot empower an individual to enjoy a fulfilling mental health experience within an inflexible regime that is incapable of allowing therapeutic risk taking.

A security world view also has the effect of diminishing the stature of the individual to the level of the other three concepts (society, health and nursing) and as the four concepts occupy the same base it follows that they may be accorded the same significance—or insignificance. If the analogy is employed that those who shout loudest will make themselves known first then it must also follow that those whose voice is weakest will be

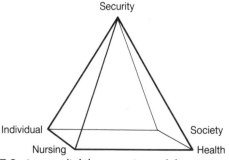

Fig. 27.2 *A custodial therapeutic model: security as the primary concept.*

heard last—if at all. This indeed is the lot of many users of the secure health care system at the moment (though other areas of the psychiatric health care system and social services also similarly disempower individuals) for the patients and clients have little say in the planning and administration of services.

Goffman (1961) has alerted carers to the fact that the comparatively weak voice of the patient has been subjugated in the past to the tyranny of the institution—which represented the requirement of society for 'security' within a stereotype of normality that excluded the mentally disordered or deviant; the European Commission of Human Rights (1981); Martin (1984); Riley (1991), and the Committee of Inquiry into Ashworth Hospital (DH, 1992) assert that many features of the 'total institution' as identified by Goffman are commonplace within parts of the psychiatric and high security health care sectors. Many believe that the first ministerial objective handed down to the then new SHSA (1989)—'to uphold the safety of the public'—propagates this collusion by elements of the state as guardians of the 'norm' against the individual's desire to be different (albeit in a criminal or mentally disordered sense).

The fundamental problem with holding a security world view as the primary concept is that it is incompatible with modern thought concerning the nature of being mentally disordered. The introduction of effective psychotropic agents in the latter half of this century, the more liberal Mental Health Acts of 1959 and 1983 (DH, 1983), the swing from secondary care to primary care, and the growth of consumerism have the aggregated effect of making Foucalt's (1965) 'age of confinement' an anachronism as we approach the millennium. Whilst it remains true that a minority will require asylum for at least some period of their lives, it is now believed that it is in the individual's best interests that that asylum will be continued not for a lifetime but for as short a period as is possible—a so-called 'revolving door' service.

Pilgrim (1989) discussed the problems associated with providing psychotherapeutic interventions in institutions that are philosophically incompatible with free choice—the assertion

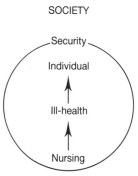

SOCIETY

Fig. 27.3 *A penal system model.*

under discussion being that psychotherapy and secure hospitals are mutually incompatible, though Pilgrim concluded that psychotherapy can be an agent of social control and still retain its therapeutic integrity. Burrow (1991) illuminates the issues associated with the role of being a modern mental health nurse in the English special hospitals and explores the many conflicts associated with the somewhat incongruent and blurred roles of therapist and custodian; and Dyer (1991) identifies some of the tensions for psychiatric nurses who attempt to advocate the best interests of their patients whilst simultaneously having to restrict the freedom of movement and choice of those same patients.

A simple and appealing solution to some of the conflicts, dilemmas and tensions of the therapy–security debate is to follow the prison service model of separate 'discipline' and 'nursing' forces working within the same institution (Fig. 27.3). This model has the advantage of allowing for a clearer differentiation of functions and no role-blurring or ambiguity for the nurse—he or she is purely a therapeutic agent.

Unfortunately this model, as it operates within the British penal system, always leads to the disempowerment of the therapeutic voice as security is perpetually accorded primacy, and the risk-taking practices that are so characteristic of enlightened mental health care are simply not allowed. A paradoxical effect also seems to occur in that nurses trained outside of the prison system do seem to acquire quite punitive attitudes whilst working in the prison system—a sort of vicarious security mindset that pervades the therapeutic culture—even within dedicated prison hospitals and hospital wings.

Clearly the security world view is out-moded and not compatible with acceptable standards of care within modern mental health care. Unless that is, the concept of security is redefined and made less absolute and restrictive to become a liberating and malleable (or 'fluid' as Dyer would have it) force for ensuring that the health care career of the mentally disordered offender is a route back into society and citizenship; rather than into the oblivion of a Goffmanesque total institution, be that in the health care sector or in a penal establishment.

Forensic nurses—carers, therapists and co-ordinators of the care of others—must rise to the challenge of the redefinition of security by being in the forefront of the debate, thereby influencing the development of thinking and securing sufficient resources in an increasingly competitive health marketplace to ensure that forensic patients are not disadvantaged by their inherent unpopularity.

A PERSON-CENTRED WORLD VIEW

Now is the time in the evolution of mental health services to effect a decisive shift in which the security world view and custodial ideology is subjected to a redefinition of construction (whilst not diminishing the public's necessity to feel safe from those whose behaviour is considered dangerous to the many) so that security is not conceptualized as an entity in its own right, but its existence is expressed via the needs of the individual. If this approach is adopted it may then be possible to ensure that the focus of security within controlled environments is directed towards the requirements of the patient or client instead of towards a blanket provision (Fig. 27.4). This redefinition of traditional thought would acknowledge the political climate and re-enforce the tenets of the advocacy movement by defining a clearer focus for health care activities upon the individual's requirements for safety and security.

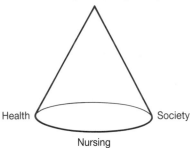

Fig. 27.4 *A person-centred forensic nursing model: the primary of the concept of the individual.*

THE INDIVIDUAL RECIPIENT OF FORENSIC NURSING CARE

What exactly is a human being—and what are human security needs? A human being (female or male) is a sentient being with unique features that characterize that individual and which set him or her apart from other individuals, and the integration of these individualizing characteristics is known as personality. Persons are, in the main, gregarious, actively seeking the companionship of others, and an individual constantly affects and is affected by the human and material environments in which he or she lives—Rogers (1970) eloquently explains the mechanisms by which the human and environmental energy fields interact.

All human beings have security needs which are required to be met prior to the human being experiencing growth. Maslow (1954) has postulated that the fulfilment of these fundamental needs—safety, affiliation and development to an advanced cognitive and/or affective level—will allow the individual to experience full personhood or 'self-actualization'. Erickson (1963) has further proposed that tensions occurring at key psychosocial stages in the development of a human being may, if not resolved, cause feelings of anxiety, insecurity and inadequacy leading to a failure to actualize or to achieve the full potential for growth. Erickson's stages of development are expressed as psychosocial crises including:

1 Trust v. mistrust
2 Autonomy v. shame and doubt
3 Initiative v. guilt

4 Industry v. inferiority
5 Identity v. confusion
6 Intimacy v. isolation
7 Generativity v. stagnation
8 Integrity v. despair

Failure to achieve, or to complete development at these stages will lead to feelings of insecurity and a form of non-maturation characterized by regression, anxiety reactions and possible mental disorder.

Bowlby (1988) linked his own innovative thinking to the more traditional evolutionary and ethological schools of thought to suggest that many innate behaviours are designed to ensure that the infant secures her/his existence, and that the needs for psychological attachment to the primary care givers are similarly innate mechanisms that activate when the infant feels threatened or anxious by a potential breech of the security afforded by the relationship with its supportive and nurturing carers. Therefore whilst an infant's cry may signal that the child is uncomfortable or hungry, the cry may also signal that the child wishes to feel the security of being touched and embraced by the carer. The feelings of reassurance and security are a necessary corollary to the physical care given to the baby otherwise the infant may fail to thrive and experience problems with coping with experiences later in life.

Human beings have the capability to afford each other rights so that minimum standards for security of existence and quality of life may be attained by all. A number of bodies set the rights of groups of people at both national and international level and some organizations codify their members' rights within their constitutions, whilst still others prefer their rights to evolve as the society evolves. In the 1990s a refreshing consensus has emerged that mentally disordered persons are citizens who retain the full rights of citizenship unless their behaviours render them incapable of exercising the responsibilities of citizenship. The following indicators represent the minimum value set to be associated with the rights accorded to persons within psychiatric care facilities:

All patients are entitled to:

Life sustaining food, fluid, warmth and shelter
Humane treatment and freedom from fear
Freedom of conscience, thought and action
Freedom of expression, suggestion and complaint
Maintenance of their liberty
Confidentiality regarding their affairs
Affiliations and relationships of their choice
Socialize with others
Information necessary to attain their rights
Organizational systems to safeguard rights
Be informed of the temporary infringement of their rights should it become necessary, recording of those infringements and regular review, and explanations being given to bona fide interested parties
External monitoring of the maintenance of their rights by advocacy agencies

---

Human rights should be limited only if the exercising of rights by an individual involves unnecessarily compromising that person's security, and/or failing to take reasonable account of the rights and security requirements of others.

By conceptualizing mental disorder as a temporary imbalance within the citizen who retains the rights of citizenship unless he or she is incapable of acting responsibly, and by viewing security as a developmental and existential requirement of the individual, it is possible to adopt a fluid rather than institutional view of service provision and to engender a more enlightened attitude to those whose behaviours are deemed to be dangerous. The nurse will be seeking opportunities to reduce restrictions and empower the mentally disordered person—rather than seeking to uphold a hypothetical norm by the adoption of security world view methods of working.

Patients are human beings currently experiencing illness events, which may necessarily include a period of detention for their own safety or the safety of others. However, whilst detained, mentally disordered patients retain their individual rights unless they fail to act responsibly whilst exercising those rights (it is important to strike the balance between the rights and responsibilities of citizenship). Neilson (1992) has described how in-patients within a controlled environment may be encouraged to participate in exercising their rights and responsibilities as a therapeutic activity.

Individuals detained in controlled environments retain their entitlement to resume their places in society at large when their illness events are over, or to be cared for in a less secure facility at the end of the acute illness event or when dangerousness is diminished. It should be remembered that individuals, whether detained by law or otherwise, are presumed to be capable of exercising informed consent concerning the services and care offered to them unless the strict criteria are met within which treatment against the individual's wishes would be permitted by the Mental Health Act, 1983.

HUMAN SOCIETY AND THE HUMAN SECURITY CONTEXT

Human beings organize themselves into communities or societies for affiliative and security reasons. The accompanying process of socialization is characterized by the harmonization of the individual's values, beliefs, customs and the creation of laws, so that societies themselves develop unique characteristics and cultural attributes. From this scenario it may be deduced that mental health will be indicated by the acquisition of socially determined and culturally acceptable forms of behaviour and patterns of thought, and that individuals not similarly socialized or encultured may be prone to being judged, and possibly be found wanting, by the host societies' standards.

As hospitals are merely microsocieties that to a large extent reflect the characteristics of the macrosociety, forensic nurses must remain aware of the situation of persons alien to the British culture, or reared within subcultures or ethnic minority groups, who may be wrongly determined as being mentally disordered. Stigmatization of individuals from abroad or from subcultures and ethnic groups on mental ill-health grounds is more likely than stigmatization of individuals from the indigenous population. A forensic nursing service alert to these pitfalls will provide guidelines for staff members to care for service users from minority groups, and will encourage an on-going dialogue with service users' representative bodies and advocates.

Individuals and societies have constant needs for security of existence, though sadly human history is a catalogue of failed attempts of human groups to co-exist peacefully, and Fromm (1975) has suggested that human beings are fatally flawed in this regard, that destructiveness is a predisposition within the very fabric, or anatomy, of human existence.

This century has seen many wars and skirmishes as well as two World Wars, during which the human potentials for dangerous behaviours and destructiveness have been given their full head. Earlier in the century, however, a League of Nations was formed in an attempt to allow national entities to co-exist peacefully, trade, and settle disputes in a non-aggressive manner, and in 1948 the League of Nations was superseded by the United Nations (UN) with the following agenda:

> 'To save succeeding generations from the scourge of war, which twice in our life-time has brought untold sorrow to mankind, and to reaffirm faith in fundamental human rights, in the dignity and worth of the human person, in the equal rights of men and of nations large and small, and to establish conditions under which justice and respect ... can be maintained, and to promote social progress and better standards of life in larger freedom ...'.

Currently 166 nations subscribe to these noble aims, which are concerned with the security of nations and individuals as the fundamental bedrock upon which growth and prosperity may be set.

The UN Charter (Europa, 1992) specifies a number of organs, one of which is the Security Council (Articles 7, 23–32) whose function is to safeguard the sovereignty of nations by the peaceful resolution of disputes, or by force as a last resort (Articles 39–43). The UN has also established its own International Court of Justice to enable the resolution of international disputes without recourse to armed conflict.

Each continental region of the world has developed its own form to minimize risks to security because of international disputes. Within Europe this takes the form of the European Economic Community (EEC) and the Conference on Security and Co-operation in Europe (CSCE). The EEC was established in 1958 by the Treaty of Rome, and the CSCE in 1972 (its tenets are to be found in the Helsinki Final Act of 1975). Whilst the EEC is principally concerned with economic co-operation, the CSCE is a forum by which threats to security may be resolved on a pan-European basis. Two judicial bodies, the Court of Justice of the European Communities and the Court of Auditors of the European Communities along with the European Commission of Human Rights exist to resolve the disputes between member nations, and between the governments and citizens of member nations.

The hope of the human family for security of existence and an increasing quality of life rests with these supranational entities as guarantors of global security, otherwise the relentless and unavoidable nature of conflict and the insecurity that is bred by political and economic instability will deleteriously affect the well-being and mental health status of every individual within this global village.

At national level each nation has its own mechanisms for dealing with internal security issues, though perhaps no group is more problematic to a government in this regard than those citizens who refuse to abide by the law without obvious reason, or whose behaviour causes great offence or concern for safety to the many. Whilst the vast majority of these problematic individuals—the mentally disordered—are a threat to no one, a small minority could be described as dangerous and therefore the requirement exists for them to be detained in secure facilities—they are largely to be found in the special hospitals, the medium-secure units and the prisons. Currently the special hospitals house 1,700 patients, the medium-secure units house circa 600 patients, and the prisons around 14,700 persons who are estimated to be mentally disordered (Gunn *et al.*, 1991). The Reed Committee (1992) is recommending an increase to 1,600 beds within the medium-secure provision. The needs for low-security provision at

district level are more problematic to estimate, but the Glancy Report (1975) recommended 2,000 beds.

Currently the low-security provision is seriously underfunded—though one or two health trusts, and some private hospitals are now starting to realize the business potential of this area of need. The funding of the current arrangements is known as an 'inverted pyramid', the majority of money being focused at the high-security end, with the medium-secure sector being relatively underfunded, and the low-security sector being significantly underfunded. A challenge for the 1990s is to rectify this situation so that the majority of funds are concentrated at the point of highest need—the low-security part of the system. Although a reduction in special hospital beds would free up some capital, a major investment programme will be necessary by the Government with monies for the capitation and 'pump priming' of the new low security or 'Glancy' type services.

MENTAL HEALTH AND THE FORENSIC NURSING CONTEXT

Health is a state of optimum functioning in the whole individual as an integrated entity and not merely the absence of disease (WHO, 1966). Illness is a state of non-optimum functioning in a part, or the whole of the individual, and permanent forms of illness are disabilities of that optimum functioning that may be found in the general population. A complex and reciprocal relationship exists between the physical, psychological, social and spiritual domains within an individual so that the health and illness status of each domain affects, and is affected by, the status of the other domains.

Mental health is a most precarious area in which to offer a definition because of its inextricable link with cultural determinants. Also, definitions of mental health do not travel easily, and it is extremely injurious for one culture to attempt to enforce its norms upon another. When deciding whether or not an individual is mentally healthy a number of factors should be taken into account including the norms for that individual and his or her family and the abilities of the individual to stay within the legal and the social boundaries of the host culture. Where the individual believes a threat to his or her security exists (without corroborative evidence), or where the individual represents a threat to the security of others (because of problems associated with his or her mental state) the individual may be experiencing an illness event that may require treatment in a controlled, residential facility.

Hershenson *et al.* (1989) offer the following useful parameters to consider when assessing the mental state of an individual, and it is suggested that positive indicators within these criteria signal a state of mental health:

The capacity for survival

The capacity for growth

Identifying with clear boundaries and contexts

An integrated personality

The capacity for adaptation

An internal locus of control

Reality-based perception and response to stimuli

An ability to learn from experience

Coherence of thought, feeling and action

Constructive activity

A willingness to accept challenges

Intellectual curiosity

A concern for others

A future orientation

A hopeful outlook

It is important to remember that whilst an individual may be experiencing problems or insecurities in one or a number of these areas people are extremely resilient and are often capable of maintaining a reasonable existence despite experiencing ill health. Mental health (rehabilitation) nursing begins with the identification of those positive

characteristics of mental health still intact within an individual and the development of nursing strategies to strengthen the positive aspects of the individual whilst treating out the disordered behaviours.

A combined rehabilitation and treatment approach allows the patient to feel secure within his or her strengths and enables the community to be reassured that the aberrant behaviours are being addressed.

All individuals, whether temporarily mentally disordered, chronically mentally ill, personality disordered or permanently disabled (mentally impaired or severely mentally impaired), have the right to health care that encourages positive coping strategies directed towards achieving the optimum quality of life for that person. Forensic nurses should seek to maximize mental health (whilst treating mental disorder with colleagues from other disciplines) by the adoption of a model of working that is designed to maximize the positive aspects of the patient's mental health rather than the traditional role of custodian of the incarcerated mentally disordered.

DANGEROUSNESS AND ITS SIGNIFICANCE FOR FORENSIC NURSING

Two characteristics immediately set the forensic nurse apart from other nurses, the first being the role concerning the maintenance of security, and secondly the role concerning assessing and caring for the dangerous individual.

Dangerousness is an ill-defined concept that is used too loosely, in part because a definitive model to predict dangerousness accurately has not yet been developed, and because the context and meaning of the word is confused. Some decision-making processes that lead to a diagnosis of dangerousness are non-rational or biased towards professional ideologies (e.g. see Pfohl, 1978; Hepworth, 1982 (sociological model); Marra *et al.*, 1987 (psychological model); Blueglass, 1988 (psychiatric model); Binder and McNiel, 1988 (medical model) for a wider discussion); the concept is 'not even admissible' (Conrad, 1983). Larsen (1976) provides a fascinating discussion upon the myths surrounding the concepts of aggression, violence and dangerousness; and Pollock and Webster (1989) give an illuminating account of clinical decision-making and the assessment of dangerousness.

Hollin (1989) reviews the contemporary literature which attempts to assert a correlation between criminal behaviours and mental disorder, and it would appear that the American literature is far more positive about a correlation than are the European writings; Hollin draws some interesting conclusions about the limitations of the behavioural sciences in what is, more realistically, a sociological domain. Tardiff (1989) has published a most useful pocketbook concerning the assessment and management of violent patients, which provides immediately accessible and applicable information for use in the clinical setting.

For the purposes of forensic nursing, dangerousness should be understood as the probability that an individual will commit a violent act upon the person of another (or others) in the near or distant future, if afforded the opportunity to do so. In the absence of definitive criteria the assessment of risk to others should encompass the following:

---

1   The severity of the antisocial behaviour

2   Previous offences or abnormal behaviour

3   The presence or assumption of mental disorder

4   Circumstances of the antisocial behaviour

5   The personality of the individual

6   The social background and life-career of the person

7   The social control and support available

8   Uncertainty about cause and unexpectedness or perceived abnormality of the behaviour

9   Intuitive feelings about the individual

These assessment criteria, proposed by Hepworth (1985) are most useful indicators from which forensic nurses can make a valid contribution to the deliberations of the multidisciplinary team. Nurses in the high-, medium- and low-security sectors must ensure their full participation in the assessment of dangerousness by developing models on which to base their opinions that are methodologically defensible and reliable in their predictability—though it has to be said that work undertaken so far, largely by colleagues from psychology and sociology is disappointing—there may in fact be no one model with true utility, and therefore professional judgement, albeit subjective and fallible, will continue to be the final arbiter in the difficult risk-taking decisions that the forensic multidisciplinary team must face.

FORENSIC NURSING

Nursing is an activity licensed by society concerning assessing, planning, implementing and evaluating strategies of care designed to assist individuals to return to a state of health, or to assist with an acceptable adjustment to a state of disability or loss. Nursing care is mediated by the therapeutic investment of self and as such is both an objective and subjective activity, a science and an art, and the process of nursing is indivisible from the interpersonal nature of human existence.

Psychiatric nursing is concerned with promoting mental health, arresting and limiting psychological disorders, and with assisting human beings in mental health endeavours (Antonovsky, 1979). Forensic nursing is about 'the employment of those skills necessary to address the needs of the ill individual who has offended, or is likely to offend, or who remains subject to detention within the terms of legislation' (ENB, 1989), although occasionally forensic nurses do care for individuals who have not originated from the clinical justice system, but whose mental state is deemed treatable within secure settings.

Patients are entitled to expect the highest standards of good health care practice from forensic nurses who are subject to professional scrutiny against set criteria laid down in the *Code of Professional Conduct* (UKCC, 1992a) and are advanced practitioners in terms of the *Scope of Professional Practice* (UKCC, 1992b). They do, however, share much in common with nursing colleagues whose names appear on other parts of the professional register and those working in high security areas in particular must remain apprised of contemporary practices within the wider health service.

Many believe forensic nursing to be an emergent specialist branch of nursing in the UK. For this to be the case the profession will have to demonstrate a clear knowledge base, and articulate a systematic methodology for delivering care. Although the first three years' experience of the ENB 770 course 'Nursing in Controlled Environments' has begun to address the identification of this body of knowledge acceptability within the scientific community will only come about with the publication of conventional research papers within professional journals both within and beyond nursing—papers published so far are few in number, but are of a high calibre. The special hospitals maintain a register of research papers and projects by their staff and it is to be hoped that nurses will play an increasing part in future research activities within controlled environments.

Three years of experience with ENB 770 at Ashworth Hospital suggest that the knowledge base to be researched and developed lies within the broad areas of core curriculum material; principles of nursing in controlled environments; forensic psychiatric nursing, and associated studies and sciences:

Knowledge base for forensic nursing

Core curriculum
  Maintaining professional roles
  Management of services and the change process
  Standards setting and quality assurance
  Teaching and learning
  Research
  Health promotion
  Use of information technology

Principles of nursing in controlled environments
  Psychiatric nursing within controlled environments
  Provision of services and security designs

Principles of normalization
Ethics, law and professional accountability
The concept of dangerousness
Therapeutic use of security
Personal stress management

Forensic psychiatric nursing
  Promotion of mental health
  Patient advocacy
  Self-awareness and reflectivity
  Communication studies
  Social (interpersonal) skills
  Values underpinning service design/delivery
  Concepts, theories and models
  Counselling
  Contemporary issues affecting care
  Psychodynamic psychotherapy
  Behavioural psychotherapy
  Social psychotherapy
  Family therapy
  Psychosexual counselling
  Drug, alcohol and substance misuse
  Victims of abuse
  Management of dangerousness
  Personal and organizational security
  Community nursing studies/Court Diversion schemes
  Control of infection

Associated studies and sciences
  European/international studies
  Social policy/politics
  Psychology
  Sociology
  Criminology
  Psychiatry/pharmacology
  Women's studies

Another area that is under-researched is the skills base of forensic nursing. Niskala (1986) identified a list of 13 core competencies about which skills are clustered:

Niskala's competencies and skills

Maintain security

Communicate effectively

Maintain records

Counselling

Perform nursing process

Plan/participate in programme

Conduct/participate in groups

Administrative functions

Diagnostic and treatment procedures

Maintain professional role

Psychiatric nursing modalities

Research

Instruct offenders

Some of Niskala's competencies are somewhat disappointing, though perhaps these reflect the status of nursing as a profession in North America. Students of the ENB 770 course at Ashworth Hospital have identified far more competencies, which seem to suggest that forensic nurses possess all the competencies listed in the syllabus of training for Part 3 (and 5 in the case of the nurses caring for the mentally impaired) of the professional register (ENB, 1982) but to a far more honed extent. Additional skill areas that are being identified concern the management of the security aspects of controlled environments and the management of dangerousness and challenging behaviours. Although the skills required of forensic nurses will vary from high- to medium- to low-security services (and indeed even within units) the core skills of forensic nursing can be related to the essential knowledge base:

Forensic nursing skills

Core skills
Study skills/information acquisition skills
Professional etiquette skills
Management of human resources
Management of services/multidisciplinary working
Management of change
Standards setting and quality assurance
Teaching and learning

Research awareness skills, researching skills
Health promotion
Information technology and use of information

Skills of nurses in controlled environments
Psychiatric nursing (refreshment of base competencies)
Environmental design and management
Application of normalization programmes
Clinical application of ethics and law
Assessment of dangerousness (to self and others)
Therapeutic use of security
Methods of physical control and restraint
Cardio-pulmonary resuscitation
Personal stress management

Forensic psychiatric nursing skills
Promotion of mental health
Assisting patient with self-advocacy/advocating
Self-awareness and reflectivity
Communication skills
Social (interpersonal) skills
Operationalization of professional values
Utilization of professional knowledge base
Counselling
Psychodynamic psychotherapy
Behavioural psychotherapy
Social psychotherapy
Family therapy
Psychosexual counselling
Working with abusers of alcohol/drugs/substances
Working with victims of abuse
Management of dangerousness (to self and others)
Personal and organizational security
Control of infection

The further elucidation of both the knowledge and skills bases of the profession will be facilitated by the adoption of a systematic process of nursing in all forensic nursing environments, computerization of nursing records to create a more readily accessible empirical knowledge base, and the switch to primary nursing and the move towards the 'named nurse' approach (Patient's Charter Group, 1991; Manthey, 1992).

The process of forensic nursing

There are two processes of nursing, the first is an intuitive, and therefore subjective approach, in which the nurse cares for and assists an individual on the basis of the nurse's feelings and experience; the second is a positivistic, systematic and objective method for analysing care needs. Whilst it is possible to nurse quite effectively using one or both of the processes, interventions formulated using the 'gut feeling' approach are hard to defend as no two practitioner's judgements, when based upon intuition, will be the same. The systematic method, however, will yield data concerning the process of care that will facilitate the identification of effective intervention strategies, and this method forms the base for the way nursing care is delivered in the UK. The systematic process of nursing, or the 'nursing process' has the following attributes:

Assessment of the patient's needs

Planning care to address the needs

Implementation of the care strategies

Evaluation of the outcome

According to Mulhearn (1989) whilst the use of artful intuition is valuable, the acceptance of the nursing process may 'enhance clinical credibility, accountability and communication, especially among novices'. If forensic nurses wish to enhance their clinical credibility they must use the data derived from the process of nursing to identify effective nursing interventions (it should be remembered that some patients will respond to interventions and treatment quite slowly, in some instances over years) and the analysis of past care plans and outcomes is a most suitable place to start. There are literally thousands of care plans from discharged patients lying under-utilized within medical records departments up and down the country. Some haste is necessary in this matter, for a number of trusts within the UK are

actively considering care programming methods of working—and unless forensic nurses can contribute with diagnoses and care plan formulations that can adequately predict outcomes, then other disciplines, which are in a position to do that, will tend to dominate the construction of care plans.

In controlled environments therefore forensic nurses should consider the adoption of an enhanced nursing process:

Particular data collection—observation of factors indicative of health/ill health

General data collection—global assessment of the patient as a whole

Nursing diagnosis

Care planning, in agreement with the patient and stipulating specific care outcomes

Marshalling of required resources and delivery of care

Evaluation of the nursing care delivered against the specified outcomes

---

An annual audit of care plans will reveal those diagnoses and types of care prescribed that are most effective within given parameters of requirement.

As each forensic facility has a different function—high-, medium- or low-security—each with a different mission (and indeed within each category different units have 'speciality' interests) it is difficult to construct a model assessment document that is applicable to all. As a profession, however, forensic nurses must agree on a common approach in order to facilitate the development of forensic nursing diagnoses. (Examples of systematically structured pre-admission and post-admission assessment documents which may be coded for computerized analysis at annual audits are available from the author.)

The methodical review of care assessment documentation and care plans will allow forensic nurses to identify commonly derived nursing diagnoses and to prescribe the appropriate nursing care to be given for each identified requirement. Some members of the profession are unwilling to go down the road of nursing diagnoses as they can limit the scope of creative nursing. However, nurses faced with justifying their practises after the event, often with inadequate written records, will attest to the value of a more systematic approach to caring—despite its more time-consuming nature.

Nursing diagnoses are clinical judgements about the individual, family, or community responses to actual and potential health problems/life processes (Kim *et al.*, 1991). A nursing diagnosis provides the basis for the selection of nursing interventions to achieve outcomes for which the nurse is accountable. The North American Nursing Diagnosis Association (NANDA) has already approved 100 diagnoses, some of which are of immediate utility within forensic nursing:

NANDA diagnoses suitable for use within forensic nursing

Anxiety
Body image disturbance
Communication, impaired verbal
Coping (various)
Decisional conflict (specify)
Denial, ineffective
Diversional activity deficit
Family processes, altered
Fatigue
Fear
Grieving (various)
Growth and development, altered
Health maintenance, altered
Health-seeking behaviours (specify)
Hopelessness
Knowledge deficit (specify)
Non-compliance (specify)
Parental role conflict
Parenting, altered (various)
Personal identity disturbance
Post-trauma response
Powerlessness
Protection, altered
Rape-trauma syndrome (various)
Role performance, altered
Self-care deficit (various)
Self-esteem disturbance (various)
Sensory/perceptual alterations
Sexual dysfunction
Sexuality patterns, altered
Sleep pattern disturbance
Social interaction, impaired
Social isolation
Spiritual distress
Thought processes, altered
Unilateral neglect
Violence, potential for (directed at self/others)

Once units have gained experience in working with NANDA and other home-grown nursing diagnoses they may then start to amend assessment materials to highlight areas for investigation that will enable accurate and efficient diagnoses to be made. Standard care plans may then be developed (see Gorman *et al.*, 1989; Fortinash *et al.*, 1991 and Haber *et al.*, 1992, for examples of systematic care plans of value to forensic nurses) and these care plans will do much to secure resources for the nursing care of patients, especially where intensive care or rich skills mixes are required. They provide a cogent base from which to make the case for extra resources, especially as they indicate performance criteria attached to each nursing intervention arising from the diagnosis.

The day-to-day work of forensic nurses concerns the therapeutic investment of security within a caring relationship which is designed to nurture a return to mental health for that patient. All patients may benefit from a given set of universal nursing interventions that may be incorporated into core and standard care plans which the patient may be offered during the initial assessment and diagnostic phase. Some, however, will require more advanced forms of nursing intervention, designed where possible by the nurse and patient in collaboration, in order to address the patient's health care requirements. A recent survey at Ashworth Hospital (Tarbuck *et al.*, 1992) has indicated that patients may benefit from up to 27 forms of specialist nursing intervention, the 10 most useful of which would be:

(*n* = 389 patients)

Counselling (one-to-one verbal therapy) 34.2%

Group psychotherapy	21.9%
Social skills training	21.1%
Anger management training	15.1%
Behaviour therapy	14.9%
Psychosexual counselling	13.9%
Reality therapy	13.6%
Cognitive behavioural therapy	11.8%
Relaxation therapy (including autogenics)1 1.6%	
Dramatherapy	8.7%

These data have clear implications for the preparation of nurses at post-registration level and also for the development of advanced nurse practitioners within a clinical nursing specialist framework.

Once a series of planned interventions has been delivered, the nursing care should be evaluated by the patient and nurse together, and the plan be amended to include new objectives to be attained. Evaluation criteria would include the attainment of goals and objectives, the time frame within which the objectives have been achieved, and the patient's level of satisfaction with the care being offered. In the rare case where a patient is incapable of understanding the care plan or contributing to its construction, or refuses to participate in the process, the patient's relatives must be kept aware of the nursing care programme and their agreement to its delivery should be sought.

Standards of care within forensic nursing

The report of the Boynton committee (1980) suggested that it is unwise for organizations to let individual practitioners set the minimum standards of exceptable performance as, presumably, each person's standards are different and therefore there will be no corporate baseline from which to subsequently measure. There exists a legal responsibility placed upon the managers of forensic facilities to set standards that not only reflect the best possible practice, but also the minimum standards for attainment by which the

performance of all members of staff may be evaluated. With this in mind, the SHSA has produced its own target standards for the special hospitals concerning forensic nursing—encompassing such areas as patient-centred practice; meeting patients' needs; assuring the service; education and practice; nursing teamwork; multidisciplinary teamwork; forging links with outside agencies, and nursing management. It is to be hoped that the medium-secure and low-security settings will similarly publish target standards to be attained within their services.

It should be remembered that true standards of attainment and quality enhancement can only occur in an environment that recognizes total quality management (Royal College of Nursing (RCN) 1991), and that a total quality service will include quality specifications at every juncture of its activities and requires constant commitment and vigilance to maintain the ground that has been gained; Clifford *et al.* (1989) provide a summary of the issues associated with assuring quality in the mental health services—the QUARTZ method.

In 1986 the RCN Society of Psychiatric Nursing published a set of standards for the profession (to their credit well in advance of other members of the nursing family). Those standards represented an enhanced version of the American Nurses' Association professional standards.

Professional standards for nursing

Professional Standard 1
The nurse applies appropriate theory that is scientifically sound as a basis for decisions regarding nursing practice.

Professional Standard 2
The nurse continuously collects data that are comprehensive, accurate and systematic.

Professional Standard 3
The nurse utilizes nursing diagnoses and standard classifications of mental disorder to express conclusions supported by recorded assessment data and current scientific premises.

Professional Standard 4
The nurse develops a nursing care plan with

specific goals and interventions delineating nursing actions unique to each patient's needs.

Professional Standard 5
The nurse intervenes as guided by the nursing care plan to implement nursing actions that promote, maintain, or restore physical and mental health, prevent illness, and effect rehabilitation.

Professional Standard 6
The nurse evaluates responses to nursing actions in order to revise the data base, nursing diagnoses and nursing care plan.

The introductory comments to the RCN document are still valid today:

'... the development of individualized nursing care plans, and the continuing debate on accountability have highlighted the need for the nursing profession to establish agreed standards of care'.

Most NHS-controlled environments are now beginning to articulate their standards of care, which the service users are entitled to examine as a result of the Patient's Charter (1991). In order to assist individuals the RCN has published its 'DySSY' system of standards setting (1990). DySSY suggests that a standard statement should be made by the workforce (to attempt to engender ownership), and then three criteria are articulated by which the standard may be addressed—structure (environment and resources); process (nursing actions), and outcomes (expected achievements). A comprehensive compilation of works concerning standard setting and quality maintenance and measurement from a variety of perspectives is to be found in Green and Lewis (1986), and the processes of standard setting, quality assurance, auditing and quality enhancement are explored.

The NHS Management Executive has been keen to encourage nurses to engage in the process of care auditing and has published a guide entitled 'Measuring the Quality' (1991). This approach follows a cyclical method of observing; standards setting; data collection; monitoring; action planning; making changes; and evaluating and reporting to give regular information regarding the quality functions of a service. Robinson (1991), breaking new ground in forensic care, developed a comprehensive auditing tool known as 'OSCAR' that is now being used in two special hospitals. It provides immediately useable information that can be used to set standards to improve the service. Robinson and his colleagues at Rampton Special Hospital are currently experimenting with more sophisticated forms of audit including the use of hand-held computers.

Whichever approach to standards setting a controlled environment decides to adopt, and whichever quality assurance and enhancement mechanisms are used to assess forensic nursing care, they must be capable of clearly demonstrating the achievement or otherwise of corporate and care planning goals.

CONCLUSION—TOWARDS AD 2000

During the last decade a new branch of psychiatric nursing has emerged relating to the care of mentally disordered offenders within controlled environments—forensic nursing. Forensic nursing has a conceptual base that is compatible with modern thought surrounding the nature of nursing within the paradigms of the individual, society, health and nursing. The paradigms can be conceptually related within a model that seeks to affirm that individuals have security needs and that the therapeutic investment of security by forensic nurses will assist with the transition of patients back into the host society after the illness event and period of dangerousness is over. Forensic nurses can do much to enrich the multidisciplinary milieu of care by the identification and articulation of an appropriate knowledge base and the development of forensic nursing practitioners with advanced roles. This new nursing speciality is currently taking its first faltering steps upon this painful, though exhilarating, path.

The areas for research into forensic nursing are becoming clearer and some areas are starting to be explored in a systematic manner, including the nursing requirements of forensic patients; the knowledge base; the competency and skills bases;

and the standards setting and quality enhancement processes.

As we approach the year AD 2000 the UK health care system is in a state of accelerated change and great uncertainty exists. Forensic nurses must not let the development of an internal market within controlled health care environments deleteriously affect the maturation of the profession, and to this end forensic nurses must unite with one accord—to offer consistently enhanced quality of forensic nursing care to patients and clients via the development of the academic base of the profession.

By the year AD 2000 all forensic nurses, be they working in high-, medium- or low-security environments, must become known for the expertise and abilities that will ensure public confidence in their activities—forensic nurses must become informed doers.

FURTHER READING

Bowlby, J. (1988) *A Secure Base—Clinical Applications of Attachment Theory*. London: Tavistock/Routledge.

Burrow, S. (1991) The special hospital nurse and the dilemma of therapeutic custody. *Journal of Advances in Health and Nursing Care*, **1** (3), 21–28.

Bynoe, I. (1992) *Treatment, Care and Security*. London: MIND.

Department of Health and Welsh Office (1991) *Code of Practice Mental Health Act 1983*. London: HMSO.

Erickson, E. (1963) *Childhood and Society*, 2nd edition. New York: Norton.

Fawcett, J. (1989) *Analysis and Evaluation of Conceptual Models of Nursing*, 2nd edition. Philadelphia: A. Davis.

George, J. (1989) *Nursing Theories—the Base for Professional Nursing Practice*, 3rd edition. London: Prentice-Hall International.

Hepworth, D. (1985) Dangerousness and the Mental Health Review Tribunal. In Farrington, D. & Gunn, J. (Eds) *Aggression and Dangerousness*. London: Wiley.

Maslow, A. (1954) *Motivation and Personality*. New York: Harper & Row.

Niskala, H. (1986) Competencies and skills required by nurses working in forensic areas. *West. J. of N. Research*, **8** (4), 400–413.

REFERENCES

Antonovsky, A. (1979) *Health, Stress and Illness*. Josse-Bass.

Binder, R. & McNiel, D. (1988) Effects of diagnosis and context on dangerousness. *American Journal of Psychiatry*, **145** (6), 728–736.

Blueglass, R. (1988) Psychiatric approaches to aggression and violence. In Howells, K. & Hollin, C. (Eds) *Clinical Approaches to Aggression and Violence. (Issues in Criminological and Legal Psychology*, **12**). British Psychological Society.

Bowlby, J. (1988) *A Secure Base—Clinical Applications of Attachment Theory*. London: Tavistock/Routledge.

Boynton Report (1980) *Report on the Review of Rampton Hospital*. London: HMSO.

Burrow, S. (1991) The special hospital nurse and the dilemma of therapeutic custody. *Journal of Advances in Health and Nursing Care*, **1** (3), 21–28.

Bynoe, I. (1992) *Treatment, Care and Security*. London: MIND.

Clifford, P. (1989) *Assuring Quality in Mental Health Services*. London: RDP/Free Association Books.

Conrad, J. (1983) *The Dangerous and the Endangered*. Lexington: Lexington Books.

Department of Health (1983) *The Mental Health Act*. London: HMSO.

Department of Health (1991a) *The Patient's Charter*. London: HMSO.

Department of Health (1992) *Report of the Committee of Inquiry into Complaints about Ashworth Hospital*, Vols 1 & 2. London: HMSO.

Department of Health and Welsh Office (1991b) *Code of Practice Mental Health Act 1983*. London: HMSO.

Dyer, L. (1991) Opinion: special hospitals. *Mental Health Supplement. Nursing Times*, **87** (39), 69.

English National Board (1982) *Syllabus of Training for Part 3 of the Professional Register*. London: ENB.

ENB (1982) *Syllabus of Training for Part 5 of the Professional Register*. London: ENB.

ENB (1989) *Outline Curriculum No. 770 'Nursing in Controlled Environments' Course No. 770*. London: ENB.

Erickson, E. (1963) *Childhood and Society*, 2nd edition. New York: Norton.

Europa (1992) *World Year Book 1992*. London: Europa.

European Commission of Human Rights (1981) *Report of a visit to Broadmoor Hospital. Case No. 6870/75*.

Fawcett, J. (1989) *Analysis and Evaluation of Conceptual Models of Nursing*, 2nd edition. Philadelphia: A. Davis.

Fortinash, K. & Holoday-Worret, P. (1991) *Psychiatric Nursing Care Plans. Mosby Year Book*. New York: Mosby.

Foucalt, M. (1965) *Madness and Civilization*. New York: Pantheon Books.

Fromm, A. (1975) *The Anatomy of Human Destructiveness*. London: Penguin.

George, J. (1989) *Nursing Theories—the Base for Professional Nursing Practice*, 3rd edition. London: Prentice-Hall International.

Glancy Report (1975) *Revised Report of the Working Party on Security within NHS Psychiatric Hospitals*. London: HMSO.

Goffman, E. (1961) *Asylums*. Chicago: Aldine Press.

Gorman, K., Sultan, D. & Luna-Raines, M. (1989) *Psychosocial Nursing Handbook for the Non-psychiatric Nurse*. New York: Williams & Wilkins.

Green, L. & Lewis, F. (1986) *Measurement and Evaluation in Health Education and Health Promotion*. California: Mayfield.

Gunn, J., Maden, T. & Swinton, M. (1991) *Mentally Disordered Prisoners*. London: Home Office.

Haber, J. *et al.* (1992) *Comprehensive Psychiatric Nursing. Mosby Year Book*, 2nd edition. New York: Mosby.

Hepworth, D. (1982) The influence of the concept of 'Danger' on the assessment of 'Danger to self and others'. *Med.Sci.Law*, **22** (4), 245–254.

Hepworth, D. (1985) Dangerousness and the mental health review tribunal. In Farrington, D. & Funn, J. (Eds) *Aggression and Dangerousness*. London: Wiley.

Herschenson *et al.* (1989) Mental health counselling theory. *Journal of Mental Health Counselling*, **11** (1), 44–69.

Hollin, C. (1989) *Psychology and Crime*. London: Routledge.

Kim, M., McFarland, G. & McLane, A. (1991) *Pocket Guide to Nursing Diagnoses. Mosby Year Book*. New York: Mosby.

Larsen, K. (1976) *Aggression: Myths and Models*. Chicago: Nelson-Hall.

Manthey, M. (1992) *The Practice of Primary Nursing*. London: King's Fund Centre.

Marra, H., Konzelman, G. & Giles, P. (1987) A clinical strategy to the assessment of dangerousness. *International Journal of Offender Therapy and Comparative Criminology*, **31**, 291–299.

Martin, J. (1984) *Hospitals in Trouble*. Oxford: Blackwell.

Maslow, A. (1954) *Motivation and Personality*. New York: Harper & Row.

Mason, T. & Patterson, R. (1990) A critical review of the use of Rogers' model within a special hospital: a single case study. *Journal of Advanced Nursing*, **15**, 130–141.

Mulhearn, S. (1989) The nursing process: Improving psychiatric admission assessment? *Journal of Advanced Nursing*, **14**, 808–814.

Neilson, P. (1992) A secure philosophy. *Nursing Times*, **88** (8), 31–33.

NHS Management Executive (1991) Measuring the Quality: Nursing Care Audit. Bristol: NHSME.

Niskala, H. (1986) Competencies and skills required by nurses working in forensic areas. *West. J. of N. Research*, **8**, (4), 400–413.

Patient's Charter Group (1991) *The Named Nurse—Your Questions Answered*. London: HMSO.

Pfohl, S. (1978) *Predicting Dangerousness: the Social Construction of Psychiatric Reality*. Lexington: Heath.

Pilgrim, D. (1989) Psychotherapy in British Special Hospitals: a case of failure to thrive. *Free Associations*, **11**, 58–72.

Prins, H. (1991) Dangerous people or dangerous situations?—Some further thoughts. *Med.Sci.Law*, **31** (1), 25–37.

Pollock, N. & Webster, C. (1989) The clinical assessment of dangerousness. In Blueglass, R. & Bowden, P. (Eds) *Principles and Practice of Forensic Psychiatry*.

Riley, M. (1991) A collective responsibility. *Nursing Standard*, **5** (33), 18–20.

Rix, G. (1988) Care plan for an aggressive person. In Collister, B. (Ed.) *Psychiatric Nursing—Person to Person*. London: Edward Arnold.

Reed Committee (1992) *Review of Health and Social Services for Mentally Disordered Offenders and Others Requiring Similar Services*. London: Dept of Health/Home Office Consultation Documents.

'Reed Two' (1992) A Committee under the Chairmanship of Dr Reed, set up by the Minister for Health to examine high security service provision for mentally disordered offenders. The Minister announced the initiative in August and the Committee first met in October 1992.

Robinson, D. (1991) *Observational Standards of Care Audit and Review*, 2nd edition. Retford: Rampton Hospital.

Rogers, M. (1970) *An Introduction to the Theoretical Basis for Nursing*. Philadelphia: F. A. Davis.

Royal College of Nursing (1986) *Standards of Care in Psychiatric Nursing Practice*. London: RCN.

RCN (1990) *Quality Patient Care: the Dynamic Standard Setting System*. London: RCN.

RCN (1991) *Total Quality Management—A Framework for Quality Health Care*. London: RCN.

Special Hospitals Service Authority (1989) *Starting Afresh*. London: SHSA.

SHSA (1991) *Nursing in Special Hospitals*. London: SHSA.

Tarbuck, P. (Ed.) (1992) *Primary Nurses' Perceptions of Patients' Needs*. Analysis undertaken by the nursing staff of Ashworth Hospital.

Tardiff, K. (1989) *Concise Guide to Assessment and Management of the Violent Patient*. Washington: American Psychiatric Press.

Torres, G. (1989) The place of concepts and theories within nursing. In George, J. *Nursing Theories—the Base for Professional Nursing Practice*, 3rd edition. London: Prentice-Hall International.

UKCC (1992a) *Code of Professional Conduct*, 3rd edition. London: UKCC.

UKCC (1992b) *The Scope of Professional Practice*. London: UKCC.

World Health Organization (1966) *Statement on Health*. Geneva: WHO.

PART

V

POLICIES AND PRIORITIES

This section explores and analyses the present and future impact of recent changes in social policy on both nursing and the provision of care services. It identifies that the philosophy of particular governments, expressed through legislation, directly affects people experiencing mental health problems as well as those who are involved in their care. Practitioners, managers and educationists therefore have to be aware of emergent trends in order to plan their contributions effectively.

Nursing should be included as one of the essential elements of national health plans . . . and nurses should take part in the debate on health policy.

Recommendation 8 from the first WHO European Conference on Nursing

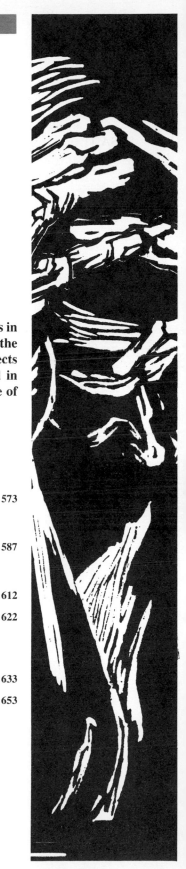

DEMARCATION AND THE PUBLIC SECTOR
THE IMPACT OF THE CONTRACT AGENDA UPON MENTAL HEALTH PRACTICE

John Brown

AIMS

i) To identify and analyse the changes taking place within the National Health Service and local government
ii) To explore the implications for nurses

KEY ISSUES

Policy parameters
Contract culture
The contractual cycle
Line-management implications
Training and education
The contract agenda

Identify, analyse and assess factors causing distress and illness	Promote health, provide direct care and make interventions	Manage care programmes and services
Be critical, analytical and accountable, continue professional development	Counter discrimination, inequality and individual and institutional racism	Work within and develop policies, laws and safeguards in all settings
Understand influences on mental health and the nature/causes of disorder and illness	Know the effects of distress, disorder, illness on individuals, groups, families	Understand the basis of treatments and interventions

INTRODUCTION

In the summer of 1992 the Government published its White Paper *The Health of the Nation* (DH, 1992a). Five priority target areas were identified, one of which was mental health. Three years earlier publication in another White Paper *Caring for People*, where proposals for community care were outlined, the only user-group to be allocated an entire chapter was mental health (DH, 1989c). Mental health, again, was the only group to have an earmarked grant. At the same time, within the National Health Service mental health nurses comprised one in six of all nurses (which increased to one in four if combined with learning disabilities) (DH, 1991a). Early in 1992 the Department of Health, recognizing the important contribution of mental health nurses, started a comprehensive review of their current and future role. Yet while factors such as these indicate the prominence of mental health in the policy arena the situation in which mental health nurses practise has changed dramatically, as it has for all nurses.

Shortly after publication of *The Health of the Nation*, a Government-commissioned report on medical facilities in London was published. In the Tomlinson Report arguments were forwarded for the merger and closure of London hospitals, a shift in resources away from acute to primary services, and suggestions made that hospital consultants might need to be made compulsorily redundant (DH, 1992b). Even a short time ago such possibilities would have appeared unthinkable.

The Tomlinson Report, more than any other recent report, reflects the dramatic changes that have taken place within the NHS and which are increasingly influencing local government. It is these changes, and some of their implications for mental health nurses, that form the basis of this overview. While the focus is upon the mental health nurse the emphasis is very much on how nursing as a whole is responding to a rapidly changing policy agenda.

POLICY PARAMETERS

Professions as trade unions

When the Conservative Party was returned to Government in 1979 it was pledged to undermine the power and influence of the trade union movement. Success in this area is probably best symbolized by the treatment of the National Union of Mineworkers in the dispute of 1984–85 and the NUM's subsequent decline. After tackling the formally attributed trade unions in the early 1980s the Government turned with undiminished vigour in the mid- to late-1980s to those occupations traditionally regarded as professions. This was not surprising.

When definitions of professions are stripped of their various elements a profession is, in essence, a trade union. While altruism and humanitarian concerns, along with aspirations to unique and highly skilled expertise, may provide the *raison d'être* of the profession it is still, none the less, concerned with the terms of employment, conditions and pay that protect its members' practice. It could come as no surprise, therefore, when the Government began to consider the situation of the professions. What has been a surprise, however, has been the speed and scope of the Government's success.

The medical profession, for example, has had a new contract imposed on general practice in spite of continued opposition from the BMA and, from what can be gleaned from various surveys, the majority of doctors. When the Government published *Promoting Better Health* in November 1987 it signalled its intention to alter the GP's contract that was to be taken forward in *Working for Patients* in January 1989 (DH, 1987, 1989a). By September of that year the press was reporting 'victory' for the Government (Smart, 1989) and in April 1990 a new contract was in place. From the initial public signals of intent to the introduction of new conditions of employment took less than two years—and this with one of the most powerful professional groups resisting the changes.

Medicine, however, was not alone in having its practices placed under the spotlight by the Government. The legal profession, like medicine well-established and with great emphasis placed upon the academic excellence of its practitioners, was told bluntly that:

> '... practitioners must be able to show their clients that they possess the necessary competence to perform the particular service sought from them ... (and that) the Government believes that it is not of itself sufficient for practitioners to belong to a particular branch of the legal profession ...'.
> *Lord Chancellor's Department, 1989*

Teaching, as will be shown below, also came under the spotlight. While nursing did not come under the same intense scrutiny as these other professions it was, none the less, an indication that no group could make assumptions about its future role.

Local salary negotiations

Excluding the armed forces, the NHS is the largest employer in north-west Europe with nursing the largest group of employees. Yet in the whole of the White Paper on the future of the NHS, *Working for Patients* there are only three references to nurses and nursing. Two of these references are to discretionary payments and local salary negotiations for the new NHS trusts:

> 'The Government has ... asked the Review Body to accept the case for more local discretionary payments to nurses to help with particular local staff shortages and nurse management problems'.
> *DH, 1989a*

and

> 'The Government also intends that NHS Hospital Trusts should be free to settle the pay and conditions of their staff, including doctors, nurses and others covered by national pay review bodies. ... NHS Hospital Trusts will be free either to continue to follow national pay agreements or to adopt partly or wholly different arrangements'.
> *DH, 1989a*

Such moves run counter to one of the main tenets of national salary scales where the same work is rewarded at the same level regardless of the part of the country where it is carried out (the London weighting being one exception to this). Indeed, one of the distinctive features of trade union history is the battle to establish national negotiating rights. This move away from tradition is well marked by the recent experience of the teaching profession.

After the dispute of 1986–87 the National Union of Teachers (NUT), the largest teaching union, lost its membership on the Burnham Committee which determines teachers' pay and conditions. As a result the Government was able to introduce an initiative, *Qualified Teacher Status*, with important implications not just for teaching but also nursing (DES, 1988). This initiative was quietly launched as a consultative document the same week that the Conservative Government announced its acceptance of Project 2000 at the 1988 RCN Annual Congress. This consultative document proposed that, along with various other developments, local education authorities could employ staff without teaching qualifications. After a two-year probationary period, if performance was appropriate, the local education authority could confer 'qualified teacher status' upon the individual. Although the NUT objected to this there was little it could do as it was no longer on the Burnham Committee and the document went on the statute book as part of the Education Reform Bill in the spring of 1989. Crucially, it was possible for the individual with 'qualified status' to be paid the same as someone with a professional qualification.

There was clear implications in this development for nursing. There was no reason why, for example, a health care assistant should not, in certain circumstances, be paid the same as a registered nurse. Such a statement may have seemed ridiculous at the time but the experience of teaching and the statements in *Working for Patients* indicated it was less ridiculous than would have previously been the case. Indeed by 1992 health visitor assistants were being paid the same as staff nurses (*Nursing Times*, 1992). This situation throws into sharp relief the importance of clarifying precisely what work a registered nurse does that is different from work done by others who have not been professionally trained. Again, it is instructive to look at *Working for Patients*.

Questioning traditional demarcation

Besides discretionary payments and local salaries the only other reference in *Working for Patients* to nurses and nursing is to question traditional lines of demarcation:

'There have been many developments in recent years in the better use of nursing staff, but the Government believes that there is still scope for more progress at local level. It has already endorsed the need to provide better training for the non-professional support staff to nurses. As part of this initiative, local managers, in consultation with their professional colleagues, will be expected to re-examine all areas of work to identify the most cost-effective use of professional skills. This may involve a reappraisal of traditional patterns and practices'.
DH, 1989a

In April 1989 the Department of Health published *A Strategy for Nursing* in which a succinct statement was made that reinforced this position: '. . . traditional restrictions on the exercise of professional and occupational skills are coming under critical scrutiny in every field' (DH, 1989b). The necessity of identifying the distinctive contribution of nursing was paramount but the difficulties involved in defining this contribution were well illustrated by the strategy document itself.

The opening paragraph to *A Strategy for Nursing* states:

'Nursing is professional caring. The ideal of caring is common to nursing, midwifery and health visiting and is central to their enduring

appeal. But this appeal is a combination of many factors: compassion for human suffering; concern for the wider health of people; the prospect of a responsible and varied career; the challenge of scientific enquiry and the quest for new and more effective forms of care. All will play a part, some more strongly with one individual, some with another'.
DH, 1989b

It is difficult to imagine any nurse disagreeing with this. Yet at the same time all references to nursing could be deleted and replaced with 'teaching', 'social work' or any one of a number of professional groups and would apply just as well to those professions. This problem of definition is a difficulty that all professions have and one that nursing has grappled with for a considerable period of time. Yet there is in the early 1990s, with the development of the National Council of Vocational Qualifications (NCVQ), the possibility of employing staff without professional training but offering alternative non-professional qualifications. When traditional patterns of demarcation are being questioned it is imperative to distinguish precisely what it is the professional does, and the way that it is carried out, that is different and better than possible alternatives.

Alternative qualifications

Shortly after the UKCC submitted Project 2000 to the Government for consideration in 1986 the DoE and DES published the White Paper *Working Together—Education and Training* (DoE/DES, 1986). The White Paper proposed a new national infrastructure for training based on the concept of competence with five levels of activity, and associated competences, outlined. Nursing as a profession was ambivalent about this development. With initial activity from the new NCVQs concentrating upon the first three levels many nurses saw little point in becoming involved in the initiative as there was the feeling that nursing would be at level 5, the professional level.

Although the RCN, with limited UKCC commitment, had been involved in the Care Sector

Consortium established to promote health and social care there was little appreciation of NCVQ. For many nurses, as NCVQ was seen as related to the training of support workers, now called health care assistants, the issue of involvement was, and is, seen in the simplest of terms—it had nothing to do with them. Although points are made about the number of health care assistants that will be recruited into professional training this is not seen by the Government and health services managers as a primary consideration.

At a time when staffing the services within the NHS continued to be difficult it was not impossible to imagine hard-pressed managers, on short-term contracts and with annual performance appraisal, turning to the new range of NCVQ courses, such as BTEC Life Sciences, as alternatives to professional qualifications in certain circumstances. As one report by Price Waterhouse recognized, such courses are cheaper, shorter and the employer can be directly involved in the curriculum and practical experience for the student gained directly on the wards (Price Waterhouse, 1987). Nursing failed to recognize that, given the points already made under new lines of demarcation and local salary negotiations, such alternative qualifications were as big a challenge for the profession as direct confrontation with the Government was for both the medical and legal professions. In one sense it was more of a challenge.

Neither medicine or law is having to cope with the prospect of doctors and lawyers being prepared through alternative non-professional routes. There has been increasing encroachment, especially at levels 3 and 4 of NVQ, into areas that nursing has traditionally seen as its preserve (Friend and Tattam, 1991). Not to be involved in NCVQ is to be excluded from the crucial discussions in these grey areas of competence between non-professional and professional. Competence and NCVQ was not restricted solely to health care assistants—as the Management Executive documents on 'Project 2000 Implementation' and 'Health Care Assistants' made clear (NHSMB, 1988; NHSME, 1990). Competence in the NCVQ, and not traditional UKCC, sense became the cornerstone upon which the new regional educational contracts were based.

CONTRACT CULTURE

Commentators have increasingly come to use the term 'contract culture' as shorthand for the wide range of management and market initiatives being introduced into the NHS. This is represented most dramatically for nurse training and education in *Working Paper 10—Education and Training* published as part of the implementation documents for *Working for Patients* (DN, 1989d). Compared to only a few years ago the vocabulary has changed—talk is now of competence, outcomes, ownership, accountability and the like. It is a vocabulary that the Government has brought to bear across the whole range of health and social care activities.

Crucially, *Working Paper 10* gave the responsibility to regional health authorities to decide the contracts for nurse education and training with the new Colleges of Nursing and Colleges of Health. It was clear that measuring outcomes, apart from crude figures of recruitment and retention, would also embrace statements about the competence required of successful students. These statements would not necessarily be expressed in the terms of Project 2000 but more in the vocabulary of competences as represented by NVQ. While it was possible to implement Project 2000 divorced from the introduction of NVQ it was not possible to develop Project 2000 without incorporating competence statements.

Contracts for nurse education were introduced in April 1991 and, with regions working to introduce first-wave self-governing trusts, the contracts were relatively simple and based on past experience. However, subsequent contracts were to be more considered and detailed tackling present and future services in a more systematic manner. The NHS is one sector of the welfare state that with the introduction of the management function, and the information-gathering technology developed since the early Körner enquiries, has a well-developed contract culture that the Government is exploiting with the advocacy of purchasers and providers (DH, 1989e, 1990a). *Working Paper 10* showed that nurse education and training was not exempt from that process and, more than anything else, illustrated dramatically how the employment context had changed since Project 2000 was submitted to the Government in 1986. This change had been accompanied by changes in the legislative framework that directly influenced the work and employment of the professions.

Legislative framework

In the summer of 1989 the Department of Trade and Industry published a White Paper *Opening New Markets: New policy on restrictive trade practices* (DTI, 1989). As the title implied the document was about competition, monopolies, takeovers and the way companies operated in the market place. However, tucked away among the appendices was one annexe entitled 'Impact of the legislation on the professions'. A range of professions was identified including nursing, midwifery, medicine, dentistry, law and teaching.

In essence what is said is that, as with the extract quoted earlier about the legal profession, membership of a particular branch of a profession, together with possession of the appropriate qualification, does not necessarily imply that the holder will meet a particular job specification. This has to be decided on the basis of competences which a qualification may or may not incorporate. It is by adopting an approach such as this that it was possible for the Government to forward an initiative such as 'Qualified Teacher Status' where employment and reward is based on competence rather than a professional qualification. Crucially, an employer can legally use non-professionally trained staff to carry out tasks traditionally reserved for those with the professional qualifications if competence can be shown. The implications on how health care assistants are used within the health service by managers were and are profound. It was a development that the nursing profession could not shut its eyes to and ignore. At the same time there were the beginnings of considerable changes in the infrastructure of services.

Service infrastructure

The main proposals in the two White Papers *Working for Patients* and *Caring for People* are well known and will not be repeated here (DH,

1989a,c). Apart from the limited references to nurses in *Working for Patients*, already referred to, there is little specifically about nursing, other than references to community nurses in general and Community Psychiatric Nurses (CPNs) and Community Mental Handicap Nurses (CMHNs) in particular. These references are appreciative of the work of such nurses but do not consider in any way the long-term impact of the introduction of changes proposed elsewhere in the documents.

For example, little is made about the emerging role of the Family Health Services Authority (FHSA), responsible for organizing primary health care, and the redefined contribution of the GP. In one paragraph reference is made to the contribution of the GP being 'ill health and social handicap' (DH, 1989c). It is difficult to see what is left for other professional workers, especially nurses and social workers. With the new GP contract giving an unprecedented boost to the employment of practice nurses by health centres and GP practices there were serious implications for the work of the health visitor. As a health economist working for the British Medical Association commented when discussing the opting out of community services:

> '… health visitors and district nurses, who were applying to opt out, were fooling themselves into thinking they could easily co-exist alongside well-organized GPs who, under their new contract, were keen to do the immunizations and child health surveillance previously done by community services'.
> *Ferriman, 1990*

At the same time, it was clear that GPs were to be more involved with child health surveillance of the under five-year-olds. Previously unthinkable questions could be asked. How long will it be before children, and then possibly the elderly, are transferred from under-resourced social services departments to FHSAs? Will primary care services begin to take responsibility for community care services on an *ad hoc* basis? It is difficult to answer such questions. But what is clear is that the changes now ongoing make it possible to pose questions such as these. The implications not just for community nursing but for all aspects of nursing as Project 2000 moves nurse training away from an illness to a health model need to be considered.

It is not at all clear, however, whether such changes, both realized and potential, will be seen by other nurses as opportunities to be grasped. Nor is it possible to gauge how far the emergence of employer-led training over profession-determined education is fully appreciated by nursing staff under daily pressure within the NHS.

EMERGING TRENDS

New boundaries

The cumulative impact of the seven issues identified under policy parameters was to emphasize the importance of the challenges they present to all aspects of health and social care. There was a need for a sense of urgency that events and developments within other professions indicated was necessary. One example, among many, was for an active and full involvement within NCVQ, and the acknowledgement that this represented a new national infrastructure in which professional training had to be placed. It was imperative that nursing clarified in contractual terms and in the appropriate language of competence and outcome the differences between professional and non-professional training programmes. Yet when, in 1992, the opportunity to become involved in discussions for occupational standards at the higher levels of NCVQ became available the offer was turned down (Carlisle, 1992). Instead, nursing became focused on the details of other developments.

In 1988 the English National Board published a circular that encouraged the development of new colleges (ENB, 1988). A significant achievement of the new Colleges of Nursing and Colleges of Health that emerged was that they, at last, began to integrate nurse education into higher education. No longer were nurse training schools isolated from education in other areas. Although in reality there may still be separation, it marked a move away from the former situation of 'standing

alone'. This move needed to be accompanied by a broadening of horizons to look across the range of policy proposals if developments within nursing were to be placed within an appropriate framework. Otherwise initiatives, such as Project 2000, would become increasingly marginalized within the wider arena of current workforce concerns as both Government and employers attempt to grapple with the issues raised.

There had to be recognition that all aspects of training, whether at a professional level or not, could not be divorced from training developments at other levels and in other arenas. The battle to get a single level professional training, represented in Project 2000, had been long and hard and limited the recognition of other training programmes in meeting the pressing demands of recruitment and retention if a viable level of staffing was to be met on hospital wards and in community units.

Project 2000 called for a change of emphasis away from an illness to a health model. What could be overlooked was that this implied a realignment between nursing and other professional groups where relationships and demarcation between them have been based on the 'old' illness model. To take social work as an example, over the years links have developed based all too frequently on antipathy between the sister/charge nurse and medical social worker, between the health visitor and the field social worker—the list could go on. Project 2000 calls into question these links and, if anything, could lead to an increase in questions over demarcation with antipathy being replaced by animosity.

Social work, like nursing and like all professions, is itself having to respond to the challenges outlined as key developments earlier. At a time when the Government was questioning the traditional autonomy of the professions across all their activities, and encouraging joint and shared training (DH, 1989c, 1990b), to perpetuate traditional distinctions and arguments over boundaries of demarcation that are going to change anyway was to fight battles that were no longer relevant. Yet if it was important to question stereotypes between professions it was also important to question stereotypes within the profession.

Ever since the Nurses Registration Act of 1919 sought to reconcile competing interests, nursing has been a broad umbrella incorporating a range of activities. Not all these activities have been seen as in the mainstream of the profession—a situation common to all professions. Mental health and learning disabilities have often been seen as marginal to the interests of the nursing profession with its emphasis upon clinical aspects of care (Salvage, 1985). Yet it is in these areas on the margin that moves have begun to be made towards co-operation with other professions and where issues over training programmes, organizational structures and administrative responsibilities have had to be tackled for the specialisms to survive. Learning disabilities, a Cinderella service in terms of resources and status, has gone further than any other area in exploring joint and shared training possibilities that are so favoured by the Government in implementing *Caring for People*. Mental health was slow to follow, yet these developments provided lessons for the nursing profession as a whole.

The nature of employment in health and social care is changing with important implications for all levels of training and education. It is no longer possible, as it has been in the past, to consider only a limited range of education and training divorced from the context of staff preparation that stretches from tasks that require the humblest of abilities to those that call upon the most sophisticated levels of skills. Unless the nursing profession, like all professions, accepts the necessity of becoming involved in debates and discussions across the training spectrum then nursing will have unwittingly colluded in the erosion of the nurse's role. This has particular urgency since the passing of the National Health Services and Community Care Act, 1990 (DH, 1990c) and, in particular, the emergence of the general management function in the NHS.

The general management function

Amid the lively debate that accompanied the controversy over the poll tax, the announcement by Michael Heseltine of a review of local government tended to pass relatively unnoticed by those not directly involved (DoE, 1991). It is clear, however, that an essential element of such a review will be consideration of whether the 'general management function' is appropriate to introduce into local government departments. For those in the health service already familiar with such a development this may lead to a rueful reflection upon how the health service functioned prior to the introduction of managers. Yet the legacy of the Griffiths management review in 1983 (Griffiths, 1983) has probably had as profound, if not greater, impact upon community care than his report specifically focusing upon care in the community (Griffiths, 1988).

When the Government White Paper 'Better Services for the Mentally Ill' was published in 1975 a commitment was made to reduce the number of available psychiatric hospital beds (DHSS, 1975). This policy built upon the community care plans of the early 1960s. Progress, however, was slow (Jones, 1972) yet, as a little publicized part of one of the final reports of the Social Services Select Committee shows, significant reductions were achieved in the 1980s. Psychiatric hospital resident numbers fell by over a quarter from 77,297 residents in 1979 to 56,200 in 1989 (Social Services Committee, 1990).

It is clear that one factor in achieving this target was that throughout the 1980s there was a Government ideologically committed to promoting the private sector. At a time when health service budgets were being squeezed and, as with previous years, local authorities could not respond significantly to the closure of hospital facilities, the movement to the private sector was inevitable. Although this was helped as welfare benefits were not cash-limited by the Treasury (a situation that was altered with the social security legislation of 1988) there is little doubt that the crucial catalyst was the introduction of the manager (Korman and Glennerster, 1990).

While some commentators questioned the style of particular managers (Robinson and Strong, 1990) the introduction of the general management function with short-term contracts allied to performance reviews has proved to be a powerful incentive to change. This change has not always been beneficial to the client '. . . as (some) hospital beds have been closed before better alternative facilities were fully in place' (Social Services

Committee, 1990). However, in trying to attain specified objectives, managers have of necessity questioned assumptions about practice and staffing. This has inevitably led to a questioning of the role and contribution of different professional groups and to a move away from reaching decisions on the basis of traditional stereotypes. This can manifest itself in a variety of ways.

To take one instance, no group can expect to assume as of right that it will be represented in the evolving structures introduced in the recent health and community care legislation. In the NHS self-governing trusts, for example, there are effectively five areas of responsibility—management, finance, contracts, personnel and quality. Of these five areas it is perhaps only 'quality' where it could be assumed that nursing would automatically take executive responsibility. Yet the number of nurses offered such responsibility has been low and led to increasing concern in the professional press with calls for 'succession' training for nurses (George, 1990; Davidson and Cole, 1991). It appears that when nurses are appointed to positions of executive responsibility it is because of their personal attributes and achievements rather than because they are nurses. The fact that they are a nurse is secondary. This is a challenge for the nursing profession. It is also a challenge for other professional groups. For mental health specialists, in particular, this must also be seen as an opportunity.

Stereotypes which are now largely out of date still present a considerable barrier to the acceptance of the skills-base of, for example, nurses in both mental health and learning disabilities. Such stereotypes about inappropriate philosophy, institutionalized practices and the like, have proved to be remarkably persistent. However, if such nurses can illustrate the relevance of their skills-base to managers then the general management function holds out the possibility of undermining the traditional stereotypes that have so hindered recognition of the relevance of their contemporary skills to meeting the needs of the client.

This is not to deny that general management can be a source of irritation and frustration to many in the health service, including those providing direct-care services. But it is important not to be restricted by stereotypes that are just as limited in vision as those applied to the psychiatric nurse. Management is the essential audience to which the claims of the psychiatric nurse, as well as other professionals like social workers, must be addressed. These claims must be supported by appropriate arguments which provide not only an overall strategy but also embrace consideration of tactics. The tactics that are identified, however, must be placed within the context of workforce planning.

Workforce planning

The development of the role of the manager has been accompanied by the emergence of workforce planning as an activity, the importance of which is often overlooked. While recognition is usually made of workforce planning as one aspect of the current situation, it is a mistake to assume that such an acknowledgement is sufficient. Significant policy developments both within and outside the NHS are having a direct and immediate impact upon workforce planning and patterns of employment. To take but one example, locally negotiated salaries are beginning to be introduced. These complement the performance-related pay and discretionary increments already introduced for some sections of the NHS over recent years. The profound implications this will have upon employment practice when allied to the emergence of the contract culture could not have been anticipated even only a few years ago. It is a development that focuses attention upon the employment setting in which all professionals will be trained and will practice.

With such developments, workforce planning, in its broadest sense, is more than just one among a number of factors that have to be considered— it provides the overall context in which any proposals will be interpreted, evaluated and implemented.

It has become important for mental health practitioners to incorporate workforce planning considerations into any proposals for the future that they forward. While responsibility for making decisions rests with managers, the information and arguments upon which those decisions are made are increasingly being provided by workforce planners, whatever their local job title may be. Some of the issues this raises are considered in the next section.

IMMEDIATE CONCERNS

The National Health Services and Community Care Act, 1990 (DH, 1990) symbolizes a period of change within the NHS that has increased in momentum throughout the 1980s. In particular, since publication of the White Paper *Working for Patients* at the beginning of 1989 (DH, 1989a) the volume of new initiatives in health and community care has been considerable. This has been matched by an increased pace in the implementation of legislation by the Government. Even though full implementation of the community care proposals was delayed until 1993, changes in the NHS continued unabated.

These changes have placed new demands on staff at all levels and in all sectors and have highlighted the vital role that training and education has to play in preparing staff to meet these demands. In the immediate and foreseeable future the continuing education of qualified staff will be as important, if not more so, than Project 2000 and the Diploma in Social Work in preparing staff to meet the workforce needs within the NHS and local government. Post-registration training and post-qualifying training have a crucial role to play in developing the contribution of the profession, regardless of setting, especially at a time of unprecedented change (UKCC, 1990, 1992). However, in the context of the contract, culture issues have to be addressed in a way appropriate to those who will have to implement the recommendations. In particular, an attempt has to be made to recognize the importance of the contractual cycle.

The contractual cycle

For mental health nurses the introduction of *Working Paper 10*, upon which the educational contractual cycle in the NHS is based, has particular significance (DH, 1989c). With responsibility for education contracts now resting with the regional health authorities it is not at all clear exactly what priority, if any, the regions will place upon maintaining present levels of mental health nurse training.

The first-round contracts introduced by the regions in April 1991 this year were, inevitably, relatively crude. Activity was concentrated upon the introduction and establishment of self-governing trusts. For the second-round contracts the following year the focus was upon nurse education, with the contracts being more considered and sophisticated than had been possible before. It is too early to discern any patterns across regions. However, it is no longer possible to assume that mental health training will persist at current levels. The drop in student recruitment figures reinforces this possibility (ENB, 1992).

While many within social services may see this as not necessarily inappropriate these are considerations that will affect local government itself in the immediate future. The training agenda now has to lock into the contractual cycle. This must also involve identification of any possible line management implications when specific training proposals are forwarded.

Line-management implications

In 1986, the Audit Commission called for professions to be used as specialist workers with a new non-professional generic worker directly under their control (Audit Commission, 1986). This was also advocated by Griffiths in his subsequent report (Griffiths, 1988). As the 1990s get under way the likelihood of this general approach being introduced in some form increasingly becomes likely as the much anticipated demographic problems begin to be experienced. In such circumstances, and especially with many health service managers and workforce planners not necessarily appreciating fully the necessity for a mental health practitioner, it has become necessary to indicate precisely what a specialist role involves. Recent Audit Commission reports highlight the importance of this (Audit Commission, 1992a,b,c). But more is required.

The implications for other levels, grades and type of staff need to be clarified where the work of the specialist impinges upon their areas of activity. Crucially, the line-management responsibilities need to be identified along with any organizational implications. Structural repercussions have to be addressed. Also for the individual member of staff it involves considering possible career paths and opportunities, especially for those who become jointly qualified as the White Paper, *Caring for People* advocates. This requires a breadth of policy appreciation allied to an approach that makes the criteria used explicit.

Explicit criteria

Training programmes have to be advocated using recognized criteria. Such criteria are already available for this using both Credit Accumulation Transfer Scheme (CATS) and NCVQ competences. Developments with health care assistants pivot around NCVQ levels, and have enabled new patterns of linkage to be established with workers covered by the residential, domiciliary and day care initiative (JAB, 1990). With NCVQ-compatible competences forming the basis of the learning disabilities branch programme it should be possible to build upon this within mental health to develop a coherent policy for training and practice across the spectrum of levels and activities involved both within nursing and across professional boundaries.

Developing ideas across such a spectrum avoids the insularity of promoting one level of training or area of practice which current workforce concerns and legislation is making increasingly untenable. The use of terms such as those expressed by NVQ provides a common vocabulary for describing the performances and outcomes that have become integral to the contract culture. Some nurse commentators are not happy with NVQ but it is, none the less, a reality that must form an essential part of developing a dialogue with managers and workforce planners. Such a dialogue must embrace all levels of activity and complement the current debates about health and social care.

Training and education

Health and social care is a distinction made by the Government in the White Paper *Caring for People* (DH, 1989b). The very terms used, though, bring to mind echoes of debates based on past patterns of demarcation between different groups. It is all too easy to equate the nurse with 'health care' and the social worker with 'social care'. However, for many in positions of responsibility the pressures of their job make it difficult to begin to find the time to appreciate the significance and importance of developments in the 'grey area' between the extremities on the continuum of health and social care. The health and social care distinction will, almost subconsciously, be the health and social care divide. Joint training has begun to undermine such stereotypes and has been pioneered in learning disabilities. This development, however, has been in learning disabilities rather than mental health.

Joint training between nursing and social work had an acrimonious start in the early 1980s. Upon the revival of attempts for co-operation between the ENB and Central Council for Education and Training in Social Work (CCETSW) from late 1986 onwards a momentum built up that meant that although the number of courses involved was small by the end of the decade learning disabilities had progressed further with joint staff training than had been achieved with any other client groups. The significance of this achievement was highlighted when, in *Caring for People* joint training became official Government policy:

'It will be important to continue to develop multidisciplinary training for staff in all caring professions, including the provision of joint training at both the qualifying and post-qualifying stage'.
DH, 1989a

Subsequent guidance notes on implementing a training framework reinforced the commitment to joint training (DH, 1991b). Yet the pioneering work in learning disabilities has gone almost unheralded.

In 1990, the Department of Health brought together the National Health Services Training Authority (NHSTA), the Social Services Inspectorate and CCETSW on a joint training project. Seven sites were selected throughout the country for work on 'organizational and individual training needs' for staff working with the elderly and the mentally ill (DH, 1990b). In a classic case of rediscovering the wheel it was hoped that lessons might be learned for those working with people with a mental handicap and those with physical disabilities. The fact that for such clients there was a reservoir of experience, greater than that either in mental illness or work with the elderly, was not acknowledged. It highlighted also that while mental health and learning disabilities are often associated in the minds of policy planners and commentators in reality they have developed independently. Both have reacted differently to being on the margins of mainstream nursing.

The future of the mental health practitioner has tended to be eclipsed by other concerns within nursing, not least the emergence of the practice nurse since the introduction of the GP contract. Marginality leads others to interpret initiatives in a certain way. This is illustrated by the reaction to the work done to incorporate NVQ compatible competency statements into the learning disabilities branch programme of Project 2000. Rather than alerting the nursing profession to the importance of NVQ, an importance that every other profession in the health and welfare sector recognized long ago, the involvement of learning disabilities has seemed to reinforce its marginality!

In such circumstances it is imperative that mental health practitioners, along with those in learning disabilities, in spite of all the pressures at present and in the foreseeable future, strive to maintain the momentum of the 1980s. The development of the contract culture and the challenge that it poses to traditional assumptions makes all professional groups vulnerable. But this threat can also be a challenge—a challenge to use the general management function to obtain recognition for the real achievements of recent years and to show, through providing appropriate patterns of care, that the mental health practitioner has a continuing role to play.

THE CONTRACT AGENDA

Such is the volume and pace of current legislation, both within and outside the NHS, that all professional groups have to consider their future contribution in ways that begin to step outside traditional patterns of expectations. This future contribution has to be built on the adoption of a broad-based perspective that is based on meeting the needs of the user. The cumulative impact of the policy changes in recent years has been to challenge the vested interests of professions. At the same time, the development of a Citizen's Charter has promoted the interests of the user. As hospitals run down and community services are built up, whether in the statutory or independent sector, structures of collaboration between the different agencies are developing in a hesitant and *ad hoc* manner (Audit Commission, 1992c).

It is clear, however, that the policy parameter, trends and issues, introduced in this chapter are being promoted on the basis of benefiting the user. This provides the rationale for the new service structures within which the techniques of the mental health nurse practitioner will be delivered. For the mental health nurse it is important to appreciate the full import of the significant changes that have, and are still, taking place.

These changes have been summarized in the area of community health services by the Audit Commission as a series of questions in seven areas:

1 *Vision and Need*—is there a vision for the future which takes account of the challenges and opportunities facing community health services, and which is shared with the local authority and FHSA? Is analysis of need being used to question historical resource patterns, i.e. are effective services being targetted on areas of greatest need?

2 *Strategic planning between districts and local authorities*—to what extent are the health authority and local authority collaborating particularly in respect of the movement of people from long-stay institutions and of preparations for the forthcoming changes in community care?

3 *Strategic planning with FHSAs*—are the health authority and FHSA collaborating to provide complementary services which

avoid unnecessary duplication and which maximize health gain?

4 *Care co-ordination*—are health services for individuals co-ordinated in such a way as to allow more people with additional health care needs to be looked after in the community?

5 *Managing service delivery*—is the field workforce being adequately managed?

6 *Information systems*—are management decisions based upon useful management information?

7 *Quality assurance*—are quality systems continually improving the services delivered to clients?
Audit Commission, 1992b

This is not an exhaustive list of questions but it does convey the issues that have to be addressed by all occupational groups in the contract culture. Mental health nurse practitioners are no exception. The crucial question for them, however, is the extent to which the nursing profession as a whole responds to the issues raised. The nature of this response will determine whether mental nursing consolidates and enhances its position or becomes increasingly marginalized as managers grapple with 'the cascade of change' (Audit Commission, 1992a). The only thing that is certain is that the NHS and local government is undergoing changes as fundamental as when the welfare state was introduced in the late 1940s. The outcome is still far from clear.

FURTHER READING

Bornat, J., Pereira, D., Pilgrim, D. & Williams, F. (Eds) (1993) *Community Care: A Reader*. London: Macmillan.

Hill, M. (1993) *The Welfare State in Britain: A Political History since 1945*. London: Edward Elgar.

Levitt, R. & Wall, A. (1992) *The Re-Organised National Health Service*, 4th edition. London: Chapman & Hall.

Robinson, J., Gray, A. & Elkan R. (Eds) (1992) *Policy Issues in Nursing*. Milton Keynes: Open University Press.

Salvage, J. (1985) *The Politics of Nursing*. London: Heinemann.

REFERENCES

Audit Commission (1986) *Making a Reality of Community Care*. London: HMSO.

Audit Commission (1992a) *Community Care: Managing the Cascade of Change*. London: HMSO.

Audit Commission (1992b) *Homeward Bound: A New Course for Community Health*. London: HMSO.

Audit Commission (1992c) *The Community Revolution: Personal Social Services and Community Care*. London: HMSO.

Carlisle, D. (1992) Governing bodies to fight NVQ incursion into nursing. *Nursing Times*, 16 September, Vol. 88, p. 6.

Citizen's Charter (1991) London: HMSO.

Davidson, N. & Cole, I. (1991) A crisis of leadership. *Nursing Times*, **87** (1), 22–24.

Department of Education and Science (DES) (1988) *Qualified Teacher Status: a consultation document*. London: DES.

Department of Employment and Department of Education and Science (DoE/DES) (1986) *Working Together—Education and Training*, London: HMSO.

Department of Environment (DE) (1991) The internal management of local authorities: a consultation document.

Department of Health (DH) (1989a) *Working for Patients*. London: HMSO.

Department of Health (DH) (1989b) *A Strategy for Nursing: A report of the Steering Committee*. London: HMSO.

Department of Health (DH) (1989c) *Caring for People*. London: HMSO.

Department of Health (DH) (1989d) *Working for Patients—Working Paper 10: Education and Training*. London: HMSO.

Department of Health (1989e) *Working for Patients—Contracts for Health Services: Operating Procedures*. London: HMSO.

Department of Health (DH) (1990a) *Caring for People: Consultation paper on an NHS training framework—Implementation Guidance, number 12* (Draft). London: HMSO.

Department of Health (DH) (1990b) *Caring for People: joint training project (specification)*. London: HMSO.

Department of Health (DH) (1990c) *The National Health Service and Community Care Act*. London: HMSO.

Department of Health (DH) (1991a) *NHS Workforce in England*. London: HMSO.

Department of Health (DH) (1991b) *Caring for People: implementation guidance note 12*. London: HMSO.

Department of Health (DH) (1992a) *The Health of the Nation*. London: HMSO.

Department of Health (DH) (1992b) *Report of the Inquiry into London's Health Service, Medical Education and Research* (The Tomlinson Report). London: HMSO.

Department of Health and Social Services (DHSS) (1975) *Better Services for the Mentally Ill*. London: HMSO.

Department of Health and Social Services (DHSS) (1980) *Mental Handicap: Progress, Problems and Priorities*. London: HMSO.

Department of Health and Social Security (DHSS) (1987) *Promoting Better Health*. London: HMSO.

Department of Trade and Industry (DTI) (1989) *Opening New Markets: New Policy on Restrictive Trade Practices*. London: HMSO.

ENB (1988) *Project 2000: A new preparation for practice—guidelines and criteria . . . and centres of Higher Education*. London: English National Board.

ENB (1992) Unpublished internal memorandum. London: English National Board.

Ferriman, A. (1990) Opt-out hospitals face bankruptcy. *The Observer*, 9 September.

Friend, B. & Tattam, A. (1991) Nurse leaders slam NVQ plans. *Nursing Times*, 22 May, Vol. 87, p. 6.

George, J. (1990) *Facilitating Career Management*. London: NHSTA.

Griffiths, R. (1983) *NHS Management Inquiry*. London: HMSO.

Griffiths, R. (1988) *Community Care: an Agenda for Action*. London: HMSO.

JAB (1990) *Introduction of National Vocational Qualifications in Social Care and Health Care*. London: Joint Awarding Bodies.

Jones, K. (1972) *A History of the Mental Health Services*. London: Routledge & Kegan Paul.

Korman, N. & Glennerster, H. (1990) *Closing a Hospital*. Milton Keynes: Open University Press.

Lord Chancellor's Department (1989) *The Work and Organization of the Legal Profession*. London: HMSO.

NHS Management Board (NHSMB) (1988) *Project 2000 Implementation*. London: Department of Health and Social Security.

NHS Management Executive (NHSME) (1990) *Health Care Assistants*. London: Department of Health.

Nurses Registration Act (1919). London: HMSO.

Nursing Times (1992) Support posts to include HV duties. *Nursing Times*, 2 September, Vol. 88, p. 6.

Price Waterhouse (1987) *Feasibility Study into YTS in Health and Social Care Programmes: Final Report*. London: DHSS.

Robinson, J. & Strong, P. (1990) *The NHS Under New Management*. Milton Keynes: Open University Press.

Salvage, J. (1985) *The Politics of Nursing*. London: Heinemann.

Smart, V. (1989) Doctors give up hope of halting changes in NHS. *The Observer*, 3 September.

Social Services Committee (1990) *Community Care: Services for People with a Mental Handicap and People with a Mental Illness*. London: House of Commons.

UKCC (1990) *The Report of the Post-registration Education and Practice Project* (second report). London: United Kingdom Central Council.

UKCC (1992) *Report of the Proposals for the Future of Community Education and Practice*. London: United Kingdom Central Council.

29

THE LAW RELATING TO MENTAL HEALTH AND DISORDER

Enid E. Wright

AIMS

i) To provide a review of the legislation which applies to people experiencing mental disorder

ii) To provide a reference to relevant sections within the legislation

KEY ISSUES

Mental Health Acts 1959 and 1983
Actors within the Act
Exclusions from definitions of mental disorder
Legislative duties and powers of health service personnel
Other statutory services (legislative base)
Children and young people
Other legislation

Identify, analyse and assess factors causing distress and illness	Promote health, provide direct care and make interventions	Manage care programmes and services
Be critical, analytical and accountable, continue professional development	Counter discrimination, inequality and individual and institutional racism	Work within and develop policies, laws and safeguards in all settings
Understand influences on mental health and the nature/causes of disorder and illness	Know the effects of distress, disorder, illness on individuals, groups, families	Understand the basis of treatments and interventions

INTRODUCTION

Many people suffer from mental disorder during some stage of their lives, either personally or through their families or friends. The relevant law varies according to the mentally disordered person's condition at different times.

There is a continuum of relevant legislative provision ranging from that which promotes good mental health, through preventive/enabling/rehabilitative measures, to statutory powers and duties relating to acute mental disorder. The application of preventive/enabling/rehabilitative legislation by social workers, nurses and others can help move the focus of their work with mentally disordered people along the continuum towards the mental health end.

Legislation can also be used to support the families of mentally disordered people and others who feel overwhelmed by traumas and personal problems. Professional support, with timely application of enabling legislation, can often prevent them also becoming mentally ill.

It is important, however, to know the difference between statutory duties and enabling powers. While all local authorities, for example, must fulfil their statutory duties, the extent to which enabling powers are used depends on the policy and resources of the particular authority. In this respect, social workers can bring pressure to bear on their employers in the interests of their clients and families.

Some legislative provisions are specific to mental health or disorder whereas others apply to mentally disordered people as they do to other vulnerable citizens. This chapter will consider both types.

Current legislation

Disabled Persons (Employment) Act 1944
National Assistance Act 1948
National Assistance (Amendment) Act 1951
Disabled Persons (Employment) Act 1958
Mental Health Act 1959
Criminal Procedure (Insanity) Act 1964
Health Services and Public Health Act 1968
Chronically Sick and Disabled Persons Act 1970

Local Authority Social Services Act 1970
Matrimonial Causes Act 1973
Juries Act 1974
Social Security Act 1975
National Health Service Act 1977
Nurses, Midwives and Health Visitors Act 1979
Education Act 1981
Health and Social Services and Social Security Adjudications Act 1983
Marriage Act 1983
Mental Health Act 1983
Representation of the People Act 1983
Police and Criminal Evidence Act 1984
Registered Homes Act 1984
Enduring Powers of Attorney Act 1985
Housing Act 1985
Disabled Persons (Services, Consultation and Representation) Act 1986
Social Security Act 1986
Access to Personal Files Act 1987
Children Act 1989
National Health Service and Community Care Act 1990
Social Security Act 1990
Criminal Justice Act 1991
Criminal Procedure (Insanity and Unfitness to Plead) Act 1991
Registered Homes (Amendment) Act 1991
Community Care (Residential Accommodation) Act 1992

Rules of the Supreme Court 1965
County Court Rules 1981
Mental Health Act Commission (Establishment and Constitution) Order 1983
Mental Health Act Commission Regulations 1983
Mental Health (Hospital, Guardianship and Consent to Treatment) Regulations 1983
Mental Health (Nurses) Order 1983
Mental Health Review Tribunal Rules 1983
Court of Protection Rules 1984
Nursing Homes and Mental Nursing Homes Regulations 1984
Court of Protection (Enduring Powers of Attorney) Rules 1986
Local Authority Social Services (Designation of Functions) Order 1989

Children (Secure Accommodation) Regulations 1991

Representations Procedure (Children) Regulations 1991

Owing to space limitations, it has been necessary to restrict the section on children and young people. However, much of the rest of the chapter applies to them and there are suggestions for further reading.

CURRENT LEGISLATION SPECIFICALLY AND RELATING TO MENTAL HEALTH DISORDER

Mental Health Act 1959

Although the Mental Health Act 1983 consolidated much of the law of England and Wales specifically relating to mentally disordered persons, certain provisions of the Mental Health Act 1959 have not been repealed, including the following.

s.8 Function of welfare authorities

This section enables local authorities to provide residential accommodation for the care or after care of mentally disordered people under the National Health Service Act 1977 even though they are required or authorized to provide such accommodation under s.21 of the National Assistance Act 1948.

s.128 Sexual intercourse with patients

This section makes it an offence (i) for a man on the staff of, or employed by a hospital or mental nursing home to have extramarital sexual intercourse with a woman who is receiving treatment for mental disorder in that hospital or home either as an out-patient or an in-patient, and (ii) for a man to have extramarital sexual intercourse with a woman who is subject to his guardianship or is otherwise in his custody or care. No offence is committed under s.128 if the man did not know,

and had no reason to suspect, that the woman was a mentally disordered patient.

Mental Health Act 1983

This Act consolidated much of the law of England and Wales specifically relating to mentally disordered persons. It applies to Scotland and Northern Ireland only to the extent provided for in sections 146 and 147 respectively, which mainly relate to the removal of patients between the different countries of the United Kingdom.

The DHSS Memorandum (DHSS, 1983a) on Parts I–VI, VIII and X of the Mental Health Act 1983 provides guidance on the Act. The revised Code of Practice (DH and Welsh Office, 1993) required under s.118 of the Act was prepared by the Mental Health Act Commission and published by the Secretaries of State for Health and for Wales in August 1993. It came into force on 1 November 1993. (DH and Welsh Office, 1993, DH, 1993c.)

The Code is not mandatory in that professionals carrying out functions under the Act are not legally obliged to follow the advice contained in the Code. However, a failure to have regard to the Code could be used in legal proceedings as *prima facie* evidence of bad practice although the effect of non-compliance will largely depend upon the nature of the provision in the Code that has not been followed. Section 118 of the Act requires the Secretary of State to revise the Code from time to time.

The Act is divided into 10 Parts and six Schedules. This chapter gives a guide to key aspects of the application of the Act and the main definitions relating to patients, nurses and approved social workers under the Act. There is no space, however, to consider the other provisions in the same detail. In any case, this would duplicate what is more authoritatively stated in the legislation itself, the DHSS Memorandum and the Code of Practice, and more comprehensively dealt with in legal manuals and law books. The *Mental Health Act Manual* (Jones, 1991) is especially useful as it both updates the legislation and comments on it, with references to Government circulars, cases and other documents. The chapter refers to relevant delegated legislation and other Acts where appropriate. It also considers the key themes reflected throughout the legislation, Memorandum and Code of Practice.

Part I (s.1) sets out the application and extent of the Act and defines 'mental disorder'

s.1(1) says 'The provisions of this Act shall have effect with respect to the reception, care and treatment of mentally disordered patients, the management of their property and other related matters'.

s.1(2) defines 'mental disorder' and three of the four specific categories of mental disorder as follows:

'In this Act—

"mental disorder" means mental illness, arrested or incomplete development of mind, psychopathic disorder and any other disorder or disability of mind and "mentally disordered" shall be construed accordingly;

"severe mental impairment" means a state of arrested or incomplete development of mind which includes severe impairment of intelligence and social functioning and is associated with abnormally aggressive or seriously irresponsible conduct on the part of the person concerned and "severely mentally impaired" shall be construed accordingly;

"mental impairment" means a state of arrested or incomplete development of mind (not amounting to severe mental impairment) which includes significant impairment of intelligence and social functioning and is associated with abnormally aggressive or seriously irresponsible conduct on the part of the person concerned and "mentally impaired" shall be construed accordingly;

"psychopathic disorder" means a persistent disorder or disability of mind (whether or not including significant impairment of intelligence) which results in abnormally aggressive or seriously irresponsible conduct on the part of the person concerned;'.

The DHSS Memorandum (DHSS, 1983a) points out at para. 10 that the term 'mental illness' is undefined in the Act and says 'its operational definition and usage is a matter for clinical judgement in each case'.

The actors within the Act

The patient. s.145(1) defines the 'patient' as 'a person suffering or appearing to be suffering from mental disorder', except in Part VII, which relates to the management of patients' property and affairs, and unless the context otherwise requires.

However, the applicability of the condition of 'mental disorder' and of the specific conditions varies between different sections of the Act. Who is 'the patient', therefore, also depends on the particular section of the Act under consideration. More than one of the conditions may, of course, affect the patient at any one time (CCETSW, 1992).

For many purposes of the Act a general diagnosis of 'mental disorder' is not sufficient and a diagnosis of one of the four specific categories of mental disorder—mental illness, mental impairment, severe mental impairment or psychopathic disorder—is required. A specific diagnosis must be made for an admission for treatment (s.3), a reception into guardianship (s.7), a hospital or guardianship order made by the court (s.37), an interim hospital order (s.38) and a transfer from prison to hospital (s.47). On the other hand, a specific diagnosis is not required in relation to admission for assessment (s.2), admission for assessment in cases of emergency (s.4), application in respect of a patient already in hospital (s.5), warrant to search for and remove patients (s.135) and mentally disordered persons found in public places (s.136).

See chapter 29 of the Code of Practice (DH and Welsh Office, 1993) for definitions and discussion relating to mental handicap/learning disabilities. See also the DHSS Memorandum (DHSS, 1983a) and Jones' Mental Health Act Manual (Jones, 1991).

A 'patient' for the purposes of Part VII—management and administration of property—is defined in s.94(2). Most patients are informal patients (see s.131 below).

Exclusions from the definitions of mental disorder.

s.1(3) of the Act says:

'Nothing in subsection (2) above shall be construed as implying that a person may be dealt with under this Act as suffering from mental disorder, or from any form of mental disorder described in this section, by reason only of promiscuity or other immoral conduct, sexual deviancy or dependence on alcohol or drugs'.

Paragraph 16 of the Memorandum (DHSS, 1983a) advises:

'This means that there are no grounds for detaining a person in hospital because of alcohol or drug abuse alone, but it is recognized that alcohol or drug abuse may be accompanied by or associated with mental disorder. It is therefore possible to detain a person who is dependent on alcohol or drugs if they are suffering from a mental disorder arising from or suspected to arise from alcohol or drug dependence or from the withdrawal of alcohol or a drug, if all the other relevant conditions are met. Similarly sexual deviancy is not of itself a mental disorder, for the purposes of the Act, which can provide grounds for compulsory detention'.

Relatives.

The terms 'relative' and 'nearest relative' are defined in s.26 of the Act. See also para. 68 of the Memorandum (DHSS, 1983a). Section 26, which defines 'relative' and 'nearest relative' for the purposes of Part II of the Act, also applies to patients who have been placed under hospital or guardianship orders by a court under s.37.

A person who has been identified as the patient's nearest relative can authorize any person, other than the patient or a person disqualified under subsection (5), to perform the functions of the nearest relative. The authority can be revoked at any time. Both the authority and the revocation must be in writing (see reg.14 of the Mental Health (Hospital, Guardianship and Consent to Treatment) Regulations 1983).

Section 27 as substituted by the Children Act 1989 defines the nearest relative of a child or young person in care. Under this section, if an unmarried child under the age of 18 years is in the care of a local authority by virtue of a care order in England or Wales, that local authority becomes the child's nearest relative.

Section 28 as amended provides for a person who has been appointed as a child's guardian (other than under the Mental Health Act) or a person who is named in a residence order (as defined by s.8 of the Children Act 1989) to be that child's nearest relative.

Sections 27 and 28 also apply to children who have been placed under hospital or guardianship orders by a court under s.37.

Section 29 relates to the appointment by a court of an acting nearest relative. The section gives the county court power to make an order directing that the functions of the nearest relative shall be exercised by another person, or by a local social services authority.

Section 30 provides for the discharge or variation of an order made by a county court under s.29 for the appointment of an acting nearest relative. It also specifies the duration of an order which has not been discharged.

National Health Service personnel.

A wide range of health service personnel is involved with mentally disordered patients in hospitals, residential and day services and the community generally. These include consultants, psychiatrists, psychologists, psychotherapists, hospital managers, doctors, nurses, occupational therapists, ambulance personnel, porters and receptionists. The legislative duties and powers of nurses include the following.

Nurse of the prescribed class.

This term is defined in s.5(7) of the Mental Health Act 1983 which says 'In subsection (4) above "prescribed" means prescribed by an order made by the Secretary of State'. The Mental Health (Nurses) Order 1983 prescribes the class of nurse for the purposes of subsection (4) of this section as 'a nurse registered in Part 3 (first level nurses trained in the nursing of persons suffering from mental illness) or Part 5 (first level nurses trained in the nursing of persons suffering from mental handicap) of the register prepared and maintained under s.10 of the Nurses, Midwives and Health Visitors Act 1979 (the professional register)'.

Section 5(4) provides for nurses of the prescribed class to invoke a 'holding power' in respect of a patient for a period of not more than six hours. Guidance on this is contained in chapter 9 of the Code of Practice (DH and Welsh Office, 1993). Jones (1991) submits that, as this Part of the Act only applies to mental nursing homes that are registered to receive detained patients, a nurse of the prescribed class who works in a mental nursing home could only exercise the power provided for in this subsection if the home in question is so registered.

Nurses generally. Nurses nurse mentally disordered patients in hospitals, mental and other nursing homes and in the community. They also have particular roles under ss.57 and 58 of the Act which deal respectively with treatment requiring consent and a second opinion and treatment requiring consent or a second opinion. Section 57 provides that certain of the most serious forms of medical treatment for mental disorder can only be given if the patient consents to the treatment and three independent people, one being a doctor, have certified that the patient understands the treatment and has consented to it. The doctor must also certify that the treatment should be given because it will have a beneficial effect. Section 58 provides that certain forms of treatment shall not be given to a patient unless the patient consents or an independent medical practitioner has certified that either the patient is incapable of giving his consent or that the patient should receive the treatment even though he has not consented to it. Under both sections, before issuing his certificate the doctor must consult two other persons who have been professionally concerned with the patient's medical treatment and one of these shall be a nurse. See chapter 16 of the Code of Practice (DH and Welsh Office, 1993) and DHSS Circular No. DDL (84)4 'Mental Health Act Commission: Guidance for Respon-

sible Medical Officers—Consent to Treatment' (DHSS, 1984a). Chapters 14–26 of the Code which relate to treatment and care in hospital are also especially relevant.

The Act also defines the responsibilities of the responsible medical officers, managers, doctors and health authorities and considers Approved Social Workers as follows.

LOCAL AUTHORITY SOCIAL SERVICES PERSONNEL

Approved social workers. An 'approved social worker' (ASW) means an officer of a local social services authority appointed to act as an approved social worker for the purposes of the Mental Health Act 1983.

Section 114 provides for the appointment of approved social workers by a local social services authority for the purpose of discharging the functions conferred on them by this Act. No person shall be appointed by a local social services authority as an approved social worker unless approved by the authority as having appropriate competence in dealing with persons who are suffering from mental disorder. In approving a person for appointment as an approved social worker a local social services authority shall have regard to such matters as the Secretary of State may direct.

In respect of approved social workers' functions the relevant sections are:

s.4 Admission for assessment in cases of emergency
s.10 Transfer of guardianship in case of death, incapacity, etc. of guardian
s.11 General provisions as to applications
s.13 Duty of approved social workers to make applications for admission or guardianship
s.14 Social reports
s.18 Return and readmission of patients absent without leave
s.29 Appointment by court of acting nearest relative

s.30 Discharge and variation of orders under s.29

s.40 Effect of hospital orders, guardianship orders and interim hospital orders

s.87 Patients absent from hospitals in Northern Ireland

s.89 Patients absent from hospitals in the Channel Islands or Isle of Man

s.115 Powers of entry and inspection

s.135 Warrant to search for and remove patients

s.136 Mentally disordered persons found in public places

s.138 Retaking of patients escaping from custody.

Other sections of the Act also involve approved social workers. Indeed, the whole Act is relevant to their role to some extent.

DHSS Circular No.LAC(86)15/WO Circular No.51(86) (DHSS, 1986) contain revised directions from the Secretary of State, made under s.114 of the Mental Health Act 1983, on the appointment of approved social workers. Paragraph 4 says:

'The new arrangements provided for in this Circular are designed to ensure that all approved social workers receive appropriate and adequate training for the statutory duties they are required to perform. CCETSW will be responsible for approving training courses and for monitoring the standard of training provided by authorities—whether singly or in consortia: no costs will arise to authorities for this. Authorities themselves will be responsible for ensuring that only staff who have been properly trained and who are competent to perform statutory duties are appointed'.

CCETSW's revised training requirements are in CCETSW Paper 19.19 (CCETSW, 1993).

Paragraph 8 of the above Circular says, in judging the number needed, full allowance should be made for the time that these trained and experienced mental health social workers need to spend on preventive work which avoids the need for compulsion.

Paragraph 14 says:

'Approved social workers should have a wider role than reacting to requests for admission to hospital, making the necessary arrangements and ensuring compliance with the law. They should have the specialist knowledge and skills to make appropriate decisions in respect of both clients and their relatives and to gain the confidence of colleagues in the health services with whom they are required to collaborate. ... Their role is to prevent the necessity for compulsory admission to hospital as well as to make application where they decide this is appropriate'.

Paragraph 15 of the Circular stresses cooperation with other services.

The Code of Practice (DH and Welsh Office, 1993) spells out in chapter 2 the role of approved social workers in assessment and paras 2.10–2.17 stress the individual professional responsibility of the ASW. Paragraph 2.10 says:

'It is important to emphasise that where an ASW is assessing a person for possible admission under the Act he has overall responsibility for co-ordinating the process of assessment and, where he decides to make an application, for implementing that decision. See also paras 2.28–2.29 of the Code on disagreements between different professionals and paras 2.30–2.31 on the choice of applicant for admission.

Other chapters of the Code are also especially relevant to ASWs including chapter 3 'Part III of the Mental Health Act—Patients concerned with Criminal Proceedings', especially para. 3.12 on the role of the ASW, chapter 6 'Admission for Assessment in an Emergency', chapter 11 'Conveying to Hospital' and chapter 13 'Guardianship'.

Social workers, residential workers and other staff in local authority social services.

Paragraph 8 of the above DHSS/WO Circulars (DHSS, 1986) says that 'social workers to be approved should be selected from amongst those engaged in the wide range of mental health work in their departments'. Many sections of the Mental Health Act set out the other powers and duties of local authority social services. These include s.14 which places a duty on social services authorities to arrange for a 'social worker of their social services department' to interview the patient and provide hospital managers with a social report on a patient's social circumstances if the patient has been admitted to hospital pursuant to an application made by his nearest relative under either ss.2 or 3. Local authorities also have a duty to provide social circumstances reports to Mental Health Review Tribunals. Other local authority responsibilities under the Act include those relating to Guardianship (ss.7 and 37, and chapter 13 of the Code of Practice) and Aftercare (s.117, and chapter 27 of the Code). Local authorities also have a responsibility to provide social work support to the Health Service, including psychiatric hospitals. HO Circular No.66/90, Annex F (HO, 1990) sets out the responsibilities of local authority social services departments in relation to mentally disordered offenders. In addition to social workers, a wide range of staff in the personal social services, including residential workers, day-care workers, home help organizers and home helps, provide services to mentally disordered people of all ages.

Probation officers.

Probation officers are particularly involved under Part III of the Mental Health Act 1983 with patients concerned in criminal proceedings or under sentence. Chapters 3, 7, 17 and 28 of the Code (DH and Welsh Office, 1993) are especially relevant as are HO Circular No.66/90 (HO, 1990) and the Police and Criminal Evidence Act 1984 and its Codes of Practice (HO PACE, 1991).

Voluntary and private sector staff.

Many social workers, residential and other staff work in the voluntary and private sectors.

Police.

The police have powers and duties under the Act, including s.135 relating to warrants to search for and remove patients to places of safety, s.136 removal to places of safety of mentally disordered persons found in public places and s.137 provisions as to custody, conveyance and detention. Chapters 3, 7, 10, 17 and 28 of the Code (DH and Welsh Office, 1993) are especially relevant as are HO Circular No.66/90 (HO, 1990) and the Police and Criminal Evidence Act 1984 and its Code of Practice (HO PACE, 1991).

Lawyers.

Lawyers have responsibilities under the Act including those relating to Mental Health Review Tribunals, both as tribunal members and as solicitors with experience of tribunal work, as well as in relation to the management of property and affairs, for example, as Lord Chancellor's Visitors.

The prison service, prison medical service and forensic psychiatric service.

These services also have responsibilities under the Mental Health Act 1983 and are dealt with in HO Circular No.66/90 (HO, 1990). The chapters in the Code (DH and Welsh Office, 1993) relating to criminal proceedings and medical treatment are also especially relevant.

The courts.

Courts, including Magistrates Courts, and the Crown Prosecution Service, have responsibilities under mental health legislation including those set out in the Act, Code (DH and Welsh Office, 1993) and Home Office Circular (HO, 1990) relating to criminal proceedings.

Generally speaking, all the main 'actors' are involved to a lesser or a greater extent in most parts of the Act. In any case, each needs to know the roles played by the others.

Medical treatment.

It is worth noting that the term 'medical treatment' 'includes nursing, and also care, habilation and rehabilitation under medical supervision' (s.145).

The Community.

The term 'Community' is not

defined in the Mental Health Act, but it is where most mentally disordered people live.

The law should not be applied in isolation, but needs to be seen in the context of social work, nursing, medical and other professional practice.

Part II of the Act (Sections 2–34) relates to compulsory admission to hospital and guardianship

Documentation must be in the form set out in the Mental Health (Hospital, Guardianship and Consent to Treatment) Regulations 1983. Many chapters of the Code of Practice (DH and Welsh Office, 1993) are also relevant. Part II contains the following provisions:

---

s.2 admission for assessment

'(2) An application for admission for assessment may be made in respect of a patient on the grounds that

(a) he is suffering from mental disorder of a nature or degree which warrants the detention of the patient in a hospital for assessment (or for assessment followed by medical treatment) for at least a limited period; and

(b) he ought to be so detained in the interests of his own health or safety or with a view to the protection of other persons.

(3) An application for admission for assessment shall be founded on the written recommendations in the prescribed form of two registered medical practitioners, including in each case a statement that in the opinion of the practitioner the conditions set out in subsection (2) above are complied with'.

This section authorizes compulsory admission to hospital for assessment (or for assessment followed by treatment) and for detention for this purpose for up to 28 days. If the applicant is an approved social worker he or she must inform the nearest relative about the application, although the nearest relative cannot prevent an approved social worker making an application. The approved social worker is required to have regard to any wishes expressed by relatives of the patient, but is not required to consult with them.

DH/WO Circular Letter of 18 February 1992 (DH and Welsh Office, 1992) removed an obscurity from the former Code of Practice on the Act which seemed to suggest that people would only be admitted compulsorily if they were a danger to themselves or others. It has now been made clear that people can be compulsorily admitted for the sake of their health alone. The amended Code could help reduce the number of mentally ill people sleeping rough.

Paragraph 23 of the Memorandum (DHSS, 1983a) points out that the conditions for s.2 admissions are not quite so stringent as those for s.3 admissions because assessment may well be used for the purpose of determining whether the more stringent conditions for admission for treatment are met.

---

s.3 admission for treatment

'(2) An application for admission for treatment may be made in respect of a patient on the grounds that:

(a) he is suffering from mental illness, severe mental impairment, psychopathic disorder or mental impairment and his mental disorder is of a nature or degree which makes it appropriate for him to receive medical treatment in a hospital; and

(b) in the case of psychopathic disorder or mental impairment, such treatment is likely to alleviate or prevent a deterioration of his condition; and

(c) it is necessary for the health or safety of the patient or for the protection of other persons that he should receive such treatment and it cannot be provided unless he is detained under this section.

(3) An application for admission for treatment shall be founded on the written recommendations in the prescribed form of two registered medical practitioners, including in each case a statement that in the opinion of the practitioner the conditions set out in subsection (2) above are complied with; ...'.

Compulsory admission to hospital for treatment and subsequent detention can last for an initial period of up to six months. Under s.3 if an approved social worker makes the application he or she must consult with the patient's nearest relative if practicable and cannot proceed with the application if the nearest relative objects. The applicant must have seen the patient within the previous 14 days and an approved social worker applicant must interview the patient before making an application.

Applications under ss.2 and 3 can be made by either the patient's nearest relative or an approved social worker and should be addressed to the managers of the hospital to which admission is sought.

Whether it is appropriate to detain a patient under ss.2 or 3 is considered by the Code of Practice (DH and Welsh Office, 1993) and chapter 5 of the consultation documents relating to revision of the Code (DH, 1992a, 1993a).

s.4.
s.4 provides for **admission for assessment in cases of emergency** for a period of up to 72 hours. Applications may be made either by an approved social worker or the nearest relative and shall be sufficient in the first instance if founded on one of the medical recommendations required by s.2 (see Code of Practice at para. 6.1 *et seq.* (DH and Welsh Office, 1993)).

s.5 applications in respect of patients already in hospital.
This section provides for applications for compulsory detention under ss.2 or 3 to be made by a registered medical practitioner for up to 72 hours in respect of mentally disordered patients who are already receiving treatment in hospital as informal patients. It also sets out the procedures that can be used if it is considered that a patient might leave the hospital before there is time to complete an application under ss.2 or 3.

Subsection (4) provides for nurses of a prescribed class to invoke a 'holding power' for up to six months:

'If, in the case of a patient who is receiving treatment for mental disorder as an in-patient in a hospital, it appears to a nurse of the prescribed class:

(a) that the patient is suffering from mental disorder to such a degree that it is necessary for his health or safety or for the protection of others for him to be immediately restrained from leaving the hospital; and

(b) that it is not practicable to secure the immediate attendance of a practitioner for the purpose of furnishing a report under subsection (2) above,

the nurse may record that fact in writing; and in that event the patient may be detained in the hospital for a period of six hours from the time when that fact is so recorded or until the earlier arrival at the place where the patient is detained of a practitioner having power to furnish a report under that subsection'.

See also the Code of Practice (DH and Welsh Office, 1993).

s.6 the effect of an application for admission.
This section authorizes the applicant or anyone authorized by him or her to take the patient and convey him or her to hospital within specified periods and the hospital managers to detain the patient once admitted. See Chapter 11 of Code of Practice (DH and Welsh Office, 1993).

s. 7 an application for guardianship.
This section specifies the circumstances whereby a patient aged 16 years or over may be received into the guardianship of a local social services authority or a person who is acceptable to the authority. Neither the authority nor individual is obliged to accept the duties of guardian. The grounds for a guardianship application in respect of a patient are that:

'(a) he is suffering from mental disorder, being mental illness, severe mental impairment, psychopathic disorder or mental impairment and his mental disorder is of a nature or degree which warrants his reception into guardianship under this section; and

(b) it is necessary in the interests of the welfare

of the patient or for the protection of other persons that the patient should be so received'.

A guardianship application must be founded on the written recommendations of two registered medical practitioners and may be made by either the patient's nearest relative or an approved social worker. The latter cannot make an application if the nearest relative objects, which can cause difficulty if the relative seems to be acting irresponsibly towards the patient (Jones, 1991). It is not possible for a mentally handicapped person whose impairment is not associated with abnormally aggressive or seriously irresponsible conduct to be placed on a guardianship order.

A patient may also be compulsorily admitted to a hospital or residential care facility under s.47 of the National Assistance Act 1948 or in an emergency under s.1 of the National Assistance (Amendment) Act 1951. In practice, the use of these provisions tends to be confined to elderly people, living alone and unable to care for themselves. Under s.47 a local authority may make an application to a magistrates court to remove a person from home on the grounds (i) that the person is suffering from grave chronic disease or, being aged, infirm or physically incapacitated, is living in insanitary conditions; (ii) that the person is unable to devote to himself or herself, and is not receiving from others, proper care and attention; and (iii) that removal from home is necessary, either in the person's own interests or for preventing injury to the health of, or serious nuisance to, other persons.

s.8 effect of a guardianship application, etc.

This section confers specific powers limited to restricting the liberty of the person under guardianship only to the extent necessary to ensure that various forms of treatment, social support, training, education, occupation or residence are undertaken. The guardian does not have the power to detain the patient, use or dispose of the patient's property, or carry out any financial transactions on the patient's behalf. The guardian is subject to the duties laid down in Part III of the Mental Health (Hospital, Guardianship and Consent to Treatment) Regulations 1983. See also para. 13.7 of the Code of Practice (DH and Welsh Office, 1993).

s.9. s.9 empowers the Secretary of State to make **regulations as to guardianship**.

s.10. s.10 provides for the **transfer of guardianship** where the guardian dies, becomes incapacitated, wishes to relinquish the function or is found to be performing his functions negligently.

s.11. s.11 contains **general provisions as to applications for admission for assessment or treatment or guardianship**.

s.12. s.12 contains **general provisions as to medical recommendations**.

s.13. s.13 sets out the **duty of approved social workers to make applications for admission or guardianship** if they consider that applications ought to be made and are of the opinion, having regard to any wishes expressed by relatives or any other relevant circumstances, that it is necessary or proper for them to make the applications. Before making an application for admission to hospital, the approved social worker must 'interview the patient in a suitable manner and satisfy himself that detention in a hospital is in all the circumstances of the case the most appropriate way of providing the care and medical treatment of which the patient stands in need'. If so required by the nearest relative, the local social services authority has a duty to direct an approved social worker to consider making an application for admission to hospital. See chapter 2 of the Code (DH and Welsh Office, 1993).

s.14. s.14 provides for **social reports** and places a duty on social services authorities to provide hospital managers with a report on a patient's social circumstances if the patient has been admitted to hospital pursuant to an application by his or her nearest relative under s.2 or s.3.

s.15. s.15 relates to **rectification of applications and recommendations**.

s.16. s.16 provides for **reclassification of patients**.

s.17. s.17 provides for **leave of absence from hospital**.

s.18. s.18 provides for the **return and readmission of patients absent without leave**.

s.19. s.19 provides for **regulations to be made by the Secretary of State as to transfer of patients**. See Mental Health (Hospital, Guardianship and Consent to Treatment) Regulations 1983.

s.20 duration of authority for detention or guardianship. This section provides for patients who have been detained for treatment or placed under guardianship to be detained or kept under guardianship for an initial period of up to six months. It also sets out the renewal criteria to be satisfied which can be for one further period of six months and subsequently for one year at a time.

These renewal provisions can only be used to renew the authority to detain a patient if the patient's mental condition requires his detention as a hospital in-patient (*R. v. Hallstrom, ex p. W.; R. v. Gardner, ex p. L. (1986) 2 All E.R. 306*). The decision in the *Hallstrom* case has generated a debate on whether there should be legislation to introduce a new 'Community Treatment Order' which would permit the compulsory administration of drugs to patients living in the community (see below).

s.21. s.21 makes **special provisions as to patients absent without leave** and s.22 **special provisions as to patients sentenced to imprisonment, etc.**

s.23. s.23 relates to **discharge of patients**. For discussion, see Jones (1991) and Hoggett (1990).

s.24. s.24 provides for **visiting and examination of patients** and the production of documents relating to discharge (see reg.10 Nursing Homes and Mental Nursing Homes Regulations 1984). See also chapter 26 of the Code of Practice (DH and Welsh Office, 1993).

s.25. s.25 relates to **restrictions on discharge by nearest relative**.

ss.26–30. ss.26–30 relate to **functions of relatives of patients** (see above).

s.31. s.31 relates to **procedure on applications to county court**. See County Court Rules 1981.

s.32. s.32 relates to the Secretary of State's power to make **Regulations for purposes of Part II**. See Mental Health (Hospital, Guardianship and Consent to Treatment) Regulations 1983.

s.33. s.33 makes **special provisions as to wards of court**.

s.34. s.34 relates to **Interpretation of Part II**.

Part III (Sections 35–55) relates to patients concerned in criminal proceedings or under sentence

It deals with the circumstances in which patients may be admitted to and detained in hospital or received into guardianship on the order of a court or transferred to hospital or guardianship from penal institutions on the direction of the Home Secretary. Guidance is contained in the Code of Practice (DH and Welsh Office, 1993) and Home Office Circular No. 66/90 'Provision for Mentally Disordered Offenders' (HO, 1990), which contains sections on the Police, Crown Prosecution Service, Magistrates Courts, Probation Service, Prison Medical Service, Psychiatric Services, Health Services and Local Authority Social Services.

The Police and Criminal Evidence Act 1984 and its Codes on Detention and Questioning (HO PACE, 1991) are relevant both to the role of the police and to the social worker's role as 'appropriate adult' for mentally disordered people and juveniles.

Section 4 of the Criminal Justice Act 1991 requires that, where an offender is or appears to be mentally disordered, the court shall normally obtain a medical report before passing a custodial sentence. It also requires the court to consider the likely effect of such a sentence on that condition and on any treatment that may be available for it.

Under common law, a person is considered unfit to plead or 'under disability' if unable to instruct a legal representative, understand a charge against them, follow evidence, or challenge a juror. These aspects of the common law are not affected by the Criminal Procedure (Insanity and Unfitness to Plead) Act 1991. The 1991 Act was a response to civil liberties campaigns which complained that under the Criminal Procedure (Insanity) Act 1964 the only option available to the court was a hospital order without restriction of time, that is potentially indefinite detention without trial. Moreover, the evidence relating to the alleged offence used not to be heard by the court, so there was a presumption of guilt. Now, where an accused person has been found unfit to be tried, the Criminal Procedure (Insanity and Unfitness to Plead) Act 1991 provides for a 'trial of the facts' by a jury.

Part IV (Sections 56–64) relates to consent to treatment

This Part, which overrides the common law, only applies to treatment relating to the patient's mental disorder. It clarifies the extent to which treatment for mental disorder can be imposed on detained patients in hospitals and mental nursing homes. It provides for two categories of treatment which have different legal consequences. These are, firstly, the most serious treatments which require the patient's consent *and* a second opinion (s.57) and, secondly, other serious treatments which require the patient's consent *or a* second opinion (s.58). Treatments that do not come within either category can be imposed on a detained patient who understands the nature and purpose of the treatment, but expressly withholds consent (s.63). The safeguards provided for by ss.57 and 58 can be overridden if the treatment is required urgently (s.62). See the Code of Practice (DH and Welsh Office, 1993) especially chapters 15 and 16, the Mental Health Act Commission's guidance in DHSS Circular No. DDL (84) 4 (DHSS, 1984a) and the Mental Health (Hospital, Guardianship and Consent to Treatment) Regulations 1983. For further advice on capacity and consent, see also the Law Commission documents 'Mentally Incapacitated Adults and Decision-Making: A New Jurisdiction' and 'Mentally Inca-

pacitated and Other Vulnerable Adults: Public Law Protection' (Law Commission, 1992, 1993).

For a discussion of supervision and treatment in the community, see 'Future Developments' below.

Patients presenting particular management problems

For guidance, see chapter 18 of the Code (DH and Welsh Office, 1993).

Part V (Sections 65–79) relates to mental health review tribunals

These tribunals are empowered under the Act to review the cases of many detained patients and can also hear applications in relation to patients who are subject to guardianship orders. They have no jurisdiction over informal patients. Provisions relating to the constitution of MHRTs are in Schedule 2. Tribunals must also follow the procedure laid down in the Mental Health Review Tribunal Rules 1983 and where the Rules are silent on a point of procedure the tribunal must follow the rules of natural justice. The function of a tribunal is to review the justification for the patient's continued detention or guardianship at the time of the hearing. It has no power to consider the validity of the admission which gave rise to the liability to be detained.

Part VI (Sections 80–92) relates to the removal and return of patients within the United Kingdom or abroad

Part VII (Sections 93–113) relates to the management of property and affairs of patients

The powers of the judge or Master of the Court of Protection are exercisable when the court is satisfied, after considering medical evidence, that a person is incapable, by reason of mental disorder, of managing and administering his property and affairs. Invoking the jurisdiction of the Court of Protection in respect of the property and affairs of patients has the effect of suspending their ability to act for themselves in all areas within its jurisdiction, even if they actually had the capacity to do so in some respects or from time to time (see Law Commission Reports (Law Commission,

1992, 1993)). The Court of Protection does not have jurisdiction over the management or care of the patient's person or where the patient should live.

Guidance to receivers who have been appointed by the Court of Protection is in a *Handbook for Receivers* published by the Public Trust Office (Public Trust Office, 1993). For information about the appointment of the Public Trustee as receiver under the Mental Health Act 1983, see Jones (1991). See also *Managing Other People's Money* (Letts, 1990).

Part VII provisions include those relating to judges' functions, wills, power to appoint receivers, Lord Chancellor's Visitors, proceedings, procedures, appeals and enduring powers of attorney. See also the Court of Protection Rules 1984.

The Enduring Powers of Attorney Act 1985 enables a donor to appoint an attorney to make legally binding decisions on his or her behalf and whose authority will not be revoked by the donor's subsequent mental incapacity. In the event of the donor becoming mentally incapable, the attorney must apply to the Court of Protection for the instrument to be registered. (See Court of Protection (Enduring Powers of Attorney) Rules 1986. See also Further Reading.)

Part VIII (Sections 114–125) relates to miscellaneous functions of local authorities and the Secretary of State
Provisions include:

s.114 Appointment of approved social workers (see above).

s.115. s.115 provides approved social workers with **powers of entry and inspection of premises** where a patient is believed to be living.

Powers of entry and inspection of mental nursing homes and residential care homes are contained in the Registered Homes Act 1984, Nursing Homes and Mental Nursing Homes Regulations 1984, Registered Homes (Amendment) Act 1991 and the Community Care (Residential Accommodation) Act 1992.

s.117 After-care. This section applies to persons who are detained under s.3, admitted to a hospital in pursuance of a hospital order under s.37, hospital order patients subject to restriction orders under s.41, or persons transferred to a hospital in pursuance of a transfer direction under ss.47 or 48, and then cease to be detained and leave hospital.

Subsection (2) says:

'It shall be the duty of the District Health Authority and of the local social services authority to provide, in co-operation with relevant voluntary agencies, after-care services for any person to whom this section applies until such time as the District Health Authority and the local social services authority are satisfied that the person concerned is no longer in need of such services'.

This section should be read in conjunction with s.7 of the Disabled Persons (Services, Consultation and Representation) Act 1986 which will apply to any patient who has been receiving hospital treatment for mental disorder for six months or more. Before such a patient is discharged, the hospital managers must send written notification of the date of discharge to the health authority and the local social services authority for the area in which the patient is to live. Following notification, the two authorities are required to co-operate in assessing the patient's need for services for which they are responsible. The assessments must be made before the patient is discharged. However, Section 7 has not yet been implemented and the Government says the National Health Service and Community Care Act 1990 has made implementation unnecessary. Many people and pressure groups dispute this.

After-care services are not defined in the Mental Health Act, but the Mental Health Act Commission has prepared a checklist of desirable features for an after-care policy (see appendix 3 to their Third Biennial Report 1987–89 (MHAC, 1989). See also chapter 27 of the DH/WO Code of Practice which includes reference to the care programme approach (DH and Welsh Office, 1993).

s.118. s.118 provides for a **Code of Practice**.

s.119. s.119 provides for the **payment of medical practitioners appointed by the Secretary of State to carry out certain functions under the Act** and for them to have access to detained patients cared for in mental nursing homes and to their records.

s.120. s.120 places duties relating to the **general protection of detained patients** on the Secretary of State who has directed the Mental Health Act Commission to carry out these duties on his or her behalf.

s.121 Mental Health Act Commission. This section provides for the continuance of the Commission and relates to its functions. The Regulations and Order concerning the functions, establishment and constitution of the Commission are the Mental Health Act Commission Regulations (1983) and the Mental Health Act Commission (Establishment and Constitution) Order 1983.

The Commission's functions are quite separate from those of Mental Health Review Tribunals which determine whether a patient should continue to be detained. The Commission has no power to discharge a patient.

s.123. s.123 provides for **transfers to and from special hospitals**.

s.125 Inquiries. The Secretary of State may cause an inquiry to be held in any case where he or she thinks it advisable to do so in connection with any matter arising under the Act.

Part IX (Sections 126–130) relates to offences against patients

Part X (Sections 131–149) miscellaneous and supplementary

The miscellaneous provisions section includes a number of very important provisions including the following:

s.131 Informal admission of patients:

'(1) Nothing in this Act shall be construed as preventing a patient who requires treatment for mental disorder from being admitted to any hospital or mental nursing home in pursuance of arrangements made in that behalf and without any application, order or direction rendering him liable to be detained under this Act, or from remaining in any hospital or mental nursing home in pursuance of such arrangements after he has ceased to be so liable to be detained'.

This section provides that patients can either enter hospital for treatment for mental disorder on an informal basis, or remain in hospital on an informal basis once the authority for their original detention has come to an end. There are no special formalities which need to be observed for an informal patient to be admitted to a psychiatric hospital and, subject to s.5, informal patients can leave hospital when they like. With the exception of s.57 provisions, informal patients are not subject to the Part IV consent to treatment provisions. Nor are they entitled to compulsory after-care services.

Jones (1991) points out that there is no legally established mechanism for reviewing either the reasons for informal patients' admission to hospital or the justification for their continued hospitalization. Once informal patients have been admitted to hospital, no person or body is placed under any legal obligation to inform them of their legal status and of the fact that they are free to leave hospital whenever they wish. Paragraph 14.1 of the Code of Practice (DH and Welsh Office, 1993) states that 'it should be made clear to informal patients that they are allowed to leave hospital at any time'. The admission is informal, and not voluntary. It is not necessary for patients to express their consent to the admission and it is possible to admit patients on an informal basis as long as they are not indicating either verbally or through their actions that they object to the admission. Paragraph 2.7 of the Code of Practice says:

'Where admission to hospital is considered necessary and the patient is willing to be admitted informally this should in general be arranged. Compulsory admission should, however, be considered where the patient's current medical state, together with reliable evidence of past experience, indicates a strong likelihood that he will change his mind about informal admission prior to his actual admission to hospital with a resulting risk to his health or safety or to the safety of others'.

In addition, many old people with some degree of senile dementia live in local authority, voluntary or private residential care homes or nursing homes. Many others are living in their own or relatives' homes.

s.132. s.132 places a **duty upon hospital managers to provide information to detained patients** and their relatives to try to ensure that they understand which section of the Act authorizes the patient's detention and the effects of that section and their right to apply to Mental Health Review Tribunals if applicable. Section 132 also places a further duty on hospital managers to ensure that patients understand the means by which their detention can be ended and the various safeguards from which they benefit, including those concerning consent to treatment, the Code of Practice, the Mental Health Act Commission, patients' correspondence and legal aid schemes which could help them obtain representation for a court appeal or MHRT.

s.133. s.133 sets out the **duty of managers to inform the nearest relative of discharge**.

s.135 Warrant to search for and remove patients. This section provides for a magistrate to issue a warrant authorizing a policeman to enter private premises, using force if necessary, to remove a mentally disordered person liable to be detained or not. In the latter case, subs.(1) provides for this, if it appears to a justice of the peace, on information on oath laid by an approved social worker, that there is reasonable cause to suspect that a person believed to be suffering from mental disorder has been, or is being, ill-treated, neglected or kept otherwise than

under proper control, or being unable to care for herself or himself, is living alone in any such place. In the execution of a warrant under subs.(1), the constable must be accompanied by an approved social worker and a registered medical practitioner. A patient may be detained in a 'place of safety' for up to 72 hours. In this section 'place of safety' includes residential accommodation provided by a local social services authority under Part III of the National Assistance Act 1948, a hospital as defined by the Mental Health Act, a police station, a mental nursing home or residential home for mentally disordered persons or any other suitable place whose occupier is willing temporarily to receive the patient. Under the Police and Criminal Evidence Act 1984 a policeman may enter and search any premises without a warrant under this section if this is required to save life or limb or prevent serious damage to property. Persons removed to a police station as a place of safety under this section are protected by the PACE Codes of Practice (HO PACE, 1991).

Local social services authorities have a duty to provide temporary protection for the property of persons admitted to hospital or to accommodation provided under Part III of the National Assistance Act 1948.

s.136 Mentally disordered persons found in public places. Subsection (1) says:

'If a constable finds in a place to which the public have access a person who appears to him to be suffering from mental disorder and to be in immediate need of care or control, the constable may, if he thinks it necessary to do so in the interests of that person or for the protection of other persons, remove that person to a place of safety within the meaning of section 135 above'.

The person can be detained in a place of safety for up to 72 hours so that he or she can be examined by a doctor and interviewed by an approved social worker in order that suitable arrangements can be made for treatment or care. A person does not have to commit an offence before the police can use their power to remove but, Jones (1991) submits, in most cases the behaviour of the persons removed would have justified their being charged with an offence against public order. See chapter 10 of the DH/WO Code of Practice (DH and Welsh Office, 1993) and the Police and Criminal Evidence Act Codes of Practice (HO PACE, 1991).

s.137 Provisions as to custody, conveyance and detention. This section specifies the circumstances whereby a person is deemed to be in legal custody and provides that anyone who is required or authorized to detain or convey a person who is in legal custody shall have the powers of a constable when so acting.

Of the **Schedules to the Act**, Schedule 1 relates to application of certain provisions to patients subject to hospital and guardianship orders and Schedule 2 to Mental Health Review Tribunals.

OTHER STATUTORY SOCIAL SERVICES

Local authorities have statutory responsibility for providing social services for mentally disordered people of all ages in their area. As well as aiding their rehabilitation and preventing recurrence of mental disorder, social services can help prevent other vulnerable people become mentally ill by supporting them in times of extra stress. Powers and duties of local authority social services authorities are listed in Schedule 1 to the Local Authority Social Services Act 1970 and the Local Authority Social Services (Designation of Functions) Order 1989. People who suffer from mental disorder and learning disabilities come within the definition of 'disabled person' in s.29 of the National Assistance Act 1948, which is also the definition used in the Disabled Persons (Services, Consultation and Representation) Act 1986 and the National Health Service and Community Care Act 1990.

In order to understand the statutory provisions,

a number of Acts need to be read together. The National Health Service and Community Care Act 1990 does not consolidate social welfare legislation by replacing earlier relevant Statutes. Many of the 1990 Act's community care provisions are based on earlier statutes which still remain in force as amended by subsequent legislation.

Part III of the National Health Service and Community Care Act 1990 relates to community care in England and Wales. Sections 42–45 relate to the provision of accommodation and welfare services and ss.46–50 to general provisions concerning community care services.

Section 46 provides for local authority plans for community care services and says in this section:

'"community care services" means services which a local authority may provide or arrange to be provided under any of the following provisions;
(a) Part III of the National Assistance Act 1948;
(b) Section 45 of the Health Services and Public Health Act 1968;
(c) Section 21 of and Schedule 8 to the National Health Service Act 1977; and
(d) Section 117 of the Mental Health Act 1983'.

The above provisions, together with s.2 of the Chronically Sick and Disabled Persons Act 1970, s.4 of the Disabled Persons (Services, Consultation and Representation) Act 1986, s.47 of the 1990 Act and the various relevant directions issued by the Secretary of State, provide the basic legal framework under which local authorities provide care in the community.

The 1990 Act provides for the Government to make specific grants to local authorities for mental illness social services. However, the Government wishes local authorities to arrange that community care be increasingly provided by the voluntary and especially the private sectors.

The Department of Health has produced much guidance arising from the 1990 Act.

Part I of the Health and Social Services and Social Security Adjudications Act 1983 also relates to community care, s.1 providing for joint financing and Part VIII permitting local authorities to make charges for certain social services.

Collecting and disseminating information

The Chronically Sick and Disabled Persons Act 1970 s.1 as amended by the Disabled Persons (Services, Consultation and Representation) Act 1986 s.9 requires every social services authority to gather information on how many disabled persons are living in its area and inform itself as to how it should plan to meet their needs. It also places a duty on the local authority to publish general information about its services for disabled persons and ensure that anyone who uses these is given information about other relevant services. The National Health Service and Community Care Act 1990 emphasizes the publication of information about the assessment process, the availability of services and access to the complaints procedure.

Assessment of needs

See Chronically Sick and Disabled Persons Act 1970 s.1; Disabled Persons (Services, Consultation and Representation) Act 1986 s.4(a) and (b), s.8; Children Act 1989 s.17 and Schedule 2 Part I; National Health Service and Community Care Act 1990 s.47. Section 4 of the 1986 Act relates to services under the 1970 Act and provides that, when requested to do so by disabled persons, their authorized representative, or any person who provides care for them in the circumstances mentioned in s.8, a local authority shall decide whether the needs of the disabled person call for the provision by the authority of any services in accordance with s.2(1) of the 1970 Act. Section 4 places a clear duty on local social services authorities to decide, when requested to do so, whether the needs of a disabled person require the provision of welfare services under s.2 of the 1970 Act. The provision in the 1986 Act relating to the authorized representative is not in force. See also DHSS Circular No. LAC(87)6 (DHSS, 87). Section 8 of the 1986 Act relates to the duty of the local authority, when assessing the needs of a disabled person who receives a substantial amount of regular care from a person other than an employee of the statutory social services, to have regard to the carer's ability to

continue to provide that care. It also requires the local authority to provide an interpretation service if the carer is unable to communicate effectively by reason of mental or physical incapacity and, in determining whether such a service is required, the local authority must take into account any views expressed by the carer. Although subs.(1) relating to carers is in force, subs.(2) relating to communication is not. Paragraph 6 of DHSS Circular No. LAC(87)6 (DHSS 87) says, although the section places no specific requirement on the local authority to provide services or support for the carer, authorities will no doubt continue as part of normal good practice to have regard to the possible need for such services and to the desirability of enabling the disabled person to continue living at home for as long as possible if this is what that person wishes.

Section 47 of the National Health Service and Community Care Act 1990 provides for assessment of needs for community care services. The local authority must assess both the needs of the local population and the social care needs of individuals. After assessing individual needs, local authorities must arrange appropriate packages of care which may include a range of options. Services provided should reflect the client's choice.

Section 17 of the Children Act 1989 relates to the provision of services for children in need, their families and others.

The provision of services in the community

These are provided under the National Assistance Act 1948 s.29 as extended by s.2 of the Chronically Sick and Disabled Persons Act 1970, the Disabled Persons (Services, Consultation and Representation) Act 1986 and the National Health Service and Community Care Act 1990 Part III. Section 29 as amended states in subs.(1) that a local authority may, with the approval of the Secretary of State, and to such extent as he or she may direct in relation to persons ordinarily resident in the area of the local authority, make arrangements for promoting the welfare of persons to whom this section applies, that is persons who are blind, deaf or dumb, or who suffer from mental disorder of any description and other persons who are substantially and permanently handicapped by illness, injury or congenital deformity or such other disabilities as may be prescribed by the Minister. Section 29(4) lists the types of arrangements that may be made under subs.(1). Section 2 of the 1970 Act extends s.29 of the 1948 Act and places a duty on local authorities to make arrangements for all or any of the matters specified.

The National Health Service Act 1977 ss.3, 21(1)(b) and Schedule 8 para. 2(1) is also relevant. Section 21(1) states that the services described in Schedule 8 in relation to care of mothers and young children, prevention, care and after-care and home help and laundry facilities are functions exercisable by local social services authorities, and that Schedule 8 has effect accordingly. The Schedule requires that local social services authorities provide necessary home help and laundry facilities for persons handicapped as a result of having suffered from illness or by congenital deformity. Local authority social services also have responsibility under Schedule 8 to provide day services for adults with mental handicap. The Schedule also provides that local social services authorities may, with the Secretary of State's approval and direction, provide preventive services, care and after-care for persons suffering from mental disorder and who are received into guardianship. Under ss.3 and 21 respectively health services and social services may provide after-care services for mentally ill and mentally handicapped persons discharged from hospital.

Provision of residential accommodation

The National Assistance Act 1948 s.21 enables local authorities to provide residential accommodation for sick, handicapped or elderly people and they must provide it to the extent that the Secretary of State has directed in DHSS Circular No.13/74 (DHSS, 74). Accommodation is also provided in voluntary and private residential homes. See also the 1990 Act and the Community Care (Residential Accommodation) Act 1992. Under the 1990 Act local authorities are responsible for assessing individual needs for residential services and for paying fees for residents according to their assessments.

Registration of residential care homes

Local authorities are responsible for registering and inspecting residential care homes. See Registered Homes Act 1984, s.48 of the National Health Service and Community Care Act 1990, Registered Homes (Amendment) Act 1991 and Community Care (Residential Accommodation) Act 1992.

Compulsory admission into residential care

See National Assistance Act 1948 s.47 and National Assistance (Amendment) Act 1951.

Protection of property

See National Assistance Act 1948 s.48(1) above.

Sheltered employment

The Disabled Persons (Employment) Act 1958 s.3 empowers local authorities to make arrangements for the provision of facilities for enabling disabled persons to be employed or work under special conditions, including sheltered employment.

Welfare of old people generally

The Health Services and Public Health Act 1968 s.45 relates to the promotion by local authorities of the welfare of old people generally.

Social work support in health settings

Local authority social services authorities provide social work support for the health service.

Housing

Part III of the Housing Act 1985 relates to housing the homeless and s.72 deals with co-operation between housing and social services authorities. Although local authority housing departments have primary responsibility for the homeless, s.72 attempts to ensure the co-operation of social services. Section 59 says a person has priority need if *inter alia* that person or anyone who lives or might reasonably be expected to live with him or her is especially vulnerable because of age, disability or other special reasons.

Access to personal files

The Access to Personal Files Act 1987 provides access for individuals to information about themselves maintained by certain authorities and allows them to obtain copies of, and require amendment of such information.

OTHER STATUTORY SERVICES FOR PERSONS WITH MENTAL DISORDER

Health services

Both specialist and generic medical services are provided under National Health Service legislation. Hospitals and local authorities are required to co-operate when mentally disordered people are discharged from hospital, as seen above. Local authority social services authorities provide social work support to the NHS.

Employment

The Department of Employment has primary responsibility for assisting disabled people find work under the Disabled Persons (Employment) Act 1944. See also local authorities' powers in relation to sheltered and other employment under the Disabled Persons (Employment) Act 1958.

Social security and welfare rights and benefits

People with mental health problems often face particular difficulties in claiming social security benefits (see Grimshaw, 1993–94). See Social Security Acts 1975, 1986 and 1990.

For further law relating to people with learning disabilities see Wright (1992). Workers with mentally disordered people also need to know about legislation relating to anti-discrimination and substance misuse.

CHILDREN AND YOUNG PEOPLE

The DH Code of Practice (DH and Welsh Office, 1993) applies to all patients including those under 18 years. Chapter 30 gives guidance of particular importance to children and young people.

There is no minimum age limit for admission to hospital under the Act. Jones (1991) submits there is nothing in the Act which prevents a child being compulsorily admitted to hospital under Part II. Provisions in the Mental Health Act specifically relating to children and young people include the following.

s.131(2) Informal admission of patients

Paragraph 30.7 of the Code (DH and Welsh Office, 1993) provides guidance applicable to young people not detained under the Act in relation to consent to medical treatment.

Children in 'secure accommodation'

The Children (Secure Accommodation) Regulations 1991 provide that s.25 of the Children Act 1989, which sets restrictions on the use of secure accommodation for children, does not apply to a child who is detained under any provision of the Mental Health Act.

Confidentiality

Paragraph 30.11 of the Code (DH and Welsh Office, 1993) says young people's legal rights to confidentiality should be strictly observed.

Placement

Paragraph 30.12 of the Code maintains the principle that it is preferable for children and young people admitted to hospital to be accommodated with others of their own age group in children's wards or adolescent units, separate from adults. Under ss.85 and 86 of the Children Act 1989 the local social services authority must be notified if a child either is, or is intended to be, accommodated by a health or local education authority, or in a residential, nursing or mental nursing home, for more than three months.

Complaints

Paragraph 30.13 of the Code (DH and Welsh Office, 1993) says children and young people in hospital (both as informal and detained patients) and their parents or guardians should have ready access to existing complaints procedures, which should be drawn to their attention on their admission to hospital. Certain children are also entitled to use the Children Act complaints procedure established in accordance with the Representations Procedure (Children) Regulations 1991.

The Mental Health Act Commission is concerned

about children with mental disorders who are outside the control of the Mental Health Act, 1983 (e.g. re. levels of dosage).

Other statutory social services for children and young people

The Children Act 1989 contains most of the other current legislative provisions relating to children except children in court proceedings or adoption. To some extent, the whole Children Act is relevant to mentally disordered children, but Part III of the Act makes special provision for 'children in need', which term includes 'disabled children'.

Section 17(10) states:

> 'for the purposes of this Part a child shall be taken to be in need if
> (a) he is unlikely to achieve or maintain, or to have the opportunity of achieving or maintaining, a reasonable standard of health or development without the provision for him of services by a local authority under this Part;
> (b) his health or development is likely to be significantly impaired, or further impaired, without the provision for him of such services;
> or
> (c) he is disabled ...'.

Section 17(11) states:

> 'For the purposes of this Part, a child is disabled if he is blind, deaf or dumb or suffers from mental disorder of any kind or is substantially and permanently handicapped by illness, injury or congenital deformity or such other disability as may be prescribed; and in this Part "development" means physical, intellectual, emotional, social or behavioural development; and "health" means physical or mental health'.

Section 17(1) states:

> 'It shall be the general duty of every local authority ...

> (a) to safeguard and promote the welfare of children within their area who are in need; and
> (b) so far as is consistent with that duty, to promote the upbringing of such children by their families, by providing a range and level of services appropriate to those children's needs'.

Section 17(2) states:

> 'For the purpose principally of facilitating the discharge of their general duty under this section, every local authority shall have the specific duties and powers set out in Part I of Schedule 2'.

This deals with local authority support for children and families including provision of services for families. This Schedule has the force of law and imposes on local authorities the following duties and powers:

1 Identification of children in need and provision of information
2 Maintenance of a register of disabled children
2 Assessment of children's needs
4 Prevention of neglect and abuse
5 Provision of accommodation in order to protect the child (i.e. a local authority may assist another person obtain alternative accommodation away from the child's home in order to protect the child)
6 Provision for disabled children
7 Provision to reduce need for care proceedings, etc.
8 Provision for children living with their families
9 Family centres
10 Maintenance of the family home
11 Duty to consider racial groups to which children in need belong.

As seen above, s.17(11) states 'health' means physical or mental health. Many of the legislative provisions of the Children Act are preventive measures which, if skilfully applied, can help prevent mental disorder and preserve the mental health of both children and their families.

It is not possible here to describe or even list all the relevant provisions of the wide-ranging Children Act. Detailed regulations and guidance have been prepared by the Government, including a document on children with disabilities (DH, 1991).

Other statutory services for children with mental disorder

Education

The Education Act 1981 places a duty on the local education authority to educate children in accordance with the assessment of their special educational needs. Sections 5 and 6 of the Disabled Persons (Services, Consultation and Representation) Act 1986 provide for the referral to local authority social services of disabled persons leaving special education.

Health services

Under National Health Service legislation, both generic and specialist medical services are provided for mentally disordered people of all ages.

Child guidance

Child guidance services are provided by local education authorities or social services.

Leisure and support services

Mentally disordered children and young people are entitled to use these as are others.

It needs to be borne in mind that children are often helped most by support of their families and therefore knowledge of legislation relating to adults as above is often needed by those working with children and young people.

RIGHTS AND DUTIES AS CITIZENS UNDER OTHER LEGISLATION

Marriage

A marriage can be void if either party did not give valid consent because of 'unsoundness of mind' or at the time of the marriage was suffering from a mental disorder within the meaning of the Mental Health Act 1983 which was of such a kind or to such an extent as to make the person unfit for marriage (Matrimonial Causes Act 1973). Any party to a marriage must be capable of giving valid consent, understand the nature and purport of the marriage, and freely give consent to it. Anyone who does not believe the patient capable of giving valid consent can object to the marriage. The marriage of patients detained under the Mental Health Act is provided for under s.1 of the Marriage Act 1983 and some such marriages have taken place out of hospital. Guidance on the procedure is in DHSS Circular No. HC(84)12/LAC(84)9 (DHSS, 84b), which points out that many patients detained under the Mental Health Act 1983 are capable of understanding the nature and purport of marriage and can consent to it.

Voting

The voting rights of informal patients are contained in the Representation of the People Act 1983. An informal mental patient may have his named placed on the Register of Electors if he or she has made a valid declaration under s.7(4) of that Act (see DHSS Circular No. HC(83)14 (DHSS, 1983b). Households are asked to include on their electoral registration form people who normally live in the household but are temporarily away as voluntary patients in psychiatric hospitals. Patients who are detained in a hospital or mental nursing home are not entitled to have their names placed on the Register.

Serving on juries

Mentally disordered people ineligible to serve on juries fall into three categories:

1 Any person under guardianship
2 Any person who has been determined by a judge to be incapable of managing his property and affairs
3 Anyone who suffers or has suffered from mental illness, psychopathic disorder, mental handicap or severe mental handicap and because of this is either resident in a hospital

or similar institution or regularly attends for treatment by a medical practitioner.

The definitions of mental handicap and severe mental handicap for this purpose are the same as the definitions of mental impairment and severe mental impairment in the Mental Health Act, but without the reference to abnormally aggressive or seriously irresponsible conduct. The list of those ineligible does not include people living in the community and not receiving regular medical treatment (see Juries Act 1974).

Driving licences

An applicant for a driving licence must disclose any prescribed disability. See Hoggett (1990) and up-to-date driving licence application forms.

Contracts

A contract entered into by a mentally incapacitated person not subject to the jurisdiction of the Court of Protection is binding unless it can be proved that the other party knew of the incapacity. The main exceptions are contracts for 'necessaries' (see also Part VII of the Act and Law Commission Reports (Law Commission 1992 and 1993)).

Wills

A testator must be of sound mind, memory and understanding. The Court of Protection is empowered to make statutory wills on behalf of mentally incapable people (see Part VII of the Act and Law Commission Reports (Law Commission 1992 and 1993)). Rules of the Supreme Court 1965 and County Courts Rules 1981 contain special provisions governing the participation of people under a legal disability in legal proceedings.

Workers and volunteers in citizen advocacy schemes enable people with mental health problems obtain their legal rights as citizens.

NEW DEVELOPMENTS

There are a number of new developments which may lead to future legislative changes.

Community supervision or treatment orders

In addition to the supervision or treatment orders for offenders referred to above, there have been various proposals for community treatment and community supervision orders for non-offenders which the Department of Health has been considering (DH, 1993b). The Secretary of State for Health has announced her intention to seek amendment of the Act to provide a new power of supervised discharge for certain patients who have been detained under the Act, and to extend from six months to a year the period for which patients may be given leave under section 17. The Code gives guidance on the Act as it stands and will need to be further reviewed in the light of any fresh legislation. The Secretary of State also proposed further guidance on the aftercare of mentally ill patients, particularly those who are a potential risk to themselves or others, covering the factors that need to be considered before they are discharged from hospital and the support they will need from the different agencies when they are (DH, 1993c).

Diversion from custody

Ministers are considering the recommendations of the final summary report of the joint Health/Home Office Reed Committee review of services for mentally disordered offenders (DH/HO, 1992). This emphasizes the need for agencies to work together to provide services in the community and diversion from custody.

High security psychiatric services and treatment for people with personality (psychopathic) disorders

The Department of Health has established two working groups chaired by Dr Reed on high security psychiatric services to consider the future provision of services for patients needing treatment in highly secure conditions and to review options for treatment of people with personality (psychopathic) disorders (DH, 1993a).

Seclusion practice

The Department of Health has been considering the implications of the recommendations of the

Ashworth Inquiry Report on seclusion practice (see chapter 19 of the Code).

Other vulnerable adults

The Law Commission has issued consultation papers proposing the extension of statutory protection to other vulnerable adults, e.g. elderly and disabled people (Law Commission 1992 and 1993).

Discrimination against disabled people

There have been proposals for a new Bill to help avoid discrimination against disabled people.

RECURRENT THEMES

There are a number of themes that recur throughout all the above legislation, Memoranda, Circulars and Codes of Practice. Paragraph 1.3 of the DH Code of Practice (DH and Welsh Office, 1993) sets out a number of broad principles to be applied when working under the Mental Health Act. These are also relevant to the other legislation and guidance outlined above. They include:

Respect for and consideration of individual qualities and diverse backgrounds—social, cultural, ethnic and religious

Section 13(2) of the Mental Health Act 1983, for example, says patients are to be interviewed 'in a suitable manner'. However, Barnes (1990), discusses the apparent unequal application of the law relating to assessment for compulsory detention, when racist and sexist attitudes seem to affect outcomes. Workers need to remember, too, that mental disorder is only one aspect of an individual's personality.

Treatment or care in the least controlled and segregated facilities practicable

The principle of 'the least restrictive alternative' is relevant at all stages of a patient's 'career', with the emphasis first on care in the community, then informal admission, the least restriction if admitted, and discharge and after-care as soon as possible thereafter. This principle applies to children as well as adults and to those involved in criminal proceedings.

The promotion of self-determination and personal responsibility

The provisions refer at times to the involvement of patients. Often this can be through advocacy schemes. Vulnerable people will need to be listened to and given information so that they can make informed choices. They need to be empowered so that the care packages provided for them under recent legislation reflect their real needs.

Legal rights to be drawn to the patient's attention

The legal rights include those relating to consent to treatment, Mental Health Review Tribunals, the Mental Health Act Commission and complaints procedures. The manager has a duty under s.132 to inform detained patients of their legal position and rights, both orally and in writing.

Concern for relatives and other carers and emphasis on partnership with them

Sometimes there is conflict between the patient's rights and avoiding risk to the health or safety of the patient or to others. In such complex cases, it is especially important for the professionals involved to understand the relevant law.

Prevention

The risks can often be reduced by early and skilful use of preventive measures to support those who are especially vulnerable.

Interprofessional co-operation

This is another recurrent theme. Paragraphs 2.28–2.29 of the DH Code of Practice (DH and Welsh Office, 1993) offer guidance when there are disagreements between professionals.

Access to information

Access to information is stressed in most of the relevant legislative provisions including the National Health Service and Community Care Act 1990.

All the above sounds fine, but lack of resources often prevents some of the potentially most useful legislative provisions either being implemented at all or being as effective as they might be. Pressure needs to be maintained to remedy this and remind those responsible that *The Health of the Nation* (DH, 1992b) includes mental health as one of its targets.

FURTHER READING

Children's Legal Centre (1991) *The Mental Health Handbook*. The Children's Legal Centre, 20 Compton Terrace, London N1 2UN.

Cretney, S.M. (1991) *Enduring Powers of Attorney*, 3rd edition. Bristol: Jordan.

Cretney, S., Davis, G., Kerridge, R. & Borkowski, A. (1991) *Enduring Powers of Attorney*. London: Lord Chancellor's Department.

Department of Health (1989) *An Introduction to the Children Act 1989*. London: HMSO.

Jones, R.M. (1993) *Encyclopedia of Social Services and Child Care Law*. London: Sweet & Maxwell.

REFERENCES

Barnes, M. (1990) Assessing for compulsory detention. Applying the social perspective. In: Cohen, J. & Ramon, S. (Eds) *Social Work and the Mental Health Act 1983 (England and Wales)*. Birmingham: British Association of Social Workers.

Central Council for Education and Training in Social Work (CCETSW) (1992) Paper 19.27 *A Double Challenge. Working with People who have both Learning Difficulties and a Mental Illness. Report of a Joint CCETSW/Royal College of Psychiatrists Symposium*. London: CCETSW.

Central Council for Education and Training in Social Work (CCETSW) (1993) Paper 19.19 *Requirements and Guidance for the Training of Social Workers to be Considered for Approval in England and Wales under the Mental Health Act 1983*. London: CCETSW.

Department of Health (DH) (1991) *Children with Disabilities: Guidance*. London: Department of Health.

Department of Health (DH) (1992a) *Letter. Mental Health Act 1983: Code of Practice and Attached Proposed Amendments*. London: Department of Health.

Department of Health (DH) (1992b) *The Health of the Nation: a Strategy for Health in England* (Cm. 1986). London: HMSO.

Department of Health (DH) (1993a) *Mental Health Act 1983: Code of Practice Revision and attached further proposed amendments*. London: Department of Health.

Department of Health (DH) (1993b) *Virginia Bottomley Announces Review of Legal Powers for Mentally Ill People. Call for Community Supervision Order Welcomed as a Constructive Contribution to the Debate*. London: Department of Health.

Department of Health (DH) (1993c) Circular No. LAC(93)19.

Department of Health and Home Office (DH/HO) (1992) *Final Summary Report of the Joint Review of Services for Mentally Disordered Offenders and Others Requiring Similar Services. Reed Committee*. (Cm. 2088, 1993).

DH and Welsh Office (1993) *Mental Health Act 1983. Code of Practice*, 2nd edition. London: HMSO.

DH and Welsh Office (1992) *Letter. Mental Health Act 1983. Code of Practice issued under Section 118*. London: Department of Health and Welsh Office.

DHSS (1974) Circular No.13/74.

DHSS (1983a) *Mental Health Act 1983 Memorandum on Parts I to VI, VIII and X*. London: HMSO.

DHSS (1983b) Circular No. HC(83)14.

DHSS (1984a) Circular No. DDL(84)4.

DHSS (1984b) Circular No. HC(84)12/LAC(84)9.

DHSS (1986) Circular No. LAC(86)15/WO Circular No. 51(86).

DHSS (1987) Circular No. LAC(87)6.

Grimshaw, C. (1993–94) *A to Z of Welfare Benefits for People with a Mental Health Problem: a Practical Guide for Service Users*. London: MIND.

Hoggett, B. (1990) *Mental Health Law*, 3rd edition. London: Sweet & Maxwell.

HO (1990) Circular No. 66/90.

HO (1991) *PACE. Codes of Practice on Police and Criminal Evidence Act 1984*, 2nd edition. London: HMSO.

Jones, R.M. (1991) *Mental Health Act Manual*, 3rd edition. London: Sweet & Maxwell.

Law Commission (1992) *Consultation Paper No. 128. Mentally Incapacitated Adults and Decision-making: A New Jurisdiction*. London: HMSO.

Law Commission (1993) *Consultation Paper No. 130. Mentally Incapacitated and Other Vulnerable Adults: Public Law Protection*. London: HMSO.

Letts, P. (1990) *Managing other People's Money*. London: Age Concern.

Mental Health Act Commission (1989) *Third Biennial Report, 1987–89*. London: HMSO.

Public Trust Office (1993) *Handbook for Receivers*. Protection Division of the Public Trust Office, Stewart House, 24 Kingsway, London WC2B 6JX.

Wright, E.E. (1992) The law relating to people with mental handicap. In: Thompson, T. & Mathias, P. (Eds) *Standards and Mental Handicap. Keys to Competence*. London: Baillière Tindall.

30

THE MENTAL HEALTH ACT COMMISSION
FUNCTIONS, REMIT AND CODE OF PRACTICE

C. Llewelyn Jones

AIMS

i) To identify the functions and remit of the Mental Health Act Commission
ii) To stimulate debate and discussion about elements of the Code of Practice

KEY ISSUES

Background to the Commission
Functions of the Commission
Composition of the Commission
Organization of the Commission
The Commissioner's role
The Code of Practice

Identify, analyse and assess factors causing distress and illness	Promote health, provide direct care and make interventions	Manage care programmes and services
Be critical, analytical and accountable, continue professional development	Counter discrimination, inequality and individual and institutional racism	Work within and develop policies, laws and safeguards in all settings
Understand influences on mental health and the nature/causes of disorder and illness	Know the effects of distress, disorder, illness on individuals, groups, families	Understand the basis of treatments and interventions

FUNCTIONS AND REMIT OF THE MENTAL HEALTH ACT COMMISSION

Before considering the above it is important to place the present working of the Mental Health Act Commission in some historical context.

Background to the Commission

Gostin (1983) states that throughout the history of the mental health legislation there have been a number of bodies with the authority vested in them to review the exercise of compulsory powers as well as the treatment and care of mentally ill offenders. As long ago as 1885, the then Lunatics Act established a Lunacy Commission. The Commissioners were appointed by the Lord Chancellor and formed a full-time inspectorate and had the power to investigate and supervise standards in institutions and to visit patients. In 1913 the Lunacy Commission was reconditioned as the Board of Control and was given additional responsibilities of scrutinizing documents relating to compulsory admission. That particular Board had powers of discharge of detained patients.

In relation to the above two points in the history of mental health legislation and pointing to the role and function of predecessors of this present commission, the Mental Health Act 1983 Commission has its relevance in the links that exist with the past, and it also opens out some of the differences.

The outcome of the 1959 Mental Health Act was that there was no longer an independent body which was specifically committed to safeguarding the rights, welfare and interests of detained patients. An interesting move, particularly as the 1960 Mental Health (Scotland) Act also abolished the Board of Control but in its place was established a Mental Welfare Commission. This body had a general duty to protect the rights of people who were mentally disordered.

During the period 1959 up to the late 1970s when the present Act—the 1983 Mental Health Act—was being drafted there were many advocates for a Mental Welfare Commission for England and Wales. The body pressurizing for a commission for south of the Border was The Royal College of Psychiatrists who continued to recommend the case for a permanent, independent commission to protect the interests of the individual psychiatric patient and to promote high standards of care.

The government of the time was not enthusiastic and felt there was little support for such a body (HMSO 1978). The argument was that they should not reintroduce a system for psychiatric patients which was fundamentally different from that provided for other patients. It was therefore proposed to introduce an experimental scheme of 'patients advisers' as an alternative way of safeguarding the position and myths of vulnerable patients (Blueglass, 1983).

The other particular advocates were MIND and the Butler Committee. MIND favoured a patients' advocacy scheme and the Butler Committee put forward the concept of a system of patients' friends. Both groups felt it was important not to set up a new institution of Mental Health Act Commissioners, but were looking towards some 'body' which would support the rights of individuals who were detained in a mental hospital against their wishes. It must be remembered that patients detained under the powers of a Mental Health Act are in a unique position because they have no right to discharge themselves, unlike all other patients (including some psychiatric patients). There was a necessity for setting up a body to scrutinize the procedures which led to the detention and renewal of the authority for detention of such patients. This body should be independent of those who had been concerned with the patient at the point of compulsory admission and detention.

'The Government accordingly decided to set up a Mental Health Act Commission with a general protective function for detained patients and the Government accepted the view of the Royal College that it should have responsibilities with reference to the Consent to Treatment Regulations'.
Blueglass, 1983

Functions of the Commission

A specific duty is imposed on the Secretary of State to keep under review the exercise of the powers and the duties under the Mental Health Act 1983 so far as they relate to the detention of patients and their subsequent care in hospital. This duty has been delegated to the Mental Health Act Commission under Section 121(2)(b) Mental Health Act 1983. In the previous historical content reference was made to the 1960 Mental Health (Scotland) Act where the Commissioners exercised their remit in relation to detained and informal patients in psychiatric units but the Mental Health Act Commission (England and Wales) have a remit only for those detained patients.

The tasks/functions assigned to the Commissioners can be collated under the following headings:

---

1   To keep under review the operation of the Mental Health Act 1983 in respect of patients detained under the Act or patients liable to be detained under the Act

2   To visit and interview in private patients detained under the Act in hospitals and mental nursing homes

3   To investigate complaints which fall within the Commission's remit

4   To review decisions to withhold the mail of patients detained in the special hospitals

5   To appoint medical practitioners and others to give second opinions in cases where this is required by the Act

6   To monitor the implementation of the Code of Practice and advise Ministers on amendments

7   To publish a biennial report

8   To offer advice to Ministers on matters falling within the Commission's remit
Mental Health Act Commission, 1991

It is important to note that in the 1st Biennial Report of the Commission presented to the House of Commons in October, 1985, it was stated, as in the Act, that the Commission had a task of drafting a Code of Practice. The Commission did much detailed work on drafting a Code of Practice but a decision was taken by the Department of Health that it would write the Code of Practice, so in the 1989 Biennial report the Commission's function relating to the Code was phrased 'the submission to the Secretary of State for Health of proposals for the contents of a Code of Practice'. The Code published in 1990 has led to the function of the Mental Health Act Commission (6) as being one of 'monitoring the implementation of the Code of Practice'.

Composition of the Commission

The Commission is set up as a Special Health Authority. It is a multidisciplinary body comprising 90 part-time members appointed by the Secretary of State for Health. Approximately 12 commission members are appointed by the Secretary of State for Wales. These members are drawn from the medical, legal, nursing, psychological, social work and allied professions and occupations involved in mental health. Some members are lay members. By part-time it means commissioners devote a day a week on average for that primary purpose of visiting NHS (and trust status) hospitals where detained patients are receiving care and treatment and special hospitals (whereby definition, all patients are detained), and meeting with social services departments.

Organization of the Commission

In order to fulfil its functions of visiting NHS hospitals and meeting social services departments, following some reorganization in 1990, the 90 commissioners are divided into seven commissioner visiting teams covering England and Wales. The geographical boundaries for each team are defined by the boundaries of various regional health authorities and Wales (e.g. CVT 7 covers two regions, that is the North West Regional Health Authority and the Mersey

Regional Health Authority, and CVT 6 works within the West Midlands Regional Health Authority and the whole of Wales). Prior to reorganization, Wales was divided by the Commission, the North of Wales going with the Mersey Region and South Wales linked with the South West Regional Health Authority! This organization of work is supported from a large centralized office based in Nottingham. The office is staffed by civil servants headed by William Bingley, the chief executive. There are seven officers who have a team of administrative officers linking in to the seven commission visiting teams.

A major part of the commissioners' work is obviously done with the three special hospitals, Ashworth, Rampton and Broadmoor, because all the patients in the special hospitals are detained patients within the meaning of the 1983 Mental Health Act. In visiting special hospitals, the commissioners are divided into 'Panels' each panel having responsibility for visiting each special hospital, for example, there are some 38 commissioners on the Ashworth Hospital panel, headed by a convenor and divided into five multidisciplinary teams each visiting a group of wards. Each CV team has a convenor.

During its existence the Commission has established 10 national standing committees. Most commissioners are members of at least one such committee. Three national standing committees take responsibility for overseeing the three fundamental operational responsibilities of the Commission, as indicated by their titles—visiting, complaints and consent to treatment. The other national standing committees take responsibility for discrete policy areas and include race and culture, Code of Practice, mentally disturbed offenders, community care, research and information, legal and parliamentary affairs, mental handicap and non-volitional patients.

There is a central policy committee, membership of which is governed by the provisions of a statutory instrument and comprises Chair and Vice Chair and 10 members of the Commission. All members are appointed by the Secretary of State for Health. The central policy committee has overall responsibility for the activities of the Commission and for overseeing the financial control of the organization.

How the Commission fulfils its various tasks and functions

The organization decided in early days, between 1983 and 1985, that there was a need for commissioners to visit/have meetings with social services department staff although this is not stated as part of the Commission's functioning. However, before 1985 it had become the practice for commissioners to visit hospitals/psychiatric units where patients were detained (under the 1983 Mental Health Act) once per year and that meetings should be held at social services departments at least once every two years. Special hospitals were visited more frequently, usually six times per year and regional secure units twice per year. All visits are recorded in a formal report which is presented verbally at the end of each visit and appears in its written form approximately one month after the visit.

Later, the Commissioners felt it was appropriate to visit hospitals and have meetings with social services departments, of the same locality, on a joint visiting basis. For example, a common pattern is a two-day visit to a hospital and social services department area spending one and a half days at the hospital base and half a day meeting approved social workers, and separately meeting police and user groups while at the social services department. Wards are visited, all detained patients seen and their records reviewed as is a selection of the documentation of patients who have been in hospital during the interim year between Commission visits. This point of the 'how' of the visit does raise issues about Commissioners' interviewing detained patients as they can only interview those who are in hospital on the given day of the visit and in so doing get but a small sample of views/complaint, issues relating to detained patients receiving a service at the time of a visit.

Joint visiting has been encouraged by both health authority/trusts and social services departments which has reflected in itself the massive changes which have taken place during the decade since 1983, of a move from institutional care to community care. Some social services departments have resented the Commissioners' 'visiting' as they receive inspection from social services inspectorate and others, and yet other social services departments have been critical of the Mental Health Act Commission 'reducing' the time being spent at social services departments to half a day but there is certainly an agreement that there should be a 'joint' view of the mental health services in a given geographical area.

Analysis of the Commissioners' role and function and issues related to their role

In any review, or reflection of the Commission's work one has to start with a reminder of the Commission's statutory functions. Its primary role is 'to keep under review the exercise of powers and discharge of duties conferred or imposed by the 1983 Mental Health Act so far as relating to the detention of patients or to patients liable to be detained under the Act'. In pursuit of this remit the Commission carries out three statutorily defined basic activities:

Visiting detained patients

Investigating complaints that fall within its statutory remit

Administering the consent to treatment safeguards set out in the Act

It was noted at the beginning of the chapter that there were hopes that the commissioners would be an independent body and that the 1983 Act would set up an advocacy-type service. Clearly the Commission is not an independent body in the true sense of the word but legally it is a creature of the Secretary of State, with members nominated by the said Secretary. The Commission is not a patients' advocacy organization (such organizations do not have a statutory complaints investigations remit). The Commission is not an 'inspection' agency like the Health Advisory Service; rather it is primarily a visitorial body (Bingley, 1991).

The remit given to the Commission of investigating complaints has been very difficult to fulfil by the very nature of the organization's services being carried out by 90 part-time commissioners.

The commissioners' jurisdiction to investigate complaints is set out in Section 120(1)(b) of the Mental Health Act 1983. This section of the Act defines two types of complaint which are within the remit of the Commission's investigative powers:

Any complaint made by a person in respect of a matter that occured while he was detained under this Act and which has not been satisfactorily dealt with by the Managers.

Any other complaint as to the exercise of powers or discharge of duties conferred or imposed by the Act in respect of a person who is or has been detained.

The Commission has been aware of its difficulties in relation to fulfilling its function and has been most mindful of criticisms which recently came to light in the Ashworth Hospital Inquiry Report published in August, 1992 which highlights such difficulties. The Mental Health Act Commission has now got a clear policy, procedure and guidelines to be used in the investigation of complaints. One of the major features of the policy is the inclusion of time limits with an intention that most complaints will be dealt with within 14 days.

One of the Ashworth Hospital's Inquiry Report's major recommendations is that the Commission should cease to investigate complaints and that it should concentrate on supervising hospital complaints procedures. This must await ministerial and legislative action. In the meantime it gives the Commission food for thought about its future role, particularly in relation to special hospitals. It is true that patients, mostly those in the special hospitals, see commissioners as powerless in relation to resolution of individual complaints. Certainly the Commission's ability to investigate complaints has been hampered by its resources. Does this 'failure' take one back to the role of the Commission—is it essentially a visitorial body? It is not an inspectorate, and it is not strictly a complaints body adjudicating individual complaints.

Look again at point (5) in the list of functions of

the Commission. The administration of Part IV of the 1983 Mental Health Act continues to be one of the most important activities of the Commission. The amount of work generated by this statutory responsibility has increased steadily. The second opinion doctors (appointed by the Commission) responded to 3,500 requests for second opinions in 1991. Whereas there have been many examples of the Commission having had a powerful and beneficial impact on the care and treatment of individual detained patients or on individual establishments or organizations that provide such care and treatment, there remains a tension between the responsible medical officers and the second opinion doctor: on the one hand the opportunity to consult in relation to difficult cases is appreciated but a minority of doctors still see this Part IV of the Act as a bureaucratic intrusion into their clinical practice. (Part IV of the Act looks at Treatment/Consent to Treatment.)

Some further points relating to consent to treatment will be raised below, but it is important to state that under Section 57 of the Act, which currently applies to psycho surgery and surgical implantation of hormones, a nominated doctor and two other nominated commissioners have to interview each person to undergo such treatment and have to be assured that the person is consenting to the treatment and that he/she understands the nature and likely effects of the treatment. Commissioners have to interview the referring doctor and two other professionals (one a nurse) who are professionally concerned with the patient's treatment. This function is carried out by commissioners regardless of whether the patient is informal or detained.

In monitoring Section 58 of the Mental Health Act, commissioners are making sure that patients are consenting their treatment, or for those who are not consenting, that there is the necessary documentation completed. Initially there were many instances where patients were receiving medication illegally but as the years have progressed so the medical officers are far more conscientious about their practice and most importantly about the rights of the detained patient.

The commissioners have produced papers on compulsory treatment in the community (Royal College of Psychiatrists, 1987). These have been consultative papers on consent to treatment and community treatment orders, both of which have made a powerful contribution to the debate about these issues.

Lastly, in our consideration of some of the functions of the Commission, function (4) is the only executive function. The powers of hospital managers to examine and withhold postal packets and their duties to exercise such powers are within Section 134 of the 1983 Mental Health Act. If a packet is withheld then the patient must be informed within seven days and also if known, the person by whom the packet was sent, that there is a right of review to such a decision by the Mental Health Act Commission. There are occasions over the years when the Commission have used its powers and reversed the decision made to withhold such mail.

Conclusions

The Commission has been successful in drawing attention to the rights of detained patients and there are many occasions and examples during the past ten years when as a result of commissioner visits, units have been closed, or care and treatment of the detained patient has been much improved. Commissioners have focused on the patient's rights within the Act, the rights to have an individual care plan, the right *not* to be held in seclusion for periods of time, and a focus on the right to have specialist nursing. Commissioners have frequently raised at hospital, at health authority and regional health authority level the sometimes low nursing staff level of some psychiatric units. The Commission has been very good in acting as a catalyst for change.

However, a question must be posed as to whether the Act is dated and whether by now the commissioners are so limited in their role by not having a remit for informal patients. For those high numbers of persons in the community placed in care, there is no independent body that maintains their rights and wellbeing. The remit of the Commission is so very narrow in looking at the rights of only those patients detained within the Act when over the last decade the service has moved towards a community-based service from being a hospital-based service. It is important to remember that there is no clear GP representation as membership of the Commission.

The Commission itself, through its Biennial Report, has reviewed its concerns about its failure to visit private nursing homes which have a facility in the registration to receive detained patients and those liable to be detained. One must be aware of the rapid major developments within this private sector and most certainly the Mental Health Act Commission has not fulfilled its remit to visit such homes on a regular basis. There has been great difficulty in the Commission being informed of such homes and it must be recognized that some such homes may indeed be larger in number of beds than the nearby in-patient psychiatric unit.

CODE OF PRACTICE

Reference was made to the Code of Practice at the beginning of this chapter where the tasks and functions of the Mental Health Act Commission were being spelt out. It was pointed out that the presentation of a Code of Practice was a statutory duty imposed on the Secretary of State:

'The Secretary of State shall prepare and from time to time revise a Code of Practice, i.e. (a) for the guidance of registered medical practitioners, managers and staff of Hospitals and Mental Nursing Homes and approved Social Workers in relation to the admission of patients to Hospitals and Mental Nursing Homes under this Act; and (b) for the guidance of registered Medical Practitioners and members of other professions in relation to the medical treatment of patients suffering from Mental Disorder'.
Mental Health Act, 1983

Detailed scrutiny of Parliamentary debates prior to the putting into place of Section 118 of the Mental Health Act does little to reveal any specific intention of Parliament as to the particular thrust or centre of gravity which the anticipated Code of Practice relating to Mental Health Legislation should have. It was therefore possible

to envisage, and to create, either a short code consisting of critically argued principles upon which particular decisions at local level could be informed, or a very specific 'action handbook' for health care professionals and others.

The first Code produced by the Mental Health Act Commission itself in 1985 (DHSS, 1985) turned out to be an uneasy and consequently unsatisfactory mixture of critically argued principles which could inform agendas for questions to be asked at local level without in any way dictating particular answers; and on the other hand offered a catalogue of instructions for health care professions and others. It should be said that with the Draft Code there was an extremely long chapter on consent to treatment which possibly led to the medical lobby against that Code. The medical opinion perceived the laying down of parameters for the guidance of professional action to be a threat to professional independence. Thus the Draft Code of Practice was rejected as a workable addition to the professional armoury in mental health care.

What has emerged is a shorter Code of Practice, published by the Department of Health in May, 1990 with a smart blue cover and a guide which is seen as eminently 'user-friendly'. In a quiet determined way this Code points out the direction that all professionals involved in the care of mentally disordered people must anticipate. Commissioners are fulfilling their present function to monitor the use of the Code and have recently prepared a document that reflects the need to consider some changes and modifications to the code. Of course, it is through this process that the Code could become a living Code of Practice.

The present Code in its introduction states:

'This Act does not impose a legal Duty to comply with the Code but failure to follow the Code could be referred to in evidence in public procedures'.
DH and Welsh Office, 1990

'The Code provides much detailed guidance,

but it needs to be read in the light of the following broad principles, that people being assessed for possible admission under the Act or to whom the Act applies should:

— receive respect for and consideration of their individual qualities and diverse backgrouds—social, cultural, ethnic and religious;

— have their needs fully taken into account though it is recognised that, with available resources, it may not always be practicable to meet these;

— be delivered any necessary treatment or care in the least controlled and segregated facilities practicable;

— be treated or cared for in such a way that promotes to the greatest practicable degree, their self determination and personal responsibility consistent with their needs and wishes;

— be discharged from any order under the Act to which they are subject immediately it is no longer necessary.'

DH and Welsh Office, 1990

'The overall tone is firmly based on the dignity due to any mentally ill person when faced with the caring professionals at any stage in his illness and not simply when formal admission is being considered'.

Travers, 1991

The above broad principles as they appear in the introduction of the Code are firmly based on basic human rights. This is a value statement. The Code of Practice could be seen as the 'quality assurance' statement related to the care of those detained under the 1983 Mental Health Act.

Commissioners have worked through a process of ensuring the availability of the Code in hospitals, social services departments and nursing homes and have encouraged the use of the Code by getting professionals to use it as the basis for professional training relating to practice and particularly in any multidisciplinary training. Refer-

ence is continually made to a respective paragraph of the Code when commissioners write their reports following their formal visits, which should encourage managers and others to familiarize themselves with the Code. Maybe this aspect is one of the Code's strengths in that commissioners can say 'This is what you should be doing, why can't you'?

What is in the Code? It has 29 chapters. Each chapter focusing on a particular practice element of the Act and is divided into numbered paragraphs. The Code opens with a series of chapters on assessment looking at practice and process of professionals' work prior to a person's possible admission under the Mental Health Act. There are a number of chapters that offer practice guidance in relation to the use of a number of sections of the legislation appertaining to admission (to hospital) under the Mental Health Act, followed by a brief section on admission under the Mental Health Act (to guardianship). A further series of chapters focuses on practice issues relating to treatment and care in hospital. At the end of the Code are two chapters on 'leaving hospital' and the concluding chapters look at particular groups of patients, people with mental handicap, and children and young people under the age of 18. It is quite clear that in the 1990 copy of the Code the section on 'consent to treatment' is short compared with the lengthy input on this subject which appeared in the Draft Code of Practice.

The nurses's holding power (Section 5(4)) is clearly explained, that it is the personal decision of the nurse and that he or she cannot be instructed to exercise this power by anyone else is reinforced. As an example of the clarity within the chapters of the Code, this chapter is broken down into 10 sub-paragraphs. It begins with a clear statement on 'the power' of the nurse within the Act, moves on to present helpful guidance notes on 'assessment before implementation', how the nurse copes with 'acute emergencies', and the writing of the report on the use of this section. 'Use of restraint' practice notes and 'management responsibilities' are two further headings informing the nurse that this section lapses upon the arrival of the doctor. There are clear guidelines on the use of seclusion, and most certainly commissioners hoped that these practice guidelines would underpin hospital policies on such areas of work as 'the use of seclusion'.

The Code is being used to inform practice in hospital units and social services departments which are continually reviewing their policies and incorporating good practice guidelines. Chapter 26 of the Code is another chapter which sets out a statement on the purpose of after-care and offers a clear checklist of who should be involved in an after-care planning meeting well before the patient goes on leave or is discharged. Practice in relation to the implementation of this section remains variable with many responsible medical officers not setting up after-care plans for patients who go on leave.

Social workers, nurses, doctors and administrators are using the Code and many 'enjoy' the 'power' it gives them in supporting their stance or debate in relation to good practice. In chapter 2, social workers and doctors are expected to have a dialogue when there are differences of opinion in relation to assessment for admission. Nurses know from chapter 9 that no one else can make them use their powers under Section 5(4) of the Mental Health Act.

There are some areas of the Code that need redrafting and some extension. Little within the Code highlights the practice issues which could be linked with special hospitals and as stated in the Ashworth Inquiry Report (1992) the special hospitals have not really begun to use the good practice notes of the Codes of Practice.

The chief executive of the Commission in a recent paper on 'Auditing the Commission' (Bingley, 1991) states that the primary focus of the Commission's work must remain protecting the interests of individual detained patients. The Commission also has a broader responsibility to protect the interests of detained patients as a group. He goes on to suggest that commissioners must look to ways of using more effectively its operational experience in the field and to make a far more substantial impact on institutional practice, professional practice and policy development. Possibly the commission's remit/task of monitoring the Code of Practice and advising the Secretary of State about possible changes to the Code may be one way of doing this (Bingley, 1991).

In a recent article, the Chair of the Commission and the chief executive suggest that no external monitoring body can reform the institution it monitors. They suggest that what the Commission can and must do is to influence and promote the management of staff to effect appropriate change, by vigorously pressing for reform, ensuring that existing procedures work and being prepared to draw to the attention of appropriate people cases where standards of patient care are falling below acceptable standards. The Commission, they suggest, must be seen by patients to be the appropriate repository of their worries and troubles (Bingley and Bloom-Cooper, 1992).

The Biennial Report is the last of the Commission's tasks to be considered within the remit of this chapter. Each Biennial Report has improved in terms of its quality, its data and its portrait to Parliament and the public of the work undertaken by the Mental Health Act Commission. The Report raises issues for debate and discussion and is the formal conveyor to Parliament of the state of the Mental Health Service in hospital, community and mental nursing homes for those patients detained within the meaning of the Act. However, this report in terms of its communication to Parliament is only as good in its value as the communication received from the Minister and the Department of Health.

Amongst a range of concerns in 1991 was the Commission's concern about the use of Section 17 of the Act, a Section whereby a responsible medical officer may grant leave from hospital with the imposition of any conditions considered necessary. This can be helpful in a patient's rehabilitation programme but, for example, the powers of Section 17 have been employed in the administration of compulsory treatment outside hospital through extended leave and, reactive recall, before the expiry of the Section; to permit removal of the long-term section, Section 3, and then to return to the leave of absence. Commissioners feel this practice cannot be supported yet the Department of Health has not incorporated this point in its response to the 1991 Biennial Report.

Several questions remain, the main one being whether such a body as the Mental Health Act Commission in its present form is able to fulfil the tasks and functions and remit as set out earlier in the chapter. I have attempted to offer a glimpse of the working thus far, of this complex organization which has such a narrow remit. One must consider this narrow remit and its relevance to the present-day scene of mental health care and treatment, which raises the question of the relevance of the body of the Commission and indeed the relevance of the 1983 Mental Health Act 10 years on—should there be a review of the legislation? Should the Commission have its remit extended to incorporate informal patients as in Scotland? Has the time come when some full-time commissioners be appointed? The future place of such a body which sets out to protect the rights of the detained patients, to be a 'watch dog' for the mental health services and inevitably a 'pressure group' for such must continue to be considered.

The Code of Practice was revised in August 1993. Principal changes include emphasizing the power under the Act to compulsorily admit in the interests of the patient's health; enhancements of the guidance about the use of restraint, particularly in relation to elderly people and the inclusion for the first time of advice about the rights of patients to visitors.

FURTHER READING

Department of Health and Welsh Office (1990) *The Code of Practice for 1983 Mental Health Act*. London: HMSO.

Gostin, L. (1983) *A Practical Guide to Mental Health Law*. London: MIND.

Hoggett, B. (1991) *Mental Health Law*, 3rd edition. London: Sweet & Maxwell.

REFERENCES

Biennial Reports of the Mental Health Act Commission (1985, 1989, 1991). First, third and fourth editions. London: HMSO.

Bingley, W. (1991) Auditing the Commission. *Journal of Forensic Psychiatry*, **2** (2), 136.

Bingley, W. & Bloom-Cooper, St L. (1992) Sharp Eyes and Keen Ears. *Policy in Mental Health, Community Care* 15.10.92.

Blueglass, R. (1984) *A Guide to the Mental Health Act 1983*. Edinburgh: Churchill Livingstone.

Code of Practice (1993) *Mental Health Act*. Published August 1993: operational 1.11.93. London: HMSO.

Department of Health (1983) *Mental Health Act*. Chapter 20. London: HMSO.

Department of Health and Welsh Office (1990) *Code of Practice for 1983 Mental Health Act*. London: HMSO.

DHSS Mental Health Division (1985) 'Mental Health Act 1983: Section 118'. Draft Code of Practice.

Gostin, L. (1983) *A Practical Guide to Mental Health Law*. London: HMSO.

HMSO (1978) The Review of the Mental Health Act 1959. Cmnd. 7320.

Hoggett, B. (1990) *Mental Health Law*, 3rd edition. London: Sweet & Maxwell.

Travers, R. (1991) *Ode to the Code*. *Psychiatric Bulletin*, **11**.

Report of the Committee of Inquiry into complaints about Ashworth Hospital. Vol. I. (1992). London: HMSO.

Royal College of Psychiatrists (1987) Compulsory Treatment in the Community. A discussion document.

Williams, J. (1990) *The Law of Mental Health*. London: Fourmat.

31

PREPARING FOR THE FUTURE

Eric Moxham

AIMS

i) To consider the implications of changes in services for the preparation of mental health nurses

KEY ISSUES

The development of community-based provision
Therapeutics
Understanding of mental disorder
Attributes of mental health nurses and nursing
The curriculum for the mental health branch of Project 2000

Identify, analyse and assess factors causing distress and illness	Promote health, provide direct care and make interventions	Manage care programmes and services
Be critical, analytical and accountable, continue professional development	Counter discrimination, inequality and individual and institutional racism	Work within and develop policies, laws and safeguards in all settings
Understand influences on mental health and the nature/causes of disorder and illness	Know the effects of distress, disorder, illness on individuals, groups, families	Understand the basis of treatments and interventions

DEVELOPMENT OF COMMUNITY-BASED PROVISION

The growth in community-based psychiatry and community psychiatric nursing has revolutionized the way in which both follow-up after-care and primary health care is provided, and it is envisaged that further growth will occur in GP attachment schemes over the next few years. Similarly, recent growth in the private sector has provided further evidence of alternative services being established within the domestic setting.

This scenario will obviously mean a complete reappraisal of future work force requirements and it is therefore important to review present and future skill mix to meet the changes in mental health care delivery. These changes, coupled with accelerated changes in nurse education, herald a new era, both in terms of user care, mental health care and nursing practice.

The advent of psychiatric day hospital provision is worthy of note and provides an alternative for the user by reducing domestic disruption and further lessening the need for in-patient care.

Psychiatric hospitals are places where some people come because they have had a surfeit of anger, fear, sadness and boredom which they cannot control or explain. They may no longer prevent these feelings running away with their thoughts. In consequence they may no longer be able to cope with life's practicalities nor with the relationships in which those feelings originated.

In the psycho-dynamic model, the mental health nurse is a primary resource in the system. When working with personal feelings, it inevitably means that the nurse is moved by the pain and hurts of the patient. Therefore, the mental health nurse must have reserves to draw upon. For example, outside of work nurses require satisfying positive relationships and should have the resources and psychological capacity to enjoy life. They must know what their limits are at work and be able to draw upon a service support system that is flexible enough to adjust to their emotional needs.

Professor Tony Butterworth, the chairman appointed to review mental health nursing in Britain states:

'Developments in the mental health field are happening all the time and it is important that we carefully identify how best to equip and deploy nurses in this changing environment to respond fully to the needs of individuals'.
Butterworth, 1992

Most nurses in the speciality (psychiatry) have in the past worked in NHS long-stay hospital and residential settings. With the closure of the large institutions, actual and planned for in the future, care is increasing in the private, independent and voluntary sectors. Where the larger institutions have clients who are unable to be supported in residential settings care is being provided in smaller units within the district general hospitals.

Inherent in the changes is of course the need to prepare mental health care staff for the future in more selective systematic ways:

'Use of treatment for the benefit of staff. Reliance on medication, use of ECT so that staff could be seen to be trying to do something; inappropriate use of MHA 1983, forced feeding of the elderly and humiliating toilet procedures with the elderly; lack of confidentiality; lack of privacy when talking or washing, favouritism to certain patients; restrictive and authoritarian approaches; power relations between patients and staff. Tendency to turn to medication and control'.
Davey, 1992

Being realistic about the possible changes in the future it must be accepted that some of the problems highlighted here might have been bequeathed, for example, by bad organization or bad architecture, and not the failings of those working in the front line of care provision.

It is not suggested that the old mental hospitals were better, even though most had flower beds, lawns and grounds. Most mental hospitals were designed during the last century and were similar to prison accommodation, with small cell-like rooms, barred windows and locked doors. The culture generated by such institutions tended to subordinate everyone, and patients in particular.

People usually require structure and small settings to feel safe and secure, but are the large institutions giving way to smaller, possibly replicated institutions?

Unless there is a constant dialogue between practitioners and users in any care setting a whole multitude of practicalities may be missed and it is important to create a climate in which practitioners, users and the professionals feel that they are being listened to and what they say makes a difference.

The major change over the last two decades in the mental health nursing field has been a move from traditional to therapeutic care. Prior to this there was a shift from custodial to traditional care. These very radical changes which have taken place and are still taking place within the mental health services have resulted in a complete reappraisal of the skill mix required in the services. Changes in health care provision and policy have already resulted in a major shift from the institution to the home or community setting.

The preparation of a workforce that is evolving and changing is challenging for both education and service providers. Project 2000 with its broader preparation and slightly higher academic input to this cause should provide the workforce with a good foundation, suited to the mental health care field and for the further development of specialisms at a later date.

Education provision and delivery should be flexible and responsive to both students following the programme and their clients. The creative pathways should offer both professional and academic achievement.

The mental health nurse is required to be prepared and able to operate in a variety of situations including domiciliary, residential, day care settings and within a variety of systems, for example, primary care, hospital care, social services, and with different users and carers including families, self-help groups and individuals. They must also be alert to factors which influence the quality of life experienced by clients who now find themselves involved in resettlement activity.

Kirkby in Ashfield Report 1990
(see Francis and Smith, 1991)

In October 1988, 23 long-stay psychiatric patients left hospital to take up residence in a group of purpose-built bungalows, located near to the centre of a Nottinghamshire town. The majority of these patients originated from that town. They were the second group of patients to 'go home' as part of the local health district's relocation programme. They followed a similar group of 15 patients who were transferred to another comparable bungalow scheme in July 1988, and whose progress has

been seen to be satisfactory. It was anticipated that smaller, domestic-style settings with access to the community would facilitate the principles of 'normalization'.

An important aspect of the health district's decision to relocate those patients resident in the mental hospital was a commitment to evaluate the psychosocial impact of the hospital closure.

This report is one of a series that has documented the effects on the patients involved, and is concerned with the progress of that group of patients who moved to the new bungalow scheme over 18 months previously. It may be useful to consider and debate the following:

No significant impact on physical health symptomatology has been observed, other than the slow deterioration which might be expected in such an aged group.

The quality of care is seen to improve significantly for all patients, particularly with regard to improved privacy, access to the community, access to education, and to choices regarding the nature of their physical environment.

However, the activities checklist has demonstrated a reduction in opportunities to participate in diversional activities. Many patients lack the resources (financial and/or physical) to avail themselves of these activities available to the general public. Additionally, the bungalow schemes have few activities on site to offer patients. This has meant that for some patients the move from the mental hospital and the relative richness of its on-site activities, has bought a more limited lifestyle. While most would agree that this limitation has been offset by other apparent advantages, many staff are concerned by the relative restrictions of the new environment, and are pursuing alternatives.

Findings like these confirm that the quality of life does not always change automatically for the better with change of location and that it is important for the nurse to be able to evaluate factors which affect clients' experience and find ways of helping clients to gain access to activities which lead to richer experiences, as well as (or on the basis of) being able to develop a direct therapeutic relationship with the client.

THERAPEUTICS

Our understanding of psychiatric conditions (mental illnesses) and therefore of the appropriateness of various diagnoses and treatment (therapies) has changed dramatically in the last 20 years. Observers with little appreciation of the finer points of psychiatric practice may be bewildered by the proliferation of approaches and be unsure about which to support and which to condemn. It is possible to argue that improved practices and approaches have been introduced and are still being developed in our generation more than ever before in mental health nursing history. The process has begun for changing the whole of our caring services in the next few years.

The mental health nurse will need to be more flexible than at present, and be able to practise in both institutional and non-institutional settings. This will require an increased emphasis on professionalism, problem-solving skills and peer support. New nurse practitioners will need support in the field, therefore continuing educational opportunities must be available to retain nurses in clinical practice as a means to decreasing wastage from the speciality.

A general nurse is often taught to observe outside of herself or himself. The focus is the presenting condition of a person. They observe, note and record subtle changes in the environment and individuals in accord with a theoretical perspective; they may apply theory and this forms their perceptual frame.

The psychiatric nurse is taught (if this can be taught) to experience fully the presence of a person and his or her own internal responding. The presence of a person changes from moment to moment and this produces a reciprocal change in response from within the psychiatric nurse. In order to experience fully the person and be aware of their own internal responses, psychiatric nurses must suspend judgement, know their own assumptions, opinions and prejudices and how

these may get in the way of a full experience of a person. In other words, psychiatric nurses should aim to strive towards non-judgemental communications and must be aware of the nature of their own responses to the person and ask themselves questions such as 'How do I feel when I am with this person? Do I want to pull away, move close, do I feel disgusted, sad, aloof, caring? How am I going to relate to this person and use these responses within me, which contribute to the therapeutic process of the relationship, enhancing the person and providing the information (my own responses) which a person may need in order to facilitate change?' This is the conscious and intentional use of self. It is not enough to be aware.

A relationship develops in which the nurse knows or learns when to intervene and when not to intervene and works with the person towards independence through the acceptance of responsibility. It is important therefore that the nurse keeps up to date with developments in the understanding of mental disorder and illness.

MENTAL DISORDER AND ILLNESS

Despite all our advances and knowledge of mental illness there are gaps. Severe mental illness remains one of the most challenging situations for mental health practitioners. We cannot always predict the course of the illness or even the extent of improvement which can be expected from treatment.

Language changes have preceded the proposed structural changes to the British health care system. 'Patients' are now 'consumers' of services which are traded according to 'market forces' (HMSO, 1989). The patient is no longer a passive recipient of treatment but is an active customer who sets out to get needs met from professionals who are there to serve (Lazare *et al.*, 1975).

Results from surveys of psychiatric disorder amongst the general population assume significant levels of un-met needs (Goldberg *et al.*, 1976). However, it remains to be demonstrated that people in the community need psychiatric treatment just because they meet symptomatic case criteria (Bebbington, 1990). Currently, no substantive research is available to inform mental health service providers which services the public would find most helpful if they were indeed 'consumers' rather than being restricted to the more usual limited role of respondents (Martin, 1986). These issues pose a real challenge to the current distribution of mental health care resources in a health service that is geared to becoming more consumer oriented.

'There they stand, majestic, imperious, brooded over by the gigantic water tower and chimney combined, rising unmistakable and daunting out of the countryside the asylums which our forefathers built with such sobriety. Do not for a moment underestimate their power of resistance to our assault ...'.
Powell, 1961

However, since Enoch Powell's statement, mental health care is now offered in a wide variety of settings, fewer clients receive continuing care in the setting of a large psychiatric hospital. Resident populations in English psychiatric hospitals were reduced by over 50% from 1960 to 1985 (Jones, 1988) and large hospitals are being run down and closed. The effects of such closure programmes upon hospital staff are beginning to be investigated. However, the effects of the proposed closures on clients is less well researched. This is a serious omission, since an increasing number of users of mental health services are wishing to be more involved in the way that services are planned and provided (Francis and Smith, 1991). Yet it is often because people are supported at home that they fail to come to the attention of the service early on in the onset of mental disturbance.

If this is the case, then we have to make our services more flexible, accessible and approachable. Perhaps these can be achieved through such innovations as the peripatetic day hospital (Higgins, 1980).

Some clients experience disabling features, such as delusions and hallucinations. Other may have acute and potentially destructive features. A proportion has intermittent illness which improves for periods of time. Others may have more

pervasive and progressive impairment—losing ground with each successive event, including for example, schizophrenic illnesses, chronic emotional disorders and organic brain syndromes. Although acute features of mental illness may subside, problems can persist during the non-acute phase of illness, often referred to as residual problems. These may also have a pervasive or progressive quality. As an emerging consequence, social interactions, family relationships, community living and self-care skills may be deeply affected.

The range of therapeutic options for care will depend largely upon the nature of the client's mental disturbance, and the extent of the family support and the skills of the mental health nurse. The trend over the last 20 years has been to close psychiatric hospitals and favour smaller community-based provision. Advocates of de-institutionalization point to a profound dissatisfaction with conditions in large mental hospitals as well as the likely benefits of 'normalization'. Sceptics have been alarmed by the inability of community provision to keep up with rates of discharge. What is clear is that the policy has been pursued in the absence of scientifically based information regarding the planning of community services, or the types of patients who might benefit from de-institutionalization (Thorncroft and Bebbington, 1989).

THE CHANGES IN NURSE EDUCATION

The Royal Medico-Psychological Association (RMPA, founded in 1841) laid down regulations for training and the examination of candidates for the certificate of Proficiency in Nursing and Attending of the Insane.

The General Nursing Council for England and Wales (GNC), set up in 1919, gradually began to assume responsibility for mental nurse training. By 1948 the RMPA had relinquished its function and by 1950 the RMPA examination (based on Brooking *et al.*, 1992) ceased. In 1952 the GNC introduced a training syllabus for psychiatric nurses which clearly reflected that they were similar to general nurses.

By 1957 an experimental syllabus for the preparation of Registered Mental Nurses (RMNs) was introduced, based on the educational concept of situation-centred teaching as a basis for learning mental nursing skills. Another syllabus followed in 1964, which included some minor amendments. It emphasized the relationship of classroom learning and the work in the clinical setting. In 1974 another syllabus was introduced continuing a similar manner, but with a new focus on sociological concepts and community care.

The latest and final RMN syllabus, known as the '1982 syllabus' emphasized skills development. It clearly demonstrated the influence the humanistic movement based on the work of Rogers (1951). The main features are stated as follows (Brooking *et al.*, 1992):

The specific skills of the psychiatric nurse can be identified and promoted

That psychiatric nursing is essentially 'human activity'

That self-awareness skills vitally underpin all therapeutic interventions.

Since almost 50 years have lapsed following the inception of the NHS, it is hardly surprising that changes have taken place in the provision of care for the mentally ill, their family and carers. The advent of the revolutionary 1982 RMN syllabus highlighted how different the scene was from that which had confronted the statutory body in the late 1940s. Experiential forms of training and changed emphasis in psychology had taken place as early as the mid-1970s. The humanistic school of thinking and the Rogerian movement challenged many of the more rigid traditions of training, and there was an explosion in counselling theory and therapies. All these influences led to a proliferation of courses and the modification of language in mental health nursing.

In the early 1960s many mental nurse training schools seemed to study little else but medicine, anatomy and physiology, psychology, psychiatry. In 1980 many were refusing to be restricted by these, since they reflected the so-called 'Medical model' and its limitations. These factors together meant that the justification for any new curriculum would face stiff questioning, as there were those who were quick to ask why, with so many changes happening, yet another syllabus was needed through Project 2000.

It was against this background that the training schools set to work on the Project 2000 curriculum. Their first step was to recognize the best aspects of the previous syllabuses. A survey of existing training programmes found that a substantial part of the content in mental health nursing courses overlapped with other branches of nursing.

It was then necessary to match the old with the new, so as to avoid the impression that one half was from the eighteenth and nineteenth century and the other half from the twentieth century. Inevitably this meant changes in language. The statutory bodies (United Kingdom Central Council for Nursing, Midwifery and Health Visiting and the National Boards of Nursing) rejected the idea of a slavish uniformity, but have influenced language, wherever possible and appropriate, through guidelines and official communications.

In general, Project 2000 courses continue the traditions of earlier syllabuses of training. Naturally, expression has been given to that which emphasizes mental health nursing, but at the same time the selection of content includes theories and concepts drawn from a wide variety of other professions and agencies.

The Colleges that offer Project 2000 courses are urged to respond to and reflect the changes in the mental life of people in modern society, and mental health branch programmes in particular must do this. In the last 30 years many mental health nurses have paid more attention to their skills development, and this change is reflected in the different arrangement of the practice experiences supporting the course.

During the same period most mental health nurses have moved further towards informality and spontaneity in their approaches, and the inclusion of greater self-awareness and relationship promotion is also intended to help inform their practice. If the mixture of both approaches in the branch programme encourages each new intake of mental health practitioners to explore what is best in the other branches, much will be achieved for our clients. Since many mental health nursing skills can be used in different situations the custom of shared learning and cross-referencing with other branches will be extremely beneficial.

The statutory bodies have endeavoured to include in all approved courses those skills which mental health nurses would expect to have developed and available to them whilst selectively introducing new ones necessary for the decade to come. They have tried to recognize the contemporary trends and styles within the mental health nursing branch.

Modern psychiatry will have to confront the cultures and sub-cultures of contemporary society and promote the knowledge and skills specifically related to these. The potential demands upon the mental health nurse can been seen to be significant. The range of clients is increasing, encompassing the whole of human experience and its problems. Consequently, the mental health nurse will need to develop self-confidence and presentation skills.

There is a set of behaviours or norms underpinning the ways in which the mental health nurse is expected to care:

Greater awareness of self and sensitivity towards others

Increased skills promoting and building positive relationships with others

Highly developed critical thinking and reflective skills

CONSTELLATIONS OF ATTRIBUTES

The development of sets of qualities or attributes enables the mental health nurses to deliver consistent behaviour related to their role or roles. The reference point is the competencies stated in Rule 18A (Nurses, Midwives and Health Visitors Act 1989) first referred to in Chapter 2.

The English National Board for Nursing, Mid-

Wifery and Health Visiting state the rationale for the constellations of attributes concept as follows:

'The identification of constellations of attributes is derived from the theory that people adopt and develop excellence of performance more rapidly, together with retaining higher levels of performance more rapidly, together with retaining higher levels of performance, if there is congruity between the role specification and established personal attributes'.
English National Board Guidelines, 1989

Roles that nurses might adopt are shown in the left-hand column below, the related competence is shown in the right-hand column.

Role	Competencies (Rule 18A) (See Appendix I for statement of competencies a–m)
Assessor	a j b
Planner	a j c g
Enabler	f i b c g j
Evaluator	e j d a
Learner/researcher	c d e b a
Teacher	m i f g
Manager	l i k m
Counsellor	i f j
Advocate	e d b h
Resource	l b i
Health educator	g i f
Professional	k h c e l m

Assessor
Each individual user/client is unique and should be assessed accurately. Training programmes must promote the skill of assessment and obser-

vation as being fundamental to mental health nursing practice.

Planner

It is important to design appropriate, realistic and individualized programmes of care for the user and family.

Enabler

Mental health nurses are agents of care delivery. Training programmes must promote the skills of motivation, encouragement and achievement within their individual style.

Evaluator

It is important for the mental health nurse to reflect upon self and to self-appraise as an on-going process. Training programmes must enable the nurse to develop ways of achieving accurate, relevant and objective evaluation. This includes the use of analytical, reflective and critical skills involved in accurate decision-making.

Learner/researcher

Each nurse has his or her own individual learning style. Learning is a continuous process and should be exciting. Training programmes must promote an openness to learning whilst the elements of challenge, exploration and novelty are included. Finding out promotes a freshness and informs practice.

Teacher

Teaching is assisting other people to learn and progress. This includes the use of role modelling, example setting, imparting information and clear communication. Training programmes must promote the skills involved in teaching others.

Manager

The role of manager includes the effective use of leadership, decision-making, delegation and monitoring skills.

Advocate

It is the basic right of every individual to be treated with fairness and justice.

Resource

The processes of care include the effective use of resources, both personal and material.

Health Educator

Valuing good health and healthy living in its broadest sense is an acceptable ideal for user and carers. Training programmes must emphasize the concept of health promotion.

Professional

The mental health nurse has a responsibility to society and must behave within standards, expectations and competencies which are acceptable to that society. Training programmes must promote the vital aspects of quality of care, codes of conduct and the need for continuing professional development.

Counsellor

Component skills in counselling underpin the functioning of the mental health nurse. A vital part of mental health nursing is being able to develop therapeutic relationships in the helping process.

PROJECT 2000 CURRICULUM—MENTAL HEALTH BRANCH

Colleges are looking anew at their nursing programmes in the light of the demand for tailored higher education. Trends in social life, health and disease are changing. Therefore any curriculum offered must be capable of taking on any change with the major development in the future. A mental health nurse needs to be able to recognize the development of mental health problems much earlier, take different approaches with different clients and know how to manage psychiatric emergencies. Nurses will be working in a situation of changing services with all the uncertainty associated with change in a modern society.

The extra demand for skilled practitioners means using more relevant and specific programmes within preparatory courses. A three-pronged approach may be useful for future courses of preparation based on:

Community care needs

Special care needs

Progressive care needs

Community care needs

Since few clients face long-stay institutional care, it is important for student practitioners to see where clients live and begin to value the lifestyle of the individual. As the community services expand and develop there is likely to be more emphasis on preventative work.

The focus is on developing the primary skills, for example, communication, counselling, relationships, group work as well as the capacity to promote mental health.

Special care needs

The major mental health problems experienced by society are escalating. Therefore the social and cultural settings of behaviour need to be explored and understood. Challenging behaviour, for example, self-injury, emotionally charged situations and crisis management, should be included in the programme.

During a practitioner's career, he or she will come into contact with groups who have special care needs or for whom specialized interventions are required, as in the instances of, for example:

1 Substance misuse (Chodse and Maxwell, 1990)
2 Prolonged exposure to stress
3 Supporting people with any mental health problems associated with their experience of physical conditions/illness
4 People who offend or break the law or are at risk of doing so
5 Survivors of disasters
6 Post-traumatic stress (Hodgkinson and Steward, 1991)

Progressive care needs

Also included should be the development of structural programmes for the prolonged care of people who experience enduring problems and who may be severely mentally ill. The programmes should include how to respond to difficult and challenging situations which require quick and accurate decisions about individuals with serious mental illness. Considerations from acute psychiatry, along with care for elders and rehabilitative care provision needs to be explored and understood.

The focus should be on the development of managerial skills, for example care management, self-management, professional management (see Chapter 19).

CONCLUSION

We need time to reflect in order to ensure that everything we attempt to do for the person experiencing illness has a true value. We also need to address what it is that will be required of mental health nurses in 2000 and this will mean not attaching ourselves too much to the old traditions. Mental health nurses and nursing will continue to adapt as ideas about the nature of mental illness and the services which should be provided change and develop.

A lot of thought is being given to the direction of national health care. It is hoped that some thought will be devoted to the future of mental health nurses who are woven into the fabric of nursing and on whom the services have relied for so long.

ACKNOWLEDGEMENT

I thank Brian Davey, Patients' Advocacy Council, Nottingham, and Val Francis, Principal Psychologist, North Nottinghamshire Health Authority, for their assistance.

FURTHER READING

Brooking, J.I. (1986) *Psychiatric Nursing Research*. Chichester: Wiley.

Brooking, J.I., Ritter, S.A.H. & Thomas, B.L. (Eds) (1992) *A Textbook of Psychiatric and Mental Health Nursing*. Edinburgh: Churchill Livingstone.

Llewelyn, S. & Trent, D. (1987) *Nursing in the Community: Psychology in Action*. London: The British Psychological Society in association with Methuen.

Simmons, S. & Brooker, C. (1990) *Community Psychiatric Nursing (A Social Perspective)*. London: Methuen.

REFERENCES

Bebbington, P.E. (1990) Population surveys of psychiatric disorder and the need for treatment. *Social Psychiatry and Psychiatric Epidemiology*, **25**, 33–40.

Brooking, J.I., Ritter, S.A.H. & Thomas, B.L. (Eds) (1992) *A Textbook of Psychiatric and Mental Health Nursing*. Edinburgh: Churchill Livingstone.

Butterworth, C.A. (1993) *The Mental Health Nursing Review*. London: Department of Health.

Chodse, H. & Maxwell, D. (1990) *Substance Abuse and Dependence: An Introduction for the Caring Professional*. London: Macmillan.

Davey, B. (1992) One user's view of psychiatric nursing. Paper presented to a Conference. Nottingham Advocacy Group.

Department of Health and Welsh Office (1990) Code of Practice: Mental Health Act 1983. London: HMSO.

English National Board Guidelines (1989) Project 2000. A New Preparation for Practice: guidelines and criteria for course development and the formation of collaborative links between approved training institutions with the National Health Service and Centres of Higher Education.

Francis, V.M. & Smith, A. (1991) The run-down and closure of a psychiatric hospital. *Social Psychiatry Epidemiology*, **26**, 92–94.

Goldberg, D., Kay, C. & Thompson, L. (1976) Psychiatric morbidity in general practice and the community. *Psychological Medicine*, **6**, 565–569.

Higgins, P. (1980) *Nursing Times*, **76**, 1062–1064.

Hodgkinson, P.E. & Steward, M. (1991) *Coping with Catastrophe. A Handbook of Disaster Management*. London: Routledge.

Jones, K. (1988) *Experience in Mental Health, Community Care and Social Policy*. London: Sage.

Lazare, A., Eisentham, S. & Wasserman, L. (1975) The Customer Approach to Patienthood: Attending to Patient requests in a walk-in clinic. *Arch. Gen. Psychiat.*, **32**, 553–558.

Martin, E. (1986) Consumer evaluation of human services. *Social Policy and Administration*, **20**, 185–200.

Powell, J.E. (1961) Speech by the Minister of Health, the Rt Hon. Enoch Powell. Quoted in Jones, K. *Experience in Mental Health, Community Care and Social Policy*. London: Sage.

Rogers, C.R. (1951) *Client-centred Therapy: its Current Practice, Implications and Therapy*. Boston: Houghton Miffin.

Thorncroft, G. & Bebbington, P.E. (1989) De-institutionalization—from hospital closure to service development. *British Journal of Psychiatry*, **155**, 739–753.

APPENDIX

RULE 18 COMPETENCIES (UKCC)

Rule 18(A)

1 The content of the common foundation programme and the branch programme shall be such as the Council may from time to time require.

2 The common foundation programme and the branch programme shall be designed to prepare the student to assume the responsibilities and accountability that registration confers, and to prepare the nursing student to apply knowledge and skills to meet the nursing needs of individuals and of groups in health and in sickness in the area of practice of the branch programme and shall include enabling the student to achieve the following outcomes:

(a) The identification of the social and health implications of pregnancy and child bearing, physical and mental handicap, disease, disability, or ageing for the individual, her or his friends, family and community.

(b) The recognition of common factors which contribute to, and those which adversely affect, physical, mental and social well-being of patients and clients and take appropriate action.

(c) The use of relevant literature and research to inform the practice of nursing.

(d) The appreciation of the influence of social, political and cultural factors in relation to health care.

(e) An understanding of the requirements of legislation relevant to the practice of nursing.

(f) The use of appropriate communication skills to enable the development of helpful caring relationships with patients and clients and their families and friends, and to initiate and conduct therapeutic relationships with patients and clients.

(g) The identification of health-related learning needs of patients and clients, families and friends and to participate in health promotion.

(h) An understanding of the ethics of health care and of the nursing profession and the responsibilities which these impose on the nurse's professional practice.

(i) The identification of the needs of patients and clients to enable them to progress from varying degrees of dependence to maximum independence, or to a peaceful death.

(j) The identification of physical, psychological, social and spiritual needs of the patient or client; an awareness of values and concepts of individual care; the ability to devise a plan of care, contribute to its implementation and evaluation; and the demonstration of the principles of a problem-solving approach to the practice of nursing.

(k) The ability to function effectively in a team and participate in a multiprofessional approach to the care of patients and clients.

(l) The use of the appropriate channel of referral for matters not within his or her sphere of competence.

(m) The assignment of appropriate duties to others and the supervision, teaching and monitoring of assigned duties.

CONTEMPORARY ISSUES IN THE PREPARATION AND EDUCATION OF COMMUNITY MENTAL HEALTH NURSING

D.T. Sines

AIMS

i) To consider the development, nature and provision of community mental health nursing services in the UK

ii) To identify the implications for the preparation and education of community mental health nurses

iii) To explore the key issues facing the community mental health specialism

KEY ISSUES

Skills and competences for community mental health nursing

Intra- and interprofessional learning

Curriculum planning, models and frameworks

Community profiling and care management

Community education

Identify, analyse and assess factors causing distress and illness	Promote health, provide direct care and make interventions	Manage care programmes and services
Be critical, analytical and accountable, continue professional development	Counter discrimination, inequality and individual and institutional racism	Work within and develop policies, laws and safeguards in all settings
Understand influences on mental health and the nature/causes of disorder and illness	Know the effects of distress, disorder, illness on individuals, groups, families	Understand the basis of treatments and interventions

INTRODUCTION

Community mental health nursing (or as it is often known, community psychiatric nursing) is recognized as an integral area of discrete practice within the primary health care team and within the 'family' of community nursing (UKCC, 1992). In partnership with health visitors, district nurses, social workers and other professionals this branch of nursing is justifiably interdisciplinary in nature.

The past 35 years have witnessed major changes in the way that social and health care needs are met and perhaps the most significant change is the context within which care is provided. Reliance on long-stay specialist hospitals has been slowly replaced over the past decade by a recognition that care is best provided for as close to the person's own home and environment as possible. This may be in the person's own home, in a family home, or in some form of supported housing other than that provided by the National Health Service. This chapter is concerned with this component of health care delivery—domiciliary or home-based health care.

Throughout this chapter you are advised to consider the essential differences between the provision of nursing care to people in their own homes and care delivered to people in hospital settings. It is suggested that the nursing skills will often be the same but the context of care delivery and the art of professional practice may differ. Some of the key influences that have shaped the context of community nursing practice are identified below.

STRATEGIC PRINCIPLES

During the course of the Project 2000 mental health branch programme, students will be expected to develop progressively and to adapt their skills to work in a range of community settings. Students will be introduced to a variety of issues related to community care both in non-hospital residential settings and in people's own homes.

The provision of nursing care in the community is dependent on acquisition and development of competence in different care environments (in fact in any area where a person may reside outwith hospital) which may not be characterized by traditional or hierarchical support and management systems. Rather, the philosophy of care operates in a client-controlled environment demanding responsive, pro-active skills, such as health surveillance, risk analysis, communication skills and social action which are needed to meet the expectations and needs of consumers. Community mental health nursing responds to a rapidly changing social context of primary health care provision and, as such, nurses will require access to a flexible curriculum to prepare them for practice.

The following social, economic and political factors are usually considered in preparing a *community-focused curriculum* for students:

1 In the Declaration of Alma Ata, the World Health Organization (1978) stated that their aim of 'Health For All' by the year 2000 should be realized through the introduction of a range of targets for the promotion of health (and the prevention of ill-health) for the population. The Government has adopted this aim within resource constraints as part of its strategic plan for mental health in the 'Health of the Nation' report (DH, 1992a) and its allegiance to a Eurostrategy. As a consequence, students must be provided with opportunities throughout the course of their educational programme to acquire competence as 'knowledgeable practitioners' in the community.

2 The publication of the NHS and Community Care Act (DH, 1990a) and its associated White Papers emphasize the importance of caring for people in the community which will be accompanied by reduced dependency on secondary health care service (hospital-based) provision. In particular the Government White Paper 'Caring for People' (DH, 1990b) noted that 'nurses working in the community ... are ideally placed to respond quickly to the needs of individuals and families'.

3 The growth of consumerism and non-statutory sector care in the voluntary and

independent sectors suggests that there will be a demand for more equal relationships with clients/patients and health care professionals. The Government Patient's Charter (DH, 1992b) with its emphasis on the rights of individuals (and the responsibility of nurses to be accountable for their practice by upholding the highest professional standards) is a further example of an emergent partnership between health care professionals and clients. There is also a growing expectation that individuals will assume responsibility for their own health and lifestyles.

4 Changes in social policy have also placed increasing continuing care responsibilities on informal carers in the home. Demographic changes and economic demands are changing the nature of the family's caring role which may be influenced by the number of women entering the labour market. Similarly the projected increase in the number of elderly persons requiring community care will demand additional nursing resources, particularly in the community.

5 Rapid technological and pharmacological developments, nurse prescribing, the emergence of new patterns of disease and disability and the emergence of 'new' diseases, such as HIV infection and stress-related disorders, indicate a need for nurses who are flexible and able to respond to change.

6 The development of primary health care teams has also provided an impetus for change. The importance of interprofessional teamwork and interagency co-operation is emphasized. Community mental health nursing teams have a major contribution to make in the assessment of community health needs and priorities for their local communities and nurses must therefore be prepared to identify, evaluate and access a range of support services for clients and their families.

7 International perspectives on the provision of community care will also demand the preparation of a more responsive and informed nurse in the future. The opportunity to consider community care programmes in a range of different cultural settings will be a necessary component of future educational programmes.

THE EMERGENCE OF COMMUNITY MENTAL HEALTH NURSING

The notion of caring for people with mental health needs outwith hospitals is not new. The first community nursing service for this client group was witnessed in South London as early as 1954 at Warlingham Park Hospital in Surrey. Experimentation with day- and home-based care was also a feature of the day hospital culture of the Maudsley Hospital in London during the first half of the 1950s (influenced by the pioneering work of Douglas Bennett, consultant psychiatrist at the hospital). These nurses were hospital-based and provided an outreach service from their wards and day hospitals and were normally engaged in following up specific individuals after admission, in organizing social activities and in the provision of out-patient clinics (Peat and Watt, 1984).

This was the era of 'infinite experimentation' in mental health care when rapid advances in physical and chemical treatments were accompanied by the recognition that nurses were able to demonstrate effectiveness in care delivery and thus to enhance the possibility of recovery from a range of mental illnesses and disorders.

The mental hospitals were overcrowded and in many cases filled to capacity. Large, isolated institutions provided places of employment for the nurses and, for many patients, a long-term home. In 1961 Enoch Powell, the then Minister of Health, announced a policy initiative which was to act as a vanguard for community care for people with a mental health need. At that time there were approximately 150,000 mental illness beds in long-stay hospitals and his aim was to halve these during the course of one decade.

At this time psychiatric nurses received the whole of their training in hospital settings. However by 1964 the training syllabus reflected discussions on community care and the advantages of the concept of a therapeutic community. This change in the training syllabus (although insignificant in comparison to the Project 2000 emphasis on community care) paralleled the Government's policy intentions for the gradual reduction of in-patient beds in hospitals.

In anticipation of the policy shift, the 1960s witnessed further development of the community psychiatric nursing services. At this time social care was provided by mental welfare officers who were employed by local authorities to undertake the role that we now associate as specialist social work. Nursing responded by introducing (in 1964) sociology, social policy and psychology into the psychiatric nursing curriculum which broadened the perspective of the nursing profession. As a result, a significant number of mental nurses sought employment with the local authority as mental welfare officers. This, then, was the era of shared skills characterized by the flexible deployment of nursing competencies in both health and social care settings.

Across the Atlantic community care was advocated within the Community Health Centers Act of 1963 and thus had a major influence on the development of community psychiatric nursing practice. Similarly changes in Scandinavia and Italy have marginalized the role of the state hospital system and have had catalytic effects on the transfer of resources to the community resulting in a predominant community psychiatric nursing workforce.

For many of these nurses no specific preparation was provided either in nurse training programmes or in the form of continuing or in-service education. In England and Wales, in 1973, the Joint Board of Clinical Nursing Studies (the Board responsible for continuing education on behalf of the then General Nursing Council) extended its remit to include specialist aspects of community nursing provision. The first approved course in community psychiatric nursing was validated in Chiswick in London in 1974 with the aim of preparing Registered Mental Nurses to work in the community as effective members of a multi-disciplinary team. The course focused on the re-orientation of psychiatric nursing skills to people in the community placing emphasis on the nurse's therapeutic and rehabilitative role. By 1966 the

Royal College of Nursing was to report that 225 nurses were working in the community from 42 different hospitals.

One other significant change occurred in 1968 with the publication of a Government review of social work services (DHSS, 1968). The Seebohm Report (the report which preceded the Local Authorities Act) recommended the assimilation of specialist social workers and mental welfare officers within generic social work teams, thus effectively reducing the availability of expertise to people with mental health needs. The gap that was left was rapidly filled by a growing number of community psychiatric nursing services.

Other developments were also taking place in specialist hospital centres such as the Maudsley Hospital where the role effectiveness of behaviour nurse therapy was being evaluated (Marks *et al.*, 1975). As a result of this work a nationally recognized course in behavioural psychotherapy was launched. The role of the community psychiatric nurse (CPN) was subsequently influenced and in addition to the provision of generic support to people with mental health needs and their families was added responsibility for specialist intervention.

The specialization of the community psychiatric nurse's role became the centre of intense debate during the 1970s. Nurses began to associate themselves with discrete areas of work which ranged from the deployment of behavioural skills for people with anxiety states and other neurotic conditions to those who worked exclusively with persons and psychoses. Others specialized with children or older people. As a consequence the nature of the CPN service evolved to become a visible and viable service which has its roots firmly established within the context of multi-professional teamwork.

Work outwith the hospital facilitated the development of a range of networks with primary health care teams and social work departments. By the early 1970s these close links encouraged the devolution of hospital-based community nursing and a significant number of nurses were to be found working in health centres, day hospitals in local towns and in social services departments. The GP became a major referral source for the nurses who in return received the opportunity to demonstrate their position as autonomous practitioners.

Community mental health nursing had, therefore, come of age and in a study undertaken by the Community Psychiatric Nurses Association in 1985 reported that there were a total of 2,758 working in the community which compared to 1,667 in 1980 (a 65% increase in five years). The majority of staff were employed as sisters and charge nurses (75%) and in the same survey it was noted that 793 nurses were working in specialisms within community psychiatric nursing.

National breakdown of CPNs who specialize by area of interest

Specialism	No.	%
Elderly	505	64
Crisis work	100	12.6
Drugs/alochol	72	9
Rehabilitation	42	5.2
Children	36	4.5
Behaviour therapy	36	4.5
Family therapy	2	0.2
Total	793	100.0

Reproduced from CPNA, 1985

Recognition of the specialist nature of the community mental health nurse's role was emphasized throughout this period by the profession and by consultant psychiatrists. During the 1970s the Joint Board of Clinical Nursing Studies (JBCNS) approved a 36-week long post-registration community psychiatric nursing course and by the end of that decade the course was provided at certificate level in 25 centres throughout the UK. It had been argued that the influence of these courses shaped the role of the community psychiatric nurse (Barker, 1981).

In response to emerging trends and developments in community psychiatric nursing the JBCNS course in community psychiatric nursing underwent several revisions during the 1980s as the English National Board for nursing, midwifery and health visiting acknowledged the evolving nature of the speciality. The final course was known as the 812 course and has recently been provided in centres of higher education as a diploma level course for a total of 56 weeks. In 1992 White reported (White, 1992b) that 42% of males and 34% of females had completed a formal post-qualifying course in community mental health nursing and that in 1990 there were 1,192 people undertaking formal courses each year. White (1992a) also reported in his 3rd Quinquennial National Survey that there was a sevenfold increase in the number of CPNs in the UK during the period 1980–90.

PREPARING THE WORKFORCE FOR THE YEAR 2000

In 1991, the United Kingdom Central Council for Nursing, Midwifery and Health Visiting (UKCC) announced proposals for a new curriculum to prepare qualified nurses to practise in community settings as community health nurses. Community mental health nursing was recognized as one of the key areas of practice alongside health visiting, district nursing, community mental handicap nursing, school nursing, occupational health nursing, community nursing in a GP setting and community paediatric nursing.

The new programme planned to commence in 1994 will build upon the knowledge and competencies acquired by nurses during the course of their pre-registration education programme and their subsequent experience.

The course will be designed to meet the needs of those Project 2000 nurses who have already completed a Diploma in Higher Education (equivalent to 120 CATS points (*Credit Accumulation and Transfer System*) at certificate level and 120 at diploma level) nursing course and will also accommodate those nurses who qualified before the introduction of the Project 2000 programme.

The course will be provided as a modular programme and will be designed to enable students to study in higher education centres and gain academic credit for each module of study that they undertake within the CATS framework (see below). Each module of study is taught and assessed individually and upon successful completion of pre-determined modules and supervised practice students may qualify as a community health nurse in one of the areas of specialist practice mentioned above and receive an award from the UKCC and the university or higher education institution within which the course is validated. The actual level of award will be determined by the individual's entry qualifications and by the number and level of modules studied within the context of the course programme.

Credit Accumulation and Transfer System

The CATS framework is recognized by all centres of higher education in the UK and the new community health nursing course will ensure that successful students attain both professional and academic recognition for their studies. Each module of study will usually require approximately 140–156 hours of effort from the student with a varying number of contact hours within these, depending on the nature of the subject. One module is the equivalent of one-sixth of a normal academic year's workload and is worth 20 credit points. The level and credit points are allocated to each module to indicate the standard and amount of study undertaken. The three levels of certificate, diploma and degree are equivalent to the first, second and third years of a normal three-year honours degree.

Students are required to obtain 240 credit points, at least 120 of them at diploma level (II), to gain the award of Higher Education Diploma. To obtain the award of an Honours Degree (BSc) in community health nursing 360 credit points are needed in total, at least 120 of these must be at degree level (III) and no more than 120 credits at certificate level (I).

Thus students have to acquire credit points for specific awards as follows:

---

　　120 credit points at Level or I
+ 120 credit points at Level or II—Diploma in HE

+ 120 credit points at Level or III—Honours Degree

or

60 credit points at Level II
　and
60 credit points at Level III
　　　　　—Unclassified Degree

The community health nursing course

Community mental health nursing has been identified as a specialist area of practice by the UKCC. The course is provided flexibly to enable students to complete their studies (and to acquire the necessary practice competencies to work as a community mental health nurse) on a part-time or full-time basis. Fifty per cent of the course is theory-based and the remainder is practice focused. Practice placements are provided for students throughout the course and students progress from taught practice placements to working as community mental health nurses under the supervision of a qualified practice teacher who also has the appropriate community mental health qualification.

The common core modules of study are provided for all community health nursing students prior to their specialization. Students will be expected to study together within the primary health team context and in association with their period of taught practice the first half of the course will precede the specialist modules for preparation as a community mental health nurse.

The *key elements* for the core component of the course have been specified as:

Care or case management

Health needs assessment and activity

Quality assurance and standard setting

Health promotion and maintenance

Recognition of unmet need

Team work and leadership

Communication skills, teaching and media skills

Professional accountability; moral and legal issues

Interpersonal skills

Team management

Issues in community nursing, research, comparative and speculative

Students will be expected to:

Organize and plan effectively programmes of professional care

Set standards, initiate quality assurance programmes to meet these standards and measure the outcomes

Initiate, collate and disseminate new research findings

Develop and modify policy and

Empower others to use available knowledge and skills to maximize health potential

The knowledge and skills that will be required of the specialist community mental health nurse will build upon the competencies that were included in the community psychiatric nursing courses that have evolved over the past two decades. Naturally the key aim will be to enable practitioners to provide expert nursing care and to act as a support and resource to primary practitioners (those nurses who have not undertaken specialist post-qualifying educational programmes) to enhance their skills and development. Other outcomes will be to support informal carers and families by developing a partnership in care and to advise them on a range of services available to assist them with care.

The specialist component of the course has been designed to ensure that the competencies required of community mental health nursing will have policy relevance within the context of the Government's strategy for the further closure of long-stay specialist hospitals and for the full im-

plementation of care in the community for this client group.

Organizational context

Many of the skills acquired during the course of the pre-qualifying programme will be applicable in both hospital and community settings. However there are a number of specific features of *community* mental health nursing practice that demand a rather different preparation and application.

The context of care delivery in people's homes requires that nurses should be able to adapt their methods of care practice with the support of a range of available and variable resources. The aim of developing a partnership with clients to promote healthy lifestyles and to prevent illness will also demand that students acquire teaching skills to transfer knowledge and demonstrate competence in nursing procedures with their clients.

Community nurses' work demands highly developed interpersonal and coping skills. In particular community nurses assume personal responsibility for their interventions without the immediate or accessible support of their peers and managers.

Specific skills

Specialist community mental health nurses must be able to respond to the health needs and expressed demands of the client group so as to:

Stimulate a healthy lifestyle and self-care

Educate the community and other care workers

Solve or assist in the solution of both individual and community health problems

Orientate their own as well as community efforts for health promotion and for the prevention of diseases, unnecessary suffering, disability and death

Work in, and with, community mental health teams, and if necessary contribute to the development of leadership to such teams

Participate in the delivery of primary health care in a mutidisciplinary care context

---

The educational programme should provide preparation for nurses to:

Organize, teach and supervise support staff

Educate individuals and communities in positive health measures, in self-care, and in the development of self-reliance

Manage and organize the environment in which care is provided

Plan, implement, and evaluate the care of individuals and groups

Communicate effectively and to collaborate with other colleagues

---

In applying their skills and practice in the community, students will also need to assess a range of social risk factors that might emerge at different times to challenge the health status of individuals and groups. For example, child and adult abuse; victim abuse and deterioration in physical and mental health may challenge the diagnostic and problem-solving skills of practitioners. Social issues such as living with elderly carers and moving from hospital to live in the community will also demand particular responses and approaches. The legal context of care delivery must also be appreciated and observed.

During the course of the community health nursing programme students will be expected to participate in the assessment of individual and community care needs and to contribute to the formulation of strategies to address identified health care needs of this client group. The compilation of neighbourhood profiles will assist students in the identification of local resources to enable the production of responsive community care plans and programmes for their clients and their families.

The organizational context of community nursing practice will demand the flexible application of a range of skills and nursing procedures in the community. Not only must students ensure that they are personally acceptable to their clients but they must understand the nature of the particular value system and culture of each individual in order to appreciate issues that might influence the delivery of health care.

Students must demonstrate a range of skills and competencies that aim to promote independence and self-reliance for their client's wellbeing. A variety of core skills characterize the community nurse's role and function but the application of these skills will demand differing responses depending upon the nature of the care environment and the resources available.

The programme for specialist preparation for community mental health nursing may be presented as three modules.

Module one

Management and practice of community mental health nursing

This module provides students with opportunities to examine critically and analyse a range of management and leadership styles that influence the provision of mental health nursing practice in the community. Students will be expected to acknowledge the role that management and political awareness plays in directing clinical practice. Students will be introduced to a range of care philosophies relating to the community mental health team practice and will utilize a range of management and leadership skills to demonstrate competence in managing change within a service that is in a state of consistent transformation. Resource management and clinical audit will be introduced as fundamental principles.

Learning outcomes

At the end of such a module students will be competent to:

---

1 Employ a range of scientifically validated assessment techniques to formulate a profile of a person's strengths, needs, wants and ambitions within the context of a care management framework.

2 Assume responsibility for the formulation, implementation and evaluation of various

care planning methodologies for a group of clients for whom they are responsible.

3   Utilize consumer advocacy skills, experiential learning and specialist knowledge to represent and empower people with mental health needs within a shared action planning context.

4   Identify, through nursing diagnosis, a range of issues and problems that influence the emotional, spiritual, physical and social wellbeing of clients.

5   Recognize, assess and respond to the support needs of informal carers.

6   Investigate and monitor the effect that community mental health nursing interventions have had on the health gains of individuals and their families.

7   Adopt and employ a range of qualitative and resource management measures and processes to evaluate the efficiency and effectiveness of community nursing practice.

8   Formulate and implement standards (in partnership with clients and other carers) in order to maintain high quality service delivery.

9   Engage in self and peer review to evaluate the therapeutic effectiveness of nursing and other care delivered.

10 Lead and facilitate a multidisciplinary team to deliver comprehensive services to people with mental health needs and their families within a defined geographical area; to act as a specialist health care resource within a multidisciplinary framework.

11 Recognize resource limitations and contribute to the collection and analysis of activity data to justify resource allocation.

12 Critically appraise the extent to which service providers meet the expressed needs of users and their families and to identify areas of deficiency.

13 Act as a peripatetic resource to residential care staff and to lead a team with a varying 'skill mix' as a specialist nurse leader.

14 Influence the process of change by encouraging the development of new community service responses by projecting personal and professional vision and by engaging in objective research.

Module two

Advanced clinical skills and practice in community mental health nursing

The importance of a specialist clinical or interventionist module is considered to be essential to build upon previously acquired competencies. Such a module will provide students with opportunities to further develop clinical nursing skills specific to working with people with mental health needs, their families and other carers in community settings. Increasing emphasis on non-institutional approaches to care requires that community mental health nurses critically examine the scope of their practice and acquire competence in the provision of specialist nursing skills in a flexible and responsive manner.

The design of the module should prepare students for their period of supervised practice and specialism. Specific role-play and care methodology will enable students to develop the skills required to practice in community settings which range from the family home to residential care *facilities outwith hospital*.

Learning outcomes

At the end of this module students will be competent to:

1   Apply and contract a range of appropriate specialist nursing interventions related to health gain areas for this client group:

to enhance the acquisition of self-help and social skills for people with recurrent mental health needs;

to enhance the successful integration (and where relevant the relocation) of people with mental health needs in the community;

to reduce the effects of specific age-related disorders and presentations;

to reduce the effects of symptoms related to dependence on substances, multiple presentations, sensory impairments and other specific clinical conditions;

to reduce the effects of acute mental illness and to promote positive mental health;

to reduce the effects and presentation of challenging or antisocial behaviours;

to reduce the effects of forensic behaviours and presentations.

2 Identify and respond to the needs of a wide range of people with mental health needs (irrespective of age or degree of learning disability) with the aim of developing personal capacity and to encourage self-reliance for their health and social status.

3 Critically analyse the theoretical basis of interventions deployed within the community mental health nursing service and to select appropriate approaches to meet specified needs.

4 Apply advanced skills in:

the design, implementation and evaluation of behavioural therapies/strategies;

meeting the interpersonal and emotional needs of clients through the use of a range of counselling and psychotherapeutic techniques including group therapy;

clinical management of conditions such as epilepsy, physical disabilities, metabolic and neurological disorders, organic presentations.

5 Demonstrate through the formulation, implementation and evaluation of shared action plans (and care management packages) their ability to negotiate, cost and facilitate high-quality care for individuals, families or groups, recognizing and articulating ethical/moral implications of their actions.

6 To communicate effectively with other professionals and to work as members of an interprofessional team.

7 Apply a range of strategies designed to promote positive health and well-being and to prevent the presentation of disabling conditions (for example, through acquisition of skills in prevention and crisis management.

8 Apply moral, legal, medico-legal aspects of care to practice and to assume professional accountability for risk-taking and the management of care.

9 Employ a range of skills to educate the local community with the aim of encouraging meaningful integration.

10 Demonstrate through the use of case methodology their appreciation and understanding of the importance of evaluation and research within the therapeutic context; to contribute to the discovery of new knowledge.

Module three

Professional development in community mental health nursing

The focus of such a module centres upon the development of community mental health nursing services within the UK. Opportunity should be provided to appraise critically and explore the major professional, political, social, economic and medical influences on the development of community mental health nursing.

Students will be expected to synthesize knowledge gained from other areas of professional study and to apply this to the community mental health perspective. It is expected that students will be able to locate their role in both the primary health care team and in the community mental health team and to evaluate their practice within the continuing development of the profession and the broader context of a changing society.

Learning outcomes

At the end of this module students will be able to:

1 Analyse the development of the community mental health nursing service.

2 Critically examine the current and future role of the community mental health nurse

within a changing political and social climate.

3 Articulate and apply the recommendations from specific reports and government policies for community mental health nursing.

4 Analyse moral dilemmas to the appropriateness of custodial or therapeutic care to a particular individual.

5 Challenge current methods of teamwork and service response and through the employment of dynamic leadership skills to engage as an active participant in the design of new responses to meet changing consumer needs.

6 Promote and articulate the rights of people with mental health needs in accordance with ordinary life principles and Government conventions (e.g. the Patient's Charter).

7 Acknowledge personal and professional development needs within a changing context of care and to participate in programmes designed to enhance skills and knowledge.

8 Apply nursing knowledge to evaluate the effectiveness of care provision and through the process of self/peer review to evaluate their own performance and potential as a specialist nurse practitioner and strive to enhance personal and professional growth.

The role of the community mental health nurse

The role of the community mental health nurse is to work as a key member of a primary health care team and to provide specialist advice to clients, their families and carers and to other professionals. In so doing community nurses must be accessible to the population they serve and to the cultural values and norms of the local neighbourhood within which they provide their care. A primary aim of the community service will be to empower clients to assume maximum responsibility for their own care and mental health.

The role of the community mental health nurse was defined by the Joint Committee of Mental Health Nursing Organizations in 1986. In their publication the authors identify the unique characteristics of this branch of the profession and acknowledge that the skill base is the direct result of the synthesis of knowledge derived not only from nursing itself but also from the professions of medicine, psychiatry, behavioural sciences, physiological sciences and from interpersonal skills training. The importance of developing a positive rapport with clients is emphasized throughout the literature on this subject and should justifiably form the locus for any preparatory educational programme.

The role might also be described within a framework which includes the following skill components.

Clinical role

The clinical role refers to the provision of a responsive service to clients and their families based on individual rights, responsibilities, needs, abilities and aspirations. This will involve the provision of specific nursing interventions to offer informed choices to clients to promote and maintain positive mental health and to prevent the occurrence of mental illness. Community nurses will require advanced clinical skills and will need to provide their services flexibly to ensure that the need and wishes of clients and their families are respected.

An understanding of the local environment and its influence on the presentation of mental health is essential and community nurses should be able to develop mental health profiles in the community and apply their knowledge to specific groups of people in need in the locality. Priority setting to ensure that those most in need receive the support of the community nursing service will be imperative.

The success of the nurse's role will also depend on his or her ability to seek feedback from consumers on their experience of the service and upon his or her ability to set standards and to measure resultant performance. In order to encourage self-reliance consumers will also require access to information, advice and support.

Nurses should also respond to the assessment of the safety needs of their clients and to employ suitable risk-taking strategies to assure the minimization of potentially hazardous or life-threatening life events. Crisis intervention services will be one response and the design of individual support packages and networks will underpin this principle.

Organizational role

Interprofessional collaboration is perhaps the most important aspect of the organizational role. The integration of all support services and multi-disciplinary team management will require the nurse to become proficient in a range of managerial skills. To be able to work and communicate effectively in partnership with others is a pre-requisite.

The negotiation of a key role in a multidisciplinary team will also demand that community nurses articulate their specific skills and rationale for practice. One indicator of independent professional status will be the extent to which referrals are taken and accepted from and to other agencies without having to defer to others. Consequently community nurses will be expected to function autonomously and to establish independent referral routes.

Setting performance objectives and measuring the outcomes of their intervention will also be key skills. This will involve the collation of workload statistics (activity data) and the design of annual performance review systems. In response to information received and research findings a problem-solving approach will also be required to translate service needs and challenges into workable solutions. Time management and an awareness of personal accountability and legal responsibility must also be acknowledged.

Case review and personal planning will be fundamental to this process. Multi-agency personal planning systems will be necessary to support this object (see below).

Leadership role

Self-discipline and acceptance of personal responsibility for keeping up to date in developments in community psychiatry/nursing are fundamental leadership functions. Self-awareness and appraisal of personal needs and effectiveness will assist individuals to work as effective team members.

Interpersonal skills such as assertiveness training, counselling, communication and stress management are examples of person-centred negotiating skills required for practice.

Contracting for community health care in partnership with others

The community nurse will also be expected to deliver responsive care to others within the context of a negotiated contract. The contract for health care (or health gain) will often be informed by the process of care management.

There will always be a need to appreciate the contribution of all professions and this principle forms the basis of the nursing profession's role in assessing needs and care with others. In so doing nurses and social workers (in partnership with their clients and their families) will be encouraged to develop multiprofessional responsibilities for providing care in a variety of settings and in response to individual and different needs.

Sir Roy Griffiths in his report 'Community Care: an Agenda for Action' (DH, 1988) addressed the importance of such flexibility:

'... I believe that the starting point has to be to identify and respond reasonably and appropriately to the needs of individuals and their particular circumstances. How these needs are to be met will call for particular responses, one of which in a given locality may be to provide special facilities for the elderly or handicapped and to organize accordingly. The emphasis, however, is that the structures have to be responsive to the local situation and there is room for infinite experiment'.

Consequently, there is a great deal of room for flexibility over who does precisely what for whom and the skills of nurses and social workers can combine to provide an excellent partnership from which a range of support networks can be offered to people with mental health needs and their families.

The principles of care management require that the individual needs, wishes and ambitions of individuals and their families are identified and acknowledged by skilled practitioners. The task of the care manager will be to match these needs and ambitions against a range of available resources in the community which will include the need to access relevant skills of practitioners to support people and their families. In order to achieve this objective, multi-agency personal planning systems will be required to which service users, their carers, nurses, social workers and other professionals contribute in a meaningful and valued way. In response to this shared process valuable information is obtained which will enable care to be contracted from nurses and social workers. The outcomes of nursing intervention may also be evaluated.

Community mental health nurses will be expected to define their skills and competencies in order to respond to the actual needs of their client group. In many cases both health and social care needs will be identified and joint working between various professionals will require sensitive co-ordination. Current Government legislation has provided opportunities for the development of a free market within which nurses, social workers and other support staff will be able to provide services to clients in response to their identified needs.

The increasing emphasis on providing individualized services for people with mental health needs demands that the systems that we use to manage those services are sensitive enough to take account of each person's needs. In many agencies the concept of life planning has provided a forum for the development of a partnership with clients and their families which has resulted in a better understanding of the needs and wants of people. However, such systems have usually been subjective and led by professionals employed by service agencies. The degree to which each system has been successful has also left much to be desired and we are only just beginning to understand the complexities involved in identifying the needs, wants and ambitions of service users.

Preparing for care management

In April 1993 the principle of care management was introduced throughout the UK and all community mental health nurses have subsequently been expected to contract their services through this process. Care management is essentially a way of ensuring that individuals are connected to all the services that they require irrespective of the source. It is a model based on the principle of providing the widest range of choice possible to clients without reliance on any one service agency. In order for this to be achieved there will be a need to prepare community workers to work as care managers.

Their preparation for practice must therefore include specific instruction and demonstration of the care management process and might be presented as:

---

1 To demonstrate proficiency in the use of a variety of assessment procedures in order to identify client needs.
2 To utilize a variety of care planning procedures in order to prepare detailed care plans for individuals.
3 To evaluate critically the effectiveness of systems currently employed to identify and to deploy resources for service users.
4 To demonstrate competence in co-ordinating services for clients.
5 To negotiate and agree (in partnership with service users and others) the optimum package of care (services) following critical appraisal of a variety of options.
6 To secure and facilitate service provision.
7 To provide opportunities for user and carer involvement and views in the process (by ensuring sensitivity, flexibility and choice).
8 To secure and maintain effectiveness and efficiency.
9 To evaluate and review the outcomes and success of all care packages.
10 To identify and advise service planners and policymakers of the results of all care plans including communication of unmet needs.

In order to meet these objectives consideration should be given to a range of curriculum topics which might include:

1 *A review of the statutory framework*; organizational issues; philosophy of care management; review of community care policy; value base and 'vision' requirements; multidisciplinary/agency collaboration; access to services.

2 *Assessment criteria and methodology*; objective care planning; consumer involvement; review and monitoring; information and communication systems; identifying service deficiencies.

3 *Roles and responsibilities of participating professionals*; professional boundaries and responsibilities; skill sharing; identifying professional competence; appointment of care managers; key worker functions; roles and responsibilities of care managers; skills for participants involved in the care management process.

4 *Care management—the components of the model*; levels of assessment; needs of specific client groups; areas and objectives for assessment; ecological assessment and resource search; methods; care planning and managment; review processes and evaluation.

5 *Delegation of responsibility including budgets*; principles of budget management; information systems; costing packages; cost efficiency and effectiveness; monitoring of outcomes; consumer satisfaction; accountability; flexibility and budget virement; charging and costing systems.

6 *Purchasing of services and contracts*; principles of an 'open economy of care'; competitive markets; introduction to the principles of quality assurance; service specifications and contract contents; activity data and outputs.

7 *Organizational requirements*; information systems; training and staff development; service development and procurement; interagency relationships and co-operation; liaison with the voluntary and independent sectors.

Care management in action

For care management to operate each person with a longer term community mental health need will require access to a named person who will be designated as a care manager. Care managers will usually be social workers, specialist community health nurses and other community workers but there is no conditional requirement that any one professional background is required. The care manager will be responsible for getting to know each individual consumer and their family and will 'map' their day-to-day needs and requirements and formulate a clear action or care plan to take account of their needs, wants and ambitions. Ideally, the care manager should be as independent from the statutory agencies as possible.

Once the care manager has agreed a package of care to meet the needs of each individual, contracts will be assigned to one or more service providers who may be selected from statutory, voluntary or independent sector agencies. Contracts will identify the exact nature of services to be offered and delivered and clear statements of responsibility and accountability will be contained within them. Each care package will also be costed and paid for from a complex system of allowances which will be co-ordinated by the local authority social services department. In order to ensure that each service provider delivers the services outlined in the contract, each agency will be required to demonstrate that they have in place systems to quantify the services that they are providing on a day-to-day basis. The systems to be used for this purpose will be determined by local social service departments in collaboration with other agencies. Independent inspection and audit will also operate to ensure that clients and public authorities receive the best value for money from service providers.

The concept of quality assurance is an essential component and agreed standards will be established by health and social service teams in order to ensure that services may be assessed and evaluated in respect of their ability to meet these standards in practice. Service users and their families will also be involved in the positive monitoring of the services that they receive and will be encouraged to participate in service audits.

In practice, the aim will be to provide individually tailored packages of care which will be subject to regular review and monitoring and which can be adapted as individual circumstances change. In some cases the community nurse may find that they act in the capacity of representative or 'advocate' for their clients to speak on behalf of those people who are unable to make decisions for themselves. This will be particularly true for those people with mental health needs who have traditionally relied on employed staff from statutory agencies to represent their needs (for example, those people who have lived for some considerable time in long-stay hospital services).

This section has considered the importance of care management a specific process for the identification of care needs and for the formulation of responsive contracts for care provision. The community mental health nurse may act as a care manager or may be involved in direct service provision. In other cases nurses may co-ordinate a range of services between primary health care nurses (district nurses, health visitors and social workers, etc.) and in so doing they may be regarded as 'key workers'. On other occasions they may account for their work to other professionals who have similar responsibilities. The allocation of care manager or key worker responsibilities will depend on local arrangements between health and social work departments and will be determined by the actual needs of the clients involved and the skills and availability of participating professionals.

No matter which method of operation is adopted community mental health professionals will require a number of requisite processes to support them in the implementation of care management:

1 A system of multi-agency personal planning based on common principles and understanding.

2 A computerized database to identify each person's needs and wants and abilities.

3 Individually designed day and residential services.

4 A flexible budget system with compatibility between health and social service agencies and which enables the transfer of money to follow clients and to meet each individual's needs.

5 Joint training packages to assist staff from different agencies in acquiring the necessary skills, knowledge and competences required to encourage service users to become equal participants in the planning of their care and future.

6 Systems to promote consumer awareness and advocacy.

7 A common agreement of agency policies, procedures, systems and structures to promote good quality services.

8 An agreement across agencies on individual responsibility and accountability in the formulation, placing and discharge of contract agreements.

9 Agreed central policy on standards against which local service should be judged and monitored.

10 An agreed system for service monitoring and evaluation.

The principles of care management suggest that people with mental health needs are change agents themselves and must be involved in determining their own futures. It relies on promoting individually designed packages for people and as such replaces traditional models of life planning. It requires that a range of opportunities is provided to service users based on the principle of integration within normal communities and requires that people have the right to adopt and to maintain an ordinary life and to have personal relationships and friendships. Finally care management requires all service providers to evaluate their own performance in respect of the quality of service that they are offering to consumers and clearly defines personal responsibility for each component of the service.

Integrating theory with practice

In order to assess the competencies acquired during the course of a programme of preparation for community mental health nursing, students will require experience in applying their knowledge and skills to real life situations. Approximately 50% of the community students' total learning experience will be devoted to periods of taught and supervised practice in their specialist areas of study (26 weeks).

The aim of each period of practice is to establish an environment conducive to learning the specialist or enhanced skills of a community mental health nurse and the provision of suitable opportunities for the students to demonstrate their level of competence and achievement which will indicate safeness to practise. This section of the course is built on and integrates with all the theoretical components and gives the student the opportunity to apply in practice in a progressive learning situation the knowledge and skills acquired in previous stages of the course. Students are expected to reflect on their own development, recognizing their own learning needs.

Students will normally receive a period of taught instruction, which is characterized by observer status, followed by a period of supervised practice where responsibility is delegated for specific clients. At the conclusion of supervised practice students will be able to:

1 Demonstrate ability to accept the role and responsibilities of a qualified community mental health nurse by:
   (a) facilitating individual and holistic care for clients/families or groups;
   (b) planning and implementing a health promotion exercise;
   (c) maintaining accurate records for clients;
   (d) applying the clinical and interpersonal skills deemed appropriate in each situation.
2 Utilize interpersonal and contracting skills to ensure the provision of a comprehensive programme of care for each client by:
   (a) establishing a rapport and partnership with clients, their families and carers;
   (b) establishing good relationships with members of the multidisciplinary team and other agencies;
   (c) utilizing referral procedures for clients in his or her care.
3 Demonstrate the management and organizational skills required of a community mental health nurse by:
   (a) the prioritizing of visits to clients/families;
   (b) managing a fluctuating caseload on a daily basis;
   (d) demonstrating the ability to maintain a high standard of care within variable levels of resource constraint;
   (e) recognizing the appropriate time to admit, transfer or discharge clients.
4 Demonstrate professional responsibility by:
   (a) maintaining confidentiality in relation to each individual client and their family;
   (b) accepting accountability for nursing actions and interventions;
   (c) acting as an advocate for clients when required;
   (d) endeavouring to maintain an appropriate level of knowledge to deliver effective and responsible care to clients;
   (e) striving to enhance personal and professional development.

During the course of their placements students will be expected to negotiate and to develop a small caseload, the precise number of which will depend on the complexity and methods of treatment being used.

Students will require support from experienced nurses who hold a recognized community mental health nursing qualification (recognized by the UKCC). Supervision in practice settings is an essential component of the assessment of student performance.

The functions of the supervisor are as follows:

To assist students to understand the neighbourhood in which they will be working thereby helping the students to develop an awareness of the particular needs of the community.

To enable the student to determine priorities and to plan everyday work effectively.

To identify areas in which the student requires additional experience ensuring that arrangements are made to meet individual needs.

To provide a negotiated level of support for the student, acting as interpreter, counsellor and consultant and to arrange regular times for contact and discussion on achievements and performance.

To supervise performance of the student in all aspects of work and to facilitate an awareness of individual abilities, strengths and needs, and to achieve a balance between freedom of action and the necessity of providing a safe and effective service to the public.

Assessment of competence to practise

At the end of the taught and supervised practice period students should be competent and confident to begin practising as a qualified community mental health nurse. The supervisor should ensure that the student has achieved a level of ability commensurate with that expected of a qualified practitioner considered competent to practise within the community nursing service.

Supervisors (or teacher practitioners as they are sometimes known) will require extensive preparation for their role as teachers, mentors and assessors. Attendance at recognized courses is a prerequisite for their acceptance as supervisors.

At the end of the placement supervisors will be expected to produce a summative report on the student's ability with specific reference to the following areas:

Provision of care, assessment, planning and evaluation of client care, teaching of client and carers, and health education.

Communication skills including: record keeping, referral procedures, liaison and consultation and the use of interpersonal skills.

Management and organizational skills.

Professional awareness and responsibilities.

Personal values and attitudes and equal opportunities.

Wilkin (1992) reports that the components of clinical supervision for community mental health nursing are:

Casework skills to assist the community nurse to:

1 Assess individual problems and needs

2 Formulate and document clinical strategies

3 Implement and evaluate clinical interventions

4 Identify alternative strategies and interventions

5 Improve therapeutic skills

6 Widen clinical knowledge

7 Identify alternative and more appropriate community resources

Personal feelings to assist the community nurse to:

1 Identify feelings aroused by his clients or work situations

2 Explore the significance and appropriateness of those feelings

3 Resolve negative feelings

4 Achieve emotional growth through self-awareness

5 Indentify sources of personal stressors and ways of dealing with them

The supervisor and the student enter into a negotiated contract which identifies the objectives of each placement. Learning outcomes should also be specified and together both student and supervisor should form a working alliance.

All of this takes time and supervisors will require opportunities to update their skills and time away from their own case-work to supervise their student practitioners.

CONCLUSION—THE STATUS OF COMMUNITY MENTAL HEALTH NURSING

Clinical specialization is not a new phenomena and early in its development professional nursing recognized certain consumer needs and settings for nursing practice. Community mental health nursing is one such development.

Benefits of specialization are said to accrue to the profession, to practice and to the practitioner (Affara and Styles, 1990). For the community nurse the clarification of their skills and methods to be employed for their preparation for specialist practice are welcomed.

This has been achieved by the adoption of a new framework for education and practice in community mental health nursing (UKCC, 1992) and by the determination of minimum standards of practice, experience and performance by the specialty itself. The UKCC has also afforded the specialism with a recordable qualification which regulates the standards and competences to practise in the community.

Affara and Styles on behalf of the International Council of Nurses (ICN) have defined the nurse specialist as:

'The nurse specialist is a nurse prepared beyond the level of a nurse generalist and authorised to practise as a specialist with advanced expertise in a branch of the nursing field. Speciality practice includes clinical, teaching, administration, research and consultant roles. Post-basic nursing education for speciality practice is a formally recognized program of study built upon the general education for the nurse and providing the content and experience to ensure competency in speciality practice.

Preparation and authorization are in accordance with scope of practice and with the education and regulatory policies and practices for post-basic specialists in other professions'.
ICN, 1986

Thus the community mental health nurse may justify the acquisition of the title community specialist and through the heightened interest in researching the effectiveness of the community nurse's actions general managers in the NHS have acknowledged the essential and pivotal role that these nurses play in the delivery of responsive health care of people with mental health needs.

During the next decade the number of community mental health nurses is set to increase as reliance on traditional long-stay hospitals diminishes. Community nurses will specialize even further as they target their skills to respond to specific needs amongst their client group.

Care management and the design of individual client contracts will further acknowledge the competencies demanded of nurses and will provide valuable case-study data against which the role and effectiveness of the community mental health nurse may be evaluated.

The Royal College of Nursing has defined community health nursing as:

'professional nursing directed towards total communities or population groups as well as individuals living in the community. It includes assessment of the environmental, social and personal factors which influence the health status of the targeted population. Its practice incorporates the identification of groups and individuals within the community who require help in maintaining or achieving optimal health.

Community health nursing contributes to health care both independently by virtue of its

own knowledge and skills and in partnership with other disciplines. Community health nurses are autonomous practitioners and as members of multi-disciplinary teams work collaboratively to plan, implement and evaluate health care programmes for individuals, groups and communities. The common factor in all forms of community health nursing is that part of the "business" of primary health care'.
RCN, 1992

Community mental health nursing is firmly enshrined within the philosophy, practice and education of community nursing. As such it possesses the characteristics of other primary health care nursing specialisms such as health visiting and district nursing. The next decade will continue to present challenges to the profession of nursing; the community mental health nurse has already risen to this challenge to emerge as a competent, confident and self-directed practitioner of community nursing.

FURTHER READING

The Audit Commission (1986) *Making a Reality of Community Care*. London: HMSO.

The Audit Commission (1992) *Community Care—Managing the Cascade of Change*. London: HMSO.

Brandon, D. & Towe, N. (1989) *Free to Choose—An Introduction to Service Brokerage*. London: Good Impressions.

Brechin, J. & Swain, A. (1987) *Changing Relationships—Shared Action Planning for People with a Mental Handicap*. London: Harper & Row.

McCarthy, M. (1989) *The New Politics of Welfare—an Agenda for the 1990s*. London: Macmillan.

Towell, D. & Beardshaw, V. (1991) *Enabling Community Integration—the Role of Public Authorities in Promoting an Ordinary Life for People with Learning Disabilities in the 1990s*. London: King's Fund.

Webb, R. & Tossell, D. (1991) *Social Issues for Carers—A Community Care Perspective*. London: Edward Arnold.

REFERENCES

Affara, F. & Styles, M.M. (1990) *Nursing Regulation: From Principle to Power—A Guidebook on Mastering Nursing Regulation*. A Report for the International Council of Nurses. Geneva: ICN.

Barker, C. (1981) Into the community. *Health and Social Services Journal*, **20**, 315–318.

Community Psychiatric Nurses Association (1985) *The 1985 National Community Psychiatric Nursing Survey Update*. Leeds: CPNA.

Department of Health and Social Security (DHSS) (1968) *Report of the Committee on Local Authority and Allied Personal Social Services (The Seebohm Report)*. London: HMSO.

Department of Health (DH) (1990a) *The National Health Service and Community Care Act*. London: HMSO.

Department of Health (DH) (1990b) *Caring for People*. London: HMSO.

Department of Health (DH) (1992b) *The Patients Charter*. London: HMSO.

Department of Health (DH) (1992a) *The Health of the Nation*. London: HMSO.

Department of Health and Social Security (DHSS) (1988) *Community Care: An Agenda for Action (Griffiths Report)*. London: HMSO.

ENB (1986) Project 2000—*Mental Health Nursing Branch Programme—Guidelines*. London: ENB.

International Council of Nurses (ICN) (1986) *Nursing Regulation: A Report on the Present, a Position on the Future*. Geneva: ICN.

Joint Board of Clinical Nursing Studies (1974) *Course Number 800: Outline Curriculum, Community Psychiatric Nursing for Registered Nurses*. London: JBCNS.

Joint Committee of Mental Health Nursing Organizations (1986) *The Role of the Psychiatric Nurse*. London: JCMHNO.

Marks, I., Hallam, R., Philpott, R. & Connelly, J. (1975) Nurse therapists in behavioural psychotherapy. *British Medical Journal*, **3**, 144–148.

Peat, L. & Watt, G. (1984) The passing of an era. *Community Psychiatric Nursing (CPN) Journal*, **4** (2), 12–16.

Powell, E. (1961) In *Emerging Patterns for Mental Health Services and the Public, Proceedings of a Conference*, 9–10 March. London: National Association for Mental Health.

Royal College of Nursing (1966) Investigation into the

role of the psychiatric nurse in the community (unpublished). London: RCN.

Royal College of Nursing (RCN) (1992) *Powerhouse for Change: A Charter for Community Nursing in the 1990s*. London: RCN.

UKCC (1992) *Report on Proposals for the Future of Community Education and Practice*. London: UKCC.

White, E. (1992a) *The 3rd Quinquennial National Community Psychiatric Nursing Survey*. Manchester: Department of Nursing. University of Manchester.

White, E. (1992b) *The Future of Psychiatric Nursing by the Year 2000: A Delphi Study*. Manchester: Department of Nursing. University of Manchester.

WHO (1978) *Internal Conference on Primary Health Care, Alma Ata*. Geneva: WHO.

WHO (1991) *Targets for Health*. Geneva: WHO.

Wilkin, P. (1992) Clinical supervision in community psychiatric nursing. In Butterworth, T. & Faugier, J. (Eds) *Clinical Supervision and Mentorship in Nursing*. London: Chapman & Hall.

33

COMPETENT TO CARE

Tony Thompson & Peter Mathias

AIMS

i) To identify and reflect on approaches to qualifications and training in the 1990s

KEY ISSUES

Outcomes of learning
Competence
National Vocational Qualification

Identify, analyse and assess factors causing distress and illness	Promote health, provide direct care and make interventions	Manage care programmes and services
Be critical, analytical and accountable, continue professional development	Counter discrimination, inequality and individual and institutional racism	Work within and develop policies, laws and safeguards in all settings
Understand influences on mental health and the nature/causes of disorder and illness	Know the effects of distress, disorder, illness on individuals, groups, families	Understand the basis of treatments and interventions

INTRODUCTION

The last decade has seen international moves to decentralize mental health care and to integrate it into primary health care services. Within this general movement it can be expected that skilled and experienced mental health practitioners will be at a premium and will work on complex mental health problems, whereas more basic support will in reality be given by health workers who are more generally competent and less highly specialized. As other chapters in this book have highlighted, adequate health care must produce more than freedom from disease, it also has to promote an individual and community sense of physical, psychological or social wellbeing.

The greater emphasis put on activities associated with maintaining and enhancing mental health by practitioners who function at the community level will continue to challenge many of the assumptions about mental health. Failure of workers to function competently in ever-changing situations will not only lead to more personal negative effects associated with psychosocial distress on individuals but, of course, in terms of health economics will also lead to an under-utilization and wastage of scarce human and material resources. The skills that have been highlighted throughout this book lend themselves to application by the diversity of practitioners working in health and social care, and will find application across a range of client groups.

Mental health practitioners can apply experience and knowledge of psychosocial and behavioural sciences to mental health problems in:

Enhancing the work of generic health services

Directly improving an individual's quality of life

Positively affecting the socio-economic development of the community

Promoting programmes of mental health

Although the above aspects have rarely been articulated in direct training programmes this is likely to change as the emerging influences in the changing European scene push for a 'new vocationalism'.

Another aspect of change in vocational preparation is that associated with the complexities of providing efficient delivery of a primary health care service. These aspects are found in the provision of maternal and child health care, the continuing control of disease, consideration of dietary factors together with reacting to environmental hazards and disasters.

Health and social care workers of the future will be presented with programmes of training which identify the importance of being equipped with skills to deal with problems associated with mental health and will be able to identify the consequences of neglect for individuals and society.

It is against this backcloth that new training principles and practices (spearheaded by the National Council for Vocational Qualifications) are emerging in the UK. It will be important to incorporate into these the development of skills which until relatively recently did not necessarily have a high value placed upon them and their application. Many such skills are lodged in the professional make-up of the psychiatric nurse including the development of interpersonal skills, advanced counselling skills, the modification of adverse behaviour, instructional techniques of relaxation and medication, accurate empathy and therapeutic listening and the use of trust and charisma in the therapeutic guidance of people who are disadvantaged by emotional disorders.

Preparation of practitioners in future is likely to focus on the outcomes of their learning as opposed to the input of a traditional academic programme of teaching.

Most noticeably the opportunity is arising whereby a number of qualifications and programmes can be made to interrelate or interlock with each other. It will be possible for prior experience and learning to be taken into account more formally and to credit it against the requirements of other qualifications, or against entry requirements for training programmes. Assessment may become increasingly independent of the mode of learning, allowing people more freedom to choose the learning route best suited to them. Assessment will be against standards perhaps expressed as units of competence, and agreed by employment and professional interests.

At its best, this movement towards outcomes, expressed in the language of occupational standards, recognizes that learning is a very personal experience and can take a variety of forms and occur in numerous contexts. It is probably a fair observation that a lot of professional teaching is based on the assumption that the learner knows very little before they start the process. However, of particular relevance in relation to mental health care is the fact that the learner must be able to make sense of the diversity of inputs which they receive and relate them to their perception of their developing professional world. The world of work associated with providing for mental health is closely related to the needs of individuals to realize their ultimate potential and to develop their skills, their knowledge and their attitudes.

This is compatible with seeking more responsible and fulfilling occupations in order to earn a better salary and to be seen as a flexible and competent practitioner.

The shortcomings of vocational qualifications in the UK were addressed in the 1986 White Paper *Education and Training—Working Together*. This paper recommended a development of standards picked up in the concept of a new training initiative, new forms of qualifications which were to become described later as National Vocational Qualifications (NVQs), and a new framework was to be created for these qualifications. In order that these proposals were implemented, a new body was set up called the National Council for Vocational Qualifications (NCVQ).

This body has already exerted a considerable influence on care sector qualifications and has done so by working in co-operation with the employment interests, awarding bodies, professional bodies and similar agencies. As part of the process of rationalizing the qualification structure in the UK, it is fair to say that there is tension in the debate, particularly in relation to the possibility of reforming the process of standard setting and qualification design associated with professional preparation.

NVQs are based on statements of competence relevant to work and intended to facilitate entry into, or progression in, employment and further learning. The statement of competence specifies standards relating to the ability to function in a range of work-related activities and the underpinning values, skills, knowledge and understanding that are required for functioning in employment (see Chapter 3).

THE NVQ FRAMEWORK

The framework of qualifications proposed by the NCVQ allows for the allocation of a vocational qualification to an area of competence and a level within a unified national system. Until recently the framework has composed of four levels which span qualifications from the most basic to those which approximate to higher levels of certification within existing systems. In March 1990 the framework was extended to include another level (the levels are numbered 1–5) and it is anticipated that professional qualifications will be incorporated into the overall structure at various levels. It is of concern to the professions that the criterion for allocating NVQs within the framework recognizes the present status of professionals. However, the higher the level of a qualification the greater number of characteristics it will need to have if it is going to be considered to be included at Level 5. These characteristics are likely to reflect:

High level of transfer of competence from one context to another

Complexity of competence

Pre-requirements for specialized knowledge and skills

Wide ranging and breadth of competent functioning

Diagnostic and planning aspects in relation to organizing work

Duty to supervise others

At the present time employers and employees who represent their occupation sector in what is known as industry lead bodies are being encouraged to take a national overview and to set broad-based standards. Within the health and social care section this has been achieved by the formation of a body known as the Care Sector Consortium which has produced a series of qualifications in health and social care over the last three years, most of which are at Levels 2 and 3. During 1993 the Care Sector Consortium will be reorganized and its constitution and remit changed in order to allow it to work with professional associations and regulatory bodies on completing a framework or series of qualifications for the care sector which covers all the appropriate NVQ levels. In Scotland, Scottish Vocational Qualifications are offered based on the same standards as those for NVQ offered in England, Wales and Northern Ireland.

Naturally, if progression and transferability issues are to be encountered diverse interests and power bases will be confronted and will probably have to be reconciled. The impact of sustained developments in this area cannot be underestimated and there will be profound implications for the future of health and personal social services and the way in which they present their programmes of professional preparation.

In order to achieve some of the aims of the new vocational structure it is likely that the practice of drawing up a 'profile' of a person before embarking upon official or informal course of study will take place. This should include the individual's competence as described in the achievement of formal qualifications, records of achievement and credits gained from a variety of sources. Of particular importance to the framework as far as the professionals who work in health and social care is concerned, is the assessment of their performance when applying their skills in the form of competent practice. Naturally, when functioning at the higher level, particularly within the relationships encountered within mental health, emphasis is likely to be placed upon the need for evidence of accurate practice under operational conditions within a normal working environment.

The ability to cope with variation in work settings as opposed to performing routine activities really provides a clear distinction between a lower level and higher level occupation which will be included within the NVQ framework. It is likely that the practitioner working within the mental health field will have to cope with unanticipated variation across diverse settings whilst undertaking sophisticated and demanding roles.

We must make sure that professional and occupational standards match, influence and are influenced by standards of services. In turn, these must reflect the aspirations of clients and advances in understanding the nature of mental disorders, and how to prevent ill-health, and to treat and support those experiencing illness and distress.

It is important for practitioners to continue with professional development and to be critically and constructively alert and active, particularly now as the changes described in previous chapters are put into place at service level.

REFERENCE

HMSO (1986) *Working Together: Education and Training*. HMSO Cmnd. 9823.

GLOSSARY

Accountability Liability; being answerable for one's own actions; the need to explain and justify decisions taken or activities performed, as the best course available within prevailing circumstances. Accountability is awarded in an authority to act, and requires detailed knowledge of the proposed course of action, the alternatives available, the potential implications and repercussions of each, to be weighed in reaching a conclusion.

Acute confusional state A sudden and rapid onset of confusion, of an alarmingly high level, usually a symptom of an acute physical illness. The duration can be short and the cause can be treated.

Affect A subjective interpretation of the feelings accompanying an idea or image. Similar in meaning to 'mood', it can be defined as a state of emotional tone or feeling which can fluctuate between range of depression and elation.

Affective disorder Disorder of mood including the commoner disturbances in emotional equilibrium which may form part of an overall clinical picture in mental disorder; depression, anxiety, incongruity and blunting of affect, la belle indifference, lability, hostility, depersonalization. There may be difficulty in differentiating the symptoms of major affective disorders from environmental causation or organic illness, therefore careful assessment and history taking is particularly important.

Alma Ata The city which was the venue for 1978 World Health Organization International Conference on Primary Care.

Alzheimer's Disease Causes of dementia due to an acceleration of the general loss of branch cells beyond the normal level. Occurs in 20% of people over the age 80. A progressive and global disorder commoner in women.

Arbitrary inference This is a type of error in logic as identified by Beck; it is characterized by the individual jumping to a conclusion on the basis of little objective evidence, it may also occur when there is contrary evidence.

Assessment Involves acquiring information about a person or situation that may include a description of the person's wants, needs, wishes and ambitions. Part of a larger procedure and service to support planning towards goals which have been separately identified.

Asylum Latin meaning 'sanctuary'; a place of refuge for debtors and fugitives from the law or other persecutors: a term used historically in relation to institutions providing relief for the 'unfortunates' of society—the blind, the mentally ill, for example.

Attention The focusing of information-collecting apparatus upon selected aspects of the environment; conscious awareness of relevant stimuli accompanied by a central nervous system readiness to respond.

Audit Commission An independent organization set up by the Government to review all aspects of the work of local government and, since the introduction of the NHS and Community Act, 1990, also the work of the NHS. Pays particular attention to issues of quality, efficiency, effectiveness, and value-for-money.

Automatic thoughts As described by Beck these

are contained in a stream of thoughts which is usually going on in an individual's head. They effect the person's feeling and inform their behaviour, but often occur without the person being aware of them. It is only when individuals are asked to focus in on their unreported thoughts that they become aware of them.

Basal ganglia Subcortical masses of grey matter embedded in each cerebral hemisphere, comprising the corpus striatum (caudate and lentiform nuclei), amygdaloid body and claustrum. Other structures have also been considered to be part of the basal ganglia.

Behaviour Campbell defines it as 'the manner in which anything acts or operates'—observable performance or overt activity; general reaction to internal or external motivating stimuli.

Behaviour therapy A therapeutic approach based on the experimental work describing classical and operant conditioning. It emphasizes the central role of reinforcement in establishing and maintaining both adaptive and maladaptive behaviour. The focus of the therapy is the observable behaviour. It utilizes a nonmediational model in arriving at a formulation of a problem (see nonmediational model).

Care Management A process introduced in the NHS and Community Care Act (1990) that provides a consistent approach for matching individual needs to services (rather than the other way around). The process depends upon the holistic assessment of individual needs and the appointment of a care manager who is responsible for the design and costing of a care package that will be systematically evaluated in respect of its effectiveness in meeting the identified needs of the client concerned.

Carer Refers to a person who participates in recognized care (formally or informally), in relation to an individual experiencing a mental health problem.

Catastrophizing This is often a feature of the cognitive style of anxious people. It is seen in the person who typically anticipates the worse possible outcome of events.

Cerebellum The part of the mesencephalon situated on the back of the brain-stem, to which it is attached by three cerebellar peduncles on each side; it consists of a median lobe (vermis) and two lateral lobes (the hemispheres).

Cerebral cortex The convoluted layer of grey matter covering the cerebral hemispheres, which governs thought, reasoning, memory, sensation, and voluntary movement.

Chronic confusional state A slow and insidious onset of confusion which is likely to go unnoticed. A symptom of chronic physical illness such as thyroid gland deficiency. May occur over a period of years but with treatment can be reversed.

Circadian Rhythm An innate cyclical pattern of activity or behaviour which operates on the timing associated with a lunar day.

Classical conditioning The early work of Pavlov exemplifies this process of learning which is the encouragement of new behaviour by modifying the stimulus-response association.

Client The lay, but equal partner within a professional consultation; a seeker of professional guidance and specialist skills.

Client centred therapy An approach to therapy which considers the client as best able to deal with their difficulties. It is nondirective with the therapist offering nonjudgemental support in the hope that given such support the individual will be able to work out and resolve his difficulties. There is no attempt by the therapist to interpret the nature of the problem for the client (see unconditional positive regard). It requires skilled practitioners clienting as part of a team who are able to provide observation and feedback associated with therapeutic interventions. Sometimes called Rogerian Therapy where lay counsellors are trained in the Rogerarian humanistic approach of recognizing the client's capacity for growth and self-regulation.

Code of Practice Was required under Section 118 of the Mental Health Act 1983. The Code offers a set of guidance notes intended, primarily, to accommodate the needs, rights and entitlements of mentally disordered persons who are detained under relevant Mental Health Act legislation.

Cognition A generic term utilized to describe those mental processes involved within collection and storage of information. This is a general term which is used to describe the mental and internal events which cognitive psychology concerns itself with. It can be used to refer to mental images and symbols, which may be reported by an individual as their thoughts about an event.

Cognitive Behaviour Therapy The approach to therapy which utilizes techniques from both behavioural and cognitive perspective in therapy. It emphasizes the importance of utilizing a mediational model in arriving at a formulation of a problem, but highlights the importance of using both aspects of operant and classical conditioning in enabling the client to overcome their difficulties (see behaviour therapy and cognitive therapy).

Cognitive disorder Disorder associated with the way in which an individual perceives and interprets the world. The underlying thought processes are seen as instrumental in determining how a person behaves and their emotional reactions.

Cognitive distortion Associated with cognitive disorder. Psychological stress is seen as a result of dysfunctional cognitions in which perceptions are interpreted inappropriate in disabling ways. Therapeutic strategies associated with the above include:
- cognitive therapy
- rational emotive therapy
- personal construct therapy
- transactional analysis
- neurolinguistic programming (NLP)

Cognitive disturbance Self defeating attitude or responses which may become habitual particularly directed towards lowered self esteem.

Cognitive psychology The approach in psychology which studies the internal mental processes. Behaviour is explained using a model which takes account of mental events (see the mediational model).

Cognitive restructuring A technique used in the practice of cognitive therapy which through a process of challenging an individual's interpretations of an event a therapist attempts to enable the client to reconsider their construction of the event and to think about it in a different kind of way, thereby encouraging a different affective response.

Community Mental Health Teams These teams have developed in the United Kingdom over the past two decades and are to be found in most areas in recognition of the fact that most people with mental health needs live in the community. Teams are based according to historical and geographical factors. Teams generally include a community mental health nurse, a consultant psychiatrist, a specialist social worker, a clinical psychologist and other members of the health care team. The function of the team is to support people living in the community and their carers. This may be done directly or by facilitation through generic health and community services.

Competence The optimum levels of performance possible within ideal circumstances. Wood and Powers indicate that competence requires the availability of detailed accurate knowledge, plus experience in performance, plus flexibility to meet changing environmental conditions and the performer demonstrating an appropriate mood, attention and motivational levels.

Congenital hyperthyroidism A condition in the new born which results in overactivity of the thyroid gland producing an excess of thyroid hormones. Results in anxiety, restlessness, increased pulse, sweating and protuberance of the eyes. People with Down's Syndrome are thought to have a slightly higher incidence than normal.

Contract Culture Shorthand term used to refer to the introduction of *purchasers* and *providers* in health and social services. Services are now to be delivered on the basis of contracts drawn up between two groups. An example is when a Regional Health Authority sets a contract for the number of pre-registration mental health students with a College of Health. In this case the RHA is the purchaser and the College the provider. An alternative term for purchasers is *commissioning agents*.

Contractual cycle The timetable that purchasers and providers work to in reviewing existing, and setting new, contracts. Usually done every 12 months so there is an annual contractual cycle.

Dangerousness The probability that an individual will commit a violent act upon the person of another (or others) in the near or distant future, if afforded the opportunity to do so.

Demarcation When applied to professions and occupations refers to the boundaries put around skills, tasks, activities that are felt to be unique, or exclusive, to a particular profession or occupation.

Dementia An organic mental disorder resulting in a lowering of the usual level of mental ability.

Depersonalization A characteristic of depression when a person is aware of a change in self and may feel that they have become so different as to have become detached from their personality. The person may describe the feeling as 'if in a dream' or 'like an automaton'. Mild depersonalization can occur in states of physical and mental fatigue.

Deviation Different from expected standards associated with a particular course or status; a movement away from the 'norm' which involves judgements being made in regard to the acceptable parameters of this 'norm' and which is often accompanied by a specific qualifying term, for example, a health deviation, sexual or social deviation.

Emotion An amalgamation of consciously perceived feelings and the objective manifestations accompanying such feelings, for example, physiological changes.

Empathy An accurate understanding or perception of another persons emotional state. It should not be confused with sympathy in which there is a sharing of the feeling of another person. Empathy is related to feeling for the other person; sympathy is related to feeling with the other person.

Errors in logic These refer to the way in which depressed people typically interpret events in the world. Beck noted a distinctive cognitive style in this group of people. He described this style and categorized several errors in logic.

Extrapyramidal system A functional, rather than anatomical, unit comprising the nuclei and fibres (excluding those of the pyramidal tract) involved in motor activities; they control and coordinate especially the postural, static, supporting, and locomotor mechanisms. It includes the corpus striatum, subthalamic nucleus, substantia nigra, and red nucleus, along with their interconnections with the reticular formation, cerebellum, and cerebrum; some authorities include the cerebellum and vestibular nuclei.

Family psychotherapy The application of psychotherapeutic techniques within a family context (see **Personal psychotherapy** below).

Functional analysis This technique is aimed at establishing a relationship between the environment and behaviour. It involves collecting detailed information about both the client's behaviour and aspects of the environment so that an hypothesis may be made regarding aspects of the environment which may be cueing or reinforcing the behaviour.

Good subject effect This refers to the fact that individuals, when taking part in a psychology experiment, may try to guess the purpose of the experiment and give the answers they think the experimenter would like, rather than the answer they would give if they were not subject to this influence.

Health Care 'Investigation, diagnosis, treatment, rehabilitation and continuing care', identified within *Caring for People: Community Care in the Next Decade and Beyond*.

Health of the Nation Government White Paper published by the Department of Health in 1992 outlining strategy for Health in England.

Health Promotion The World Health Organization's definitions of health promotion: 'Health promotion is the process of enabling people to increase control over and to improve, their health'. There are seven major areas of health promotion activities: health education programmes (primary, secondary and tertiary); preventive health services; community based work; organizational development; healthy public policies; environmental health measures; economic and regulatory activities.

Human information processing The general model used in cognitive psychology which argues that cognitive processes occur in stages. These stages are often likened to computer programs in which there is an input of information followed by some internal processing of the input during which the message is coded. The input can then either be stored or used straightaway to guide and inform behaviour.

Hypothalamus The portion of the diencephalon lying beneath the thalamus at the base of the cerebrum, and forming the floor and part of the lateral wall of the third ventricle. Anatomically, it includes the optic chiasm, mamillary bodies, tuber cinereum, infundibulum, and hypophysis (pituitary gland), but for physiological purposes the hypophysis is considered a distinct structure. The hypothalamic nuclei activate, control, and integrate many of the involuntary functions necessary for living. The various hypothalamic centres influence peripheral autonomic mechanisms, endocrine activity, and many somatic functions, e.g. a general regulation of water balance, body temperature, sleep, thirst, and hunger, and the development of secondary sexual characteristics.

Individual Programme Plan (IPP) A system for making plans for one person based on the strengths and needs of that person as an individual with the assistance of people who are well known to him/her. A meeting is held to formulate the IPP at which objectives are set to be achieved within a specific time span. The person responsible for each of their needs is identified. Any service deficits which prevent the need from being met are also identified and managers are informed. In this way service provision can be based on the needs of clients.

Individualized patient care Care focused upon the unique requirements of the individual in pursuit of a state of wellbeing, that includes the targeting of resources to that end.

Infradian Rhythm An innate biological cycle which occurs on a schedule exceeding a lunar day, that is, monthly or annually.

Institution A designated establishment approved by a Local Health Authority to receive and care for mentally ill people.

Institutionalization (i) Described by Martin (1955) as the loss of volition and individuality apparent in many long-term psychiatric patients. Often used in conjunction with the term Institutional Neurosis coined by Russell Barton in 1959. This describes the constellation of adverse effects of protracted institutional living. (ii) The habituation of an individual to the patterns of behaviour and routines associated with, and expected in, an institution: this requirement to conform is associated with restrictions in personal freedom and choice, creating loss of individuality and the uniqueness of the person.

Joint training Training programmes where staff from different occupations train together, such as nurses and social workers, and obtain joint qualifications approved by the professional bodies. This can be at either the pre- and post-registration levels of training. If staff from different occupations train together but do not receive the qualification of the other profession this is referred to as *shared training* or *shared learning*. In such circumstances, students from different occupations may cover only part of a course together whereas with joint training the whole course has to be covered.

La belle indifference A term sometimes applied to an apparent lack of concern commonly associated with symptoms of hysteria. Its presence may indicate removal of anxiety by hysterical mechanisms. If anxiety is not completely removed emotional detachment or disassociation may result.

Labelling Grouping according to general or specific characteristics: categorization. Within a sociological perspective, labelling has been considered as one of the methods by which individuals who are 'different' or who fail to conform to societal norms and expectations are segregated from that society. A special status—criminal, schizophrenic, prostitute—is awarded by an authoritative body and this label generates a stigma and often weighty moral condemnation. Pickerill asserts that differentness has been recognized and responded to prior to the award of the official label and that the latter may merely confirm society's view.

Lability A rapid change in mood which can occur especially in elderly people with a mental disorder.

Language A system of symbolic communication by which thought and activity are made available to conscious awareness and which provides the basic vehicle used to both structure experiences and share these structures with others. Language similarly provides facility for a shared conjecture about the non-immediate world.

The Law of Effect As described by Thorndike this law demonstrates how if an event results in 'good' consequences it is likely to be repeated, but if the results are 'bad' then there is less likelihood of it being repeated and the relationship between stimulus and response is unlikely to be maintained.

Lymbic system A system of brain structures common to the brains of all mammals, comprising the phylogenetically old cortex (archipallium and paleopallium) and its primarily related nuclei. It is associated with olfaction, autonomic functions, and certain aspects of emotion and behaviour.

Mediational model A way of explaining behaviour which takes account of cognitive factors. It was proposed as a result of experimental work done by Tolman, who although a behaviourist he argued for the recognition of mediating factors in the establishment and maintenance of behaviour (see stimulus response model).

Memory Encoding, storage and retrieval of mental representations relating to current experiences for use at a later juncture.

Mental disorder A temporary imbalance within the citizen who retains the rights of citizenship; the imbalance may be recognized by various forms of malfunction in behaviour.

Mental health A term used in a broad, general sense to imply some optimum level of psycho social functioning.

Mental Health Act Commission Is a body of 90 persons appointed by the Secretary of State to work on a Part-Time basis. Members are lawyers, doctors, nurses, social workers, psychologists and lay persons. Their remit is to care for the Rights of patients detained in Hospital and Nursing Homes, within the meaning of the 1983 Mental Health Act.

Mental health nurse An appropriately qualified and experienced nurse who practices by virtue of their qualification in the maintenance and promotion of mental health and the treatment of mental illness.

Mental health nursing The identification of those positive characteristics of mental health still intact within an individual undergoing an illness event and the development of nursing strategies to strengthen the positive aspects of the individual whilst treating out the disordered behaviours.

Metaparadigms Concepts fundamental to an understanding—in the discipline of nursing these are human being; society; health/ill-health; nursing.

Mood A general overview of predominant feelings: includes past and current affective experiences.

Multi-infarct dementia The second most common cause of dementia. Patchy loss of brain cells occur due to an impoverished blood supply to parts of the brain because of the thickening and narrowing of the arteries. Occurs in 55% of all cases of dementia. A progressive but intermittent disorder.

Needs Things that can be identified or assigned. They are presented as statements of fact which can be deduced by someone else.

Non-institutional An establishment which is outside of the Local Health Authority provision for the care of mentally ill persons.

Nursing model A way of representing concepts

and relationships which feature in the act of nursing.

Nursing process A systematic approach to providing nursing care, including the collection of data indicative of health/ill-health; nursing diagnosis; care planning, in agreement with the patient; marshalling of required resources and delivery of care; evaluation of the nursing care delivered against specified outcomes.

Operant conditioning After the work of Skinner there was a recognition that if an organism emits a behaviour and this behaviour is reinforced then the behaviour is likely to be emitted again. The behaviour is seen to have an effect on the environment and depending on this consequent effect the behaviour may or may not be reinforced.

Optimum health The concept associated with the desirable state of mental and physical wellbeing. WHO defines health as a state of 'ideal physical, psychological and social wellbeing and not merely the absence of disease'.

Overgeneralization This error in logic is exemplified by the individual who, on the basis of the outcome of one incident assumes all other similar incidents will have the same results.

Paradoxical intention A technique used in a range of psychotherapies in which an individual is goaded into doing what they most fear. It is argued that the use of humour is important in this approach. It is a technique which should only be used by those who are trained in its use.

Patient A passive recipient and focus of professional illness-orientated, nursing, medical and paramedical personnel.

Perception The organization and interpretation of stimuli into meaningful knowledge.

Performance The levels of skilled activity observable within the realities imposed by everyday personal, professional and environmental constraints.

Personal Construct Theory Frames of reference which differ between individuals and professionals are included in the problems associated with using conceptual definitions interchangeably and sometimes wrongly. Of particular significance in this context is the way in which an individual may hold negative and distorted perceptions about their body or self image. Factors which influence personal constructs include, internal such as how are facts about ones self as a person; and external such as the reactions one individual experiences from the people with whom they are in contact. The self construct is made up of abstractions built upon the individual's own behaviour and subsequent observations together with other responses for attitudes and performance.

Personal psychotherapy Treatment of emotional or psychosomatic disorders based on the application of psychological knowledge rather than on physical forms of treatment. Explores inner feelings and encourages the exploration of 'inner' coping strategies to deal with stress and life events.

Personalization As an error in logic this is seen in individuals who interpret the outcome of events by only making reference to themselves. They have a particularly egocentric view of the world and assume that all the negative events that befall him are in some way his fault. This cognitive style should not be confused with ideas of self reference which are a symptom of psychosis.

Phenylketonuria A condition resulting in brain damage caused by a deficiency of an enzyme (phenylalanine hydroxylase). The disorder is routinely tested for in the UK and USA and early treatment results in normal development. Treatment is with a low phenylalanine diet.

Pineal gland A small, conical structure attached by a stalk to the posterior wall of the third ventricle of the cerebrum, believed by many to be an endocrine gland. In certain amphibians and reptiles the gland is thought to function as a light receptor. In most mammals, including man, it appears to be the major or unique site of melatonin biosynthesis. The effect of melatonin on the body and the exact function of the pineal body remain obscure.

Positivism A predisposition to focus and build on

strengths and positive points rather than weaknesses and negative points. A philosophy of approaching situations positively, which encourages favourable attitudes, policies, solutions and self images.

Psychiatric nursing An appropriately qualified and experienced person who has received preparation for ensuring that relevant care is provided for mentally ill persons, in all stages of the life cycle.

Psychiatry A branch of medicine that deals with the study, treatment and prevention of mental illness.

Psychological situation Rotter's term used to describe how an understanding of not only the physical setting in which an event occurs but also the person's interpretation of that situation.

Reality orientation A technique in which the repeated presentation of facts with positive reinforcement and encouragement is used to help dementia sufferers to make use of their remaining faculties: unlikely to help those suffering from severe dementia.

Reinforcement This term suffers from over use to the point that it has almost lost its meaning. It stems from the original use in psychology as part of learning theory where it was used to describe something which has an effect of strengthening a bond of association which has developed between a stimulus and a response. It should *not* be used as synonymous with the term reward.

Reinforcement value Rotter argued that humans attach different values to various activities and rewards and that this has an influence on the way people behave in response to stimuli.

Reminiscence therapy Stimulations of the memory to recall past and pleasant events which has the therapeutic value of helping elders to improve their confidence.

Responsibility An onus; an obligation; a duty one is charged with conducting.

Rogerarian therapy Therapeutic input based on the expert theorist Carl Rogers who expounded the view that the whole task of psychotherapy is the task of dealing with a failure of communication.

Role A conspicuous part played in life; a more or less prescribed pattern of activity with associated parameters: may be ascribed at birth—woman, son, Queen—or may be acquired in relation to social function—teacher, student, Pope. The professional nurse assumes a variety of roles within care provision in negotiation with the client, his significant others and professional colleagues. Associated roles include care manager, care collaborator, interventionist, resource manager, health promoter, facilitator, researcher, adviser and energizer.

Schedules of reinforcement The delivery of reinforcement varies in time, an individual action can be reinforced immediately after it happens, after a given period of time, or at a time which is independent of the action. Depending on when the reinforcement is delivered there will be a different schedule of reinforcement. A schedule may be simple or compound, *intermittent reinforcement* is an example of a simple schedule. Under the condition of intermittent reinforcement an action is literally reinforced intermittently. For a full definition of schedules of reinforcement see Reber (1984).

Secondary gains A gain derived from being ill. This is especially associated with the gains derived from avoidance of conflict and should be seen as a potential reinforcer not just for the victim of the illness, but also for those associated with the individual.

Security A developmental and existential requirement of the individual related to feelings of safety.

Selective abstraction This refers to a persistent error in logic which is demonstrated by the individual who takes details of events out of context and as a result misinterprets them.

Self disclosure Part of a stage used in Rogerarian therapy where there is an increasing ownership of self-feelings. Eventually feelings are expressed or experienced with full immediacy and flow to full results. Any problems expessed are perceived as subjective and not as an object external to self and divorced from feelings. As counselling relationships develop the client feels more confident in disclosing more intimate details about themselves.

Self instructional techniques A general term used to refer to a variety of techniques which employ self talk. This is the process whereby the individual literally tells himself what to do in a situation. It is based on the experimental work which demonstrates a guiding link between motoric behaviour and the emission of verbal self instruction.

Sensory ganglia Any of the ganglia of the peripheral nervous system that transmit sensory impulses; also, the collective masses of nerve cell bodies in the brain subserving sensory functions.

Setting events Those events in the environment which prompt a response. They can be manipulated in order to alter behaviour, they may be equated with unconditioned stimuli in classical conditioning which through a process of association become conditioned stimuli. In operant conditioning they are assessed as antecedent behaviour which prompts behaviour.

Shaping A technique widely used in behaviour therapy in which an individual is taught to perform new behaviours through a series of approximations to the required outcome.

Shared action planning A system based on the IPP approach which emphasizes the importance of relationships and friendships as the core principle for the development of care plans. It ensures that service users share in all aspects of the process as joint decision makers. It involves goals, aims, assessment and provides strategies and actions to ensure that outcomes are evaluated in accordance with prescribed action plans.

Skill A learned or developed ability to perform to a prescribed standard.

Social Care 'Help with personal and domestic tasks, such as cleaning, washing and preparing meals, with disablement equipment and home adaptations, transport, budgeting and other aspects of daily living' is the definition provided within *Caring for People: Community Care in the*

Next Decade and Beyond. Mental health care personnel, including nurses, encounter deficits in an individual's daily living skills as both a precipitating factor and a resultant feature of mental health problems. Currently, therefore 'social care' is an integral part of the mental health nurse's focus of attention.

Social cognitive theory An elaboration of learning theory which takes account of cognitive elements in the establishment, maintenance and exhibition of behaviours. It highlights the importance of anticipation of the value of reinforcement and the belief in one's ability to reproduce the behaviour.

Social psychiatry The practice of psychiatry based on a social model of mental health and illness. The model is one in which relationships and the context of the environment are viewed as crucial to mental wellbeing. The primary focus is on family and group relationships.

Social Skills Training Focused training aimed at generating and maintaining competent social skills which are culturally appropriate. Often includes the reinforcement of interpersonal interactions. The types of social reinforcers which may be used as part of a structured programme include attention, assertion, praise, approval, smiles and physical contact. It can be inferred that social behaviour involves complex cognitive, personal belief and emotional processes.

Standard questionnaires An assessment tool that has been developed in such a way as to ensure both validity and reliability. There are numerous commercially available assessment tools which may be used to assess a range of behaviours and cognitions.

Statutory bodies Bodies i.e. United Kingdom Central Council for Nursing, Midwifery and Health Visiting and National Boards for Nursing, Midwifery and Health Visiting set up by statute and responsible for the formal education for professional nursing practice. They are responsible for the standard, kind and content of practice and are accountable to the Government and public.

Stimulus response model This model disregards the notion of an intervening variable in the acquisition and display of a behaviour. It is the model which is favoured by behaviourists who argue that observable behaviour is the only legitimate object of study and that it can be explained by a consideration of the establishment of the links made via association during the learning process (see classical conditioning and operant conditioning).

Systematic desensitization As described by Wolpe this refers to a method of treating phobias. It is based on the practice of pairing a feared object or situation with relaxation; the relaxation will have the effect of inhibiting the physiological response which leads to the experience of fear; in addition there will be an element of learning via classical conditioning in which the feared object becomes paired with the feeling of relaxation. The treatment of phobias is often done in a systematic way through a series of stages during which the client is exposed to the stimulus which is increasingly more fearful for them.

Therapeutic alliance Refers to the interpersonal process which is central to the practice of mental health nursing. It emphasizes the interpersonal interactions with individual groups coping with current or potential mental health problems.

Thinking The skill in manipulation of images and symbolic representations to arrive at strategies by which changes in status may be managed. This is achieved by the utilization of previous knowledge and current understanding of the presenting situation, and involves patterns of activity such as reasoning and problem solving in an attempt to make sense of data available.

Total institution A term introduced by Goffman in 1961 as part of his attempt to identify those institutional forces and practices which combine to erode individuality and self esteem.

Transactional analysis A term introduced by Eric Berne in the 1960s which broadened the humanistic approach to psychotherapy. The technique focuses on the interpersonal 'transactions' of the client. It is best viewed as a communication tool and therapeutic approach which helps the practitioner consider their own responses as well as those of the client.

Ultradian Rhythm An innate cyclical activity which is seen to occur on a greater frequency than daily; that is, seen several times a day.

Unconditional positive regard As described by Rogers, this refers to a central element of the behaviour of a therapist involved in client centred psychotherapy. He considers it to be vital in practice of psychotherapy. It describes an approach in which the client is not challenged in their revelations or attempts at resolution of their difficulties.

User An individual who requires access to the mental health services in relation to treatment for a mental health problem.

WHO Targets for All by the Year 2000 (TFA) Targets in support of the European Regional Strategy for Health for All.

Workforce planning The collection of statistics on all aspects of staffing services. This includes figures on recruitment, retention, qualifications, hours of work and the like. Used to be called *manpower planning* or *manpower studies*. A particular emphasis is placed upon projecting future workforce needs as services evolve.

INDEX

Note: Names of people mentioned only once in passing are omitted.